REPAIRING THE "MARCH OF MARS"

Repairing the "March of Mars"

The Civil War Diaries of John Samuel Apperson, Hospital Steward in the Stonewall Brigade, 1861 - 1865

Edited by

John Herbert Roper

Transcribed by
Jason Clayman, Peter Gretz, and John Herbert Roper

Mercer
University
Press
2001

ISBN 0-86554-779-3
MUP/ H586

6316 Peake Road
Macon, Georgia 31210-3960

First Edition.
∞The paper used in this publication meets the minimum requirements of American National Standard for Information Sciences—Permanence of Paper for Printed Library Materials, ANSI Z39.48-1992.

Library of Congress Cataloging-in-Publication Data

Apperson, John Samuel, 1837-1908.
Repairing the "March of Mars" : the Civil War diaries of John Samuel Apperson, hospital steward in the Stonewall Brigade, 1861-1865 / edited
by John Herbert Roper ; transcribed by Jason Clayman, Peter Gretz, and John Herbert Roper.
p. cm.
Includes index.
ISBN 0-86554-779-3 (hardcover : alk. paper)
1. Apperson, John Samuel, 1837-1908—Diaries. 2. Hospitals—Confederate States of America—Staff—Diaries. 3. United States—History—Civil War, 1861-1865—Medical care. 4. United States—History—Civil War, 1861-1865—Hospitals. 5. United States—History—Civil War, 1861-1865—Personal narratives. 6. Medicine, Military—Confederate States of America—History. 7. Virginia—History—Civil War, 1861-1865—Personal narratives. 8. Confederate States of America. Army. Stonewall Brigade—Biography. I. Roper, John Herbert, 1948- II. Title.

E625 .A67 2001
973.7'42—dc21

2001004786

In Memoriam
Mack Sturgill

CONTENTS

Means and Ends
viii

Introduction
1

Part One
15 January—2 July 1861
"We Must Take Hold in Earnest"
17

Part Two
3 July 1861—20 March 1862
"A Desperate Attempt at a Place Called Bull Run near Manassas"
87

Part Three
8 October 1862—15 April 1865
"The Sad, Blighting March of Mars"
From Sharpsburg to Appomattox Court House
247

Epilogue
619

Index
626

Means and Ends
An Explanation of Process and Technique

There is a schoolboy's tale about "turtles all the way down," and it says that beneath one turtle is another, and beneath it another, ad infinitum. The tale is offered as a humorous and off-putting answer to some persistent school teacher's question about the origin and nature of things, but it shows a trace of an old native-American story about creation as understood by the Creeks. In their version, the Creeks said that the world rested on the top of a turtle's back, and that that turtle in turn rested atop another, and on and on, ad infinitum. Since learning the Creek myth, I have found turtles to be especially worthy, and I love the image, for it describes aptly the processes by which we have transcribed and edited and finally proffered this diary to readers. It has been a slow process, but a very steady process, and Marc Jolley of the Mercer University Press and the very patient descendants of the diarist have all encouraged this last turtle to move at my own pace. Certainly, the whole project involves more than one turtle, for there are turtles all the way down, and each is sacred to me.

The diarist himself, John Samuel Apperson is the first turtle, and his stately march to an education and a career is something to behold. Growing up in Orange County in the piedmont of Virginia, he was part of a large family of small-time, freeholding farmers, in their own words, "middling" farmers who hoped for more for themselves. A local planter established a field school, which consisted of a college-boy tutor working in a one-room building with all comers, regardless of age. Instruction could not have lasted more than a few seasons of one hundred and eighty day sessions, and probably not that long, and even those sessions were interrupted often. Still, John Samuel fell in love with reading and with writing, and he spent much time with the family's Bible and with a religious publication to which they subscribed. He loved novels and poetry, and consumed both when he could find them, and he tried his own hand at writing verse. But in time he had to realize what many acknowledged during the economic downturn of the late 1850s, viz., that a hard life was going to get harder, and there were too many boys on a small farm in tough times.

Thus, John Samuel started walking, ironically in steps that he would retrace at the end of the Civil War, but with different ends in view: In 1859 he marched resolutely westward from the old piedmont, aiming toward Georgia and perhaps even Mississippi, for to make his fortune in a Deep South or New South cotton plantation; in 1865 he marched with unsteady step westward, along the same route, mostly dodging Federal patrols and trying to figure out which surviving Confederate regiment he could join up with. The antebellum boy, despite his personal poverty, found a world penny-bright with promise and hope, and in his words he had "every good prospect" when he fetched up in Smyth County beyond the Blue Ridge and in the distant southwestern highlands of the vast commonwealth. Taking up with patron physician William Faris, John Samuel not only continued his work at reading the Bible and literature, but he also began serious study of chemistry, "physick," pharmacology, and medical treatises and journals. With a kindly sponsor and some savings, he intended to enroll in the Medical College of Virginia in Richmond, attending lectures and then standing the medical board examinations. He began keeping his diary with these hopes before him.

When the War came, he suspended his medical training, or rather entered a kind of apprenticeship as a steward, or surgical assistant, to Confederate surgeons, and his diary records both his passion for the Confederate cause and his regret at postponing the medical lectures. As the diary continues, we see him teaching himself about medicine, as he records what he studies and reads, and we also see that he learns on the job in the bloodiest conflict then seen. He resolved to write everything in his diary, and he kept at it, although sometimes he had to write recollections covering previous events instead of daily entries. When the War mercifully ended, he lay his diary aside, finally attended the medical lectures and began practicing medicine; but he later wrote "Reminiscences," looking back at his life, and to do so he obviously consulted the wartime diary. After a long and full life of service to his adoptive Smyth County, he left both the diary and the "Reminiscences" to his heirs and assigns. His wartime and New South benefactor Harvey Black was a Blacksburg man, and John Samuel's descendants are Blacksburg people devoted to their land-grant university, and thus it was propitious that Virginia Tech University receive the diary and "Reminiscences" for the school's special collections. "Reminiscences" has passed into private hands outside the family. Full rights to the diary remain with the descendants, and Greer and Mary Apperson Kent Elliott arranged for the materials to be available to scholars, and the couple also sought actively to find someone to transcribe and edit the diary. Ellen Apperson Brown, Harland and Nita Apperson Little, and Don and Fanny Apperson

Mason, and Dr. Eugene Bane made material and spiritual contributions to this editorial cause.

Professor William Gleason Bean of Washington & Lee University, an able student of the Civil War and biographer of CSA staff adjutant Sandie Pendleton, worked with the diary for long years, through much of the 1960s and the early 1970s, producing a fascinating transcription and a valuable set of notes explaining who some of the characters were and where the action was taking place. Professor Bean proceeded with the then-standard editing technique of silent-editing, correcting punctuation and spelling and grammar and smoothing out sentence structure and word syntax. The diarist's hand is a fine one, but he wrote in small spaces under flickering light of candles and gas lamps late at night, and much of the original manuscript is quite difficult to read. Despite heroic efforts, Professor Bean did not complete the project as he had wished before his death in 1974, and the Elliotts arranged to have his transcription and the original diary both put onto microfilm as well as manuscript and typescript for some other student to finish. Evidently a number of the fine students of the matchless Civil War historian James I. "Bud" Robertson also took a hand to some transcriptions, and one of Dr. Robertson's students and young colleagues Dr. Glenn McMullen produced some fine essays concerning Dr. Harvey Black and John Samuel Apperson based on a careful reading of the original diary, the "Reminiscences," and Professor Bean's transcriptions.

Still the diary was not fully transcribed, and Dr. McMullen warned this correspondent and others rather sharply, but accurately, that a transcription must needs start all over again, from the beginning of the handwritten manuscript. Greer and Mary Elliott the persisting turtles in this story, met with the late Mack Sturgill, a close student of Smyth County, and asked his advice; and the historian brought the couple to me. Mack Sturgill knew the John Samuel Apperson and Harvey Black stories, and all other Smyth County stories, fully, and he had used the diary and the "Reminiscences." He told me the story, and the story of the story, and I marveled at the patience of the Elliotts and agreed to climb atop the other turtles and try to get this thing done.

How simple life seemed at first, and sometimes in looking back on the whole process I find myself to be considerably more naive than that young steward who thought he would go off to war a few months and then wrap up his medical studies in a few more months. I decided to take most of Dr. McMullen's advice, but to alter it somewhat, so that I do in fact stand upon broad shoulders of the late Professor Bean as well as upon so many other shoulders. I set up a microfilm reader with the orignal manuscirpt diary and next it set up another microfilm reader with Professor Bean's transcription. In between these grey boxes I set up an Apple Macinthosh computer into which I typed the transcriptions and behind the barricade of machines I set up two long tables with a map of the Commonwealth and a score of Civil War and local history books. I should say too that the machines needed constant attention, provided generously by David Baber of the Kelly Library staff; and my own lack of knowledge of Smyth County needed even more attention, provided generously by then-librarian Thelma Hutchins, who kept finding and giving me books and by Mack Sturgill, who knew everything about the area. How difficult it became once Mack Sturgill passed on and once Thelma Hutchings took another job in another state!

I arranged for a wonderful student, Jason Clayman, to work with me in transcribing the diary. The original plan was that he would do transcribing, and I would edit, explaining who was who and what was what in footnotes. I would follow behind his transcriptions, correcting any transcription with which I disagreed and answering the queries that he left in his neat hand on a legal pad. At first, Jason Clayman was about a month ahead of me in terms of what he was transcribing and what I was editing, but soon it became a full year. Moreover, before he could transcribe more than two years of the diary, he graduated from Emory & Henry College and began teaching with distinction in the public schools of Sullivan County in his native upper east Tennessee. I gladly give him credit for transcribing, for he was a genius at reading a difficult handwriting (that is, not only John Samuel's, but my own in instructions I left him).

Then a young administrator Peter Gretz of the Washington County, Virginia public schools, agreed to pick up the transcriptions where Jason Clayman had left off, and he too proved adept at figuring out what the diarist was trying to write. In time, Peter Gretz too had to attend other duties, but I am delighted to credit him as one of my other transcribers in this project. In the spring of 2000, I finally faced the fact that I was transcribing and editing alone, albeit of course on top of that marvelous stack of steadily moving turtles who had gone before me. Accordingly, I cranked the microfilm back to the very first page, ran the computer diskettes back to the first page, cranked Professor Bean's transcription to his first page, and moved forward, sideways and clumsily, looking at all three things at once and occasionally drawing in passing students or library assistants to stare at some word on the three screens. I have done the opposite of silent editing, trying hard to type exactly what John Samuel himself wrote; if it is hard to understand, I have put things into brackets, and I have probably over-documented things, but have tried to keep the documentation out of the way of those readers who simply want to read a corking good tale, which this diary certainly is. Two more fine students, Willie Bordwine of Emory University and Jennifer Nicole Stewart of Emory & Henry College, did much of the work of indexing for me.

These processes of transcribing and editing ended propitiously late in April one hundred and thirty six Aprils after the War, and quite a number of turtles since the diarist first resolved to keep a record of his doings.

In terms of scholarly guides, I stand on an even larger mountain of turtles. The local history of Smyth County has been wonderfully covered by five publications: Goodridge Wilson, *Smyth County History and Traditions* (Kingsport, TN: Kingsport Press for Centennial Celebration of Smyth County, 1932), which is especially helpful for lists of clergymen, political office holders, and corporation board members; Joan Tracy Armstrong, *History of Smyth County: Ante-bellum Years through the Civil War* (Bristol, VA: McFarlane Graphics for Smyth County Historical and Museum Society, 1983), which has wonderful word-pictures of personalities and many compilations of anecdotes and recollections as well as astute summaries of events, some of which are drawn directly from John Samuel Apperson's diary and some from his "Reminiscences"; James Presgraves, *Alexander Smyth, Smyth County Families and History*, ed. and comp. and arr. Presgraves (Pulaski, VA: B.D. Smith Printing for Presgraves, 1972) includes reprints of Confederate regimental records, municipal records, and contemporaneous biographical sketches of Smyth County persons; Smyth County Heritage Book Committee, *Heritage of Smyth County Virginia, 1832-1997* (Waynesville, NC: Don Mills for Smith County Heritage Book Commitee), is a genealogical compilation of submissions of family histories by Smyth County residents; Mack H. Sturgill and Kenneth L. Sturgill, *Smyth County Virginia Cemetaries*, 2 vols. (Marion, VA: Dean Tucker for Sturgill, 1994) tells exactly where residents have been buried and includes the tombstone inscriptions, a useful way to check birth, marriage, and death data, as well as Civil War service.

My home of Washington County, neighbor to John Samuel's adoptive Smyth, and nearby areas including Smyth County have been well covered by Lewis Preston Summers in his magisterial *History of Southwest Virgina* (1903. Reprint ed.; Johnson City, TN: Overmountain Press, 1989). For John Samuel's native Orange County, W.W. Scott, onetime state librarian of Virginia and a veteran of the Black Horse regiment in The War, produced *A History of Orange County, Virginia from its Formation in 1734 to the end of Reconstruction in 1870; compiled mainly form Original Records* (Dayton, VA: Ruebush-Elkins, 1907), a very charming summary with full rosters of Orange County regiments and partial rosters for Orange County soldiers (such as John Samuel Apperson and W.W. Scott himself) who served in regiments outside the county, and with fascinating word-pictures of the churches and courthouses of the antebellum and wartime eras.

The names of towns in Virginia have changed over the decades, and in some cases towns have been shifted from one county to another, and our diarist was not always precise in his spelling of places he traveled through, but all of this is straightened out nicely by two publications: Ray O. Hummel, Jr., *A List of Places Included in 19th Century Virginia Directories* (Richmond: Virginia State Library Publications, 1960) and N.E. Warriner, *A Register of Military Events in Virginia, 1861-1865* (Richmond: Virginia Civil War Commission, 1959), which does a good job of keying the Federal and Confederate records of battlesites to the 19th century directory names for those places. In those rare instances when neither Ray O. Hummel's compilation nor N.E. Warriner's made sense in the diarist's context, I have been happy to find corrections in the lists, chronologies, and detailed maps of the Virginia Place Name Society in their own valuable *Occasional Papers*, Nos. 1-14 (Charlottesville: University of Virginia for Virginia Place Name Society, 1961).

On the medical practice and practitioners, Dr. Steven Stowe of Indiana University has kindly shared a soon-to-be published manuscript concerning antebellum and wartime history, and he has talked to me at length; and I have found that this diary confirms his insights from his many other studies, especially concerning the highly personal, holistic, female-centered, and associational nature of wartime medical care. H.H. Cunningham prepared the very useful *Doctors in Gray; the Confederate Medical Service* (Baton Rouge: Louisiana State University Press, 1958), which includes ripe insights into problems and performances and a full list of hospital directors and partial lists of staff-grade doctors and some of the physicians of the line. For medical terms as then used, there are two reference books of great service: *Taber's Cyclopedic Medical Dictionary* (16th ed.; Philadelphia: F.A. Davis, 1989) and Roderick McGrew, *Encyclopedia of Medical History* (New York: McGraw-Hill, 1984).

John Samuel Apperson was quite interested in religion, especially evangelical and pietistic churches, and I have benefited from Charles F. Pitts, *Chaplains in Gray: The Confederate Chaplains' Story* (Nashville, TN: Broadman Press, 1957). I have also learned much about wartime religion in personal conversations over the years with my onetime fellow graduate-student Dr. Gaines Foster, now of Louisiana State University, with my onetime teacher Dr. Donald G. Mathews of the University of North Carolina, with Dr. Ralph Luker of Atlanta, Dr. James Dawsey of the religion department at Emory & Henry College, our archivist Robert Vejnar, and of course Dr. Eugene Dominick Genovese, emeritus professor at Emory University.

In efforts to identify military personnel, especially conscripted and volunteer noncommissioned soldiers, I am indebted to H.E. Howard, who commissioned and edited and produced the marvelous *Virginia Regimental History Series*, most of which volumes were produced between 1982 and 1990; and of course he and all those involved in that worthy project owe thanks to Dr. James I. Robertson, who provided the regimental history for Apperson's original 4th Infantry regiment and who set many of his own able students to work writing individual regimental histories. Before that, and after that, Robertson set the standard very high for all students of the Civil War in Virginia. There is also of course the *Official Records of the War of Rebellion*, which I employed as the final authority on questions of casualties; although I do find several documented incidents in which the diarist quite obviously is tending to many more wounded men in one field hospital than the official records acknowledge for all field hospitals on the day in question.

Besides a number of specialized reference and individual monographs cited in footnotes, I have to salute Everette Beach Long's *The Civil War Day by Day: An Almanac 1861-1865* (1971. Reprint ed.; New York, Da Capo Press, 1985, 1999) for its unerring accuracy and unflagging thoroughness, as well as the cogent summaries of events and occasions. To keep track of the Federal and Confederate officers, I have relied on the biographical sketches from the team of fine historians assembled and directed by the late Patricia L. Faust in *Historical Times Illustrated Encyclopedia of the Civil War*, ed. Faust (New York: Harper & Row, 1986).

Besides Thelma Hutchins's personal knowledge and private collections of books and materials about Smyth County, her Emory & Henry College library staff, especially Jane Caldwell, Patty Greany, Claudine Daniel, Sherry Lyttle, and archivist Robert Vejnar have been remarkably patient as well as unfailingly helpful. And, in addition to the heroic mechanical and technical efforts of David Baber, I have benefited from the computer expertise and good will of Bart Di Pietro, Max Powers, and Joy Dunbar. Marsha Luttrell ably led a team of diligent and patient people in the production process.

Having noted my many kind helpers and guides, I of course acknowledge that errors found herein are completely the responsibility of the last and slowest turtle John Herbert Roper.

As noted, the entire volume is dedicated in memoriam to Mack H. Sturgill.

John Herbert Roper
Emory, Virginia

INTRODUCTION

It was springtime in 1863, and John Samuel Apperson was a twenty-six year old hospital steward in the Army of Northern Virginia. He served all comers, not to exclude troopers from other posts, nor even civilians, slaves, freedmen, and enemy soldiers; but he was attached to the First Virginia Brigade, a mountain unit of highlanders generally known as the Stonewall Brigade. On this day, 2 May 1863, he had paused on his march through Orange County, Virginia to stand at a spot in The Wilderness. The place was self-consciously named by pious Methodists and Baptists and more independent and self-contained evangelical congregations; and they had taken the Biblical images of a wind-swept desert land that gave their Hebrew heroes temptation, privation, and tension but above all it showed them a God who breathed on them in the wind and performed miracles to save them and made them suffer in order to teach them.

Physically, this Virginia Wilderness was no desert at all, but in fact sparkled with the verdant grace of a piedmont springtime. It was more of milk and honey than miasmal winds and acerbic sands, and the locusts here were not a horde of insects eating the fruits of the farmers' labors but rather a grove of hardwood trees sheltering the home of the steward's parents Alfred and Malinda Jones Apperson. He wrote in his diary:

> Passing the old Hawkins place [two miles west of the battlesite of Chancellorsville], I could but notice a great change. The fields had grown smaller and the road seemed shorter. Trees had sprung up and grown up since last I saw the place; the old [Hawkins] house was gone. The little mounds still stood in the yard, though, marking the resting place of the old people who lived so long ago. The old free Negroes' house looked familiar. When we reached the Plank road cannonading had commenced in direction of Mrs. Jones' old place. I supposed it was [at that house] but I afterwards learned better. We passed the old schoolhouse where I studied the rudiments of spelling and arithmetic in 1845—almost 18 years ago. My feelings were such that I seem not able [to] discuss them. The firing grew desperate—Dr. [Harvey] B[lack] was ordered forward to establish a [field] Hospital [at Wilderness Township of Orange Co.] and

> send the ambulances on the field. When we reached the old turnpike [where his father Alfred Apperson had once driven wagons for hire] the ambulances were sent down and the loaded wagons went to Wilderness. Our tents were pitched along a Guly [gully] where I enjoyed many, many plays at "Gully Keeper" [a game something like "King of the Hill," but with the would-be "king" standing above the gully and "keeping subjects" down in in the dredge of the depression instead of keeping them at the base of a hill].

He had come a long way and he had done many things in order to get back here to the gully where once he aspired to be keeper and king. The passage of time had marked its own subjects, whether keeper or kept, and things were different on this day, as he noted next:

> The wounded commenced coming in—and we went to work.

On 15 January 1861 John Samuel Apperson had written down two resolutions:

> Resolved this day that I will prepare myself a journal for the purpose of writing a few lines, at least, every day—giving account of how the last day was spent—at what engaged, also feelings & c.
>
> Resolved, also, that I will carry out the above mentioned resolution by writing in the evening of each day (if possible) giving in as few words as possible each day's work.

This resolved young man was from the middling class or plain folk of the Virginia piedmont, and he was newly come to the Virginia highlands when he started his diaries. Born in Locust Grove on 21 August 1837, he was eldest son of Alfred and Malinda Apperson, a freeholding family that was farming in the Wilderness on the border between Orange and Spotsylvania counties. John Samuel Apperson as a teenaged boy was slender but deceptively strong, for he quickly grew accustomed to hard work on the family's acreage plus equally hard labor at odd jobs for the neighbors. He had managed to learn to read and write and do elementary mathematics by studying at a local "field school," a few months of wintertime education paid for by an Orange County planter.

The Orange County farms Elmwood and Hoodville, both managed by Alfred Apperson, were in good land, but even this sparsely peopled piedmont of the Old Dominion was too confining for John Samuel, who was determined to make his own way. There were three brothers and three sisters who could help on the two farms, and there was actually little to keep the oldest boy on either farm, especially when times grew hard.

Eighteen-fifty-seven was such a hard time, a year of economic downturn for the United States, although some of the cotton states came through the recession relatively undamaged. The Commonwealth was not as fortunate as the states of the lower South, and the Appersons endured some privations; unlike slaveowners of their region, they could not raise money by selling off their human property to the so styled New South of Alabama and Mississippi. Instead, the Appersons had to make do with less after some seasons of relative comfort. There was thus no land or slaves to stake John Samuel Apperson to a future as he came to his legal majority, but he heard of opportunities in the cotton lands beyond his native Virginia. In particular, he heard about Georgia, which had lured William Apperson—his Uncle Bill; and he heard about Mississippi, to which Charles Jones—his Uncle Charles—had emigrated. These "western" uncles told of an almost golden prosperity; and each offered to help John if he too set out west. And so on 2 February 1859 he began heading west and south.

He gathered up as much money as he had, apparently about $20 in gold, which represented some ten weeks' wages for low-skilled labor in a Virginia piedmont town for work that he had done such as chopping wood. Taking this modest sum, he literally packed his carpetbag, threw it over his shoulder, and set off for his new career. He walked much of the way across the piedmont and through the Shenandoah Valley, but he occasionally hired a stagecoach or rode short distances on the rails of local railroad carriers. Thus, he proceeded in a very meandering path westward. Along his route, he was overwhelmed with the physical beauty of Nelson County, admiring especially the hill country, and he began to write in his 1859 diary about making a career in the mountains. This 1859 diary, really a trip journal, is eighteen pages long and describes the trip from the Wilderness to Seven Mile Ford. Dated from 2-11 February 1859, the manuscript is in Special Collections, Library of Virginia Polytechnic Institute and State University, Blacksburg.

Staying with hospitable country people, he did not pay for lodging, and he spent only loose change on food. Even so, he faced a daunting walk of at least

500 miles during a hard winter, and he had only enough money to ride the stage or rail for 100 or so of those miles. Although still bound for the cotton-rich New South of Georgia or Mississippi, he began to contemplate at least a winter's stay in the valleys and ridges of the Blue Ridge, or perhaps the highlands beyond the Blue Ridge. Meeting talkative traveler John Holt in Lynchburg, he learned of day labor and cheap rooms in Seven Mile Ford in Smyth County in the highlands at the gateway to Virginia's two mile-high mountains, Mt. Rogers and White Top. He decided to spend the rest of his money on a railroad trip from Lynchburg to the far western community. Fetching up in the "Ford" on a snowing and bitter evening, he went to a boarding house with twenty-eight cents in his pockets, and he registered as a guest for the evening. Since the room and breakfast cost around $2.00 and he simply could not pay that bill, he briefly considered slipping away in the early morning to elude his proprietor. He confessed this thought of deception and theft in this 1859 diary, punished his errant thoughts in that same venue, and then went to the proprietor and told him everything, offering his twenty-eight cents and also offering to work to pay the remainder of the charges. This proprietor, never identified then or subsequently, was also hospitable, forgave all his debts, and fed the traveler a good breakfast. More important, Apperson learned from him that Dr. William Farris, a county physician with a sprawling practice in Smyth County, needed help and was willing to offer room and board and some money.

What he found was not a respite but a career. Dr William Faris hired him to run errands and do odd jobs in the town of Marion in exchange for room and board at the doctor's home in the nearby village of Seven Mile Ford. The good doctor also began teaching his assistant the arts and science of pharmacology, and very soon Apperson was not only treating patients according to Dr. Faris's instructions but also making preliminary diagnoses for cases that were simple—if not in any sense easy. The ambitious young man worked hard at his tasks. Back in the Wilderness he had briefly and unsuccessfully worked as a clerk, but this time around he was more mature, his mathematical skills more developed, and he demonstrated a real facility for the book work. Dr. Faris for his part made available his pharmacological library and his medical library and told the assistant what books he should buy to understand medical practices.

The Faris library included *Materia Medica*, a classic multi-volume pharmacy guide then the standard for questions about drugs and treatment with drugs. It also included *Stethoscope*, a recently defunct Richmond periodical named for what was then a wonderful new device made more useful by development of new designs and the deployment of new materials. The discontinued Richmond journal (not to be confused with a later, London-based, journal of the same name) was still consulted by practicing physicians when surgery was thought necessary—and this was a time when surgeons enjoyed no special status at all and when any country physician (or his assistant) might be called upon to perform an operation. There was also *Davis's*, a standard reference for childhood diseases and treatments published by an English pediatrician who was a pioneer in serious attention to that age group. Dr. Faris, and his eager assistant, were both running hard to stay up-to-date—and neither man wanted to be accused of butchery or backwardness in serving his patients.

In no time Apperson was keeping the doctor's account books, arranging many of the doctor's appointments, mixing the prescriptions, and organizing the Marion offices while also going on the road to the little towns in the high hills of this countryside filled with Scots Irish farmers and craftspeople. These places included Marion, Seven Mile Ford, Mount Airy [now Rural Retreat], Glade Spring, and Chilhowie. Apperson enjoyed the travel associated with this work. He delighted in meeting the patients and coworkers and customers of Dr. Faris, and he became very much a citizen of his adoptive Highlands.

He no longer talked about Georgia, but instead talked about finding money from relatives and friends and his own savings in order to attend lectures at medical college in Richmond so to serve in the spirit of Aesculapius and Hippocrates—and Dr. Faris. He also determined to teach himself enough science and mathematics to pass the entrance examinations at Richmond. But the capital city was only for his professional training. He saw a future for himself in these very hills as a country doctor traveling in these same towns and villages.

Back in The Wilderness of the piedmont, Apperson had been baptized, and he had eagerly read his Bible and *The Religious Herald*, a Baptist magazine received at his father's house. There had been little else to read in that parlor, but even in Dr. Faris's well-stocked library, Apperson always took time to read from the Bible and from evangelical Protestant religious tracts. He also visited other Protestant denominations, especially the Methodists and the Presbyterians, and he recorded in his diary his many observations about local congregations. He formed friendships with several young men studying at the Methodist sponsored Emory & Henry College, a "hilltop" school that sat on farmland in Washington County at a site about fifteen miles south of Dr. Faris's offices. Simple and fervent in his piety, Apperson was very much like his neighbors, an evangelical Protestant who took the Bible with a dead literalness and expected Jesus Christ to return all at once without warning to render judgments and establish a heavenly kingdom for those judged righteous. Above all, he felt a deep need, almost an aching, to claim Jesus Christ as a living presence in his life—a being as close and as real as any of his patients and neighbors.

His pietism was always with him, and the King James version of the Bible provided the vocabulary for much of his diary. As such, his religion was not unrelievedly judgmental and prophetic, but also included a goodly portion of forgiveness and fellowship. He met people, including single young women, at Sunday services, Wednesday prayer meetings, week-night church suppers, and "protracted" outdoor preaching services during long weeks in revival season. Of course he was sincere in his professions of faith, for Evangelical Protestantism was his moral index in a world of rapidly changing situations, and Christ the Comforter was present when he sinned or when he contemplated a sin. All the same, fellowship in the different churches was vital to him, and his faith brought him joy as often as it led him to condemn. Church friends clustered about him like family members, and after all, he was still very young and his own biological family was far, far away across the ridge and the valley. When he mentions loneliness in his diary, he often subsequently attends a service or meeting at church, and these apparently never failed to comfort and succor at many levels of his life.

Besides studying the Bible, Apperson mastered Dr. Faris's library, and he taught himself organic chemistry in the evenings after the doctor's work was done—and sometimes he undertook such studies even in the oddments of time between his assigned rounds. As a second year in Seven Mile Ford rolled around, Apperson began to worry that he was too narrowly focused on applied science. Thus he began teaching himself English grammar and he began reading literature, especially *Jerusalem Delivered*, an epic poem in heroic couplets written by Torquato Tasso. The latter was a sixteenth century Italian who had glorified the medieval Crusades, and Apperson was reading the English translation recently gotten up by J.H. Griffin.[1] The sense of a holy mission, even though it was Roman Catholic and ritualistic rather than Protestant and pietistic, yet appealed to this energetic, idealistic reader.

---

[1] Torquato Tasso, *Jerusalem Delivered*, trans., J.H. Griffin (ca. 1580. New York: Doubleday, 1855).

So too did the high sense of romantic duty and service: Horsemen sworn to serve Jesus Christ do noble deeds against worthy foes, often on behalf of beautiful but vulnerable ladies. Apperson did not seem to know that this stylized depiction of the Crusades had little to do with the sordid reality in which Jerusalem was not saved but destroyed; nor did he seem to know that those crass and grubby processes had more to do with power than piety and brought about as much damage to Jews and Christians as it did to the powerful Muslims who successfully defended their empire.

If he had known about Tasso's exaggerations, he might not have cared, for he was then a romantic willfully innocent of history. It was a romantic era in the South, and many such boys found in Griffin's Tasso their own declaration of faith and expressions of service to God and damsel and homeland. If cantos were not their style, there were the historical novels of Sir Walter Scott in which still more medieval knights fought on behalf of virtue against still more infidels. And when such boys closed their books, they found in front of them the enemy. In this case the foe was not Muslim at all, and indeed Christian: The Abolitionists. What was most galling, some of the more prominent Abolitionists insisted that the truly righteous Protestants were going to stop slavery in the South, even if it took a war to do it. Under full flight of rhetoric in debate, some Abolitionists insisted that anyone associated with slavery could not be a Christian—and the poet John Greenleaf Whittier had even written a poem making his onetime hero Daniel Webster into a devil because the New Hampshire senator was willing to compromise on slavery issues in order to hold the union together.[2]

Of course Abolitionists ran the gamut of opinion, style, and intentions. There was a small and self-styled Gideon's Band ready to fight in a crusade to stop slavery, but there were much larger numbers of those who, like Abraham Lincoln, intended to stop its extension into the unlikeliest territories of the Great Plains and the Rocky Mountains and the Far West and otherwise to let slavery in the South die a very slow death, perhaps generations long. Had there been public opinion polls, it seems entirely unlikely that the northern public would answer such queries by pronouncing a clear majority to be ready to fight to end slavery. Yet Apperson believed such was the case, and he was mad as a hornet that Gideon's Band

---

[2] See "Ichabod" in Whittier, *John Greenleaf Whittier's Poetry: an Appraisal and Selection*, ed., Robert Penn Warren (Minneapolis: University of Minnesota Press, 1971), text of poem, 79-80; notes, 25-30, 79.

Abolitionists, to his mind large in number and titanic in political influence, dared to talk about the same Jesus Christ as did the southern Methodists and Baptists.

With the judgment of history, certainly, it is the northern Protestants who were morally correct in that day, and Apperson himself after a bloody war would come to see the evil of slavery. Although it goes down hard for today's reader, this young man is yet one more illustration of the fact that believing Christians can in all sincerity choose the wrong side in a moral issue, a fact demonstrated redundantly but not one that has ever slowed down the young John Samuel Appersons of any era when they think they know what is right. Of course Apperson's people held no slaves in the piedmont Wilderness, and he had no prospects for holding slaves in his adoptive high hills. If his brightest prospects in 1861 could be realized, then he would become what he one day became: A medical doctor in a highlands county of diversified agriculture with nascent industry and commerce. To his thinking, the Abolitionist threat was not to slavery, but to Virginia itself, and his diary is filled with the call to arms on behalf of southern independence. With cruelest irony given the bloody results, he misspelled *secession* as *succession*, and he marshaled everything from Torquato Tasso to the Bible on behalf of this *succession*.

Also given the bloody results, it is sometimes as hard to remember that southerners were not generally enthusiastic about secession in 1861 as it is hard to remember that the average northerner of that day was not an ardent Abolitionist with flaming sword in hand. Apperson was upset by the large number of Unionists in the Commonwealth, and even more antagonized by the handful of Abolitionists in the hills. He records travels to hear and see the debates in Richmond, and he records briefer—but much more intense—trips in the highlands to hear and see public discussions. He writes also that he debates by mail with friends in the Virginia Southside, a place long dedicated to slavery and the place most notable for producing proponents of local rule, whether Patrick Henry in one era or Edmund Ruffin and George Fitzhugh in another. Yet there they were, young and honorable men of his own age who wanted Virginia to stay in the Union. Closer to home, there were quite a few Unionists, and the most prominent were members of the Faris family, people mercifully not related directly to his boss and benefactor. Patriarch of these Faris Unionists was William Faris of Marion, a bold speaker who not only fought Apperson's *succession* but declared himself an Abolitionist. As Apperson shows in his diary notes of 5 February 1861, William Faris was in fact set upon by a mob of secessionists who administered the painful shaming called *tar and feathers*. They bound and gagged Faris and literally laid hot tar onto his quick flesh before they sprinkled chicken feathers over him. Then the mob paraded him in this state through the streets of Marion. This punishment, object of humorous cartoons, was in fact extremely painful and quite dangerous—and it was certainly treatment at odds with the values of a young fellow who was learning to heal and to cure. The diarist calls it "a hiddeous [sic] sight."

More, given the thuggish and bullying qualities of the mob action, it was hardly the kind of fair fight celebrated by Tarquato Tasso or Sir Walter Scott. In truth, Apperson was upset by the nature of the punishment. Nevertheless, he was happy with its results, for he wanted all Abolitionists to leave Virginia and he wanted all slaveowning Unionists to hush or leave. On the same 5 February he writes, "I presume I cannot say that I am very much in favour of that kind of punishment. Thus I am for punishment, and it makes but little difference."

Such hot talk could not confine itself to his diary, and Apperson spoke out with much heat in many public places. Once he almost talked himself—or really, *shouted* himself—into a duel; and on several occasions he records having to be restrained from fist fights with Unionists, sometimes even with people who merely suggest that Unionists had the right to express an opinion. Most telling, he chides himself on 30 January 1861 for disturbing the sleep of an elderly patient with one of his loud arguments. In that same passage, he even hints that he may have misapplied a "blister treatment" causing his patient an uneasy and erratic sleep because he was focused on political issues instead of his medical tasks. The bathetic coup de grace is that his long suffering patient was his *host* that winter's night, and so the steward in so misbehaving is not only breaching Aesculapian rules but also the etiquette of the proper Virginia guest.

While Smyth County residents included Unionists, the *seccessionists* of the diary won the day politically and voted to send pro-secession delegates to the state convention that debated and resolved the issue. Events moved quickly after those January and February meetings, and war seemed imminent. Before the April crisis at Fort Sumter produced a declaration of War, boys in Smyth County had created a volunteer Confederate unit, the Smyth Blues. Apperson was quick to join up, presuming at first that he would be a foot soldier rather than a member of the medical unit. He did so despite the advice of his benefactor Dr. Faris, who wanted to sponsor

Apperson for lectures at the Medical College of Virginia; indeed, Dr. Faris had his serious misgivings about the plausibility of the entire Confederate States of America (CSA) and he urged that his young charge complete training as a country physician in the one *cause*, medicine, that the Seven Mile Ford patriarch respected above all others. The resolved young man thus set aside his self-professed "aspirations" to become "an ornament" to his family; instead, these personal goals would take second place to the collective needs of the CSA and the Commonwealth.[3]

When the War did come in April, the Blues became Company D in the First Virginia Brigade, which comprised not only the Blues but also the Smyth Greys, the Grayson County Daredevils, a unit from Wythe County, and other companies from the mountains. Their commander was Thomas Jonathan Jackson, then a relatively unknown professor of artillery at Virginia Military Institute who held the baccalaureate degree from the U.S. Military Academy at West Point and who had been breveted major for valor in the Mexican War. In time, because of courage at the battle of First Manassas (21 July 1861), the brigade won the nickname *Stonewall*, and that name subsequently attached to Jackson himself. The general would go on to greater things, but the First Virginia would be always with him, and indeed it would fight on in his memory after his death. Thus the diarist would always call it *The* Brigade, as if there were no other, even and especially when he was officially in service to a hospital unit serving an entire corps of the Army of Northern Virginia.

The First Virginia demonstrated some unique features, as befit mountain folk generally noted for their will, determination, and eccentricities. Their organizer was Albert Gallatin Pendleton, a businessman of Marion who ran the county newspaper *The Visitor*, who invested broadly and boldly in the fledgling businesses of the old hills, and who was the prototype for the kind of Old South middling-class professional and New South business-elite that historian C. Vann Woodward immortalized in his studies.[4] There were the Grayson County Daredevils from the highest hills that included Mount Rogers, and they formed a regiment of young hellions with short tempers and long memories. All of these Daredevils could shoot a gun accurately, could

---

[3] "Reminiscences." Greer and Mary Kent Apperson Elliott have also shared relevant portions of the ms. and of their family memories.

[4] Comer Vann Woodward, *The Orgins of the New South, 1877-1913*, vol. 9, *A History of the South Series*, ed., Ellis Merton Coulter and Wendell Holmes Stephenson (Baton Rouge: Louisiana State University Press, 1951) passim, but esp. chapt. 1.

drink you under the table, and could fight without fear or reason, although not necessarily confining their battles to the Federal foes.[5]

There were also in the regiment two "freedmen of color," duly registered as such in the Smyth County census, and these were James Cooley and John Ross, both of whom carried guns and shot them on behalf of Virginia, if not for slavery. Cooley was a skilled bricklayer who had founded his own bricklaying company, and his descendants in the New South after 1865 would carry on his contracting firm with notable successes in building homes and business offices for blacks and whites in the county. It was Cooley who arranged for the first "school for colored" in Smyth County after The War. Less is known of John Ross, except that he had skills, had a savings account, and was well-regarded by local-historian Goodridge Wilson who notes that he typified those of "color" in the county who were "industrious, thrifty, and well behaved."[6] Rising rapidly to leadership over this rather odd admixture of folk was the young officer Robert H. Dungan, an Emory & Henry College student and longtime correspondent and friend of Apperson's.

Apperson was almost immediately transferred out of the marching regiment and into the field-hospital unit run by Dr. Harvey Black. This physician came from Blacksburg, and indeed was member of the family that gave the little hill-town its name. Dr. Black was a Calvinist and an Augustinian of the oldest and highest southern sort: He presumed very little good of most people, he was profoundly skeptical of things made by man, he brooked little democracy among the presumed commoners and less autocracy among the self-professed "talent"—and he was faithfully dedicated to a vision of *noblesse oblige* service to the suffering as a call to mission from a God who would teach His elect by testing them, probing them, all but tormenting them while commanding dutiful service from them to all of His creatures. Dr. Black's Calvinism, seen also in such leaders as Stonewall Jackson, Robert Edward Lee, and eventually in John Samuel Apperson, produced no arrogance and indeed produced instead the most humble of service even on behalf of persons that Dr. Black was pretty sure were knaves and fools.

---

[5] James I. Robertson, Jr., *The Fourth Virginia Infantry*, Virginia Regimental Histories Series (Lynchburg, VA: H.E. Howard, 1987) introduction.

[6] Goodridge Wilson, *Smyth County History and Traditions* (1932. Reprint ed. with corr. and rev.; Radford, VA: Commonwealth Press, 1976) 260-65.

Dr. B, as the diarist usually styles him, disliked Abolitionists, disdained northerners, detested Lincoln, and feared the growing power of the Federal government. Yet he also disliked slavery, scoffed at State Rights, doubted the political leadership of the CSA, and even questioned the vaunted field generals of the southern military. This man repaired bodies broken by knaves and fools who ordered young boys into doomed situations; he did so because such repair was appointed for him by a predestinated mission or call or selection. Dr. B required no less of his steward Apperson, whom he marked for elected and dutiful service and then held to that task. He fully intended that Apperson become a great doctor and a great servant to those who needed it most—the desperately mentally ill of the southwestern hill country. But on the route to that improbable service, Apperson would be tested by the demanding patriarch who interfered with the boy's romancing if Dr. B disapproved the ladies involved, who denied him leave for fun or for study, and who lectured him not to believe in slavery, secession, the CSA, War, or any other thing builded in sands by sinful man. Even medicine was not to be believed in, but rather to be practiced in the light of faith in God and duty to people. Dr. B insisted on his insight that physicians must be humble because little was known about medicine, really, and much harm ensued from arrogance among those who assumed otherwise.

Apperson squirmed and chafed under Dr. Black's supervision, often recording his anger and his frustration that lesser talents who did less work than he were sent off to medical-college lectures—and every enlisted man seemed to enjoy more days off, more leave time, than did the hospital steward who was sometimes left virtually in charge of things when Dr. B himself took his own leave. Apperson began this War completely disagreeing with Dr. Black about the worthiness of the Cause and about its chances for success. When the hammer blows came to the Cause and to his hopes—when Stonewall Jackson was killed, when the wild charges at Gettysburg were repulsed and followed by an implausible retreat of ambulance wagons through the gap of the South Mountain, when the privations of a depressed region worsened with the misfortunes of war—then Apperson too lost faith in the Cause and its Confederacy and he begged to be released from further service so that he could be about the business of becoming a competent country doctor. Here too Dr. Black was the resolute rock, demanding service to the undeserving CSA exactly because no human could possibly tell who was actually chosen and thus no human could possibly know who was actually deserving. Dr. Black firmly reproached his steward, reminding him that more and more young men were going to be wounded and that Apperson knew how to repair those wounds. That service, repairing the acute wounds from the march of Mars the crazed wargod, was his task now. When the wargod was at last quiet, then Apperson could study how to repair the more chronic wounds and sicknesses that came with civilian life. That is, Apperson could do so if God willed that *any* of them now serving were to survive this travail—no sure thing at all, for of the 1,487 men who signed the rolls of the Stonewall Brigade, only 46 reported for the final duty at Appomattox Court House (and only five men stood at attention for Company D on that April day).[7]

Much has been made, and rightly so, of the butchery of the War. One million soldiers were killed, were wounded, or disappeared in the bloodiest war fought in America. More distressing is the observation that many more, perhaps twice as many, died from sickness as from bullet, shell, or bayonet. And most distressing is the observation that many, probably most, of those who died of sickness then would not die now because today's doctors understand germs and their role in the spread of disease. It is easy to write off the doctors of this enormity as hapless bystanders in an unprecedented tragedy; they can be made to appear clownish or sinister, as you choose.

Yet there may well be another way to look at this tragedy of failed American politics. Looking at the Civil War in its own day and on its own terms, one is drawn to the pioneering work of Clara Barton in developing an international and nonpartisan standard for treatment of the wounded, a standard of transcendent professionalism that would eventuate in the International Red Cross. And, if the Civil War doctors were ignorant of the relationship between germs and disease, they certainly sensed that something was wrong, and they tried mightily to address that problem with observations and record keeping in processes at least accomplishing the elimination of the wrong answers—no small achievement in any research in any field. Finally, we must remember what they faced: When General Robert Edward Lee ordered the charge up Cemetery Hill, when General Ulysses S Grant ordered the march through the Wilderness thicket, they produced not only thousands of deaths in a few hours, but also thousands of wounded men to be treated by nineteenth century resources—a lot to lay before any hospital ward and even more to lay before a tented center in the battlefield.

---

[7] Robertson, *The Fourth Virginia Infantry*, 34.

In any case, this is no brief for the success of the medical treatment in what was the largest war to that date in the world's history. The casualties came in such volume and with such force that they overwhelmed the medical practitioners of that day. Of course they failed. Of more interest is the nature of that failure, and especially the unique feature of the personal history of a hospital steward who did his work with the First Virginia Brigade—the Stonewall Brigade—at Manassas, Fredericksburg, Chancellorsville, Gettysburg, and Appomattox Court House. This hospital steward John Samuel Apperson, author of "[a] journal kept by myself containing synopsis of each days's occupations," is a sensitive and painstaking observer of the details of the medical treatment during and after the great pitched battles. For all periods of the war his detailed personal records supplement and correct official army hospital records, and for certain periods *only* his personal records have survived to tell the medical story at all.

This Apperson is also a barometer of the common citizen's fortunes for a time and a place. At war's beginning he is *plain folk*, but very much *on the make*, with bright prospects. Then he is seen eagerly laying aside personal goals in order to serve the Confederacy. By 1863 he is so depressed by the reality of the late phase of the conflict that he rebels against his benefactor and mentor who will not let him escape the onerous—and obviously futile—duties to the losing Confederate army. Finally, he is seen in the postbellum South triumphantly rebuilding by providing up-to-date medical care facilities for the emotionally afflicted in his adoptive Virginia Highlands—and in that phase he takes to wed Lizzie Black, the very seed of his tyranical and unbending benefactor, thereby becoming patriarch to the very family that once sponsored him.

This immense Civil War, even and especially in Virginia, is too complex to generalize without damaging the historical record, and Apperson's diary must not be treated as being typical. His literary sensitivities, his passions for science, his curiosities and energies are no more representative of the era than Hollywood's celluloid butchers. Yet its very singularity, the intensity of the individual's response to the particular, is still more proof of the artwork that poet Wystan Hugh Auden found in the "muse of the unique historical fact."[8] As the hospital steward makes his way, his own keen observations about life in Civil War era Virginia teach us much about what happened

[8] Wystan Hugh Auden, "Homage to Clio," *Collected Poems*, ed., Edward Mendelson (New York: Random House, 1976), s.v.

and why, at least in one life. In that life, we find bright promises, overwhelming challenges, overburdening defeats, and then an epiphany of service to family and community in an impoverished but hardly poor world. There is yet much to learn from the story that he records.

Part One

15 January–2 July 1861

"We Must Take Hold in Earnest"

AN APPRENTICE WITH EVERY BRIGHT PROSPECT

Seven Mile Ford is a community in Smyth County in the Virginia highlands of the "Southwest" beyond the Blue Ridge. The Ford, as Apperson often calls it, is a natural spot for crossing the Holston River whose valleys and ridges and forks provide place names for much of the Virginia highlands and the Upper East of Tennessee. Dr. William Faris, a surgeon and general practitioner in the highlands, lived at Seven Mile Ford but based his practice in Marion, the county seat located about five miles east. Marion was the county's center of commerce and trade as well as law and political activities. For instance, James P. Strother's hotel, The Continental (after the war renamed Hotel Marion) was often scene of political debates and discussions, including the interesting occasion of 22 January 1861 when Apperson heard pro-secession speeches by local leaders such as Strother and James White Sheffey and by more renowned leaders such as John Buchanan Floyd, former governor and onetime cabinet member.

Apperson did some "odd jobs" and day labor, but quickly became Dr. Faris's steward, that is, a kind of assistant to the surgeon. Some stewards served a period of apprenticeship and then went on to medical school and became practitioners, and the diary makes it clear that such was Dr. Faris's plan for his young assistant. The inquisitive and energetic youth was soon reading the physician's journals and studying pharmacological books as well as observing Dr. Faris treat patients. Besides delivering medicines and collecting fees and carrying back reports from patients, Apperson soon was trusted to diagnose simple cases and prescribe treatments and medicines for those cases. Even in difficult cases diagnosed by Faris, Apperson was trusted to "mix" the medicinal compounds and generally to administer them; he was also trusted to do some of the bone-setting and other physical treatment. It does appear from the record, however, that only Faris himself performed any surgery, albeit often with his steward at his side.

In this section of his diary entries, Apperson has shown the modern reader much about highlands society in 1861, its camp meetings, its social gatherings in parlors and at the county courthouse and at "squire's courts" (such localized legal proceedings were at least two parts social and political to every part judicial), and the nature of its business dealings, which were essentially face-to-face and often "barter" or trade in kind rather than formal transactions involving cash. Although this county was dominated by the plain folk or "middling farmers" and small-business and tradespeople and craftspeople, there was a clear majority in favor of secession. There was certainly majority opinion, occasionally becoming mob action, that militated against abolitionism. The county was namesake of Alexander Smyth, a political leader in early national days and himself a large-scale slaveowner; when the county was formed, the census marked more than eight hundred slaves and more than one hundred and forty "free colored" in its 1840 enumeration. Slavery was economically important to most residents, if only indirectly through trade and services provided slaveowners. Note that Apperson himself was in his own words "hot" for secession and southern nationalism, certainly more so than his benefactor Dr. Faris. Apperson is honest enough in his diary, however, to note that the minority view opposing secession is not insignificant in size, stature, or moral fervor.

Of medical practices, perhaps the most interesting things to note are some characateristics demonstrated by Steven Stowe in his studies of nineteenth century medicine. The antebellum practitioner is neither a butcher, nor a superstitious clown; but rather one who studies the available scientific literature and applies the techniques most recently published in professional journals. Of course, it is an era before the role of bacteria was understood, and an era before the "knowledge explosion" of late nineteenth century. The practitioner of this era made house calls, obviously, and when he did so, he joined a team of people, always including the members of the patient's family, ministers, and midwives and other women in the community who often serve as care-givers. The doctor was primus inter pares, rather than an isolated and absolute authority; he listened eagerly and attentively to the observations made by other members of the treatment team. The antebellum doctor was a close observer, as a scientific practitioner should be, but his form of expression was less technical than literary, and the notations occasionally attained a form of art.[1] Above all, without being superstitious at all and certainly without being fatalistic, the practitioner is deeply spiritualistic, intensely and intently aware that he is in the

[1] Steven Stowe, "Medical Practices," address, 10 October 1998, Southern Historical Association meeting, Birmingham. Stowe has also shared with the authors sections of a forthcoming publication concerning antebellum and wartime medical practices.

presence of forces larger and longer-lived than the merely mortal. The exhortations that Apperson made to the Lord God on behalf of patients were as sincere at the bedside as they were in the church pews--and they were as sincere, if less perfervid, as his prayers would be on the field of battle.

Finally, at the level of personal history, Apperson in this section balanced himself on the point of a delicate irony, almost a bit of dark humor. He was eager to the point of anxiety to enter studies at the Medical College of Virginia in Richmond in order to become a country physician ("attend lectures" is the language of the diarist and of the day). To that end, he was saving money and he was relying on a letter of recommendation to the faculty's lecturers from Dr. Faris. He was hopeful that one of his two "rich uncles," Uncle William or Uncle Charles, would serve as benefactor for tuition charges. Yet he was also most eager for the Commonwealth of Virginia to join other southern states in secession, a cause for which he was entirely ready to enlist. He did not seem to acknowledge that he could not simultaneously serve the Confederacy and attend medical lectures, and so throughout this section he was hoping and praying for two conflicting—and mutually excluding—things to happen. Of course, in his small way, Apperson was exactly like most youth of the day, busy with their plans for a personal future of every bright promise while also preparing for secession and war, both events less promising than foreboding.

A journal kept by myself containing synopsis of each day's occupations & c.

John S. Apperson
7 Mile Ford
Smyth Co.

RESOLUTIONS

JANUARY 15TH, 1861

Resolved this day that I will prepare myself a journal for the purpose of writing a few lines, at least, every day—giving account of how the day was spent—at what engaged, also feelings &c.

Resolved, also, that I will carry out the above mentioned resolutions by writing in the evening of each day (if possible) giving in as few words as possible each day's work.

Jno. S. Apperson

WEDNESDAY MORNING JAN. 16TH, '61

Rose about 6 o'clock this morning—had company—ate breakfast about 8 o. Studied chemistry in the morning. About 11 o. Dr. [Faris][2] was called to see a man who had been struck by the falling of a tree and as we were told had both legs broken. Dr. requested me to accompany him—I did so. We found the man very bad; but only one leg broke or rather thigh about the middle 3 fo^{rths}[3]. Several scars on the forehead—complained of pain in both shoulders, right side, and back. Pulse good, notwithstanding he had been bled by one of the neighbors, which was contrary to all law and reason. We prepared our apparatus for the fractured limb—the long straight splint. Left him complaining very much.[4]

---

[2] *Dr.* and *F.* always refer to Dr. Faris, unless otherwise indicated.

[3] Apperson's symbol for fractions. In this case 3/4.

[4] Bleeding, or venesection, was a surgical technique used in the day to remove "bad humors" in the blood, as when an infection had set in. A fracture of this kind would not be bled by a practitioner, but instead would be set with a splint, as described above. Bonesetting, even if done by a surgeon, was not a surgical technique; and would seldom involve more than a splint. In this case, Faris directed Apperson to apply a long vertical splint, another splint along the leg called a gaiter, and some kind of shielding pads, in this case, so-styled brand pads. Faris and Apperson are

We scarcely expect him to survive long, especially if there is much injury done the body, which we could not ascertain. We arrived home after night [.] I studied the proper treatment for the case before us and prepared to retire about 11 o.

THURSDAY JANUARY 17TH, '61

Rose about 1/2 past 6 this morning, prepared some medicine for a patient & then made ready to visit our patient of yesterday. We had a muddy ride—arrived about noon found the patient better than I expected—no fever—leg in same position it was put in yesterday. After we adjusted a gaiter and some brand pads, dinner was furnished. After dinner we left. Dr. went to see some patients and to settle some bills with the neighbors—did but little in that line.

One thing I witnessed to-day that proves very conclusively that man cannot be depended upon. Probably a month and a half ago the citizens of ________ [sic][5] neighborhood had a meeting to take into consideration the propriety of allowing a Still-house to be erected in their midst as they have nothing of the kind among them and have just finished a beautiful house of worship; and indeed have a very *moral* neighborhood. The still-house was to be built by a gentleman who had lately bought real estate adjoining that of many of [sic] neighbors. Dr. F addressed the meeting forcibly against a step so pernicious to their happiness. Others were called upon for remarks among whom was myself—I of course responded as best I could. The vote was taken and the still-house-erection was disapproved almost unanimously. But what a different picture is presented to-day. The man who contemplated building the house, caring, very little perhaps, for the meager disapprobation of mere man, determined to build the house. To-day the house is being erected—and who are the builders—why the very men who a few days ago declared their hatred for it in word and action. How fickle! How mistaken! Remember man: "you knew your duty but did it not". Fathers of the growing generations in Chilhowie—when will you regret the step you have taken, in giving aid to the erection of a hell in your midst? When will you be led to see your error?— It will

---

not here attempting to practice osteopathy, and they probably knew little of that emerging field. "Osteopathy," Rodereick E. McGrew, *Encyclopedia of Medical History* (New York: McGraw-HIll, 1985), s.v.; hereinafter *McGrew's.*

[5] The town is Chilhowie, in Smyth county near Seven Mile Ford; the exact neighborhood is unknown.

be when you see your children leaving the standard of morality you have erected—then you will regret it. When you see your children reeling home-ward beneath a load of intoxicating liquor—their brains racked with insanity, their hearts giving birth to thoughts of which the mouth speaketh— then you will regret it, and I fear too late.

I predict for your beautiful church many interrupted congregations—many difficulties with inebriates [that is, persons who are inebriated]—many worse than are an influence in counteracting the most sacred influences of the church.

We returned home about dusk. After making a fire in my room, I read a passage from the sketch of the life of Tasso by J.H. Griffin[6] . I am writing at 9 o. Will study a lesson in chemistry and retire.

FRIDAY JANUARY 18, 1861

Rose about 6 o'clock—ate breakfast and prepared to visit a patient—young lady who has sore throat. I started about 11 o'clock—found it to be a case of diptheria (pseudo membraneous angina). I prescribed for her and went to see the case of *fractured thigh.* Found him in a "bad fix"— bowels caustic and have not been moved since he was hurt—urine muddy—a dull aching pain about the chest and bowels. The apparatus had been thrown out of fix altogether by some effort of his own.

I immediately dispatched a message for Dr. F giving him the symptoms with the request to come immediately. He came about 8 o'clock. Patient worse—delirious—passed water unconsciously. Dr. bled him immediately which seemed to relieve him for a time. We gave him a dose of C. [castor] oil—readjusted the apparatus and gave him a dose of sulp. morphine. Left him half past 10 o'clock in a delirious stupor. We have no hope of his recovery.

We arrived home about half past 12 o'clock—very tired and sleepy. I am or have been impressed with the idea to-day that the life of a Doctor is one of responsibility and trouble. The pay of a physician is but a meager compensation for the mental and physical labor, and in fine the feelings he must of need experience in seeing his fellow being suffer without the skill or power to relieve

---

[6] Torquato Tasso, *Jerusalem Delivered*, ed. with introd., J.H. Griffin (J.H. Griffin, English tr., New York: D. Appleton & Co., 1866). Tasso was born 11 March 1544 in Sorrento, Italy, and died 25 April 1595 in Rome. He wrote cantos in heroic verse celebrating the Crusades. Griffin edited an English language version and provided a biographical sketch of Tasso in his edition. Apperson, like many young men of the era, was drawn to this romanticization and apparently carried Griffin's translation with him and consulted it often.

him. It is bad! But when we take hold of any avocation by which we are to obtain a sustence [sic: sustenance] we must take hold in earnest.

SATURDAY JANUARY 19TH, '61

Owing to the lateness of the hour that I retired I did not rise this morning until about 1/2 past 7—I guess.

Rode a few miles this morning on business for Dr. F and on my return home met Dr. He requested me to visit some patients for him this evening, it being out of his power to see them. I arrived at home about 3 o'clock, prepared some medicine and went to visit the patients among whom was Mr. _______ [sic] who was wounded by the fall of a tree. I heard before I got to him that he was supposed to be dying. I found him speechless—head hot—mouth dry—breathing very laboriously—the action of the heart fluttering—pulse *small and quick*, stopping almost entirely at intervals—eyes fixed. I think he was dying, but how long he will or can live in that condition I am unable to say. I left him altogether ignorant of the direct cause of his suffering, or any treatment therefore.

I went to a house where the case of *diptheria* I visited yesterday lay—found her better. I then came home and prepared to retire about 1/2 past 10 o'clock.

My feelings were somewhat aroused to-day. A little boy and girl— children of the wounded man—were standing over their dying father, weeping bitterly when I left him. They did not weep as children weep generally, but as old persons would when grief "deep and wide" assailed their breast. They wept not loud and frantic, but low and still with stifled sobs. The little girl placed her face near her father's; but poor thing! her father unconscious of all around him regarded her not; her tears fell upon his cheeks but he felt them not. Ah! little girl, the blood will soon cease forever to flow through the veins of those arms that once clasped you with fatherly affection.

Little boy, the voice of your dear parent is hushed probably never again to sound in your hearing, his ears are deafened by pain; his eyes bedimmed by agony; his brain is racked with delirium that benumbs every other sense. The rough breathing of his breath, that startles you at intervals, will soon cease those desperate efforts to draw life from the air around and settle down still—still in death!

Your mother has gone before, your father follows now. They have entered eternity's domain—a land for which ere long you and I and the whole of Adam's race are bound.

Go forth then to the world and for the short time you are permitted to live here do your duty—act well your part! And God will be to you a father and friend.

SUNDAY JANUARY 20TH, '61

Rose at 7— breakfast an hour later and dressed as it is usual to dress to go to church after breakfast. Sometimes, however, I finish my toilet before breakfast. Read a few pages of Tasso—company coming and remained all day nearly. We had no news for about a week, so I concluded to walk to the post office as we expect mail at 7 o'clock. The R-Road has been filled up with a "slide", consequently the cars have been very irregular. Mail came tonight— I had the pleasure to get a letter from a friend at Emory & Henry College (R.H.D.)[7] He tells me that he is doing well— has been examined on the studies of his first session and passed all his studies which was gratifying to me as I esteem him very much. I hope he may pass through his college life successfully.

I remained at the post office all night with Mr. E. A.S.[8] for the first time since I had been in West Va[9] . I like Mr. S very well.

MONDAY JANUARY 21ST, 1861

Came home this morning about 10 o'clock— wrote some and prepared to go to the Glade Spring neighborhood on business for Dr. F. Had a cool & muddy ride going and coming back I had a very cold one. Nothing of interest transpired. I saw the improvements made at the Washington Springs. They are very—very pretty. The mountains and country around have rough appearance as though nature had endeavoured to give it *drollness*: but the buildings are very

---

[7] Robert Henry Dungan was then a twenty-five year old sophomore at Emory & Henry College. From Seven Mile Ford, he left school to join the Confederate army, eventually commanding the 48th Virginia Regiment with rank of colonel. Unlike Apperson, he surrendered at Appomattox Court House. After the War, he became a teacher in Chilhowie, where he and Apperson continued to see each other. *Student Register*, 16 August 1860; *Emory & Henry College Catalog*, 1860-1861; *Emory & Henry College Catalog*, 1887 [with alumni information], Emory & Henry College Archives.

[8] E.A. Scott was clerk of circuit court, serving from 1852 to 1860. Clerk of court was a political stepping-stone, since both circuit-court and county-court sessions were as much political occasions as judicial hearings. Wilson, *Smyth County History*, 92.

[9] Apperson is referring to Virginia west of the Blue Ridge; there was not then a state of West Virginia.

artfully and beautifully erected. [10] In the whole nature and art are necessary concomitants to beauty here, at least. I was too tired and sleepy to study to-night and will retire now about 10 o'clock.

TUESDAY JANUARY 22ND, 1861

To-day being our court day I, as usual, was off about 9 o'clock—had a cold, disagreeable ride. Business dull owing to the crisis that is now upon us. I mean the revolution that has convulsed our country with excitement.

The North has injured and insulted the South and refused to make amends. The South has determined to bear it no longer. Eight states are now out of the Union— Virginia is making preparations to *snap* assunder the bonds that bind her to the Union. We all look: "wonder fraught" as to what will be the issue of the move in progress.

Ex Secretary of War, Col. [John Buchanan] Floyd adress [sic] the people of Smyth to-day on the affairs of our country. His appearance is a very imposing one, considering the times. His hair is grey and hung in locks that often received a sudden stroke from his hand while he was speaking. His hands trembled very much— his voice clear and audible—his manner was everything that could be disired [sic]. I never saw a more attentive audience for a political meeting. But really the times demand attention and attention was not out of place nor lost while listening to Floyd. He gave a full statement of facts as they had occurred at the Capitol. He gave General [Winfield] Scott some giant strokes in the mildest manner possible—milder if possible than did Mark Anthony Brutus[11] . He says that he can see no other chance for us but combined action of the South in rearing up a confederacy. Mr. Floyd took his seat *[illegible]* I might say a still applause after a speech of three hours length.

The effect he had worked upon the audience was too deep. J.W. Sheffey[12] was called for loudly he arose deeply affected amid the cheering of crowd who had

---

[10]A hotel built in Glade Spring in Washington County south of Seven Mile Ford; the hotel was built after the rail lines were extended to connect Glade Spring to other towns.

[11] Apperson seems to quote ironically William Shakespeare's version of Mark Antony's funeral oration for Julius Caesar, in which the orator slyly attacks Brutus while claiming "to bury Caesar not to praise him." *Julius Caesar*, act 3, sc. 2, lines 72-117. Of course, neither Floyd in this speech nor Shakespeare's Mark Antony on stage was in any way *mild.*

[12] James White Sheffey was a prominent businessman and major landowner in Smyth County. He was active in politics, serving as one of the first circuit court judges; briefly he joined the Know Nothing Party, but he returned to the Democrats by 1859. He was elected as the Smyth County delegate to the 1861 convention in Richmond that voted to secede from the Union. After the War, Sheffey was a partner in the Bank of Marion, serving for a time as its director; and he was elected

apparently waked from a deep feeling that Floyd had imposed upon them. I had been in the house for three hours and the diner room had become very oppressive, so I left. I returned however in time to hear the last words from Sheffey. They were "I am for a new declaration of independence and a Southern Confederacy." He sat down among the wildest applause. Mr. Strother called for the attention of the people a few moments.[13] How many staid [sic] to hear him I know not. I for one left immediately. J.W. Sheffey will be our candidate for delegate, and if nothing prevents me I shall support him. I came home more a secessionist than ever. Not being very well I did nothing but sup and retire.

WEDNESDAY, JANUARY 23RD 1861

Rose at usual hour. Nothing of interest occured to-day. I was engaged in fixing this journal & writing in it. I wrote a letter to my friend [Robert Henry Dungan] at Emory & Henry. I studied chemistry in the evening. The weather has been very boisterous. Commenced snowing about noon—the wind blew very violently. Snow fell sparingly. Every prospect for a bad night.

THURSDAY, JANUARY 24TH, '61

This morning my windows are covered with ice. It rained, hailed, & snowed last night. Not so cold this morning considering 10 o'clock the ice & sleet are thawing, the clouds seem to be scattering away. I hope we may have some fair weather: for we have, in our estimation, had one of the worse sort of winters for rain & mud & snow have been plentiful. Nature seems to have determined to give us our share of weather inconveniences at once. However it is not ours to murmur. He who holds the winds and clouds in his fist and who governs nature and natures [sic] works knows what we need and will govern everything in his kingdom here below as will be best. I studied chemistry to-day. In the evening I

---

as the county's representative to the state House of Delegates in 1875, but died before serving out the full term. Goodridge Wilson, *Smyth County History and Traditions* (Kingsport, TN: Kingsport Press for Centennial Celebration of Smyth County, 1932); Elizabeth Lemmon Sayers, *Smyth County, Virginia*, ed., Joan Tracy Armstrong (Marion, VA.: Smyth County Historical and Museum Society, ca. 1983-1986).

[13]James P. Strother was a business and political associate of Sheffey. In 1823, he built the first important hotel in Marion, The Continental, a wood-frame building on the corner of Main and Church streets. Throughout the antebellum and the war years, the Continental served as an important meeting place for political gatherings, both formal and informal. "Hotel Marion," Smyth County Heritage Book Committee, *Heritage of Smyth County, 1832-1997* (Waynesville, NC: Don Mills for Smyth County Heritage Book Committee, 1997), s.v. This meeting itself was likely in The Continental.

went to Mr. Jno L. Sanders to settle with him but did not do it. I read Tasso's "Jerusalem delivered" i.e. commenced it; but I am candid, I do not understand it yet. The figures as well as the characters are, or seem to be remote. Tasso was a great genius I suppose from the account I read of him. Although he seemed to be a man of powerful mind, and stamina enough to bear everything but he was only a man, and to say that a person is a man is saying enough to prove to us all that he is defective in some shape or form. Tasso's most obvious fault was jealousy or the disposition of thinking that he was slighted. Not envious rather; but mere apprehension that others were sharing the affection of his friends more than himself. He loved as all poets have done and the object of his affections was far above him in *society*—This I suppose was the reason why his eccentric jealousy was more easily noticed than it would otherwise have been.

10 o'clock found me writing. I shall retire soon. The weather is moderated in temperature but not in appearance for fair weather. The snow & ice have melted and the ground thawed making the mud pretty deep indeed.

FRIDAY, JANUARY 25TH, 1861

The weather seems as unfavourable this morning as usual. Foggy, wet, and muddy. I have been engaged all day settling up business for Dr. F.: but have not been very successful. I got home about 1/2 past 8 this evening.

I rec'd a letter from my Uncle Charles Jones, now in Miss. I wrote to him some time ago asking him if he was willing to let me have some money to go to the Medical Lectures next fall. His answer is as much as I could wish—He says if he can get the money he will let me have it—at any rate I can count on him for it. Times are so hard now it looks like folly almost to foster such notions as those of going to College next session. But I have confidence in my Uncle Charles and think if it is possibly in his power he will let me have the money although it may cost him some effort. Uncle Bill has promised to help me so often and done so little for me that I have lost confidence in him. I hope Uncle Charles will be as good as his word. He wrote me sometime last year that he wanted me to have some boots made for him. I contracted the making of them with a shoe-maker in Marion (Turner) who has promised to have them done every week for two months but had made only one pair at court [by the time that district court was in session]. However I do not want them now. My uncle might have involved me by ordering them and then not taking them. I wrote to Mr. Turner to-night not to make any more—& sell what he had already made.

Excitement in regard to our governmental affairs is growing more intense every day. Secession is gaining ground very fast even here among the mountains. There are some stupid as not to know that the tax paid by them goes to support the state government and not the general government as they suppose.

At nine o'clock to-night I was writing— retired about 10.

SATURDAY, JANUARY 26TH, 1861

Was up this morning at 6. Weather, worse and worse— snowing rapidly and wind blowing from the N.E. I had a disagreeable ride this morning to see a case of diptheria. Found patient improving. After I returned Dr. came home from a case of poisoning to which he was called last night —a Mrs. Cole. Found her almost lifeless from the effects of about an ounce and a half of *Laudanum.* [14] She had past [sic.; passed] recovery. Poor woman, what could have given birth to the idea of self destruction! She leaves a husband and four children to mourn her loss, besides many relatives. It is reported that she and her husband did not agree as well as they might. However, this is not for me to discuss. She is now in the presence of her maker who will judge according to the deeds done in the body. Nothing occuring [sic] worthy of note to-day. I wrote a letter to my Uncle Charles and took it to the P.O.

I studied chemistry this evening and then commenced reading over some letters that I had rec'd from my correspondents since I came to West Va. Few I think can appreciate this pleasure mingled with pain wrought by reading over old letters. They are little speaking mementos telling us of little occurrences all along the path of life. I was studying chem. at eleven o'clock—am writing since—will retire in a few minutes.

SUNDAY, JANUARY 27TH 1861

This morning passed as usual. I feel rather lazy, so lazy indeed that I got asleep sitting on my chair. I have been reading Tasso's "Jerusalem delivered". Find in it many good things some of which I have been constrained to take a

---

[14] Laudanum was tincture of opium; it appeared in bitter and colorless crystals and was used as an analgesic, that is, to relieve pain by deadening the feelings; it was also used, as here, as a sedative to induce sleep. This relatively large dose could be fatal, and evidently the woman deliberately took this amount to commit suicide. "Laudanum" and "opium," Clarence Wilbur Taber, *Taber's Cyclopedic Medical Dictionary*, ed., Clayton L. Thomas (1940. Rev. ed.; Philadelphia: F.A. Davis, 1978). Hereinafter cited as *Taber's*.

special note. By by [sic] far the greater portion of his writings is too mysterious for me, or rather, not mysterious but the names of persons spoken of by him seemed hard to distinguish from each other while they [sic] performing their part of the Crusades which is the object of Tasso to represent. In my opinion the Crusades were a rather *drastic* move anyway. I do not think that there is really much music (jingle) about Tasso's poetry when I suppose it is realy [sic] good poetry. There is portrayed in it depth of thought, at times wild and enthusiastic—now all is hope and then dispair [sic]—love one moment & hatred the next. But realy [sic] thus it is with life. Its fleting [sic; fleeting?] scenes are ever changing—each moment gives birth to some new pain or pleasure.

A friend called on me this evening an hour or so. It is great pleasure for me to receive friends—it seems to be one of my objects of life to make friends.

Reading at 9 0'clock—nodding at 10—& in bed before eleven.

MONDAY JAN. 28TH 1861

This morning I was somewhat loath to leave my bed. I to [sic] slow to rise every morning anyway. There is another thing that presses very heavily upon my mind, it is this: I am not half as studious as I ought to be. I spend too much time with my own musings, a thing which I regret very much without the power to overcome it. If I expect to be ready to attend lectures next fall I must certainly be up and doing; for I have three branches to study yet.

I went to widow Sanders to see Robt Goolsby on business for Dr. F— was gone some two or three hours—transacted my business. I studied chemistry & wrote a letter to Mr. P.F. of Tenn. I did more studying to-day than I have done for several days or several weeks. I read Tasso this evening—Tancred goes to hunt Erminia fails to find her—he fights—conquers and is lost in darkness which causes him to fall inside the walls of false Armida's castle. The prince pagan, Argantes demands a fight from the christian [sic] ranks. Fear seems to have seized upon them—no knight is brave enough to encounter the savage pagan Old Raymond, brave as he is old goes out to meet Argantes-—.[15]

I am writing at 11 o'clock. I will rise earlier than usual on the morrow morning.

---

[15] Canto 19 of Tasso's *Jerusalem Delivered.* This passage seems to attract the young medical steward and would-be student because the Crusader hero Tancred is attended to by the fair damsel Erminia, whom the dying knight calls "my kind physician,"Stanza 113.

TUESDAY JAN'Y 29TH, 1861

No better about rising out of bed yet. Seven o'clock found me in bed this morning. I studied chemistry this morning and read Tasso a short time. He is as hard as ever to understand. I went to the P. Office. Found there a letter from my esteemed friend Dr. Quisenberry.[16] The contents made me feel like seeing the Old Locust Grove and surrounding country and the country's people. My friends seem to be doing very nice which is somewhat gratifying to me feeling as I do an interest in every friend's welfare. His letter reminds me of many with whom I once could enjoy a great deal of fun and worthy sport.

Secession is gaining ground in our midst.

I performed venisection [bloodletting] on mr. Williams for, neuralgia[17] — a queere [sic; queer, that is, very odd] treatment I am sure!

Evening has here closed in upon us. Night still and sombre reigns in nature's bosom now. Ten o'clock has pass [sic] some time ago—I am expecting eleven will chime soon. I am dull—too dull indeed to indulge in any of those vagaries that often cause us to lose many hours that should be spent in useful study.

I will wrap up my fire
and prepare to retire —-
Then bid sweet Morphious to come
and stay each billow
That'll rise o'er my pillow
'Till morn's gray light shall peep in my room.

WEDNESDAY, JANUARY 30TH, 1861

This morning I made some improvement on rising (i.e. about rising) early. I was up about 6 this morning. Ate breakfast at the usual time and started on business for Dr. F and met in passing him the person whom I was going to see. I returned of course. I studied chemistry afterwards until the afternoon when I

---

16 Apparently Quisenberry of Locust Grove in Organe County; a licensed physician, who served as the family's doctor. Quisenberry's family was listed with the first national census for Orange County; members of the family held between four and ten slaves, and thus ranked as slaveowning farmers rather than planters. During the War, the doctor's nephew J.N. was listed on the roster of the 6th Va. Cavalry, Crenshaw's Battery. Quisenberry himself was exempted from duty. W.W. Scott, *A History of Orange County, Virginia* (Dayton, OH.: Ruebush-Elkins, 1907), "Appendices: Confederate Rosters," hereinafter cited as Scott, *Orange County*.

17 Neuralgia was any severe pain associated with a nerve ending. Venesection, or bleeding, was the remedy applied to remove the "bad humors," but note that Apperson regards the standard treatment very dubiously. *Taber's*.

had to go to see a sick man about 7 miles from home. I started about 1/2 past four— dark before I got to him. I did not think that there was much the matter with him. He complained of a strange burning sensation in the region of the stomach— probably more in the epigastrium[18] — headach [sic] at intervals. I applied a blister to the chest, oppisite [sic] xiffoid[19] cartilage and gave comp[ound]. cath[artic]. pills[20]. I think he will have jaundice.

I remained overnight as I had to go to Marion next day. I was much troubled with the sick mans noisy moaning about the blister hurting him. I had never applied one before and consequently knew but little about it. However, I suppose it was done as well as some others. I retired to bed after two o'clock. One thing I regret today I got in conversation with a man in the political questions of the day. He was for union any how and I was for secession. Our conversation warmer and warmer until I forgot my patient entirely and commenced discussing the parts in dispute with some degree of excitement. The patient requested us to talk a little lower if we pleased. This brought me to my knowledge of my whereabouts— and that i [sic] acting in the capacity of a helper of the sick and not a bar-room politician.

THURSDAY, JANY. 31ST, '61

This morning I was up early, more from necessity than otherwise. My patient grunting and growling about the blister as though it were killing him or nearly. I clipped the vesications [blisters] and put him to bed, ate breakfast and left for Marion where I arrived about 10 o'clock. After transacting some business I had on hand I returned home. I am writing about 8 o'clock with my eyes in a swing with sleep.

One thing I omitted in my sketch of yesterday's business. I recd. two letters—one from an Aunt the other from an Uncle in Ga. I spoke of losing confidence in my uncle Bill somewhere in my journal. I wrote to him some time ago about money to go to college next session. He has again promised me money on conditions that he can get it himself. He says that I shall have it if he can get it; but complains very much about "hard times".

---

[18] Epigastrium is the region over the pit of the stomach, "Auenbrugger," *Taber's*, s.v.

[19] Xiphoid is the lowest portion of the sternum; it is sword shaped cartilagionous processes supported by bone. No ribs are attached to it; it ossifies in the aged, as seems to have happened to this patient. *Taber's*.

[20] Chemical compound designed to produce purging of the bowels. *Taber's*.

I hope he will not allow me to look to him in vain again. But realy [sic] he has promised me so often that I do no know what to think.

I thought when I wrote my last letter that I wrote it in such a manner that if he did not intend to let me have the money he would be bound to say "no"; but I failed in bringing him to the point I fear. Well he can do as he thinks proper of course. I will get along somehow whether I get help or not.

I shall retire pretty soon tonight.

FRIDAY, FEBRUARY 1ST, 1861.

Weather is bad yet. Hailed and rained slightly last night and this morning it was exceedingly cloudy. About 12 o'clock it commenced raining.

I studied chemistry a while this morning and wrote a letter to my brother & sister. I promised a friend to prepare a piece of composition for declamation. I have made several attempts at it but they have proved failures. I attempted it to-day again and made the worst failure that I have made yet. I cant [sic] get the frame or outline of my subject although I have implored the muses scratched my head and endeavoured & took an idea or two from the bottom of my inkstand but all seems no use. I am almost ready to give it up though if I were to give it up I should have to give a reason for so doing: and to say that I could not do it would be rather coming down; I will make a few more attempts at it if I fail. Nothing more than usual has passed to-day. Nine o'clock and it is raining rapidly.

SATURDAY FEBRUARY 2ND, '61.

I rose a little earlier than usual this morning. This day two years ago was one of the most to be remembered of any of my life. Two years ago I left home for where I hardly knew[.] I never once thought of being in Virginia to-day but it seems as if fate decided that I should follow the course I have taken. However, I have had no cause, as yet, to regret it. I hope the Great God whose [sic] holds the destinies of men in his hands will do whatsoever seemeth good in his sight.

This morning is a very rainy morning. The whole face of the earth and especialy [sic] the water courses show that there was a heavy fall of rain last night.

Dr. F and myself prepared to go to Sinclair's Bottom to hear an address by Mr. J.W. Sheffey of Marion Va. on the affairs of our country. Notwithstanding the inclemency of the weather we went, and had the pleasure of meeting some seventy five or a hundred soverigns [sic] of the county. Mr. Sheffey is our candidate for delegate to a convention which is to meet in Richmond on the 13th inst. He is an able and eloquent speaker—and I suppose did his "prettiest" for us. For my part I am for him and with him in sentiment.

He spoke of the occaision [sic] that brought us together and of the present distressed conditions of our country. Giving us a historical sketch of the emigration to and the settling of our country by the pilgrims and aborigines of an early date in the history of the United States. He spoke of the trials and difficulties our forefathers encountered with the savages, the beasts and inclemencies of the climate. Then the steps taken by the settlers to raise themselves from abject want to an independant [sic] condition. The cause of the war of the revolution was also spoken of in a clear and conclusive style. He then spoke of the aggression of the northern states to the southern people, and drew a contrast between the right of one and right of the other.

The tax imposed upon the American people was but a mite in itself but the principal [sic] of right and wrong was the question. And the people of the colonies could never submit to bear a wrong, though it were only a trifling tax on tea but it was wrong and therefore the colonies refused to submit—so with the state of affairs. Northern aggression is wrong, we care not for their "Personal Liberty Acts" as they call them nor for ditto [sic, that is, personal liberty acts for] the slaves that have ever crossed Mason & Dixon's lines and been harboured by northern fools, but the right and justice is the thing taken into consideration. The northerners have ignored southern principals [sic] and treated them with as much disrespect as it is possible for them to do and their treatment to southern principals they nullify the constitution. Hence we have grounds for discontent. Again Mr. Sheffey says that the government of Virginia & U.S. is founded upon a great principal [sic] that that [sic] : *Ours is a government only at the consent of the governed.* Before the sages of Virginia ratified the Federal constitution they expressed their determination not to be subject to it an hour after it became oppressive. It is evident now that something is oppressive.

Mr. S. is for united action of the south in regard to erecting a new confederacy. "Virginia" he says "must go with the south" and when she declares herself for one party and against the other we have no more to fear.

He closed his speech by declaring himself to be southern in sentiment and feeling and pledged himself to protect her interests.

I was engaged after speaking with some business for Dr. F. I started home through the mud—which was more plenty than, I think, I have ever saw [sic] it.

I got two letters from my sister M. to-day—all are well.

I arrived at home about half past seven o'clock—retired early.

SUNDAY, FEBRUARY 3RD, '61

This morning I was out of bed about quarter 'till seven—a little earlier than usual Finished my toilet and ate breakfast. Then I contented myself reading Tasso. A coloured woman came in that wished to be bled. I performed the operation of venesection [bloodletting] and then walked to the Baptist church. Rev. Wm. Lewis preached. It was the first time I ever heard him—he preached much better than I expected. His sermon was somewhat a "money sermon" He teaches that a man that preaches for money is not Christ's servant, and those that preach the gospel are to live by the gospel— that they must [not] be paid for services. This I endorse. I had company—Mr. Brunot (a Frenchrman) & Mr. N.C.B St. John. Mrs. F. & Miss Kate F. [Dr. F's wife and daughter] staid [sic] a few hours in my room to-night.

Nine o'clock, writing—will close in a minute or two and retire. Raining rapidly.

MONDAY FEBY. 4TH, '61

This has been an exciting day to me. I was up at six this morning. After writing some for the piece of composition which I was to prepare for a friend (I concluded to get a piece already written as I could not concentrate my mind in any subject that I could make fine enough for declamation) I prepared some medicine and walked to the place where the Election was to be held—three gentlemen were also along. The Election is for delegates to represent us in a convention to be held in Richmond on the 13th inst. The crowd was very small when we arrived. As it is usual politics were discussed pretty freely and more especially at this exciting time. I forbore having any argument or dispute with any of any party. This however did not last long before two young men seemed to disagree on some point or other and by some argument one says to the other: "You are a liar"! This of course was a thing that no honourable man could take and language that no gentleman would use to another unless it was intended for an insult. This breach of good breeding was of course *resented* by a blow from Mr. A.J. Sanders the insulted man.

He was a young man that I had regard for and esteemed. Before I thought or even had time to think I was pulling men from side to side to get to the scuffle that was ensuing. I was for fighting until Sanders gave Faris (the name of the other man) a good thumping for so gross an insult. Faris was a very stout man and Sanders was weakly and would have rec'd from Faris a severe beating had they not been parted. I was insulted and disappointed in my hopes of seeing Faris whipped and I immediately became enraged. The principles that Sanders had declared was the principals [sic] I endorsed; that any man that would not fight for the south in case it were necessary at this juncture they were not worthy of the name of a man! This I declared aloud boldly and openly. Several took insult at it, which I neither cared to evade or tried to prevent. I was about to get into a fight but was *prevented* by some of the folks quashing the difficulty. I voted for J.W. Sheffey which received a handsome majority —63 to 4. Mr. Barton was the other candidate in the field. There was also another vote taken which was for reffering [sic.; that is, holding a referendum election specific to the issue of secession] and the *other* against refering—I was against refering because we have not the time for a convention—an election and then probably be upon the same ground that we are now.

The remainder of the day passed as might be expected. I was at Mr. Rectors this evening until 8 o'clock. Writing about 10—will retire now.

TUESDAY FEBRUARY 5TH, '61

I was up as usual late this morning. After breakfast I visited Mr. S.D. Sanders who has diptheria. Found not very bad. Studied a lesson in chemistry and went over to Mr. J.V. Dungan's[21] sale to settle some *ps* [sic; bills] for Dr. Faris but failed to do much. I returned home about sundown.

The affairs of our country are growing worse and worse and here in our county excitement is nearly as high as it can get I suppose. I have long since been aware that there were a great many abolitionists here among us and I find out there are persons whom I did not think.

A Mr. Wm Faris gave public expression of his sentiments so derogatory to Southern Wellfare [sic] that the citizens of Marion and surrounding country treated him with a coat of tar and feathers—a hideous sight. I presume I cannot say that I am very much in favor of that kind of punishment, but I am for punishment and it makes but little difference how.

Men that live in our country and that have lived here all their life and now speak sentiments against it does not deserve to live.

Faris was in jail when I heard from him last, what will be done with him I am at a loss to know—some of the persons that took him proposed sending him

---

[21] James V. Dungan of Seven Mile Ford was father of Apperson's friend Robert H. Dungan who was then a sophomore at Emory & Henry College. *Student Register*, 16 August 1860, Emory & Henry College Archives.

north to Horace Greeley[22] or some other hard headed abolitionist—and by the way a very good idea.

Company at our house to-night—retired about 10 o'clock.

WEDNESDAY FEBUARY [SIC] 6TH, '61

I was up about six this morning. A beautiful morning indeed. I hope we'll have some good weather now. I do long to see some dry weather very mutch [sic].

I visited Mr Sanders again this morning—found him something worse—prescribed for him again and came home after dinner.

Studied chemistry this evening—The excitement at Marion has not abated yet. Faris is in jail and will not retract anything he said. What they will do with him, I know not. It is certain he can never live in Virginia and declare himself in favour of abolitionism. The people of Va enjoy the happiness that is allowed every citizen of the Virginia Commonwealth— are nurtured and sustained by Va.: and must yield to her laws or leave.

I think the caution that is given by the treatment Faris received will suffice for a warning to all who sustain such feelings towards the *north*.

I am writing between eleven and twelve o'clock—will retire pretty soon.

THURSDAY, FEB. 7, '61

I was out of bed early this morning. After breakfast I went over the mountains into rich valley [sic][23] on business for Dr. F. The wind *blew very hard.* I stoped [sic] at *Snapp & Graham's* store at Lyons Gap[24] and paid them fifteen dollars on my *d/c* [debit/credit account]. They have been very kind to let me have goods as a credit when I did not know where I could [sic] the money to pay them. I went further. When I returned Mr A.J. Graham insisted that I should stay all night with him. I agreed to stay. He was taking an inventory of his goods—I helped him with receipts until midnight. We had a very merry time joking & c. If there is anything to regret it is our being so wild and bad.

---

[22] Horace Greeley (1811-1872) was editor of the *New York Tribune.* A presidential candidate in 1868, Greeley was early in demanding immediate abolition and also early in demanding a vigorous military campaign featuring an aggressive approach to Richmond. His most famous editorial was "The Prayer of Twenty Million."

[23] Rich Valley is a community in Smyth County northwest of Marion.

[24] Lyons Gap is a community in Smyth County southeast of Marion.

FRIDAY, FEBUARY [SIC] 8TH, 1861.

This morning I arose tollerably [sic] early and went to work again on the goods.

I proposed going home after breakfast but Mr. G. insisted that I should stay until evening anyhow [.] I concurred.

We could not do much because so many persons came in to buy goods. Among others several very pretty Ladies condescended to show their lovely faces. I think that a pretty, modest woman can do a great deal of good in the world if they are disposed to do so. I am sure that I am never in the presence of one unless I feel that she is a being destined by the Creator to soothe and quell the turbulent nature of man and that her presence demands of the male portion of humanity honor & respect amounting almost to reverence. However I am expressing my feelings towards the fair sex in rather an idle way I fear; but I have feelings towards woman that I cannot exactly discribe [sic] and can not account for it in no [sic] way unless it be from the love I have for them. I have no notion marrying any of them soon if ever[.] I love all. Yet my feelings have never been concentrated on any particular Lady. Hence it may be my lot to live an old batcheler [sic].

I left Lyon's Gap about 1 o'clock and arrived home about 1/2 past two. Studied chemistry during the remainder of the day—retired early. We learned to-day that Wm. Faris who was in jail was served with the notice to leave the State in 10 days.

SATURDAY, FEBUARY [SIC] 9TH, '61

This morning I was exceeding loth [sic] to leave my bed. I am afraid lying in bed late is growing on me. I wrote a letter to my uncle Bill this morning and studied chemistry. I will finish chemistry in a few more lessons—I am very tired of it anyhow. I have been longer at it than I anticipated when I commenced it. After dinner I brushed up the shop—a dirty job. I then went to the "ford".[25] I recd. a letter from cousin Bettie Apperson of Culpeper Co. I love Cousin Bettie. She is such a good hearted woman, lively and social in her manner: Though not gay and thoughtless. I would be glad to see her and all Uncle Tom's family. Aunt Livia was always so kind to me that it was a feast to go to see her. Uncle was good to me also. He was more discreet than Uncle Joe.

---

[25] "ford" refers to Seven Mile Ford where Apperson roomed; it is several miles south of Marion .

News from headquarters of our government is no better, war seems more and more inevitable as time rolls on. Virginia will meet in convention Wednesday. The state voted for the action of the convention to come before the people, a thing which I think is superfluous altogether, in fact wrong. We have appointed delegates to this convention and entrusted in their hands our destiny, giving them the power to set Virginia wherever they think proper that she should stand and I say let their decision be final. If they do not know what Virginia should do I am sure the people who have never studied the question do not. The brightest intellects and purest patriots of Virginia's sons are sent to mark out a course for her to take but after the course is marked out and the signboard pointed to by Virginia's best it is then optional with the mass whether they follow directions or not—they are thus asked to do as they pleased. Probably the decision of the convention will be voted down and then where will we stand? Where we are now but worse off; for the 4th of March [inauguration day for newly elected President Abraham Lincoln] will be but a few days off; Virginia's most inteligent [sic] and the masses are differing—Lincoln takes his seat at the helm of this government and the consequences are or will be such, I fear, that will startle us from our mountain homes and bid look athwart the gloom that enshrouds our once happy country.

I read the "Marion Visitor"[26] after I came home until 11 o'clock then wrote awhile. Will retire now about 1/2 past 11 o'clock.

SUNDAY, FEBUARY 10TH, 1861

I arose and dressed myself this morning and after breakfast I read Tasso's "Jerusalem Delivered" awhile. I then walked over to the camp ground to prayer meeting. There were but few persons in attendance although it was a very fine day—a little windy. Prayer meeting over and the minister was holding class meeting when I left. I came home and spent the evening with Mrs. Faris. She is good company *sometimes* when ________________ [sic]. She was somewhat inquisitive this evening about my belief of baptism & c. I gave her no satisfaction for I don't think it would be proper for me to express my feelings to

---

[26] *The Marion Visitor* was a weekly founded in 1858 by George J. Curtis and James W. Kennedy. The first newspaper in Smyth County, *The Visitor* described itself in prospectus as "A Family Newspaper Neutral in Politics, and devoted to Literature, News, Science, Agriculture, and General Intelligence." A weekly, it appeared each Friday, in "Double Medium size," but it did not survive the War. Kennedy developed another newspaper in 1869, and there were at least two competing newspapers in Marion during the decades after the War and until World War II. Wilson, "Newspapers," *Smyth County*, s.v.

any one especially when everybody is so prone to find fault with each others church. I do realy [sic] believe that the people are building a barrier up between the churches here that will in time prove impassible. I suppose it is indicative of zeal to see each one trying to build up their own church; but they should not attempt to build up their own at the cost of others; they should not eulogise their own beliefs and abuse others— such is too much the case among them. I fear there are some who had rather see their friends and relatives live estranged from Christ, an alien to God—a devotee' of Satans insidious works than to see them unite and live in a church not their own. I may be mistaken—hope I am, but I fear such is too much the case.

I wrote a letter to my Aunt Malinda to-day. I do not know whether she cares much about my correspondence or not—I wish I knew. I read Tasso after I came to my room—fell asleep in my chair and lost an hour— retired about 10 o'clock.

FRIDAY. FEB. 11TH

On the morning of this day two years ago I walked out upon the streets of Marion for the first in my life. My feelings were such then that I cannot now describe them. I knew not then what I would do for a single day ahead. No one seemed to care aught for me—and I probably cared but little for no one. I was thrown exclusively upon my own exertions for support. A twain [sic, viz., *no*] friend to confide in—no adviser to admonish or direct but alone and unnoticed I passed the frozen streets to find employment. After a long time I found it—I am now and have been ever since breasting the boisterous storms of life. Sometimes my hopes are bright as a noonday sun, my fears gone down like the clouds of an evening. But soon again they rise and threaten to blast every fond hope that filled my doubting brain. Although I have battled with difficulties some of which are imaginary and others magnified I have never had a cause to regret my course in the main. It is true there are many minor things that I regret. I am here forced to make a few remarks on "borrowing trouble". How prone we are to dread some difficulty ahead, and as it were commence climbing a hill before we get to it. When I commenced my present avocation I counted far ahead and all looked dark and gloomy, numerous little plans did devise to extricate myself from what I was almost forced to believe was an entanglement. I lived continually between fear and hope and even after I had the assurance that I should have assistance I still entertained some presentiment of difficulty. Now I see those little things that troubled my mind then have "gone glimmering through the past" a trouble borrowed for nothing a hill climbed where realy [sic] no hill existed. But now I am looking forward to a higher point—for more and more a disappointment is, in my imagination, ahead sure. So it is with all of us. There is no satisfying our craving minds nor allaying our timid fears.

I studied chemistry to-day—got along very well—will finish it to-morrow if nothing prevents. I read some speeches this evening which were spoken in congress by Sherrard Clemens—T.A.R. Nelson and A.H.H. Stuart. [27] They are forunion—union man meaning one is "submissionist" I am sure Stuart made false statements in regard to the financial difficulty of S. Carolina [which had already seceded]. He made mountains out of molehills— will study chemistry a while after 11 o'clock and retire.

---

[27] Sherrard Clemens (1820-1881) was an attorney and U.S. Representative from Wheeling, then in Virginia; he supported the Union, resisted secession, and practiced law in the new state of West Virginia after secession, eventually settling in St. Louis. Thomas Amos Rogers Nelson (1812-1873), from Knoxville, Tennessee, represented eastern Tennessee in the U.S. House of Representatives and also supported the Union. When secession came, he remained loyal to the Union, serving in U.S. congress; he was arrested by Virginians while traveling through the Commonwealth on his way to the U.S. capital, but was eventually released. Still later, he served as defense attorney for fellow eastern Tennessean Andrew Johnson in the impeachment proceedings. Nelson was from a very prominent Virginia family that had settled the Shenandoah Valley. Alexander Hugh Holmes Stuart (1807-1891) was an attorney from Staunton and a member of Millard Fillmore's cabinet. In this period he was in the Virginia Senate, where he opposed secession. Stuart, unlike Nelson and Clemens, did join the Confederacy once Virginia seceded. He was active after the War in Virginia's rapid restoration to full statehood. These figures, all college-educated men from very old Virginia families, were well-respected by Virginians.

Apperson clearly resents their status as well as their opinions. Stuart, Nelson, and Clemens joined others, including prominent judge George William Summers, in the abortive Peace Conference held in Washington in which Unionist southerners attempted to develop a compromise that would keep Virginia and the Upper South in the Union even though the Lower South had already formed the Confederacy in Montgomery, Alabama. All of these figures were old-time Whigs who emphasized the development of industry, banking, and commerce. Their economic policies would eventually become quite attractive to Apperson when the War was at last over. Arnold A. Sherman, "Thomas A. R. Nelson" and "Nelson Family", *Encyclopedia of Southern History*, eds., David C. Roller and Robert W. Twyman (Baton Rouge: Louisiana State University Press, 1979), s.v.; Selden Nelson, "Nelsons of Valley of Virginia," *Virginia Magazine of History & Biography* 18 (1910): 202-03; "George William Summers," "Alexander Hugh Holmes Stuart", and "Thomas Amos Rogers Nelson," *Biographical Directory of the United States Congress, 1774-1989* (Washington: U.S. Government Printing Office, 1989), s.v.

TUESDAY, FEB. 12TH, '61

This morning I had to visit a patient for Dr. F- a married lady. I did not think her very sick, a cold probably. I prescribed for her. I intended yesterday to finish chemistry to-day but failed—owing to other business on hand. I went to the post office this evening—nothing new. When I returned I found a young lady at Dr's— I lost some hour and a half or two hours in prescribing her. I came to my room about 9 o'clock. I read Davis on colic [28] for an hour and fell asleep in my seat—after I awoke I studied chemistry awhile and retired.

I am a strange natured fellow. When I was at the post office this evening there were several persons there among whom were three or four of the Faris' who I understand were very much insulted at me on the day of the Elections. When I saw them I felt bad—I was not mad nor afraid but was really unpleasant. I don't care to have any communication with any of them and indeed do not intend to have any. If they interfere with me I shall certainly defend myself to the best of my ability. I take them to be little or no account and hope they will never interfere with me or mine—if they do both parties might have cause to regret it. I hate difficulties as bad as anyone can and I may never have another. This may lead me into many [sic: difficulties] but at all events I am resolved to see them out honorably. What I said I shall not retract. What I did I do not think was wrong under the circumstances and therefore shall not seek to make any amends for it. Acting as I always try to do upon right and honor and if this involves me into a difficulty I enter it with a bold heart and determined purpose, hoping for my character and deportment to clear me out honorably.

WEDNESDAY FEB. 13TH, '61

A beautiful morning this. Great is the contrast between the weather of the last few days and that for several months before. I hope we will be favoured with some good weather now. This morning I was not out of bed as soon as I ought to have been but I retired late and am late rising.

---

[28]John Bunnell Davis, *An Inquiry into Some of the Principal Causes of Mortality Among Children* (1817). Davis is credited with starting "the modern approach to child hygiene and public health nursing" by opening a children's dispensary in London. Convinced that most childhood disease resulted from mothers' ignorance of healthy pracatices, he used the dispensary "as a comman post from which trained volunteers went out to counsel and assist new mothers." His 1817 text was a standard for treatment of childhood illnesses and other maladies. See "Pediatrics," *McGrew's*, s.v.

I studied chemistry this morning and I was going to say finished it. I got through but but [sic] that is not a finish with me. I am ignorant of its intricacies now and fear I shall always be. I have some strange forbodings in regard to my studies. I fear that I do not study enough and am going over the books without knowing enough about them. It is true a person need not expect to know every thing at once but I am afraid that I don't know half as much as I ought to. I do not know how it is with others who seem to go through a branch of study in short order and to all appearance know something at least about it while I try to study while I am at it and when I get through I feel that I know nothing.

I commenced Materia Medica to-day. [29] I hope to finish it in a month from the time I commence. I am forced to hurry up things to get through by fall.

The day passed as usual. I read Tasso awhile after night and retired about 11 o'clock.

To-day is the day for the Virginia convention to meet. To-day has witnessed the meeting of Virginia's *greatest* and best, whose decree will settle the fate of V[a] probably and with her's [sic] that of the whole South. What a momentous time! A Time that generations to come will look back to with pleasure or regret. No one can tell what will become. The act of the convention will come before the people.

THURSDAY FEB. 14TH, '61

This is one of the celebrated days—Sacred to memory of St. Valentine. To-day, according to an old notion prevalent many generations far back, the birds couple together in happy pairs. The dove choses [sic] his mate and retires. The blue-bird chirps and flutters around the darling of his affections and woos her to some hollow, where they can safely build their own cozy nest and fill it with lovers brood. To-day the loving send their fair Dulcinea presents and many tokens of affection. And while man and birds are thus preparing for the future bliss and happiness man in the bonds of love and the birds in instinctive sense of the *passion* given them by their Creator, there is one man of my acquaintance who it is reported will close in with the offers of Cupid, and allow the bonds of wedlock to be as Law between himself and the fair one who has been chosen by

---

[29] Dioscorides, *Materia Medica in Five Books* [ca. 60 C.E.; trans., 1665]. Dioscorides was a so-styled pharmaco-botanist who studied herbs and other plants and catalogued them with special attention to their medicinal uses. Translated into English in 1665, *Materia Medica* remained a standard in pharmacy literature in the mid-nineteenth century and was routinely studied by medical students and routinely consulted by those such as Apperson who were "prescribing" for patients. "Pharmacy," *McGrew's*, s.v.

himself to launch out with him upon life's ocean deep and dark. Peace, happiness and prosperity attend them! May they bear each other up over the shoals and quick sands of this Mammon—May no storm arise to mar the blissful moments that are in store for the happy [couple] in wedded Union—May she be to him a warm counselor and adviser, a friend and companion to smooth down the turbulent billows that oftimes assail the bosom of man; and may he be to her a guard and protector— a good husband that will ever study her tastes and wishes and gratify them prior to gratifying his own. And then may all the smiles of providence find abode in them combined is my prayer.

This was a most beautiful morning but it did not remain so long. Before noon clouds had overshadowed the earth and drops of rain were falling. By 3 o'clock it was raining rapidly and continued until nearly night—It then cleared off. The sun went down behind the western hills clear and beautiful. We had the pleasure of seeing the most beautiful rainbow this evening. Studied M. Medica—to-day Am writing at 9 o'clock—will study some and retire.

FRIDAY, FEB. 15TH, '61

This morning I was out of bed earlier than usual. Raining slowly— prospect for a wet, foggy, dull day. I studied M. Medica. Nothing new on hand to-day. I have done a good deal of reading to-day whether I know anything about it or not. Not much though I fear (I commenced writing one line in a space and am not satisfied with it and have commenced writing two.)

The clouds passed away about noon to-day leaving the upper deep clear and beautiful. I resolved to-day to devote a part of my time to the study of english grammar. I know I can study that as well alone as I can study other things and I am determined to do it. I hate when I I [sic] read a newspaper article to be lectured about the grammatical constructions of words and sentences. I have commenced Tasso and must finish reading it before I undertake anything else besides my main studies, and imperative duties. If I could master English grammar I would feel much more comfortable in regard to my knowledge of things in general. I always feel that that is one thing I lack and without which I can never get along as I would desire to do.

I am not aware of the hour now but I will read Tasso a while and retire. Every human being about the house is in the land of dreams where Morpheus has robed them in her mantle of forgetfulness.

SATURDAY FEB. 16TH, '61

I was up an hour earlier than usual this morning. I do really wish that I could make it a habit.

I spent the day not so well I fear. I wrote a letter to sister M.E. This far was spent very well. I have no fault to find of it. I have been trying to compose an accrostic [sic] in a lady's name to-day and have made almost a failure I think[.] I wrote some three or four imperfect lines.

After chopping wood for fire in my room to-morrow I went to the Post Office hoping to hear something from the Richmond convention and Washington "Peace Conference" but failed to hear anything valid from either. It is reported that a compromise has been consummated by the *Peace Conference* [30] but failed to hear anything valid from either. It is reported that a compromise has been consumated by the *Peace Conference*, but I have no faith in such report and believe it has been gotten up and circulated by some calling themselves *Conservatives.* I have no doubt that it will wield considerable influence over the convention now in session in Richmond. I think the time for compromise has passed—the seceded Southern States have organized a Southern Congress and adopted a constitution. President and Vice President for the Southern Confederacy have been elected and this confederacy will soon be on the move. I do not think that any compromise that the North will make will be sufficient to make the Southern States recall what they have said and loose what they have done. If then these states will not return but remain in league with themselves what should Virginia do? I say it will behoove her to leave the North compromise or no compromise!

I am writing at 9 o'clock. Will retire soon.

Weather is very bad to-day—commenced snowing about noon and rained and snowed alternately until sunset. For a while there there was hardly a cloud to be seen. When I retired it was snowing very fast. Did not snow much however.

---

[30] A number of prominent Virginians met at this conference, including Stuart, Clemens, Nelson, and Summers, whom the diarist has already mentioned. Dominated by slaveholding Unionists, the conference revived the old Crittendon Resolutions that sought to preserve the Union by guaranteeing protection of slavery from federal action. The proposals may have been close to popular sentiment in much of the nation, but they were moot when issued since the Confederacy had already been formed in Montgomery.

SUNDAY FEB. 17TH 61

Bad weather seems to be on the increase. This morning was partially cloudy and by ten o'clock it was snowing rapidly—it did not snow incessantly though—

Toward evening it snowed more—I don't know how it will be. This morning a friend NCB St. J[ohn] called on me. He had a piece of composition for *Miss C.C.*— a sort of burlesque on some of our opinionated ways. By the way a pretty good thing. He said it was original but I am not sure of that. He gave it to me to mail— I shall do it.

I can't say that I am much in favour of what is called *quizing*, or in other words writing anonymous letters. I have never known any good results directly from it but on the other hand have seen some bad results from them. It looks rather low and cowardly for a person to do such a thing. But however there are some folks who think they are superior to every thing around them and those are they whom I would have told of the sphere in which they ought to revolve without questioning how it was told them. Miss C. is a good girl in her own estimation I have no doubt and may be in the estimation of others also but I think she did me injustice to some extent. But she is a lady and it is not becoming in me to speak reproachful of one of her sex.

I spent the larger portion of to-day in reading Tasso and composing for a *thing* similar to a quiz—a valentine. I had promised to fix one and of course I had to do it. I finished it a short time ago but I am not well pleased with it, it is rather too comic.

Dr. Barbran was to see us to-day. I do not know how to express myself in regard to him. He seems to be a good *disposed* frenchman and a gentleman in his deportment. I am somewhat shy of the gentleman until I find him out well. I wrote a long letter to cousin Bettie Apperson to-day. It has been a busy day to me. It is now 1/2 past 9. I will read a chapter in the scriptures and retire.

MONDAY FEB. 18TH, '61

Snowing yet. Although it has been snowing at intervals for three days the snow is not over three inches deep now. It it [sic] is rather cold to snow much.

To-day has passed without anything interesting or worthy of note. I studied M. Med.—did not get along very well. The snow stopped falling by evening—still remains cloudy.

Retired about ten o' clock but not until I had taken a sound nap in my chair—bad habit. Nearly clear.

TUESDAY FEB. 19TH, '61

This morning was pretty sharp—indeed last night was a cold one. Cloudy & hazy—I hope it will clear up to-day. I rose from my [sic] somewhat reluctantly this morning—more so if possible than usual owing to the coldness of my room. To-day is court day. I, as usual went up. Had a very disagreeable ride—facing the wind and of course felt the snow rain & hail in front—pretty sensibly indeed. Times rather dull in everything except politics—that seems to be all the go now. I was "within an ace" of joining a volunteer company to-day—I resisted the temptation until I came home and spoke to the Dr. about it—he says it would be best perhaps for me not to join—that I would gain nothing and probably loose [sic] much. I am sure now that such is good advice—at any rate I shall not now join unless my services were needed to defend my country[.] then I would not hesitate a moment. The Court appropriated one thousand dollars toward furnishing the company with uniforms—the company is called "Marion Blues." Other, individual appropriations were made by gentlemen—I wish the enterprize [sic] much success.

I went to Widow [illegible] to-day on business for Dr. She is a very nice lady and there were some very nice young ladies there—visitors I suppose. I accomplished nothing by my trip.

There is much excitement in town this evening caused by the vigilance committee arresting Wm. Faris who was ordered a few days ago to leave the state which he failed to do and made his appearance to-day at court, as though he bade defiance [to] committees and laws of committees. He was warned of the intention of arresting him and he left town but was followed and brought back to await his doom. I left ignorant that they anticipated taking him again and consequently saw none of it. I have learned since I came however that he was to be sent North this evening in the cars—the report may be false. I am for punishing him some at all events, because he had been set free once and had the privilege of saving himself—he would not but showed contempt for the authority over him. He was armed to-day and made a feeble effort to use them but was prevented. I presume that he is either sent off or will be hung one or the other.

I had an offer to-day to do a job of writing. I do not know what I will do about it. I have referred this matter to Dr. he will give me the best advice about it. It is true I do now and then need all the money that I can possibly raise to keep me on but time is as precious as money to me now: hoping as I am to go to

Richmond Medical or some other next fall. I do not know what I shall do about it[.] So far as every thing else is concerned beside my studies I would rather do it than not.

Left town about four—had a very muddy time. I came home ate supper and commenced making pills.

It is now about 1/2 past 11 o'clock & will retire now in a short time. Rainy very much out of doors.

WEDNESDAY, FEB. 20TH, 1861

Clear and cool this morning. I read a while and then commenced preparing some medicine. I had a good deal to put in the process of making. Mr. A.J. Gouchon called on me to-day—was here some three or four hours. I learned from him that Faris was [not] sent off last night but was to be sent to-night. I think it more than probable that he will be liberated again. If they send him off it will be at the risk of the committee that would accompany him, for he would be taken from them before they got to a northern state and hung probably, and if they arrived in a northern state unmolested then the committee would be in danger. If Faris is taken off he is so [illegible] to all sense of honor and dignity that he would return at the earliest opportunity. I studied but little to-day—I will try and make it up to-morrow—will retire about ten o'clock.

THURSDAY, FEB. 21ST, '61

This may [be] ranked among the pretty mornings. Frosty and clear. I was up not very early—but as early as usual. I studied some to-day. No news astir now. I went to the post office this evening for the purpose of hearing from Marion and Richmond but failed to hear anything deffinite [sic] from either place. The last I heard from Marion was that Faris would be sent off last night; how far this is true however, I know not.

I returned home about 8 o'clock, came to my room made a fire and am writing about 9 o'clock . I will study some and then retire. I am drowsy now.

FRIDAY, FEB. 22ND, '61

I arose this morning as usual about six o'clock. I commenced writing a letter to my friend Dr. V. Q.[31] but did not complete it—the tenor of it does not suit me—I laid it aside. I do not know when I shall resume it again. I studied some. Mrs. Sanders was here to-day. I entertained her a short time. She is a very wise lady, I think.

This evening I studied M.M.[32] I resolved some time ago to commence the study of Eng. Grammar with the determination to go through with it and if possible learn something about our language. I commenced to-day ahead one lesson. I think I can manage four pages per day.

It is a saying; "Now this world is given to holiday living[.]" So it would seem by giving our political world a moment's thought. The convention under significant name of *Peace Conference* is now and has been in session some time considering our national difficulties and to devise some measures for adjustment. They have done nothing. When the convention of Virginia met, members from the *Peace Conference* reported that a compromise had been agreed upon—that peace would assuredly be brought about; but this is the only assurance we have of peace or compromise. The convention of Va. has been waiting for the reported action of *Peace Conference* and is still hoping; but, now alas! how I fear they are following a will o' the wisp! and ere they are aware the 4th of March will be here, and like the Ides of March to Ceasar [sic]—will welcome Virginia to an untimely grave.[33]

War seems more and more inevitable every day. I have no idea that a secession *ordinance* will pass the convention and if it should there will be another difficulty to contend against. I mean in the shape of the right of suffrage. Every legal voter of Virginia will say whether they will endorse the action of the convention or condemn it.

Let the convention pass ordinance for secession or let her consent to remain as she is [.] We the sons of the Grand Old Dominion should consider where she

---

[31] Dr. Quisenberry, the Apperson family doctor from the Wilderness subregion of Orange County, was a warm correspondent with whom the diarist often debated secession; Quisenberry was a most reluctant secessionist.

[32] *Materia Medica.* See previous note.

[33] Lincoln was to be inaugurated on 4 March, the old date for inauguration. The Ides of March refer to the old Roman calendar, a portentous time when Julius Caesar was assassinated. Generally, Apperson takes a Whiggish republican position, that is, in favor of assassinating Caesar, who is here compared to Lincoln. Lincoln and his supporters, of course, used the same analogy, but compared themselves to the republican forces of Brutus—and the southern secessionists to Julius Caesar.

ought to stand and when satisfied that we are right then exert all the influence we have in support of what we claim as right.

To me it seems in no wise difficult to decide where Virginia ought to stand. She should break of [sic; off] all social relations with our arrogant and sectional North—rend assunder the bonds that now hold her to a people who would rob her of her honor & virtue and trample her to death by downright, outright oppression. She should "come out from among these"[34] and unite herself with a people whose interests are her interests and let their destiny be her destiny. She can never, never live peaceful and happy in connection with the North: and how then will it do! The southern confederacy has done its own work, organized a congress and has now a government of its own. Then think that they will recall what they have completed and come to unite again with the North only to be abused in terms that no nation, people or individual can bear. Never! Thus I think Va. will stand apart from the North who can expect no mercy from the South We can never hope for help. Thus our national affairs are growing more gloomy every day. We can only look [to] the great omnipotent God who reigns in Heaven and judgeth on earth and who holds the destinies of man and nation in his hand and ever [will] hold them as well, for protection.

I retired about 11 o'clock.

(Written Saturday night)

SATURDAY FEB 23[D], '61

This morning I arose with the intention of taking a trip to Marion on business for Dr. F. It was late before I was ready to go. Wm. A. Sanders promised to go up with me—I got to the ford about 10 o'clock—Mr. Sanders had concluded not to go as it was so late. Setting out fair this morning at sunrise, soon after I got to the ford it commenced raining, clouds thick and heavy as if it would be a wet day. News has come from Marion that Wm. Faris who was arrested by the mob on Tuesday had been started the day before *en route* for Ohio, and that his brother was also arrested and would be tried to-day in Marion. This prompted me to be more desirous to go and I endeavor to go

---

34. Words of exorcism for unclean spirits spoken by Jesus Christ, probably from Mark 1:24; other possibilities, Mark 5:8; Matt. 8:28-34; Luke 8:26-39. The image is not entirely successful for his purposes, since Jesus Christ was calling unclean spirits out of an otherwise clean person, and Jesus's words thus address demons or other evil beings. Apperson in quoting words of exorcism thus actually says that the southern states are the unclean or evil beings who should be exorcised from the otherwise clean person of the nation!—probably not his meaning, given his principled Christian support for secession.

also. Tho' rain was considerable the whole trip—arrived in town about 1/2 past 11 o'clock. No excitement—Faris was not in town but was brought in an hour or so by an official. He had no trial, but was bound in a bond of $500—to appear before a court of magistrates on Tuesday next. I am not of the opinion that the civil law can do anything with him for the want of proper evidence.

I am at a loss to know whether to approve of this course or not. Between the two I believe that this Faris is the *more* [sic; that is, better] of the two, and it is hardly right to punish one man for an offense and leave another unpunished who is equally guilty. If the Southern people do not do not [sic] suppress incendiary sentiments wherever they are uttered, She may expect ere long to have her country overrun with such men. But still, they have made an example of one aggression which will serve as a warning to others and now it ought to rest a while. It continued raining all day—my friends and I had a wet, disagreeable ride in returning home. I arrived at home about dark. I read the *Marion Visitor*, wrote for yesterday, studied grammar, and retired about fifteen minutes past 1 o'clock.

(Written Sunday evening)

SUNDAY, FEB. 24TH, '61

This morning I was not in any great hurry to rise—ate breakfast and prepared to go to church at S. Spring [Sulphur Spring] to preaching. Dr. F. and myself rode out— the roads were excessively muddy.

We heard a good sermon preached by Mr. Jno Boring a Methodist minister from the words: "This world also, and all its works shall be burned up!"[35] He is somewhat an eccentric preacher, any how in his illustrations, which are droll and odd yet they are well applied—always give a lucid and easy view to what he would teach.

His sermon was based principally upon the question— "Where will you stand sinner when this world is consumed?" He compared the Bible to a great compass encircling three worlds, viz., Hell or the world below, the Earth or the world we inhabit, and Heaven or the world where Christ and the angels live.

He took grounds and proved from the Bible that all three of these worlds are inhabited. Hell was proved to be inhabited by the rich men. Man lives and as to the inhabitation of this world (inhabited) by real and animated beings with but our materialist world questions; that Heaven or the upper world was inhabi-

---

[35] Text is from Rev., probably Rev. 20:9-10; similar words, 8:6; 14:10; 16:8.

ted[,] proved conclusively by the ascension of Enoch, and two thousand years after[,] the ascension of Elijah, and two thousand after Elijah's ascension, Christ was taken up into Heaven to dwell with God the Father and with all the redeemed of himself forever and ever.

The ascension of Enoch represented the Patriachal age, the ascension of Elijah represented Prophetic times of the world, and the ascension of Jesus Christ represents the Gospel dispensative. Thus there are representatives in Heaven from the three great divisions of the existence of the world.

Thus Hell Earth and Heaven are inhabited by beings of like passions with ourselves. Who walked as we walked and ate as we eat, who wore clothing as well as us, and were essentially rational and animated beings as we are, and we like them must sooner or later leave this world; where then will we go? Admitting that the stars and planets are inhabited by beings also like us as many philosophers contend they are can we go there? No! When the great day shall come the stars will fall from their places in the upper deep like figs of an untimely growth, the moon will turn to blood and fire arise in mighty streams. The sun the Great King of Day will be wiped out of existance [sic]. Then again where will you stand? Either in Hell beneath or Heaven above.

He spoke of the godly man as being in Heaven looking down upon the breaking up of the fabric as a man in N Carolina who was on one of the highest mountains in that state. He saw in the distance a mighty cloud rising, it was dark & angry. He dismounted from his horse to seek shelter and prepared for the worst. Onward and still onward came the cloud boiling and raging, thunders loud and terrible filled the air with colors—lightning flashed vividly and frantic across the dark mass. He shuddered. Presently the cloud struck the mountain on whose top he was, and the mighty cloud divided into two great masses (and with their raining and lightning in their course far below him). So with the Christian in Heaven. We will see the flaming billows rolling by us; star after star will quit its place and fall into the rumbling chaos; the moon melted and gone; the sun blotted out by one terrific word; yet the Christian is safe in Heaven with God and angels.

We came home and ate dinner. I amused myself with reading and writing secession & c. until night when I made a fire and have been writing ever since. I will study my lesson in Grammar, read a Chapter in the Bible, and retire .

FEB. 25TH, MONDAY

This morning I was up late. A beautiful morning. I went to Mr I S Sanders & L N Tate's for Dr F on business. I have not done much studying to-day. I have been nearly all morning writing to a friend of mine in E. Va (Dr Quesenberry) He was always a warm friend of mine and highly esteemed by myself. I wrote him a long letter, two sheets such as I am writing on now. I am not sure that is right for me to write him so long a letter—the perusing of it may prove a boring task to him.

Nothing has transpired to-day worthy of note.

I am writing at 11 o'clock—will study a lesson in English Grammar and retire.

TUESDAY, FEB. 26TH, '61.

I went on business for Dr F to Mr L N Tate & I S Sanders. Came home about 11 o'clock. I read Davis "History of Menstruation" to-day. I was led to read by being told by Madam Faris that a girl in the neighborhood had commenced menstruating at 12 years old—very precocious.

I studied M. Medica part of the time this evening. It is about 10 o'clock while I write. I have been reading Davis on the diseases of childhood [36] for half an hour before I commenced writing. I will read it a while longer, study my grammar lesson and prepare to retire. To-day was a beautiful day but I am afraid rain will fall before morning as it is clouding over now.

MONDAY, FEB. 27TH, '61

We were favoured by the Giver of every [good] and perfect gift with another beautiful morning. Dr F requested me to visit a patient for him—a young lady who, it was supposed, had *diptheria.* I went to see her—found her not very sick—had common *angina* and *catarrh.*[37] I prescribed for her . I read a letter

---

[36] John Bunnell Davis, *Cursory Inquiry into Some of the Principal Causes of Mortality Among Children* (1817) suggests the modern understanding of child hygiene and public health nursing. Davis operated a children's dispensary in England and published this text, "in which he laid down his conviction that infant mortality owed in great part to mothers' ignorance of sound health practices." The text became a standard source for general practitioners and for students of pharmacy. Quotation from "Davis, John Bunnell," *McGrews.*

[37] *Angina* in nineteenth century refers to any disease marked by sensation of choking; *common* agina distinguishes it from *angina maligna contagiosa,* the term for diptheria; *catarrh* refers to inflammation of mucous membranes. McGrew, *Encyclopedia of Medical History,* s.v.

from my cousin Jas. Apperson— he was famous as a good fellow but rather wild. I promised A.J. Sanders that I would come up on tomorrow evening and we would go to see some girls and we would have some fun at a camp. After I can see [illegible]. I studied M. M. a while—I was made very angry by a man to-day—a Mr Thom Faris[.] I had reported that Jno Faris who was taken before a magistrate on last Saturday to answer for charges made against him for uttering at a store near his home, [38] had no trial. This young man wrote me a note stating that if I said Jno Faris had no trial I was a liar. This of course was cowardly and ungentlemanly and above all grossly insulting. I replied to it in the *roughest* manner possible. What may be end [sic], I know not. I am determined to defend myself to the best of my ability.

I am determined to give satisfaction in a meeting that was held over on Seven Mile Ford on Tuesday; and I wrote until after midnight to-night and retire.

(Written on Friday, 1st March)

THURSDAY, FEB 28TH, '61

This morning I was up late. A pretty morning. I was busy helping the carpenter raise a frame for another room in Dr. F's house until 2 o'clock. Then I went to "the switch" [39] to fulfill my promise to A.J. Sanders. We met—I enjoyed myself very well with a young lady. We will not go to the same camp tho'. We got sugar to eat and returned to the store about 10 o'clock & staid [sic] all night (Written Mch 1 st)

FRIDAY, MARCH 1ST

This morning I rose and ate breakfast and walked home. After writing a while I went up to Thomas & Summer's Factory on business for Dr. F. I visited a lady also who was severely attacked with pneumonia—she is not out of danger yet. She is badly salivated—her mouth is exceeding sore, with red gums and a white streak around the root of the teeth. I extracted a root of an old rotted

---

[38] *Uttering* was a term for deceiving a creditor, the nineteenth-century equivalent of writing a bad check; this incident involves the same pro-Unionist abolitionist family, but the alleged crime involves credit rather than political opinion.

[39] "The Switch" was apparently a building that served as gathering point for drinking and playing cards and otherwise socializing; Apperson claimed never to drink or to play cards, but often writes of meeting at "The Switch," as in this case to meet a young woman on a date arranged by his friend A.J. Sanders. Likely, this building was called "The Switch" because it stood near a switching point in the rails on the line of the Tennessee and Virginia Railroad, chartered in 1849 and extended into Smyth County after 1857. Wilson, *Smyth County*, 228.

tooth with my fingers. One of her cheeks was very much swollen—I apprehend it will form an absess and probably sloughing of part of the cheek.

I was at the factory to-day for my first time. I hope Mr. Thomas will have good luck with the enterprise. I came by Mr.Dungan's [40] to settle up but failed to do so. I came home about dusk. I had head ache and therefore did not study much. Retired earlier than usual.

(Written Sunday evening)

SATURDAY, MCH. 2ND, '61

This morning I was up and ate breakfast before light. I then went to Mr. D. Copenhaver's on business for Dr. F. and from there to Humphrey's Mill & home. On my return home I found I had to go over the mountain to attend a trial at Squire Kesner's for Dr. Faris against Mr. Whitaker.[41]

The trial was to take place at noon and I arrived about 11 o'clock. I found Mr. Kesner's daughters at home—two very nice girls. I had the pleasure of their company until dinner which was very agreeable to me. After dinner we went into the parlour and I played several games of draughts with Miss Maggie. Prior to this time the def. [defendant] in the case came[.] We talked the matter of our case over and agreed to postpone until next Saturday when Dr. F. will be present himself. The plea brought up by the defendant will do him no good. He says that Dr. F insured the case on which he (Dr. F) tended—and that if he did not effect a cure that he would not make any charge. Let this be as it may I do not think that Dr. F would digress from what his duty as a medical practitioner so far as to make such a catch penny agreement. I hope I shall never have to regret such an agreement.

I remained with until about three o'clock and left for home where I arrived about sundown. I found Dr. Barbran at our house when I arrived. I entertained

---

[40] James V. Dungan of Seven Mile Ford, father of his friend Robert H. Dungan.

[41] Squire's Court involved civil cases tried by a jury of landholders called squires. The jury functioned almost as a panel of judges, and squires of the court could ask questions of the litigants or of the attorneys (if there were attorneys present). Decisions were as often based on common sense and community mores as on statutory law. The courts were social occasions as much as legal occasions, and the sessions attracted large audiences from the countryside. The institution was loosely based on English custom, but attained its own highlands patterns different from its English origins and even different from other parts of Virginia. Squire's Courts were still being conducted in Smyth County in the 1930s, when novelist and memoirist Sherwood Anderson memorialized a session in which he was involved. Anderson, *Southern Odyssey: Selected Writings by Sherwood Anderson*, eds., Welford Dunaway Taylor and Charles E. Modlin (Athens: University of Georgia Press, 1998) 60-63.

him and made some pills—retired about 11 o'clock: after writing some in my journal. Zounds, I have been so busy for the last few days that I have neglected writing. I must try & do better in the future[.] My grammar lesson has been neglected also.

(Written Sunday Evening)

SUNDAY, MARCH 3RD, '61

This morning like all we've had for a week is a beautiful one. I prepared to go to church at Middle Fork (Mr. Neuff Preston) Several friends called in this morning on their way to church. We went and a large congregation was in attendince [sic]. We had a good sermon—rather doctrinal to be generally popular. However, this I allow all denominations. Each one has his belief and believes in his heart that the Bible sanctions and strengthens that belief. So I am for allowing Baptists, Methodists, Presbyterians and and every other denomination believe as they please. His (the Pastor's) text was 18 chapter and 36 verse of St. Johns—"My kingdom is not of this world".[42] We found out the difference of Christ's Kingdom and the Kingdom's of the world. Christ's Kingdom is not made with hands but is a spiritual kingdom. He spoke of the inhabitants of those kingdom's [sic]—the contrast between them. The the [sic] necessary qualifications for entering those kingdom's. And in giving a description of the qualifications for entrance he made several illusions to infant baptism and "probation". He spoke of what would be the probable ruin of Christ's Kingdom when infants are taken into the church there will soon be bad [.] All the people will have their children baptised and then religion will not know her own. He gave Germany as an illustration where they are born into the church and had an established a [sic] religion so that all are in the church as soon as they are ushered in the world; but the ministry of the Germanic States is tainted with and interfered with [.] Some of their ministry is as good as any I suppose.

I had the pleasure of walking with Miss M. F. Sanders to-day from church. She is a good girl—I like her very much . She is lively as a bird and mischevious as possible. She and A. T. Sanders took dinner with me to-day. Also Barbran & Brunot — two frenchman [sic].

I suppose I shall have some difficulty with this Faris crowd spoken of before. A friend advised me to arm myself and be ready for an attack—he also loan me

[42] John 18:36.

a five shooter which I shall use if necessity requires it. I do not advocate carrying arms and believe much harm has arisen from it but when they are needed in self defence as they would be in my case then I have nothing to say. I am determined if attacked to defend myself to the best of my ability.

I am writing at 8 o'clock [sic; punctuation] will write some on an article that I am preparing for publication.

I omitted to say on yesterday's paragraph that I read a letter from R. H. Dungan at Emory & Henry. We are opposed to each other in politics and have been writing a good deal about the politics of the parties to which we profess to belong. I have tried to give no offence but I do not like his political expression with the expressions as appendages to his letter. I shall reply rather rough.

MONDAY, MCH. 4TH, '61

This is a beautiful morning. Sky is clear and calm. No threatening clouds are hovering around to warn us of the attack from the regions of Jupiter. To-day is the day of the inauguration of the President of the United (Disunited now) States; but how great is the contrast between the natural sky and the political sky. The one calm and serene while [the other] is filled with howling demagogues and maniacal fanatics which have torn our union in twain and are now seeking to devour section after section until nothing of our once glorious and happy country will remain to tell of its unprecedented existence. To-day Abraham Lincoln becomes president of a part of the United States. Virginia still stands as if paralyzed— incapable of moving in self protection.

This morning I was warned by the road overseer to help make a road from Jas. Rector up to Livinard's. I refused to help from the fact that I did not think it right. The persons who are interested ought to make the road. I do not care to help make the road anyway for it is of no use to me. I may have to pay a fine but they cannot make it out of me. Dr. Faris requested me to visit a patient for him this morning and in line of which he sent William to work in my place.

I visited the patient it had been threatened with pneumonia but was something better. It had a distressing cough for which I prescribed. I returned home about noon. The evening I spent writing on an article which I am preparing for publication.

I was unusual sleepy after night so I retired very early.

(Written Wednesday Morning)

TUESDAY, MCH 5TH, '61

This morning looks rather unfavourable in regard to the weather. The clouds are thick and snowing slightly. I was up as usual this morning. I was engaged on my article again to-day and finished it. The contents of the article is, I fear not very laudable. There has been some funny attempts to have an indignation meeting in our neighborhood expressing contempt for the cause of some of the citizens of our county. I do not like such proceedings and will continue against them. The article is a burlesque and I do no know if the Editor will give it a place in his paper or not— I am rather doubtful.

I went to the post office this evening. I heard that "Peace Conference" had accepted the "Crittenden Resolutions". [43] This will do no good for the C. Resolutions will not give a sufficient guarantee to the South.

I came home about sundown. Studied M. M. a while. I was drowsy—took a nap with my head on the table and retired about 1/2 past 11 o'clock.

I have neglected my grammar lessons altogether for some days. I must do better soon.

(Written Wednesday Morning)

WEDNESDAY, MCH. 6TH, '61

This morning I was loth [sic; loath] to rise as I was anxious to get to sleep last evening for you [the diary]. I studied a grammar lesson this morning. I studied M. Medica the ballance [sic] of the day. I am simply reviewing M.M.—will finish it entire this week. I am somewhat neglectful of grammar

---

[43] Senator John J. Crittenden of Kentucky presented compromise plan to forestall secession: Let slavery be prohibited in national territory north of the line 36 30', but let it be established and maintained by Federal protection south of that line; let future states, north or south of the line, come into the Union with or without slavery as they wish; restrain Congress from abolishing slavery in places within national jurisdiction which may be surrounded by slave states; where intimidation prevents Federal officials from arresting a fugitive slave, let the United States fully compensate the owner, recovering equivalent damages from the county in which the "intimidation, or rescue, was committed;" let the fugitive slave law be rigorously enforced, and let Congress earnestly recommend the repeal of the personal liberty laws, which, though null and void by the provisions of the Constitution, have "contributed much to the discord....now prevailing." Compromise articles were to become amendments to the Constitution, with prohibition against any future amendment authorizing Congress to "touch slavery" in any of the states. Quotations, James Garfield Randall and David Herbert Donald, *Civil War and Reconstruction* (1937; rev. ed.; Boston: D.C. Heath, 1961) 150. See also *Congressional Globe*, 36 Congress, 2 sess., 114. These preexisting Crittenden Resolutions were adopted again by the figures at the Peace Conference already mentioned in the diary, that is, Sherrard Clemens, George William Summers, Alexander Hugh Holmes Stuart, and Thomas Amos Rogers Nelson.

lesson. Mr. C.W. Peake called to-day to have his throat examined. He was fearing that he had diptheria. I examined his throat and found no diptheria but he has a very sore throat. If he'd had diptheria yet I would not be surprised.

Mr. B. is a surgeon.[44] He spent some two or three hours with me.

I am writing at 9 o'clock and am very sleepy although I have already had two naps—

THURSDAY, MCH 7TH, '61

This morning I was up sooner than usual. I have been engaged to-day in reading and preparing medicine. I read Wood and Watson on inflammation of the brain.[45] I studued M. M. this evening. My grammar lesson I studied about dusk and after. I am rather hopeful about that lesson this evening—I think I can study it without much trouble.

Dr. Barbran came this evening. He is a presumptuous old chap. Why I draw this will be evident from what he says in regard to American ladies. He says our ladies are stupid—they make too free with the gentlemen—much freer than the ladies do in France. How far this is true or false I am not prepared to say but I have always heard the reverse. I am sure of one thing. Our ladies have shown to the world that they are as virtuous as ladies of any country or clime. He (Barbran) fancies in his head that he could marry almost any girl in our county—that the *title* of Doctor would prompt them to love him and desire him for a husband. But he says he is too old and therefore will not marry; though it is his fault and not our American girls' that he is [not] tied by matrimony's cord to some fair one. Vain presumption— *child of the Devil!* You are much mistaken. As free as our girls seem to be with some gentlemen, who are probably their intimate friends, I guess when you attempt to make one of them your bride (if respectable & nice) you will find yourself a victim of their stupidity. You will find your title of but little use, and that like a jug handle it will only serve to carry you about and when the handle breaks off a string around the neck will answer every purpose. I do not question his being popular among some of the ladies but he can give his oddities and eccentricities the credit for that. I like the old gentleman very much; but I think it is assuming

---

[44] Probably Barbran, the French physician.

[45] George Wood, professor at the University of Pennsylvania and later president of American Philosophical Society, wrote the especially influential *Treatise on Thereapeutics*, with much focused discussion on therapy, including discussions about opium; his text was a basic one for nineteenth century pharmacology and medicine where any brain inflammation occurred. I can locate no text on such subjects for this period by anyone named Watson. See *McGrews.*

much to say that he can get any one of some five or six of the prettiest girls that our county can afford. This is something more than any man has a right to say.

I am writing at 9 o'clock. I must study some before I retire. We are having fine weather now. Rather finer than is usual for March. I have some fun with Dr. Barbran about the girls!

FRIDAY, MCH. 8TH, '61

I arose this morning somewhat earlier than usual. I read M. Medica and studied my grammar lesson in the evening. Nothing occurred to-day worthy of note I believe.

There is a report afloat among the papers that the small pox is spreading in Lynchburg rapidly. Dr. Barbran started from here this morning and went into rich valley [sic] and returned this evening. He said that the younger Dr. Goodwin was down with small pox—how far this is reliable I am not able to say. I fancy it is some of Dame Rumor's work alone.

There is some excitement in the neighborhood about small pox—many are wanting to be vaccinated. I will make an effort to procure some vaccine vials if I can to-morrow. I have been reading Wood on small pox this evening.

I am writing at 1/2 past 9 o'clock and am very drowsy although I have had one nap. I am and have been very sleepy for several days at night. I shall retire pretty soon.

The weather is very good—I hope it may remain so for a while at least.

SATURDAY, MARCH 9TH, '1861

The weather was very fine yesterday but not so fine this morning. Some rain fell last night. Cool and cloudy this morning.

I studied M. Medica some to-day and read several articles in the "Stethoscope".[46]

---

[46] *Stethoscope* was a journal published for surgeons in Virginia; based in Richmond, the periodical merged with another and changed its name and mission in 1859. A more famous surgeon's periodical of the same name was published in London after 1862. Country doctors such as Dr. Faris would be likely to retain their old copies of the Richmond publication. Note that the stethoscope was still being perfected in this era; the design with the practical "yoke" for the ears was in place, but the microphone was not yet invented, so that the stethoscopes used by Dr. Faris and physicians of his day remained fairly crude.

I finished M. Medica to-day, or rather have gone through it and know comparatively nothing about it. I guess I will have to open [title of text illegible] on Monday.

I studied a grammar lesson and chopped wood for Sunday afternoon and then went to the Post Office in search of news. I got some however, both private and public. Privately I received a letter from my brother. He and all at home are well. My brother has but little education and hence writes a very indifferent letter. He never had any taste for books or study and never will I presume. It is greatly regretted by me too.

Public news is rather of an exciting character. Abe Lincoln took the action prescribed by law necessary to his becoming chief magistrate of the United (now disunited) States and according to custom delivered his inaugural address which predicts no good times for us in the future. He is in favor of coercion. Will enforce the collection of the revenue from the states that have already seceded and will wrest all the forts now in possession of the seceded states from the hands of those that now hold them. This speaks an ill omen to our distracted country. The conservatives or Union men are beginning to give way—Lincoln's course has struck them dumb. Memorials for secession are being sent to the delegates at Richmond demand [sic] secession of our state. We got a speech from our delegate of our county this evening. It is excellent and merits applause from every Virginian—whether male or female.

Preparations are being made for a conflict between the contending parties. Realy [sic] war seems almost inevitable. Virginia seems to stand on bad ground now[.] If she gets out now she will have to fight, and if she remains she will be forced to fight.

I am writing about 1/2 past 11 o'clock—will retire soon. The wind is blowing very hard, but that is March's privilege.

SUNDAY, MARCH 10TH, 1861

Late up—very cold and clear. Dr. asked me to visit a patient with him to-day—a case of miningitis or something similar. The patient was a child some 1 1/2 or 2 years old (a little girl) pretty and interesting. The child had been sick some two weeks before a physician was called in and had been sick three weeks when I saw it. Pulse was almost imperceptible, at times entirely so—extremities cold, breathing very short and quick—eyes very much crossed. I was impressed with the idea as soon as I saw it that it was not long for this world. Dr. recommended warm pediluvia first and afterwards ground mustard mixed with the bath.[47] Cold cloths to its head to keep down fever as much as possible. The poor little child continued to grow worse until about 1/2 past noon when its little spirit left its frail tenement of clay and went to live with angels in a bright and glorious world. Its parents were doatingly [sic; dotingly] fond of their tender babe and although they must know that it went to its Heavenly Parent; yet, it appeared like rendering [sic; rending] their hearts assunder to give it up. Who but a parent knows a parents love?

When I was, I may say, a boy rambling about hedge and bush to find some poor bird's off-spring, how elated I was to find some fledgling just able to fly from bush to bush, and evade my attempts to strike it with a stone or pierce it with an arrow long enough to give me a victim when it was finally my captive! Little did [I] think that the chirping of the [sic] of the old birds was the outbursts of a feeling equal in nature to that of the human family. It was but the wailings of a parent's heart for the life and security of an innocent and tender offspring; but how often it fell unheeded!

I met with Dr. Baker to-day who has just returned from a course of lectures in N. York. I think he must be pretty well posted [that is, *kept up to date*]—his opportunities have been good and therefore he ought to be. He follows the order of a gentleman in the way of dress. I dined at Mrs. Gollohon's with Dr. Baker & E. Gollohon. I got home a couple hours before night. I could not concentrate my mind upon anything. My friend E. P. Umbarger called on me this evening. It is now ten o'clock. I will read a chapter in the bible & retire.

Monday, March 11th, 1861

I stated on Saturday that I would commence the study of midwifery to-day but I did not. Having changed his notion Dr. told me that perhaps I had better study the practice before I studied anything else. I commenced "Woods Practice of Medicine"[48] this morning. I think it will be a pretty hard study at any rate. I find the first part—the preparatory remarks very hard to comprehend.

Nothing has occured to-day that I need to record—The weather is very good, tho' a little cool. I am exceedingly drowsy all day and night. I do not know

---

[47] Pediluvia, or foot baths, were thought to help with respiratory diseases, including miningitis. The grounds of a mustard plant were applied, especially to the chest and neck, to improve breathing for respiratory problems; mustard grounds were also applied as a stimulant, and applied in still other cases as treatment for wounds or abrasions. "Pediluvia" and "Mustard," *McGrew's*.

[48]This book is written by the same George Wood described 57 ff.

how to account for it or what remedy to apply—it makes me feel unpleasant besides I am loosing [sic] some precious time.

I studied my grammar lesson this evening or part of it and will finish it and retire —I am getting along well with it.

TUESDAY, MCH. 12TH, 1861

This was a lovely morning—I was up 1/2 past 5 and after dressing, making a fire in my room, and sweeping the floor I sat down to my studies. After breakfast I was engaged making pills and preparing some medicine for some patients. I made an axe handle for Uncle Dave. (a colored man belonging to Dr.)

I did not study much to-day. I helped Dr. to find saddle tree in the latter part of the evening. After night I took my seat with the intention of making up for lost time during the day, this I failed to do because I went to sleep in my seat—was so drowsy that I retired sooner than usual—I did not finish my grammar lesson or write in my journal. I am very sorry that I cannot study after night as much as I ought to—it is a dead loss to me.

(Written Wednesday morning)

WEDNESDAY, MARCH 13TH 1861

I was up about five this morning. After breakfast finished the job I commenced on yesterday evening. I commenced a lesson in Grammar but stopped when I found I had to go to Marion this evening for then I could take the book in my pocket and study as I went along—which I did. I studied my daily study until about noon when I went over to Mrs. Rector's to borrow a horse to ride to town. Wm. Sing loan [sic] me his provided I would hunt her up: I found hunting her up a smart job. I found her however and went to Town. I purchased a lot of medicines and returned home about 9 o'clock. After putting the medicines in their proper places I wrote a part in my journal but fell asleep and retired leaving the finish for this morning (Thursday).

I stopped at the post office this evening hoping to hear something about our government affairs. Times are becoming more and more serious every day. Preparations are being made (if reports be true) for coercion. The Convention of Virginia has been in session a month without affecting anything except spending the people's money. Reports are being made by some of the members of that convention for another convention of all the states—Consultation, Consultation!! is the perpetual cry. And I think the people ought to put a stop to monotonous strains. We have already had too much consultation; too much talk and no action. Civil War is almost inevitable now.

THURSDAY, MARCH 14TH, 1861

We have had some pretty weather for a week or so past but I think we will have some bad now. It is very cloudy this morning and raining some little. I commenced my studies early this morning and the consequence is I have done a pretty good day's work at it. I studied my grammar lesson about noon i.e. after dinner. I got along with it fully as well as I expected. The lesson I finished to-day was one on the *Tenses.* When I commenced it I was almost out of heart but now it seems comparatively easy. So it is with every lesson we learn during life. Not only with lessons but with everything destined to be accomplished by the action of man. We look at a journey ahead—it is to be performed but it seems so long and tedious that our hearts almost falter and give back. We have a job of work that we are wanting done; yet it seems so monstrous to our unwilling eyes that we are loth to commence—a failure is ahead in our imagination sure we can never do half as much. But after commencing and giving it our whole soul, mind and strength the apparently formidable barriers are removed one by one disappointment seems to vanish and the hope of success takes its place.

The journey is ended, the work is finished, and the lesson learned, are more aware of it. And after it is done we look back in wonder over the ground we have passed all seems easy—the obstacles that threatened to oppose and overcome every hope of success are gone down into insignificancy.

I was called on to-day to prescribe for a chronic case of Gonorrhea which I have been treating for some time but the patient will not take care of himself and it seems that he can never get well. He is a married man. I am surprised at men who are married and have families when they indulge in a habit that places their health and honor of a married man in jeopardy. I say honor of a married man because there are bonds binding a man to honor his wife and I am sure this is not honoring her. I believe it is as bad morally for a man to break over the bonds of connubial chastity as it would be for a woman—a wife—to do so. And what man, I care not how unusual he may be, who would or could countenance the same in his wife?

I am writing about ten o'clock—will read a while in Wood and retire.

I think Mr. Wood is rather hard to comprehend—he is to me so far sure. I am afraid after I go through with the course that I shall know nothing about it. Sometimes I have bright hope and at others I am disheartened almost. What I read is not impressive enough and until I see someone sick I can never appreciate the value of *knowing.*

FRIDAY, MARCH 15TH, 1861

This morning I awoke very early but did not rise so soon as I ought to have done. I was reading until about nine o'clock when Dr. F required me to visit a patient of his—a child who has inflammation of the brain; the patient at Mr. L[illegible letters] Tate. I admit that I felt some delicacy in going to Mr. T's as he is such a dignified old gentleman and his wife is notorious for her opinionated selfishness. But after I had gotten there and had gotten some chat with the old lady I thought I would like the old critter very well. As to the old man I have the highest sense of regard. I never got acquainted with his lady before—the reason was as much perhaps for want of inclination as anything else.

I found the patient much better than expected I thought. I was so well pleased (I reckon it was that) that I did not leave until after dinner, which was on the fashionable order—late. The old man invited me to come see them—a social visit.

I came home in the latter part of the evening. Chas. Brunot a Frenchman was to see us this evening—he is incessant talker.

I read a portion of a work on diptheria by professor Greenhow. I think it a good thing perhaps.

I am writing at ten o'clock. I had a very tedious job making pills to-night (2400). I will study until I get sleepy so that I cannot hold my eye open then I'll retire.

SATURDAY MARCH 16TH, 1861

This morning I was up tolerably early—I read a while. About 10 o'clock I was requested to visit a case, Dr. Faris not being at home. I felt some delicacy in going as it was a lady about to be confined. [49] I refused first. Not that I cared particular about what I was expected to do but I have never studied that branch of medicine and would have to follow the directions of the old woman that was there—and—if I should make a blunder although I did it at her sanction I would have the blame to bear. The woman who was sick was exceeding poor folks and I know they could get no physician from a distance to go to see her though she might die. I concluded to go and run all risks. All I had to do was to

49. *Confined* in this era was a euphemism for *pregnant,* with connotation, *ready to give birth.*

perform venesection and so on—I was afraid that she might no [sic] need it and therfore I might do damage by blood letting. I went and with boldness enough of an experienced physician I bled her pretty freely—I hurried the thing—and left before any thing came off. I told the ladies who were there—some were very nice ladies too—that they were done with me and I would leave.

I got home about 1 o'clock. I had the burlesque I wrote on the meeting in S. Fork to be published and come out this week but it did not as we got our paper to-day.

Dr. Barbran was to see us this evening—he performed vaccination on me to-day. I read some in Greenhow on Diptheria this evening. After night I was closely engaged writing a letter to my friend RHS [Robert H. Stainback] at Emory & Henry College. I answered a part of it to-night—I am afraid I answered too rough—I spoke of the letter on 3rd of the present month. I retired about midnight.

(Written Sunday Evening)

SUNDAY, MARCH 17TH, 1861

This morning was a very bad morning—raining & foggy. I rose about six and dressed and ate breakfast by 8. I intended to go to church but it was too wet—I was engaged until 12 o'clock finishing a letter I commenced last night. Dr. F came home about two with a very severe nervous headache. He went to bed and requested me to visit a case of his. The child I was to see on Friday at Mr. Tate's. I went but was not pleased with the symptoms. I got home about night. I read a few pages of Tasso's "Jerusalem Delivered". I became very sleepy and retired soon.

(Written Monday Evening)

MONDAY, MARCH 18TH '61

This was a cold disagreeable morning. I hated to get up very much—to leave a good warm bed and plunge into the coldness of my room. I had to ride to-day for Faris —down in Washington County to Mr. Wm. Allison's. It commenced snowing soon after I started from home and snowed all day—I had a disagreeable ride.

I left McCall there. I came home about 4 o'clock cold and tired. I was at work on an old saddle the balance of the day and am writing about half after eight. Will study some and retire.

TUESDAY, MARCH 19TH, '61

This morning I was up about five. I prepared to go to Marion to court. I started about 1/2 [past] 9 o'clock. It is very cold this morning but clear.

Times are dull about Marion—politics is so especially. The people seem to have become tired of politics and turned their attention to something else. This perhaps may be better for them. We were very successful in business to-day—more so than usual. It seems as tho [sic] money is getting something more plenty in our country than it has been for some time past.

We got home about sundown. I am writing about 9 o'clock. I do not feel so well as usual. My arm where I was vaccinated troubles me some and I feel some uneasiness about the throat—not like common sore throat, but an aching and dull feeling on the right side. I have already had a nap. I wil try to read some and retire. It is clear and cold this evening.

WEDNESDAY, MARCH 20TH, 1861

This was a very pretty morning. I read a while and prepared to go over to Lyon's Gap store. I rode Wm. Siry's mare. I have come to the conclusion that I will be obliged for decency's sake to have some new clothes. I went to the store on purpose to get some. I bought to the amount of thirteen dollars worth. I was bound to have them charged to my d/c. [credit and debit account] although I know it is a bad plan to do so. I will pay for them if I live. I promised Wm. Siry to purchase a pair of pantaloons for him if I could get them to trust him. The principal (Gollehan) was not at home, and his clerk (Taylor) did not know what to do. I promised to stand good in case Siry was a delinquent. I came home about four o'clock.

Studied Wood &c. I became very sleepy—so sleepy that I deferred writting in my journal until morning, which was wrong really. I retired about 9 o'clock. It snowed very hard—cold. Written Fri. morn.

THURSDAY, MARCH 21ST, 1861

This morning I should have written in my journal but put it off for some more convenient time until late when Mr. Wm. Lynan came and sat several hours with me. He wishes to get a school for a female teacher and wants the teacher to board with us. If she is good working and smart and nice I have no objection sure. I have been reading Greenhow on diptheria.

Dr. came home before Dinner and asked to visit a very sick patient with him. The patient was an old man some 80 and upwards perhaps who had a severe attack of pneumonia. I think doubtful whether the old man will recover again or not.

Poor old man, he has breasted life's turbulent waves by more than is allotted to him by the Creator. The Doctor requested me to stay with him all night. I remained all night without sleeping once. So I could not write in my journal. Clear, Windy, & Cold.

(Written Friday noon)

FRIDAY, MCH. 22ND, '61

I left my patient this morning after an anxious night. I thought him no better — perhaps worse. His pulse intermittent, or rather complicated to me. Skin soft and warm. Eyes glassy and covered with a matter of some kind. Breathing difficult, very delirious—sleeping incessantly almost and murmuring all the time. We gave him Doan's powders 4 [illegible] every four hours and Aro. Spts ammonia 15 gtt every two or three hours to [illegible] up the system.

Poor old man he has about run his race—his pilgrimage on these mundane shore is near over—his grey hair and superannuated limbs will soon return to the dust from whence they came; and his spirit will enter the forever of a just God who will decide the deeds done in the body. He has a good many children several of whom were there.

After coming home I knocked around a little, read some and repaired a door lock for Mrs. Faris. Then I took a good nap. After dinner I was reading. Mrs. Faris came into my room and conversed awhile. I went to the Post Office after sundown. I got a letter from my esteemed cousin Bettie. She is *well.*

I am writing between 10 & 11. Will retire soon.

SATURDAY, MARCH 23RD, '61

This morning I was up as usual. Dr. Faris came to my room soon after I got up and told me that he had made made [sic] arrangements for me to go over in Grayson Co. on business for him. Dr. Beatie was going over there to-day—place is located at the Mouth of Wilson. I was taken rather by surprise in regard to going, although we had spoken about the trip several times before. I had now not more than an hour and a half or two hours to prepare for the trip which was between thirty and forty miles. I had no clean shirt—not shaved—did not know whether to dress in my best (which was bad) or go in my every day clothes. I concluded to put on my *best.* I was ready by the time Dr. B. called—we started—Dr. Faris went as far as Bartens with us. Dr. Beatie had a snack of cold vituals [sic] in his pocket. We sat down on the road side and ate it. We started *heavenward* (I mean upward on the mountain) up, up, around, around hills, gorges, and ravines. We reached the top of a large mountain lying south of Rye valley about 1/2 past twelve o'clock. I am unable to explain my feelings when traveling over these mountains—the proudest and most sublime works of nature. Our road lay along a stream called "Conner's Creek["]—a tributary of the South Fork of Holston probably its main branch. Gigantic pines stood on either side of this stream as if patiently awaiting the tide of emigration to march into those ravines and with the help of the stream to convert them into lumber and ship it off to become part of some village or town or perhaps a city. I am sure a great deal of lumber might be supplied from this hollow running some five or six miles. As the ascent became greater and the stream smaller the cascades more beautifully grand. Leaping down, down among the rugged rocks, foaming and boiling.

We two were enjoying ourselves as best we could joking and relating anecdotes. I think Beatie can stretch his [tales?] a good deal, especially about himself. We passed by a house at which we had business—Mr. Wm. Lovelace. I took his note. Then we went to another man's house (Mr. Reese Dalton). I took his note also and gave him an act. to collect on Allen Hams.

We arrived at Mouth of Wilson about dark. It is a droll place—droll people. The folks seemed glad to see their doctor. I think Dr. Beatie has an excellent location—a location that he ought to stick to. I [verb missing; context is *fear*] greatly his expensive habits will sink him—I fear more too that he will become intemperate; for I believe every person old and young, rich & poor, high and low drinks in Grayson.

We retired very early because we were tired.

(Written in Monday evening)

SUNDAY, MARCH 24TH, '61

This morning we did not rise until after sun up. It seems to be the custom with a great many professional and literary men not to rise until a late hour—I do not think it right to lie in bed so long, especially when breakfast is ready and on the table—it is troublesome to the lady of the boarding home and I was somewhat puzzled to know how I was to spend the day. Dr. B. was compelled to visit some patients of his and I did not care to go. I had no acquaintance and the folks were so rough I did not care to make any. I went to his office and amused myself reading a novel called "While it was Morning".

About one o'clock Dr. returned. But before he came I had made up my mind that the people were a hard lot. The Dr. asked me to visit a patient with him this evening which I promised to do and did. I saw a very good country. We got back about a while after sundown. After supper Beatie read and I listened for some two or three hours. We retired late.

(Written Monday evening)

MONDAY, MARCH 25TH, 1861

This morning I was up about 7 o'clock. I must leave for home. I become [sic] to like Beatie tollerably [sic] well for the time I was over there. He is very profane and I am sorry to say that I was weak enough to utter a good many profane words whilst over there. I almost envy Beatie's location for many reasons. I bid him adieu and turned homewards about 1/2 past or ten o'clock. The serene hills met my view that met my view on Saturday but they did [not] seem so noble & grand as it was raining on Saturday. And when a person has company those solemnisations[50] of nature are never half so beautiful as when we are alone.

I traveled on—my mule was very tired about the time I got home, about sundown. I am writing at 8 o'clock. Will retire pretty soon.

My trip was a tiresome one but I do not regret it. I saw some of the largest mountains that I have crossed yet. The Grayson country is a rough country and the people are the roughest folks I ever saw.

TUESDAY, MARCH 26TH 1861

This was a pretty morning—I rose about as usual. I read Wood and then read several articles on female diseases from the different authors we have. I did it on Mrs. F's account. She is complaining and has been for some time. I could find nothing that suited her complaint. I planted a tree (Holly) in the yard to-day. I hope it will live and furnish a memento of the patient.

After dark Dr. Faris was called to Mr. Jno. Sanders to see a child that had been poisoned by swallowing a brass button. I suppose the Gastric juice of the

---

[50] The usage is obsolete even for nineteenth century. He may be quoting from Alexander Pope (1688-1744) or Edmund Spenser (1552?-1599), both of whom use *solemnise* as a verb to mean, *to mark something for a special occasion with due and fitting honor*; Spenser also uses *solemnise* as a noun instead of *solemnisation*; but he too uses the word in all forms as a positive and propitious ceremonial act of observance. *OED.*

Stomach acting on the copper formed acetate of copper[51] causing the child to vomit violently. Dr. asked me to accompany him. I did so. He prescribed the white of an egg. It is now after 10 o'clock. I shall retire soon.

WEDNESDAY, MARCH 27TH, '61

This was a fine morning although rain fell last night. I read &c to-day—nothing transpired worthy of notice I think. Dr. commenced building a *hen house* to-day. I am opposed to his style and place. It is no use to oppose him though; for he will do as he thinks proper in defiance of all else. It is his privilege to do so I guess.

I am getting along badly I fear with the work that I am studying. I am drowsy and dull of comprehension some how or other. I do wish I could concentrate my mind upon my books more than I do—it will be to my sorrow if I do not. I am neglecting my grammar lessons too—breaking another resolve. Thus it is with frail man.

THURSDAY, MARCH 28TH, 1861

The weather is fine. I have nothing to record of myself except being lazy to rise at morning—a habit that I fear will be more that I can manage.

I was closely engaged with my book until after dinner when I went to see Mr. Lewis for a settlement of his bill. He was not at home consequently I did [not] effect anything. I got back a short time before night. A patient called this evening who has gonorrhea. His is a bad case. I have been treating it for some three months but it baffles me. I applied to Dr. F for assistance.

I am writing at 9 o'clock after having had a good nap. I have played a trick on Luther F. He had been saving eggs for Easter for some time and to prevent any of them being for domestic purposes he hid them out in a corner of the lot by making a hole in the ground and covering it with grass. I went out to-night and robbed his nest. I do not know what he may say in the morning, at any rate I'll try him for the fun whether commendable or not.

Dr. and Mrs. Faris have gone to Mrs. Sanders to-night. I will study a while and retire.

---

[51] *Acetate* in this era means a "salt of acetic acid"; *acetic* is from the Latin *acetum*, or vinegar. Not always scientifically measured in the day, the old term means almost any aqueous solution that becomes a reagent or caustic and induces vomiting. *Taber's*.

FRIDAY, MARCH 29TH, 1861

I was up as usual this morning. We are having fine weather—Though it seems as if there might be rain soon.

I have studied some to-day and worked some—Worked in making stile[52] at the road in front of the door. I went to the Post Office this evening. I have been looking for a letter from my Uncles for some week or so but have looked in vain. Why it is they have not written to me I know not. I do hope they will not forsake me now that I need their help most .

I have spoken often in my journal of our political affairs and feel disposed to make a note to-night. I am forced to say that I fear things are no better. Our convention is acting outrageously. It has been in session now over a month and a half. Their time has been spent in speechifying and consulting trivial things; nothing of any importance has engaged their time. Speaking and and [sic] offering resolutions seem to be the object of their sessions. Why not make some move—carry out some action and let the people endorse or condemn that action. I fear Great Men are ruining our country. I would like for the session to come to a close. If we must fight let us not put it off any longer—if on the other hand that we are to have peace and reconstruction then let its consummation be rapidly brought about. I am still for secession—Secession grows with me as I get older.

I am writing between 9 & 10. Will bring some wood and water to my room— study a while and then I'll retire.

SATURDAY, MARCH 30TH, 1861

This morning I arose at 6. I have done but little reading in my regular course to-day. I was engaged part of the morning in making a box to plant some orange seed in —by way of experiment I planted the seed and set the box in my room. I was then called to see a patient—a child of Mr. Jas. Rector. I went and found it sitting up and apparently easy. I found on examination that its tonsils, especially the one on the left side very much enlarged. The outer side of its neck and throat, extending from from [sic] the helix[53] of the ear to the chin was somewhat enlarged—I prescribed castor oil internally and Liniment as a

[52] A step or set of steps, especially arranged in front of a wall or a fence for ascending and descending from a road through a fence and to a house (Middle English, obsolete). *OED.*

[53] The margin of the external ear. *Taber's.*

rubefacient[54] applied often to external parts. I returned home and dined. I was reading to see if I could find anything that would enlighten me on the subject, when I was summoned in haste to see the child again. It had been somewhat accustomed to having spasms and one had come on now. I found the child staring wildly about—taking no notice of scarcely anything. Pulse strong and hard—quick. Smacking its mouth too continually was another of the many symptoms. I put some salt in its mouth to arouse the nerves of taste some at least and: applied cold water to the head and hands. I soon had the pleasure of seeing the convulsive little creature better—except the swelling of the jaw and neck which seemed to grow worse. I prescribed a poultice[55] to be put to the swollen parts immediately. Its bowels were move about 5 o'clock. I came home and sent Dr. F down to see it—he went but done nothing. He requested me to visit the child and give it some physic.[56] I did so; but did not find the patient any better—I fear—swelling increased—fever up some. I came home about 10 o'clock.

Am writing about 11—will retire. I omitted to say that I rec'd a letter from Aunt Malvina. There are several questions she asked that I do not care to answer directly.

SUNDAY, MARCH 31ST 1861

I arose this morning about sunrise. After I dressed I sat down and wrote part of a letter to my cousin James—it being too early to start to church. I started to church about 10 o'clock. I overtook a crowd of several persons going from Mrs. Susan Sanders, Miss M.F.S., Miss Sue Alen, Miss F. Duff, and A.J.S[anders] — and others a very lively crowd that.

Our preacher today was Mr. Barr from Abingdon, Va. Associate editor of the "Abingdon Virginian". He is a Protestant Methodist by profession. I am strange in regard to preaching and preachers for I did not think he did anything extra.

---

[54] Liniment, or Linimentum [Latin for a smearing substance], was a liquefied solution of a medicament and oil, alcohol, or water to be rubbed on externally; sometimes it was smeared on a bandage, and the bandage was left on the spot on the skin. Rubefacient, from the Latin for making red, was an agent producing a local congestion of blood, the vessels becoming dilated and the supply of blood increasing in the area where rubefacient was applied. Mustard was also used as a rubefacient. *Taber's.*

[55] Poultice, from the Latin for thick paste, was a hot, moist mass of linseed, mustard, or soap and oil; the mass was held between two pieces of muslim applied to the skin to relieve congestion or pain. *Taber's.*

[56] Physic is any so-styled *cathartic*, from the Greek for purging, and was designed to move the bowels; castor oil was often used as a physic. *Taber's.*

He preached from Mat. 7th 13 & 14—: "Broad is the way &c."[57] I do not think he had much system about his sermon—nothing he said would apply very well to the text. He said the phraseology of the text presents a difficulty to the mind by saying that many went the broad way because the other way was narrow &c. That man was prone to do evil was a fixed fact and that the great enemy of the human race was was [sic] allways of pointing men to barriers and laying difficulties before men was enough without its being done from the pulpit[.] then he commenced on another branch of the argument he intended to discourse upon and left me to conjecture as I pleased about this *broad* and that *narrow way.* He said, to him, there appeared to be four concomitants to repentance 1 Conviction of sin 2 Sorrow for sin 3 A desire to leave of[f; leave off, that is, quit] sinning 4 Forsaking of sin. He spoke of the workings of the two first but the two latter so complicated that I do not know what he made of them. It may not be the fault of the preacher but my own incomprehensive mind that I did not understand him.

He promulgated a doctrine that he called *The Doctrine of Restitution.* As to its merits I am not prepared to comment. It is this, and I believe it is partially scriptural at least. That before a man can become a christian or a child of God he must make restitution for every evil that he has done as far as it lies in him to do so. If he has got gain by fraudulence or a deception he must immediately return to the loser. If he has lined his coffers with dishonest gold he can never obtain entrance into the new Jerusalem along the strait [sic] and narrow way while he possesses this gold of fraudulence. If he has robbed some fellow man of fair farms and ruined his character restitution must be made before he can ever enter the presence of his master in peace and listen to the words "Well done good and faithful servant"[58] — I think perhaps this is all right —it is scripture but how wide that is [a] course pursued [in] the world of christian I'll say, and the course this [that is, the narrow way] no other points out [the sense is that the preacher did not make application of this principle to real life, that is, he failed to show which way is "this" narrow Christian way and which "that" broad non-Christian way].

---

[57] Matthew 7:13-14. "Enter by the narrow gate, since the road that leads to perdition is wide and spacious, and many take it; but it is a narrow gate and a hard road that leads to life, and only a few find it." Words attributed to Jesus Christ.

[58] Matt. 25:23. A parable attributed to Jesus Christ. The phrase, or its alternative in verse 21 (*Well done, thou good and faithful servant*) was often quoted as epitaph on tombstones in southern cemeteries of the nineteenth and early twentieth centuries.

I had company this evening. Mr. N.C.B. St. John, the two frenchmen and J.S. Gollohon. [59] All left about night. I finished my letter to cousin Jim after reading Tasso's poetry a while retired about 10 o'clock.

I omitted to say that this is Easter Sunday. Those holidays are spent very much unlike they are in Eastern Virginia. No one regards Monday as a holiday at all. They think strange when they are told that in E. V[a]. we keep Monday. Though they do not keep holiday it is neverless a great time aong children and some old folks too. They are great for "coloured eggs." Every child and a good many old folks has a coloured egg—died [sic; dyed] with something some are jet black some red some yellow and others striped and speckled in fine every conceivable colour. I am not acquainted with its origin.

MONDAY, APRIL 1ST, 1861

I rose this morning about 6. There was every appearance of rain when I got up — rain was falling pretty fast about 10 o'clock—clear at 12. Nothing to write of importance. I studied some to-day.

Before night I went to the Post Office. I had the pleasure to receive letters from R H Dungan and my uncles Charles and Bill. Dungan seems satisfide [sic] with the letter I wrote him some days ago. (See Sat. March 16th) if he is satisfide [sic] I am. Uncle Charles writes me that he has bought a livery stable (Uncle Jake is with him) and will speculate on stock &c. I hope he may do well. But he says that he has gone in debt some $6000 which is a pretty large sum for a poor man. However I think he is a pretty good trader and will make money perhaps. One thing I am afraid his trade will break into my arrangements about going to the lectures last fall [sic; he means to say, this coming fall] as I was expecting money from him, in part anyhow, to go. Uncle Bill writes me very encouraging. He seems to think that he can let me have two hundred dollars of the three hundred that I want. This will do if I can raise the other hundred any where. I must acknowledge that I have not so much confidence in Uncle Bill as I would like to have. The hope of getting money stimulates me some. I have not been sleepy tonight, I am writing between 10 & 11. I will study a grammar lesson next which will take me to syntax.

---

[59] St. John, mentioned often prior to the fighting, eventually joined Co. A of First Virginia Bde; three Gollohons joined the brigade: this man, apparently James S.; John M., a lieutenant captured later in the War who eventually died in prison; and Robert M., sergeant major, who was captured at Winchester but later released and survived war.

TUESDAY, APRIL 2ND, '61

I rose this morning earlier than usual. I read the "Home Circle" some. I have so far made good progress with my studies today. Or that is I have passed over a good deal of matter whether I made any progress or not. I have nothing of note to personalize this morning. I spoke to the Dr. about the letter I rec'd from my uncle last evening. He seems to think that perhaps I may get a free ticket to [illegible] Med School in Washington City. I fare [fear] though that my uncle is a bad one. [illegible] he will get some friends to do all they can for me.

I am writing about 9 o'clock. Will read a while then study a grammar lesson and retire.

APRIL 3RD, WEDNESDAY

I was up this morning before sun rise [sic]. Yesterday I did a good day's reading but to-day I have done nothing scarcely. This mornig I wrote letters to my Uncles Charles and Bill, also part of another to cousin Bettie.

This evening I attend the burial of Old Mr. Stuffle Aury. He was some 80 years old. Poor old man, he outlived the time allotted to friends and family. He has been from what I have learned a stout and brave man. He was and has been afflicted with rheumatism for several years which crippled so that it was with a great difficulty that he got about at all. He has surely seen his share of the ups and downs, but he has seen his last on Earth. A little over a year ago his wife was laid beneath the cold sod of the Church Graveyard and, he was then too decripted to attend her burial. She seemed to be a kind hearted christian woman. Reverence the Proverb: "The old *must* die the young *may* die."

Man though he is clothed in purple and fine linen and fares sumptuosly every day, should remember that Death is abroad in the world, which is his harvest field—he is gathering up those whom God has destined to live no longer and welcome them to a pyous [sic] Heaven or bid them depar [sic]! depart! Though Mr. Aury has lived a long while yet I fear his course on Earth can not justify us in hope of his peace in the next world. I saw him soon after I came to West Va. and was with him daily for a month afterwards, seeing him often since. Peace be to his ashes. Let us leave him with his God—Let us leave him with the untried scene of the spirit land. Let us hope that that [sic] the merit of the atone in blood is sufficient to secure him heaven. I am writing at a late hour— have been asleep.

THURSDAY, APRIL 4TH, 1861

I was up some what earlier than usual this morning. I wish I could rise sooner than I do usually. Indeed I am so drowsy at times during the day that I do not know what to do with myself. I have read a good deal to-day. I went to Bishop's shop this evening to have Dr's mare shod for him .

I have been reading to-night. Dr. & Mrs. F. were in my room until 9 o'clock. I spoke to-night against the "Know nothing" party[60] and I ought not to have done it. Dr. is a "Know nothing["] and I am not the person to find fault and detract any thing from any sect or party. We live in a free country. Every one has the prerogative to belong to and support any doctrine he pleases if not in opposition to the Constitution. But as much as I know of "Know nothings["] I can not believe it the true Christian doctrine. Though to the man that does I say defend it and I shall not oppose unless it comes in contact with me or mine.

I am writing between 9 & 10. I will study awhile and retire.

FRIDAY, APRIL 5TH, 1861

The weather is very fine now. I enjoy the cool mornings very much when I am out of bed earlier enough to walk a piece before breakfast.

I did but little studying to-day. I read a while this morning and was engaged fixing some "Scrap Book". I rec'd a letter from M.E. She tells me that Grandmother is dead. I do wish I could see her once more. She seemed always to love me as though I had been her own child. She has passed through a tumultous and harassed life— her eyes have been failing for some time. I expect, ere this, she is well nigh blind. I wrote not a letter to-day and went to the office.

---

[60] The Know-Nothing Party, officially called the American Party, existed between 1849 and the late 1850s, and had particular strength in urban areas of the Northeast where large numbers of Irish and other Roman Catholic immigrants had recently taken up residence. The party was characterized by *nativism*, that is, a strong prejudice against immigrants, with especially strong prejudice against Roman Catholics. Originally clandestine, the party asked its members to reply, "I know nothing," if asked about what the organization did. However, by 1852, it was very much an open and well-organized party, and by 1855, 43 congresspersons of the U.S. House styled themselves Know-Nothings or American Party members. In 1856, former president Millard Fillmore of Maryland joined the party, and ran again for president on its ticket, carrying his own state and gaining some support in border states. Local historians also note the presence of the Know-Nothing Party in Smyth County, something of an anomaly since there was very little ethnic immigration into the Virginia highlands and since the area was otherwise not particularly like the border states. Besides the prominent physician Faris, the highly successful Democratic delegate James White Sheffey was for a time a member. However, Faris's continuing membership, in 1861, is atypical both for nation and region. See "Politics" in Wilson, *Smyth County*, s.v.

Nothing new. I saw Miss Garland—a school-mistress that is to teach at S. Spring Church.[61] She is a good looking woman. I was introduced by Mr. G.W. St John to old Mr. Boyd, this evening.

There is a little circumstance that occured that perhaps may be worthy of note. As I stated somewhere else in my journal that a friend had loan me a pistol. To-day I fired at a muskrat and I suppose the strain on the pistol was to[o] great and a part of the iron hold the barrel in contact with the breeches.[62] I was at a loss at first to know what to do. Own [admit] that I injured it and pay for it or just give it to him without telling the fault. The first I am resolved to do, for I had as well [illegible phrase; context is *to steal or cheat for a large sum of money*] as to deceive my friend for the sake of a few dollars, and then the character of such a thing.

I am writing between 10&11. I have made a great lot of pills to-night.

APRIL 6TH, SATURDAY

I had to go to town to-day on business for Dr. F. Started from home about 10 o'clock—in Marion at 12. Transacted my business (Gave A.G. Pendleton, a lawyer, an act. on the Estate of Rev. Robinson Gannaway.)[63] I went across towards S. Fork to see Thos. Dungan and others[.] some I saw and some I did not see. I met with Ex. Gov. McMullin to-day—had the pleasure of riding with him a few miles.[64] He is a candidate for the next term of Congress, and it is

---

[61] Sulphur Springs was site of many camp meetings for Methodists in Smyth County, some dating back to 1819. Apparently a permanent church building was there briefly in this period. The Miss Garland cannot be identified by Smyth County historians, and she does not seem to be the school teacher of the same name known to some citizens. Wilson, *Smyth County*, 144.

[62] *Breeches* is the obsolete term for the rear part of the firearm. *OED*. Apparently the gun in some way overheated and fused the rear of the piece to the barrel; however, the "injury" was not readily apparent, unless someone pointed it out.

[63] The Rev. Robinson Gannaway (sometimes recorded as Robertson Gannaway) was a Lutheran minister in Chilhowie who had died in 1859 "of an affliction of the heart," and his estate was still being settled. Armstrong, *Ante-Bellum Years*, 61. The attorney Pendleton was prominent in local politics and organized the Smyth County Blues, the first company to volunteer for the Confederate army. After the war, Pendleton remained very active in politics and business, but was unsuccessful in campaigns for office.

[64] LaFayette McMullen (often misspelled *McMullin*) was one of the most colorful of local poltiicians between the 1830s and the end of the Civil War. Usually called Old Fayette or Ex-Gov., he was said to have kissed more babies and delivered more speeches than any candidate in the country. Briefly governor of the territory of Washington, he married and divorced in the Pacific Northwest and then returned to Virginia. It is said that once he interrupted a hanging in order to give a speech while running for U.S. Congress; the story is that he stopped the hanging long enough to ask the sheriff formally for permission to take the time normally allotted for a

easily imagined how polite and gentlemanly he was to every body. That's the way with the candidates. I got home between 5 & 6. I am writing at 9 o'clock—will retire soon to my room [;] mend shirts some to-night. I shall try to read a while and retire.

SUNDAY, APRIL 7TH, '61

Like other Sundays that I have seen this morning is a very rainy one and of dull days a rainy Sunday is the dullest. However about 9 o'clock the clouds showed an inclination to clear up, so by 10 it was clear enough to ensure clear sky enough for going to church. Mr. Boring preached to-day at S. Spring: "To attack the opinion of great men however erroneous they may be is seldom condoned in the eye of the world" and criticise the eloquence and logic of a member of the pulpit where expounding [illegible] erudition might merit the critic the name of *Faultfinder*. But really Mr. B's sermon was as droll a sermon as I ever heard from a reputed sharp or smart man.

His text was the last verse of the 40th Chapter of Isaiah.[65] He seemed to be trying to tell the progresion that a Christian makes, or ought to make. He dwelt long and largely upon several features of the text and had it mixed at last (to me). I would [verb missing; provide or give?] the outline of his service but I did not come home this evening therefore I have not the time to write as much as I could wish. Among other invitations to go to dinner I [chose?] to go to Mr. St. John's. Quite a crowd was together and enjoyed ourselves very well. I became acquainted with Mr. Jame P. Sanders from Missouri. I staid at Mr. L. Sanders all night. Was treated very friendly

I have one thing to say—a quiz was written Mr. Geo. W. St. Jno by 2 persons—I saw it to-day—it has fulfilled its mission.

(*Written on Monday Evening*)

MONDAY APRIL 8TH, 1861

I came home this morning about 9 o'clock. Read awhile made some medicine and ate dinner at 1. I went to the Switch this evening for Mrs. Faris—she is expecting company tomorrow but from the appearance of the

---

condemned man to say his final words. Successful in politics before the war, he was unsuccessful in running for the Confederate congress in 1861, but he did win a seat in 1863. Wilson, *Smyth County*, 108-112; Armstrong, *Ante-Bellum Years*, 38.

[65] Isaiah 40:31. But they that wait upon the Lord shall renew their strength; they shall mount up with wings as eagles; they shall run, and not be weary; and they shall walk, and not faint.

weather now everything will be delayed before that time. Rain is falling very fast. I am writing between 9 & 10—but am one of the sleepiest fellows out—I cannot keep my eyes open.

TUESDAY, APRIL 9TH 1861

This is an ugly morning—rainy, drizly [sic], and foggy. I read several pages before our expected company arrived. They came about 10 o'clock. (Miss M.F.S., Mrs. Lauren Sanders and a Mrs. (Kennaman?) were the guests) I read no more while they were here. I like Miss M.F.S. very well—think she is a good girl. The other ladies were nice ladies. Mrs. (Kennaman?) is a very sensible lady. Mrs. Sanders seems to have less education than the other but not behind her in common sense and pleasantness of company. I came to my room and commenced writing. Wrote, or rather finished a letter to Cousin Bettie and commenced one for Aunt Malvina.

I have oft spoken of our national affairs since I commenced this book. I think times are more ominous of evil now than ever—The Convention of Va has [not] accomplished anything yet. Our last news was to the effect that all supplies were cut off from Maj. Anderson in Fort Sumpter [Sumter] and that Fort Pickens had been secretly reinforced: The next we perhaps will be pregnant with the thrilling scenes of the battlefield; may the Great God avert it, may He stop the tide that will stain American shores with fratricidal blood.

10 o'clock

WEDNESDAY, APL. 10TH, '61

We are having some very ugly weather now—foggy, drizly, muddy, and occassionally a little windy. There is not much fog either but the clouds look gloomy. I have done but little reading to-day—I was making a "Telling needle" for Miss Laura. I am studying Intermediate for now—it is rather dull. I am writing @ a few minutes after 10. Having studied a good Grammar lesson. Will retire soon.

THURSDAY, APRIL 11TH, '61

I rose this morning about 1/2 past 5, ate breakfast at 7. The weather seems to have intermitted for a while, or until another paryyxism [sic; paroxysm][66] comes

---

[66] Medical term in nineteenth century denotes any recurring spasm and connotes a fit or seizure. In applying the term to weather, he is being metaphorical. *OED.*

on. I was engaged a while this morning preparing some medicine, [illegible] [illegible] at [illegible] and then read Wood. After dinner I had to go over on S. Fork on business for Dr. F. I transacted the most of what I had to do. Some men have no heart at all. I settled with one man (Wm. (Dungan [parentheses sic]) he endeavoured to make his account to come within a fraction of Dr's. act. If it were me I should try to make it back the first time I had visit [sic] his family and make him pay immediately. There are many who think because it's a Doctor's bill they will pay it with as little as possible. And when they do that the only alternative for the practitioner is to make it up in charges. I returned home about 8 and retire (after a nap) at 10.

(Written partly Friday Morning)

FRIDAY, APRIL 12TH, 1861

Up this morning very late—later than usual. I was studying Wood to-day. Raining occasionally—There is a great deal of rain, mud & c in these diggins [sic].[67] I wrote, or finished, two letters to-day—I read some 24 pages in Wood. After dark Rector's boys came in and remained 'til 9 o'clock. They bothered me a good deal— brought lots of mud in on there [sic] big feet—I hope they will not call again soon. If they do I hope they will find another room. I was too sleepy to write last night.

(Written Saturday morn.)

SATURDAY, APL. 13TH, 1861

The weather is unsettled yet. Sunshine, clouds and rain are the modifications for the weather this morning. To-day was muster day at our place of military display. This malitia [sic] mustering is a humbug anyway. It will never discipline the farmers and plow boys to take the military step. Some step long, some short—some wheel right [,] some left and some are running and some standing—pretty soldiers to put upon the field of battle.

We mustered upon a very prominent hill and the wind blew very furious and cool. We were very glad to leave the grounds; but did not however until many a maneuver was cut many an evolution was gone through and I fancy as far from being tactical as one can immagine [sic]. There is a probability that military men will be in demand soon. From the signs of the times the Federal

---

[67] Diggings, usually treated as singular, means any place of excavation, usually by an archaeologist. Colloquially, especially with the *unsounded-g* ending, the word means any peculiar place or region. *American Heritage Dictionary.*

Government and provisional congress [of Confederacy in Montgomery] will soon welcome each other or parts of each other to a bloody grave. Every preparation is being made by the President Elect to push coercion to its fullest extent. If he does war is as inevitable between the two powers as death is to fallen man.[68] Virginia is still holding out for a reconciliation—Wo[e] be unto her [illegible]. Abraham Lincoln shall seize two forts and place fetters of free-negro tyranny upon her sons!

There is some difficulty in our neighborhood in regard to the teaching of a school. The neighbors, or rather certain individuals of the neighborhood have erected a school-house nigh unto completion, and a school has been made up by Mr. Leonard for a young lady to teach. Mr. Rector and others are opposed to a female teacher and hence they have split up. To-day there was a meeting of the neighborhood—the patrons and subalterns[69] to decide the matter. I was requested by Dr. Faris to go and represent his interest as he was so indisposed that he could not go. I did not feel much like having anything to do with it for there might be harsh feelings on one side or the other. I went however. There were not a great many there. They proceeded to business in regular form. I was asked to preside as chairman. Afterwards, P.J. Heninger, Robert S. Bonham, Jas. M. Rector, David Ready, and William Leonard were appointed trustees to watch over and protect the interest of the school house property. There was some discussion in regard to the teachers. One says if its exclusively a male school he is out, another says if a female teacher teaches there he is out. So they can never come together on these terms. Finally, they agreed to leave it [to] the subscribers the building of the school-house to say who is to teach. I did not think that right—I thought that the patrons should have the privilege of saying who should teach their children.

I think it would be to the accomodation of the greater portion of the neighborhood to have a female in summer and a male in winter.

---

[68] In theological language, he speaks of spiritual *death* for people who have not accepted the salvation offered by God's grace and forgiveness. All are "fallen" from grace in Eden, but only those who willfully refuse grace suffer "death."

[69] French word with Latin root, literally an alternate one beneath another; historically, the servant serving one who is himself or herself a servant. Militarily, any office beneath rank of captain. *OED*. In legal sense for a privately incorporated school, patrons would be the major contributors who organize and run the institution, subalterns would be the principal and teacher[s] and others who work in the school. Subscribers would be those paying fees for their children to attend the school.

I went to the P.O. this evening returned about 10 o'clock—after reading a while I retired. Written Sunday Evening.

SUNDAY, APRIL 14TH 1861

I was up this morning at 5 o'clock. I read Tasso's "Jerusalem delivered". I went to S. Spring to church to prayer meeting. There were but few in attendance.

As we have been expecting and some wishing—fort Sumpter has been attacked and taken by the forces of the S. Confederacy. We have not learned the particulars; but its being taken is a fact. What will be the issue I know not.

Mr. N. C. St. John called this evening—I went to the P. Office with the intention of hearing from headquarters—however I heard nothing of interest.

Some time ago Uncle Charles wrote me to have some boots made for him—I had the boots making when he wrote me not to send them- that he did not want them. I got a letter from him this evening containing the half two 10$ notes and stating that he wished me to send them to him immediately. Queer request! I did not take the boots and they were sold. Now if he wants boots he must wait 'til I have them made. I am writing about 10—will retire.

MONDAY, APRIL 15TH 1861

Up at 5. I was engaged writing letters this morning. I wrote one to Uncle Charles and one to the Dean of Faculty of Medical College Washing [sic] City D.C. My object in writing him is to ascertain something about Congressmen giving medical students free tickets to that institution. I know of no better way to find out. I read Wood on Yellow Fever to-day. I am not as well as I have usually have been. I am drowsy and have a dull headache—have had it for several days. Raining to-day. I am writing about 9 o'clock. Will study a while and retire.

[TUESDAY] APRIL 16TH 1861

To-day was court day. I, as usual, went. Very bad day—raining snowing and blowing. Excitement is at its pitch in regard to national affairs. Every house in Marion nearly has a secession flag floating over it—men are excited to the highest pitch of their animal power. And well they may. Abe Lincoln has demand [sic] of Virginia 9000 soldiers to be at his disposal to subjugate the South—to whip her into submission to his rule. God forbid that any Virginian may take up arms against the South—J.B. Floyd made a speech of four hours length—a happy effort. I am more and more for secession. I have a flag that I shall, if God spare me, launch in the breeze to-morrow. I wish secession God-Speed. May the tide roll in until the South shall be acknowledged free and independent—loyal to one creed or section one in sentiment one in heart and one in action.

We read news to-day that our state had seceded—may it be so is my prayer.

I am writing at 11 o'clock. My room is cold and I will retire.

[WEDNESDAY] APRIL 17TH '61

This is a bad spell of weather—snowing again this morning. I fancy we will not have the pleasure of tickling our palates with this year. I prepared my flag staff this morning and adjusted the flag and threw it to the breeze.

"Long may it wave in the land of the free and the home of the brave."

I have been reading over some pamphlets to find something applicable or applicable [sic] and use it to speak at the raising of our flag at the "switch" on Saturday next. I found nothing of any note. Dr. Barbran was to see me to-day. Dr. [Seates?] was here also—he is a case—I have often heard of his disposition but people should not judge from what they hear—though if I had never heard anything about him I think I would have known that he was small potatoes. He talks more than anybody and with as little sense I think. He pretended to give me some "good" advice about some girls (M.F.S.) In all events—he says she will fool me if I ain't mine—well let her rip. Company all left about 3 o'clock. I read an account of the battle at Charleston S.C.—the evacuation of Fort Sumpter. No one killed I think.

I suppose [illegible] disturbances of the mind occur with every moment. Heretofore I have been in the habit of going to the switch occassionally and sometimes stay all night and at others I have come home late. I have mistrusted that Dr. did not like it a great deal which I found is true. I proposed going to the "switch" this evening and Mrs. F came into my room and told me that Dr. was saying that he wished I would not stay at the "switch". I know those Sander's men are bad men in regard to drinking and gambling but perfect gentlemen in other respects. And this is the cause that Dr. objects to my staying therefore. He is afraid I might contract the habit.

I must say that I hardly know what my feelings were when Mrs. F spoke to me about it. She saw I was affected or felt it and wanted to apologised [sic] to me for telling me. I respect her for her goodness to me but I felt towards the Dr. like he had no confidence in me. But for this however I may be wrong and ought to think he is zealous of my welfare. But he ought to have more confidence in me than that since [illegible] that I have expressed my sentiments to him about drinking but I have not about cardplaying—as to cardplaying I have no taste for it all and therefore do not think that I shall ever become addicted to the vice of gambling and for the man who has not the stamina to breast boldly those little temptations is but badly prepared to try the whimsy and boisterous storm of life.

[illegible] speech I do not know whether I shall be called upon to speak or not.

10 o'clock and after.

Part Two

3 July 1861-20 March 1862

"A Desperate Attempt at a Place Called Bull Run Near Manassas"

Manassas to Kernstown

Although Smyth County included some Union sympathizers and there were many people who wanted to avoid war, there was general dislike of northerners and a particularly strong antipathy to abolitionists, as shown in the disgraceful treatment of the local antislavery family the Farises (5-6 February, pp. 34-35). When the Fort Sumter crisis escalated into a battle in April, majority sentiment in Smyth County—at least the sentiment declared openly in very public words and actions—swung in favor of immediate secession for Virginia. Thus, President Abraham Lincoln's call for nine thousand volunteers from the Commonwealth to fight for the Union and against the Confederacy was of course defied; indeed, his official call for the volunteers was only the public occasion for the country and the townspeople to rebel against the United States. Most had already decided that their cause lay with the states of the Lower South, and most of that majority understood that breaking away would not be permitted peacefully. [1]

Apperson approached The War with the passion of youth, although he finally understood that serving in the Confederacy would postpone for long years his plans to matriculate at a medical school. The first troops were organized as the Smyth County Blues, whose Company D was commanded by A.G. Pendleton, and Apperson wanted to join this group. However, he was dissuaded by his benefactor Dr. Faris, and probably Mrs. Faris as well, for that couple often functioned almost as parents for him; and each was convinced that he should serve in a medical rather than a military capacity. Another group, the Smyth County Grays, was soon formed, and the Blues and the Grays, together with other companies, were gathered into the First Virginia Brigade commanded by Thomas Jonathan Jackson, an instructor at Virginia Military

[1] Apperson's diary reports on public sentiment fully support the conclusions of the careful historian Goodridge Wilson, whose insight that the highlands included deep pockets of rabid pro-Confederacy sentiments and actions was recently reaffirmed by John C. Inscoe, *Mountain Masters, Slavery, and the Sectional Crisis in Western North Carolina* (Knoxville: University of Tennessee Press, 1989) and acknowledged for the highlands South by James Munro McPherson, *For Cause and Comrades: Why Men Fought in the Civil War* (New York: Oxford University Press, 1997). See Wilson, "the War Between the States," *Smyth County*, s.v.

Institute, which lay in the Blue Ridge north and west of the Highlands. Although Jackson was little regarded as an instructor, he of course became legendary as a military leader, and this entire brigade would gain the famous nickname Stonewall because of its performance at the First Battle of Manasas; the nickname attached as well and as famously to their commander.

No one could have known how renowned the First Virginia Brigade was to become, but Apperson the reader of Torquato Tasso and the latter-day Crusader was certainly anxious to join the campaign. In May, what was only a few weeks that Apperson regarded as a purgatorial delay, Dr. Harvey Black formed a medical brigade to serve the First Virginia Brigade. This physician, whose people had settled Blacksburg and established a sectarian college in that village in the highlands some seventy miles north and west of Seven Mile Ford, was delighted to bring Apperson into his field hospital as a steward. Field hospitals were established behind the lines of the major brigades, and of course Jackson's penchant for quick marches over considerable distances without much forewarning gave the medical brigade plenty of challenges. Black knew of Apperson's dreams, and he consciously treated his steward as an apprentice surgeon and physician and loaned him books and journals to read as well as lecturing to him as they treated patients. Like Faris, Black was patriarchal with his young charge and was never reluctant to give personal advice and counsel as well as professional instruction. Also like Faris, Black was a most reluctant secessionist, and he often confided in the steward his skepticism that the Confederacy was possible. Above all, Black tried to explain to the steward how bloody the war was going to be, but it would take the first great charges at Manassas for Apperson to apprehend emotionally what his patriarch was trying to tell him about the casualties to be produced in this war with its Napoleonic dashes against troops dug in with weapons that shot far more accurately than anything Napoleon or his chroniclers had ever imagined.

Besides these field hospitals serving the hard-charging Stonewall Jackson, there were also hospitals established in cities like Lynchburg and Richmond and there were hospitals established in relatively safe havens such as the college campus of Emory & Henry College. Notes in his diary make clear Apperson's disdain for these practitioners who did their work far from the battlefields.

As he treated soldiers, Apperson was much more likely to be fighting diseases rather than wounds, and it was to these diseases, especially those carrying unknown germs bred exponentially in the unclean conditions of the field hosptials, that the medical corps lost their own hard charges. Unlike any latter-day stereotypes, Apperson and his mentor Black read all that they could find about treating diseases, but they were years ahead of any discovery of how germs operated; dimly aware that filthy conditions were generally bad for the troops, the surgeons and physicians and their many helpers did what they could to clean up—but of course they were outdoors, and cleaning their instruments and washing their hands was simply not the same as sterilizing everything.

In these field hospitals, Apperson assisted Black in the operations on wounds, and then he joined other stewards, nurses of both genders, slaves, and various volunteers who treated the recuperating patients. The field hospital life paralleled the cavalry, infantry, and artillery, that is, there were long periods, sometimes even months, of boredom punctuated by a few hours of absolute chaos and terror. The work was humbling in any case, and not just because disease so frequently defeated the physicians after they had triumped over a wound. A steward like Apperson, and indeed even a licensed physician like Black, enjoyed none of the twentieth century standing of the medical doctor; instead, the practitioners were only players on a team injected into a context of three parts mystery and two parts doom. Bewildered by the unstoppable diseases in their tents, Apperson the apprentice and his elder professionals turned often to the women who volunteered to help and even to the slaves who came around to help. The pride, if not arrogance, associated with doctors of a later era simply could not be their part to play in this tragedy. For all that, Apperson and his fellow practitioners often knew an affection and a warmth with their patients and friends and family members and even the slaves who were there, as all stood together in the just but hopeless cause of fighting diseases they could not begin to understand. In particular, Black the Calvinist instructed by words and above all by actions the lessons that God had called them to try to help the wounded of either army, that there was no personal choice in this matter, that they would probably fail, but that a just and all-seeing God would demand their most sincere efforts—their arété, or principled struggle against an evil fate—in this cataclysm. Apperson thus absorbed a sense of Calvinist mission and a pre-Christian sense of Stoic duty to station and place, and these teachings of Harvey Black would carry him through this hell and through happier days to come.

For all the irresistible challenges assailing a young steward in a field hospital, Apperson was yet part of the Stonewall Brigade, and of course this period of time, from the Battle of Manassass to the Battle of Kernstown, was a time of military success for that brigade and generally for the Confederate forces in the eastern theatre. So successful was Stonewall Jackson—and so unknowing were Apperson and his friends about the very different story in the western theatre of the New South—that the steward could easily imagine himself emerging from this vale of tears into a time of peace in Richmond where he could attend medical lectures. And so successful was Stonewall Jackson—as noted in these diary entries he was regarded as virtually invincible—that the steward could easily foresee a quick end to the war, horrible as he had to concede that it was even in this first phase of its fighting.

In this section, Apperson begins with some notations about medicine dosages prescribed for soldiers, apparently according to company. The names and the units are extremely hard to decipher, and this is in a period when the Army of Northern Virginia is still being organized. The units include his own 4th Va., but also include some South Carolina units serving in the area. Although his diary begins again on 3 July, these notes date to May, and are his first records for his service as military steward, in this case making prescriptions and filling them for an assistant surgeon, Dr. Joseph S. Crockett of Wytheville, a man with who he would serve in the ANV medical corps until the Battle of Gaines Mill (27 June 1862). At that battle, Dr. Crockett—originally judged by the yound steward to be "wrathy" and "impatient" but later judged to be hard-working and fastidious—would himself perish.

[16 MAY 1861]

Capt [Liptung?] Aron Monroe 8 a [illegible letters—dosage]
[illegible name] D. Allegheny Ref
Brown [illegible first and last name]
Robinson [illegible name]
Dennis

MAY 16 '61

W.G.

Company A [cavalry, South Carolina] Capt. [W.R.] Terry
Rx [prescription]
Maj. Hyde [illegible, dosages?} XXX
x Peter Op. ' " ' [ditto marks?]
Plumbs Acct. ' " ' XX
Mc F. Pel No. X
xOne very four hours, amlet.
1 discharge ceases. For F. Spiller
Rx
Comp[any] Cathan Petes No. 32

x//Take two — at bed time
2For Inman
//Rx

xPulse Down Gms [grams?] XXX
D. Ghent No. VI
3For Jas. L. Pattison
One every 4 hours in Molasses
Joseph Gweltillo
Asst. Surgeon
Col. [illegible; Proctor's?] Bat.

These notes apparently were taken from prescriptions rendered by an assistant surgeon named J. Crockett

[Pluants?]

Comp. C Capt. Walker [possibly R.L. Walker, artillery]

MAY 16 - 1861

RxFr Kramerian & Zi

RxFr Opit [possibly opium] " Zij

[marginal note: Nance]

NO

SijA teaspoonful every four hours in sweetened water

4For Crockett

"

XRx Maj Sulph Zi

Take immediately

5For Carper

" Rx

xFor [Map?] grms. X

xRx Sulp diag [nosed] Zs

5Take the pill and in four hours afterwards the salt

6Crowel

IN Vials

RxSgr ScillComp. Zi

5Twenty drops every four

7Drops in water. For Darit

J. Crockett

Asst. Surgeon

Comp. A. Capt. [W.R.] Terry [S. C. Cavalry

RxSyn Scale Camp

Camp To opir. ea f zi

ziTwo spoonful every 4 hours in water, S Williams

RxCamp Catlete Pelts h/i 4

[marginal note, None]

Take immediately

J.R. Crockett

MAY 17 61

Company C
RxComp Syr Scill Zi
xThirty drops every 4 hours in water, Carper

"G leave 6 Pet No 4
Take immediately
[marginal notation: none]

Crowell, D.

Rx
Comp Syr Seele Zi

s/xTwenty drops every 4 hours in water; for Sovlan

//Rx
Blue mag grs x

xPulv oill/c fs

MTP
xRxMag & Sulp 1 Zi
none

SiPill immediately & in first hour take salts
To Roy
//RxComp C. Pills No. 4
Take immediately [marginal notation: none]
RxVin Speear
" ' " Ant. aa Zifs
[marginal notation: none]
Azzymen 2 Zy

M/SrTea spoon full every 4 hours in water [illegible letters] Craig
xLanga.
J Crockett, A.S.

Comp A Cap P[endleton?]
Rx
Comp C Pill No 4
Take immediately [marginal notation: none]
For I.M. Morris
Rx
C.C. Pill No 4 [marginal notation: none]

RxCl. Olivar
Aqua Ammon[ia] ea Zi
m
s.Pills immediately
Apply the liniment to face twice [illegible]

[illegible] Sexton
[Dr. T.L. Sexton was in original Blues, and
survived the War into the twentieth century]
[marginal notation: normal]
Rx
Vin AntZij
Comp To Opi Zi
M
Tea sponful every 4 hours in water
Bates

Rxnone
R C Pil no 4
Rx
AblumenZij
[marginal notation: none]
Take the pills immediately.
Allum as directed

Bear
//RxPulv. 2vv Gms xxx
[Giv?] chart no.
XOne every four hours
YCastor oil
[illegible Wilmoon]

MAY 17 - 61 J CROCKETT, A.S

[Apperson's double black lines]
Com C18[May 1861]
RxBAl Co L
[marginal notation: none]
Spt Nit Bal ae Zi
m
Tea spoonfull 3 times a day

Hammond

Comp C

MAY 18

RxAmt of Pob Tart gsvry
x[illegible] Special Zi
Sulph.Morph. gsr ry
2/o gera
M
A tea spoon [illegible] every four hour
For Kent Glen[letters illegible]
Carper & Farmer

RxBlue Mapazjs
Op. Pulv. grs. V

In G. Pill no. 12
Take one pill every four hours;
imel 3 are take, [illegible] in 4 horus
each [illgible] Take [illegible]
For Johnson, Vermillion, Lyon & Ray

RxVinci Sulph grms VI
" ' "Fr Opiumgm VI
MnAgua
To be dropped upon the eye ball three times a day
For Crowel
J Crockett, A.S.
Company D

Rx
Amt it P of Tant grms Vi
xPulv Specas1 Zi
Morph sulpgms VI
AquaZi

2n
Tea spoonful every 4 hours
To Bates & Overby

Rx
Blue Mapgrms x
xPill no. 2
S/one at bed time to-night & also to-morrow night

Bishop

//RxBlue Map grms. xvi
x[illegible] as Pi8lls [ditto marks] i/
sOne every 4 hours, [illgible] in the morning
John Williams

xx/RxBal Copy

[marginal notation: none]
Spt Net Ovl at Zi
Comp For Opn
m
S.Teaspoon full e times a day
McGruder

Comp F
RxCastor Oil Zi
For Stone
rxBlue Map at Op pills
No. 4 [illegible: possibly proper name]
John Bennington

[marginal notation: illegible]

RxTannan Op. No 4
[illegible, possibly proper name]

Comp A
RxBlue Map L{?] Op No 4
[illegible, starts with letter E]
RxComp Syx Seele Zip
[illegible: possibly Drops] Sulp grms [number illegible]
AguaZp
//[illegible word]
Pills two No 6 square
[illegible, possibly starts with letter N]

[check mark] Neff[illegible, possibly proper name]
[check mark] Bailey [ditto marks]
[illegible, possibly proper name] ditto marks
[check mark] James [ditto marks]
[check marks]Jones [ditto marks]

Comp C
Rx
Blue Map No 2
[illegible: possibly proper name beginning with R]
[illegible—seems to be five or six letters]

" ' "

R S S Czi
aquaZi
Morphz grms
[illegible letter] Glands [?]
Ammon.
1)Rx Mor leng {?]
[Illegible, possibly rank] Harper
Comp A [perhaps not A]
Rx
RxM at opin
Spence Ozenby [possibly not Ozenby]
RxComp [illegible, seems to be four letter, beginning with capital M or W]

[illegible: seems to be two proper names connected by ampersand; first name possibly starting with B and consisting of five or six letters; second name possibly starting with PR and consisting of seven or eight letters]

Continued: from a memorandum

Book filled

[WEDNESDAY] JULY 3RD

We are at an encampment near Buckles Town, Berkely Co. Va. [2] We were expecting to be ordered in the direction of Martinsburg Va., where it is said a large force of the enemy is posted. We expected a fight all day but night came on and we were still on the ground. Long columns of troops were moving about 10 o'clock. It is reported that Gen. [Joseph Eggleston] Johnson [sic; Johnston] sent 5,000 Mississippians & Alabamians to cut off the enemy between Williamsport & Martinsburg.[3] We expect to move to-night. Our medical wagon was taken from us to-day. I think it a bad move. The med. were put in a wagon that was to contain baggage of a company.

Provisin [sic; provision] very scarce. The soldiers "ate one man out of house & home" near the encampment. I was sorry very sorry to see the [illegible word in parentheses] the ladies of the home exercised when several hundred soldiers were swarming around her house anxious to get something to eat. She gave all she had cheerfully. I can but praise the women forever for their noble conduct during this campaign.

---

[2] Buckles Town was the old name for a tract of land, also called James Town in what was then the colony of Virginia; one of the colonial deedholders was James Buckles, and it was called by either of his names *James* or *Buckles* until 1779, when it was designated as *Darkesville*, apparently in honor of Revolutionary hero General William Darke. It is odd that Apperson has picked up the obsolete name for the place. Florence Thompson Wright, "James Town—alias Buckles Town—alias Darkesville," n.d., n.p., Martinsburg Public Library, Martinsburg, WVA.

[3] Prior to the pitched battle at Manassas, there were skirmishes and small battles in what is now West Virginia. George Brinton McClellan won these skirmishes and sealed off most of West Virginia from the Confederacy; the way was then both militarily and politically clear for the non-seceding territory to apply for recognition as the State of West Virginia. Joseph Eggleston Johnston was commanding Confederate troops in the area, and he concentrated on preparing troops for the move east for a major pitched battle. Meanwhile, this much larger engagement was shaping up in the Virginia piedmont, and Thomas Jonathan Jackson was to bring the First Virginia Brigade eastward from the Shenandoah Valley into the battle at a crucial time. Apperson seems unaware that these are separate engagements, and he also seems unaware that the Federals sought a strategic end by sealing off most of West Virginia. Instead, he discusses the emotions of the loss of Virginia territory in Berkeley County. During this phase of the war, the Federals succeeded in securing most of the border states in such skirmishes and small battles; the Confederates won some spectacular successes in major pitched battles and the diarist is typical of the Confederates in celebrating the victory at Manassas while missing the fact that vital strategic ground was already being lost in West Virginia, in the border states, and in the Confederate west.

I pity the citizens of Martinsburg and especially some ladies with whom it was my fortune to became acquainted. I know if they are there they feel severe pangs of distress. [4]

[THURSDAY] JULY THE 4TH, 1861

We are still at the encampment. This is a memorable day to the once happy American people and from the signs of the times it will be made a day of solemnity to us of the 19th century. Perhaps we go to battle to-day. While I write the command "fall in" is given and we will assuredly march in the direction of Martinsburg. Martinsburg is filled with Northern troops I understand. If this is so, we will probably have a hard battle to take it. I can not say really in what direction we shall move. My medicines have been moved again. This time I am transferred to the Ammunition Wagon. a very dangerous perch[5] I infer. I have been closely engaged all morning making pills & c.

All day we have been on the alert. Expecting to receive orders to march every hour but no such orders have yet come. From the most reliable information that we can get, the enemy, which is composed almost entirely of "low dutch", is committing the most outrageous depredations in and around Martinsburg. The unionists are pushing out the secessionists and urging the unfeeling soldiers onward to the most detestable crimes. I need not predict what will, or what is to be, the most probable programme to-morrow or during the next 24 hours, but let come what will there will be something developed within the next 24 hours. Our men seem sanguine as to the result of a battle if we have one and I fear the enemy will be underrated. We should have confidence in our arms it is true, but we should prepare for the worst—as we know not what odds we may have to run against. Our force now is reported to be 8,000 and that of the enemy between 9,000 & 20,000. Several men heard cannon firing in direction of Martinsburg—no one can account for it.[6]

---

[4] These ladies were from families previously known to the diarist: Harrisons, Levys, and Alburtises. Patriarch of the latter family was in charge of a battery in J.E. Johnston's Army. Notes, Glenn McMullen, shared with author.

[5] Word is almost illegible; it appears to be *perch*. On such a wagon, perch was a technical term for the pole connecting the gears, an unlikely application. It also was a technical term for the pad on the wagon where a person could sit, which seems to be what Apperson is talking about.

[6] General W.H. Heim of the Pennsylvania Volunteers won a battle in the Shenandoah Valley at Martinsburg. Most of Heim's troops were German-Americans, or "low-Dutch" (so styled because they spoke of the *deutsch* langauge and *deutsch* land, and southerners generally heard and pronouned these words as "dutch" even for that very large group of German-Americans living in the Valley). Apperson's rumors of Pennsylvanian atrocities in Martinsburg are not corroborated

The Regiments are on drill this evening. Provisions have been so scarce that we got nothing to eat to-day until about 4 o'clock. We are ordered to draw rations for 3 days and cook enough for one.

I expect we will be in a march to-night.

[Friday] July 5th 1861

We are yet on the same ground, but were up very early, which made us believe that we would be on the march pretty soon. It is now about 11 o'clock and we are still enduring the hot sun expecting and impatiently awaiting orders. I begin to feel that all our expectations will be deceiving our preparations useless and our efforts to have a go at our enemy futile. But *several and perhaps* the major part of the Army believe that we will have a go at them yet. As I am attached to the medical department several think that I am not in much danger of becoming a victim to the guns of the Yankees and hence they have deposited some valuables in my care. J.W. Kennedy deposits his pocket book—the contents not known to me and a gold pen and holder which he wishes given to his wife in case of an *accident.* Capt. Pendleton gave me 28 dollars to keep until the fight is over. Jno. M. Williams gave me his purse and watch—contents of the purse not known to me. A mark was fixed on our men to-day by which they may be distinguished from our enemy. It consists of a narrow strip of white domestic *joined* or *fastened* around our caps. Our regiment has no flag and it was thought advisable to have one. Col. Preston sent to Col. Duncan of Ky., or rather Col. Dungan [sic; Duncan] offered Col. Preston one for the use of the Reg. for a while. Col. P. sent for it and got it with the compliments of the Capt. Crossman to whose company it belonged accompanied with the message that he was not afraid to trust that or anything else in the hands of Virginia's sons.—A private said in commenting that we must defend it with honor for their sweethearts gave it to them.[7]

---

by others. Jackson, working with J.E.B. Stuart's cavalry, claimed victory near Darkesville at this same time, and J.E. Johnston recommended that both leaders be promoted, Jackson to general, Stuart to colonel. The results of the activities described here are strategic victories for both sides: The federals were in excellent position to hold West Virginia, while Jackson and Stuart were in excellent position to move up and down and across the Valley as needed in the eastern campaigns then just starting. Official correspondence of both sides claims victory at Darkesville [Buckles Town]. *The War of the Rebellion; Official Records,* Ser. 1, vol. 2, Reports 8, 9, 10, 11.

[7] James W. Kennedy was originally First Lieutenant of Smyth Blues and retained rank when it became part of 4th Va. Reg. in 1st Bde. A.G. Pendleton was original organizing captain of Blues

The cannon which we heard firing yesterday were fired at Martinsburg by the Federals in honor of the 4th of July. I think in candor and sincerity that they have perverted the intention of the products of the 4th of July 1776, and ignored the honor of that day and now are banging in lunacy over their pretended triumph.

Last night, about dark, a beautiful meteor shot across the (pper set) from North to South—maybe it betokened something—. A blazing comet suddenly made its appearance a few nights ago. It looks very beautiful with its tail stretching from its orbit about half-way above the horizon to the zenith.

I am not well—I fear that this way of living will prove to[o] much for my health. The day passed like the last two or three—all suspense. I understand the force of the enemy is about 15000, with two pieces of artillery. A young lady left Martinsburg yesterday and came to "Head Quarters". She gave an account of movements at Martinsburg. [8]

[SATURDAY] JULY 6TH

We are still on the same ground. I cannot see for what we are waiting. The enemy has invaded our [illegible] and they shall now pay the penalty. The opinion [illegible] in favour of a fight. Men of the South—and Virginia especially pledged ourselves to stand by Virginia's burden and die if need be—rather than allow her soil to be poluted [sic] by the unhallowed tread of Northern fanatics; but now we must live in six miles of an army of armed men with their bayonets (pointed) to the bosom of our own State without the power to make effective the pledge of other days. We are under subjection now and if

---

and retained rank in 4th Va. Reg. of 1st Bde. John M. Williams was perhaps with Co. D, 4th Va. Inf. of 1st Bde., a Smyth County volunteer wounded at Sharpsburg and discharged near Orange Courthouse.

Col. Robert T. Preston commanded 28th Va. Infantry of 5th Bde. at Manassas, but was once with 1st Bde. Col. Blanton Duncan was with one of four companies of Kentucky infantry, and Capt. Crossman served in Duncan's infantry. Wilson, *Smyth County*, s.v.; *War of Rebellion*, Ser. 1, vol. 2, s.v. Jim Presgraves, ed., *Smyth County Families and History* (Pulaski: B.D. Smith, 1974), s.v.; hereinafter Presgraves, ed., *Smyth.*

[8] Prof. W. G. Bean speculates that this woman is the famous spy Belle Boyd (1843-1900), notes Bean. Boyd, a native of Martinsburg, was called by French correspondents "La Belle Rebelle" and by New York newspapers "That Secesh Cleopatra." Unafraid of Southern public opinion or of Federal forces, Boyd traveled alone and often stayed with enemy officers in their tents in order to gain intelligence about troop movements. Theatrical and flamboyant, Boyd was twice imprisoned, but was released with warnings—after which time she spied again. She was active in this West Virginia campaign, reporting to Jackson, and she may well be the "young lady" visiting with news. Faust,"Belle Boyd," *Historical Times*, s.v.

the enemy prove victorious we may expect to feel the galling yoke of merciless tyranny. May the God of Heaven avert it!

We soldiers are seeing a hard time. Our baggage has been curtailed time and again until now nothing but one blanket, one suit of clothes, our guns & equipments are left us. Not even are our cooking utensils left—they being taken this morning. The men have to lie upon the ground at night without anything to protect them from rain or dew—will this not prove a loosing [sic] game to our cause? There is some dissatisfaction among the men.

Raining this morning.

I am very well fixed—having received wagon to stay in. About 3 o'clock to-day an alarm was given and a line of battle formed. But after waiting some hour or so and no enemy came and we were ordered to return to sleep again on the same cold damp spot as before. Generals Johnston & Jackson came on the field and rode around the troops—the several Regiments and were received with enthusiastic cheers. The line of battle formed present a formidable appearance. The night shows an appearance not very pleasant to those who have to sleep on the ground uncovered.

I am not well.

[SUNDAY] JULY 7TH, 1861

I was very unwell all last night—took some medicine. Reville [sic] was sounded very early this morning making it very obvious to the soldiers that some move would be made to-day.

We soon found that Winchester is our next point of destination—"any where" says the soldiers "to get away from this hot, dirty camp." We took up our line of march with many feelings of regret that we must leave upon our soil the enemy of our honor and liberty—those who would filch from us all that is near and dear to us—unmolested.

With all due deference to the skill and tact—good Generalship and far-sightedness of our just commander in chief—I bow in submission to his command, having confidence in his knowledge of military matters and believe it our duty to obey all his commands— but it does seem to my finite mind that we are leaving to the merciless invader that for which we should have protected or died in the attempt. They lie to secure peace. Four months ago the cry went to peace with the enemy, and so wait until Virginia's soil sees death at every stroke—'till Virginia is invaded—wait for some mercenary armies through our fields[;] open demonstration of it [hostile invasion] or to throw down our arms unfired before the enemy to Southern Rights—the enemy victorious in the field—wait until our border is threatened by the tread of *Lincoln's* armed hosts—wait until they set their feet on this sacred soil and then and there we will meet—then we will rally around the old flag, hear in the inspiring motto "*sic semper tyrannis*" and welcome "with bloody hands to hospitable graves". We have waited until all this has been done. To a man. The hired mercenaries of Northern *vituperation*[9] have approach [sic] our border, have crossed it and are now upon Virginia's sacred soil. Her army has been ignored, her interests disregarded, her rights *trampled* under foot, the property of her citizens destroyed and themselves persecuted and abused and where is the retribution or even the effort of retribution. Farther and farther into our country comes the enemy farther and farther back we go. Will we retreat—back into the very heart of our state and bend to the tyranny of a relentless enemy and offer up fair ones and their pure, undefiled virtue.

God forbid it! Let us meet them and invoke the God of battles to our aid. If our cause is a just one and we believe it is He will surely aid us in the fight [illegible] [illegible]. The excuse for our retreat seems to be inferiority of numbers on our side—we had never expect[sic] to meet them otherwise. They have the numbers over us and we must fight them as they are, and not as we wish them to be.

The order of General Johnston for our retreat was gentlemanly, patriotic, philanthropic. It reads thus: "The general announces to his gallant command that for four days he has offered battle to greatly superior forces and it has been declined. To attack the enemy in their position would make a sacrifice too heavy for the object to be obtained. Our men are patriots and freemen, theirs hirelings and mercenaries. We will resume our previous position where the health and comfort of our command can be preserved and where we can seve with the assurance of striking an effective blow. The General expects the same cheerful obedience to his orders which they have ever showed and claims the confidence which they have always accorded him".

This shows feeling and respect from General Johnston for his command but I fear we will loose [sic] ground that will be hard to recover again. I understand

[9] Vituperation is from the past participle of a Latin verb meaning to abuse with words; it is related to the legal term of uttering, which is falsely representing in a transaction. Apperson is saying that northern politicians and publicists have not only criticized the southern institutions harshly, but have consciously and deliberately lied in their denunciations. *OED.*

the R Road engines & *track* & bridges that were destroyed by us at Martinsburg are being repaired by the enemy.

The Northern Congress is in session now—the great issue now at hand will engross their time and attention I guess. We may look on with almost breathless interest—it is the only hope we have for an adjustment of the difficulty now on our hands. And, indeed we have but little to hope for from them.

"O my country's wintry state
What sacred spring can renovate
What powerful call can bid arise
The buried nobility & the wise"[10]

Our march to-day was a truly hot one—many of our men became too sick to walk and we had no way of transporting except the ammunition wagon. This served the purpose of hauling ammunition, medicine and the sick and their baggage.

I was sick a greater part of the day—medicine acted freely. I met with Tazewell Richards to-day. I was glad to see him. We walked several miles together.

We went into camp about 5 o'clock some 4 3/4 miles from Winchester. Nothing new occurred among the night.

[MONDAY] JULY 8TH, 1861

We left camp this morning about 7 o'clock. Where we will go I know not.

We did not go far before we turned into a wood where in all probability we will stay some time. I understand that fortifications are being erected at Winchester—the militia being very closely engaged at their erection. Winchester is four miles from us now and if we have a fight we can easily fall back upon the fortifications erected there.

I learn that we will get tents in a day or so. This is gratifying to the soldiers indeed. Nothing occurred of any note to-day—I was unusual drowsy all day—slept half the day at least. The weather is very warm—prospects for rain to-night.

---

[10] Apperson does not reveal the name of the poet.

JULY 9TH, 1861 TUESDAY

It did not rain last night as I expected. Nothing new occurred today. It is reported that 15000 troops are on the way from Manassa [sic] Gap to this place. If this is a fact the probability is that we will go back to Martinsburg and give *Abe's men*[11] a rout. I trust our force will be sufficient to cope with him.

I wrote a letter to Dr. F. to-day. And this evening I rec'd 3[:] one from Mrs. F one from Mrs. Tomlin and one from N. [C.] B. St. John. It is truly sweet to get letters from friends.

I am writing at 8 oclock and must stop writing as an order has been given for us to pack up.

[WEDNESDAY] JULY 10TH, 1861

We did not leave the encampment last night as we expected. I slept on the wet ground and I fear it will give me a severe cold. We left the encampment this morning at an early hour. At first I thought perhaps we would be marched in direction of Martinsburg again, as we heard of strong enforcements being sent us, but we went to Winchester and the Regiment is formed in close columns of mass on a field and ordered to cook dinner.

I understand that the enemy is coming—I am doubtful of the truth of the statement.

Evening—The above statement is false as many others of the same nature are.

A tollerably [sic] hard rain fell this evening and the soldiers have to take it without shelter. I pity them. It is injust too that they should so suffer. There are tents enough lying in sight to furnish the whole Regiment with shelter.

The men express a great deal of displeasure at being thus treated when there is no cause apparent for it. It is not right and I fear the rigidity with which the soldiers are treated will be a loosing [sic] business to the South and our cause. They can expect nothing but the wet Earth for a bed to-night. I saw Dr. Beatie of the mounted rifle men from Abingdon—I was glad to see him. his company belongs in Stuart's Boys.

THURSDAY, JULY 11TH, 1861

A great many were on hand to be prescribed for this morning. I had to go to town to-day to see about receiving the quarterly supply of medicines for our

---

[11] The Federal troops.

regiment. I did not do anything. I went to the Hospital and saw our boys. They do not seem to be doing as well as they ought. The medical attendants are too careless I fear. In fact I shall have to give up the place I occupy as Hospital Steward—Dr. Black says he will leave the Hospital in Winchester and come to the Regiment.

He has a prior claim to my place and if Dr. Black says give it up I will do so without a murmur.

A.T. Sanders seems very despondent—I am very sorry for him. [12]

Camp near Winchester.

FRIDAY, JULY 12TH, 1861

Nothing unusual occurred to-day. I wrote a letter to Dr. Quisenberry and read some. Fortifications are going on at this place. All for a fight but we will have to leave if *omens* from the North can get a show at [sic] with the superior numbers.

Dr. Black sick today.

Camp near Winchester, Va.

SATURDAY, JULY 13TH, 1861

Nothing unusual to-day. A very hard rain fell last night which dropped through the cover of the wagon in which I was asleep making everything damp. I covered up my head and let it rain.

Raining at intervals to-day. I found our boys in the Hospital improving. I went into the Dr's office. Dr. Reamill & Bean. They took plenty of *drink* and seem to enjoy it. *I never partake.* I ate supper and afterwards had a smart discussion with Dr. Reamill in regard to our national affairs. We do not differ much. He says we must be careful that we do not find a Napoleon Bonaparte in a Davis or a Beauregard. The Dr. is a very smart man but evidently not the man for that place. I would not trust any *drinking* Dr. with my health.

It rained while I was there and I was compelled to stay 'til night. I came back after dark and found several prescriptions on order and filled them all. [illegible sentence].

---

[12] Andrew T. Sanders of Smyth County was from a family that Dr. Faris and Apperson often traded with. Sanders was one of the first to volunteer in December of 1860 for patrols formed in Marion in preparation for possible war. When Virginia seceded, he joined the brigade. Wilson, *Smyth County*, 235.

WINCHESTER, VA, JULY 14TH SUNDAY

I understand that there will be no drill to-day except batallion drill this evening. I intend going to preaching to-day as there was preaching in camp but I was deprived by a young man in Capt. [James J.] White's co.—"Liberty Hall Guards" [—] name of [William] Brooks becoming very ill.[13]

When I saw him he was breathing short and quick—pulse very high[,] fever— face flushed—carotid throbbing—[two illegible words]—arteries full and bounding—face is red.

I was at once impressed [by] the idea that the danger was in the brain. Dr. Black [illegible; the sense is *applied* or *performed*] cupping on the neck[14] —the patient was entirely delirious and almost unmanagable. 16 oz. blood was taken from the arm—Linimentum saponis et chloroformis[15] was rubbed freely upon the bowels and back—cold sponge being applied to the head. A dose of ten gram Chlo[roform] with 1 eighth gram morph[ine][16] was given and followed by

---

[13] Liberty Hall Guards were apparently the students from Washington College in Lexington (now Washington & Lee University). This company of students was originally called Liberty Hall Volunteers, and its captain was James J. White, professor of Latin at the college. White was the son of the Rev. Dr. William S. White, Presbyterian minister and friend of Jackson. William Brooks, from Augusta County, was enrolled at Washington College, was member of the Liberty Hall Volunteers, and died on 16 July 1861 of wounds. Notes from Glenn McMullen.

[14] Cupping was a method of drawing blood in order to purge the blood of disease; it was also used to "draw" boils or other surface eruptions, as there appear to have been on this patient's neck. A cup was heated, its rim was greased, and the cup was then placed "bottoms up" over the area after the boil or eruption had been "scarified," either by a wound or deliberately by the physicians applying linimentum.*McGrew's*, 23. Sometimes heavy bleeding was used to make the patient "pass out" of consciousness in order to undergo an operation. Philip Syng Physick (1768-1837) had demonstrated this bleeding technique, and it was thought that Physick's bleeding left patients insensitive to and even unaware of any pain. Ibid., 15.

[15] Linimentum was any kind of liquid preparation containing a medicament with alcohol, oil, or water. Strictly for external use, it was rubbed on. Saponis, from the Latin for soap (French saponin, often also used in era), was an unabsorbable glucose from the roots of some plants; saponis formed a lather, especially when mixed with linimentum. The linimentum saponis was intended to attack problems involving the blood; it broke down red blood cells, a process called hemolysis; the saponis liniment caused great damage, especially when combined with the venesection, as here described. Chloroform was a green gas formed from plants; it had a numbing effect, and was generally used from the first third of the nineteenth century to anesthesize, or put to sleep patients prior to operations. On the eve of the Civil War, many surgeons were already suspicious that chloroform was dangerous, and many chloroform deaths were recorded from 1847 until aftter the Civil War, when other anesthetics were developed and used. *Taber's*, s.v.; *McGrew's*, s.v.

[16] Morphine was identified as a specific therapeutic narcotic in 1806. It was used to kill pain, especially after a traumatic wound. Medical people recognized its addictive qualities, and in 1860 cocaine from the coca plant was identified as a pain-killing narcotic. Throughout the Civil War, it

castor [oil][17] in 1 hour. The symptoms seemed better in some three hours from commencement of treatment though at no time was the patient rational.

He was taken to the Hospital in the evening something better. Dr. Black remarked to me that giving the morphine in combination with *calomel*[18] was one of the newest things in practice—a point that should be noted. The case as he said showed some disposition to convulse and cramp. After bleeding and the blood vessels became unloaded the probabillity is that aerophagia[19] would have been severe and caused termination of life; but, though morphine & opium is contraindicated in diseases of the brain yet the administration of it in this case was imperatively demanded. While bleeding unloaded the blood vessels and relieved the brain; morph[ine] quieted the nervous system. He told me to notice this which I will and thank him too.

CAMP NEAR WINCHESTER[20]

MONDAY, JULY 15TH, 1861

The day passed off as usual until evening when the report came that the enemy was advancing. After night the Regiment was ordered to "fall in". We were soon in a line. We then marched up to "Headquarters" and remained an hour or so[;] then returned. I suppose the enemy is certainly on their rout [e] towards this point. I wrote a letter to-day to Mrs. Faris—or commenced one.

---

was thought that cocaine was less addictive and less dangerous than morphine, and it was heavily used, as this diarist shows us in later entries. "Pharmacy," *McGrew's*, 256.

[17] Castor oil was used internally as a cathartic or purgative; in this case to induce bowel movements in order to flush out presumed "problems" "loaded" in the blood. *Taber's*, s.v.

[18] Calomel was a granular medicine. The word was from two Greek words, meaning literally *beautiful black*. It was so called because the grains were white, but they came from a mixture of black mercurous chloride. Calomel was "strong medicine" designed to "attack" certain diseases; three grains could induce diarrhea, known as "opening the bowels." *McGrew's*, 217. The morphine was administered to ease the considerable pain of the purging.

[19] Rapid air swallowing associated with hysteria; what is today called hyperventilation. The danger comes from carbon dioxide depletion (acapnia) with drop in blood pressure. *OED*; *Taber's*.

[20] Winchester as a gateway to Virginia's Shenandoah Valley was strategically crucial; and because of the place it occupied geographically and strategically, it was captured often by the two sides. Three major battles were fought at Winchester between 25 May 1862 and 19 September 1864; and the Confederates were not officially driven from Winchester until the Third Battle of Winchester, 19 September 1864. However, the city itself was taken and retaken many times by the competing forces, and even while it was "held" by one side or the other, it was subject to raiding. *Historical Times Illustrated Encyclopedia of the Civil War*, ed., Patricia L. Faust (New York: Harper & Row, 1986), s.v.; hereinafter, *Historical Times*.

CAMP NEAR WINCHESTER

TUESDAY, JULY 16TH, 1861

I was closely engaged all day and until a late hour at night pack[ing] medicines and fixing up a medicine tent. I am very simply fixed now. The reg. was called out again this evening—The enemy is still advancing slowly. To-morrow morning we may expect some ammunition. We are receiving large reinforcements every day—the yankees[sic] will be somewhat surprised to find so many southrons[21] here I guess. Dr. Black told me to-night that I was permanently appointed to this place—that he should retain me here at least.

I am glad to get it so that I can advance myself some. He also told me that he had some books that I could read. I am thankful to him for such a favour.

I rec'd a letter from Cousin Bettie to-day.

CAMP NEAR WINCHESTER VA.

JULY 17TH, 1861 WEDNESDAY—

The [day] passed as usual—The probabilities for a fight seem to be on the increase. It is now reported that the enemy is moving upon us in three division by a flank movement of some four or five thousand on right and left and the main body is coming directly forward. the regiments have been ordered out twice to-day to throw down fencing. I suppose a great deal of fence is laid close with the ground. Whether what we hear can be relied upon or not I of course can not say; but every preparation seems to be going on for a big fight soon.

I finished my letter to Mrs. Faris to-day and wrote one more. I am well as usual. I think I can stand this life tollerably [sic] well. I have been reading some to-day but very little time is left me for reading after doing my duty to the sick. I learned to-day that the young man [William] Brooks who was sick on Sunday and spoken of in this journal, died to-day[22] —Poor fellow he *knew* not a rational moment after we saw him.

---

[21] Scottish word originally applied to those living in England; Civil War connotation is someone partisan to the Confederacy regardless of where s/he lives. *American Heritage Dictionary*, s.v.

[22] Official records list his death on 16 July 1861. Personnel Directory, Historical Data Systems.

NEAR WINCHESTER.

18TH JULY, 1861, THURSDAY.

This morning during "sick call" Col. [James F.] Preston[23] told Dr. Black that we would have to leave soon. I packed with more than usual difficulty—having more baggage than before.

We were ready in an hour or so perhaps—our impression was that we would go to Charlestown [West Virginia] as the enemy had came there. We left camp about noon, 4th Regiment leading the way. After passing through Winchester, much to the surprise of the citizens we found that we were not going to Charlestown. We took the road leading to Berry's Ferry [Clarke County].

After leaving Winchester the columns were halted and informing [sic] why we we[re] going. General [Pierre Gustave Toutant] Beauregard[24] at Manassas had been attacked by an overwhelming force and call[ed] upon us for help. And our General appealed to us that we would now cross the Blue Ridge and join our gallant southern friends at the point of conflict and do or *die in* defence of our homes. The order was received with loud shouts of applause . We marched by Millwood [Clarke County] and crossed Shenandoah River about mid-night. The troop waded the river. The 4th Regiment was some 8 or 10 miles in advance of the train of wagons. I was with the wagons and travelled the whole night. Was at Paris in Fauquier Co[unty] about light in the morning. From the Shenandoah River to Paris the road sides were lined with soldiers who [had] fallen asleep. My wagon was loaded with soldiers—the team was nearly worn out—having nothing to eat since the morning before myself and several friends were lucky enough to find some ladies who gave us a good breakfast. Our stay here was short. We had heard before that there had been a desperate attempt on the part of the Yankees to take our fortification at a place called Bull's Run near Manassas but they were repulsed by our soldiers three times and did not make the third [sic; fourth?] attempt. The loss was reported to be 200 killed & wounded on our side and 3000 on the other.

This report was in circulation at Paris again. We left there for Piedmont Station [Fauquier County] where we learned we were to take the [railroad]

---

[23] Col. James F. Preston was from Montgomery County and served with 4th Virginia Infantry in 1st Virginia or Stonewall Brigade. Personnel Directory, Historical Data Systems.

[24] Beauregard (1818-1893) was a Louisianan of Creole family who spoke French before he spoke English. He graduated from West Point, number two in class of 1838. At Manassas he was second in command to J.E. Johnston. "Perhaps no other southern general was involved in so many pivotal military events...." John D. Kallman, *Historical Times*, s.v.

cars.[25] I stopped at the house of a Mr. Gibson 3 miles from Paris and got some breakfast for some sick men I had charge of. A young lady prepared it for me. We found the 4th Regiment at the Station ready to take the cars. My medicine chest and baggage were put on the cars there and the Ambulance left a corpse with the [wagon] train. When we took the cars I was very tired and my feet very sore—having walked from Shenandoah River the night before. We were well treated by the citizens at the several Stations that we passed. Buttered biscuits and sliced ham were thrown in promiscuously and a general "grab game" played by the soldiers. When we got to the Gap [Manassas Gap] we found some strong looking fortifications there. We heard also that the battle at Bull's Run was not as disastrous as reported. Some 50 or *60 killed* & wounded on our side and an estimate of 500 on the other. The enemy was allowed the privilege of burying the dead to-day.

At night 2nd Reg.—the 27th & 4th—were ordered out to Bull's Run and formed a line of battle. stacked arms and laid down to rest. The only *impression* is that we will have a fight to-night, and to-morrow morning the batt[le] will open at its fullest extent.

Troops are still coming from Piedmont Station. I suppose it would take all night to transport them up here. The Mississippians and Alabamians will hardly get to Piedmont to-day unless they march better than they did on Thursday. Our men seem very much fatigued.

I am very uneasy about my brother Nat. He was in the engagement yesterday I expect.

P.S. The foregoing paragraph is for two days.

NEAR MANASSAS, VA.

SATURDAY, JULY 20TH, 1861

This morning we marched in an easterly direction from where we camped last night and stopped near the field of Thursday's engagement. I saw and spoke to Gen. Beauregard to-day. I was standing in the road when he got out of his carriage and came along and asked me if I knew where Gen. Johnston[26] was. I

---

[25] The cars were in a train of the Manassas Gap Railroad. The line ran some sixty miles from Manassas in the piedmont to Strasburg in the Blue Ridge. Military historians believe that this was the first instance "in which a railroad was used to achieve strategic mobility." Jeffrey D. Wert, "Bull Run," *Historical Times*, s.v.

[26] Joseph Eggleston Johnston (1807-1891) was born in Farmville, grew up in Abingdon, and was a distinguished graduate of West Point in 1829. A brilliant engineer and strategist, Johnston

told him I did not and [he] passed on. I thought he was some sub-officer or other. He is very mild and affable in his manner. His size is about medium, with fine black mustache.

We spent the day in the shade which did very well if provision had been [a] little more plentiful.

We slept under the pine trees

NEAR MANASSAS, VA

[SUNDAY] JULY 21ST, 1861

This day is set apart for sacred things—it has been consecrated by God for divine purposes and has been a day of rest and thanksgiving by us for many years, but this sabbath has been a day never to be forgotten by me and many others of my age.

The history of this generation in future ages will speak of this as a bloody day—a day of war and bloodshed.

I was awakened this morning by several sharp reports of muskets in direction of our picket guard and in the direction that the enemy would have to come. A troop passed afterward rather rapidly[.] I knew something was up. The *long roll* was soon beat & the Reg. took its place. a detail was made from the companies to cook breakfast. About 1/2 past 7 o'clock several cannons fired in a north easterly direction of Manassas. The enemy seemed disposed to make an attack there but the command was unnoticed.

It was *presumed* at the time, and proved so afterward, that the enemy wished to distract our attention in that direction while a more important [target] was attacked.

Johnson's [sic; J.E. Johnston's] brigade was marched up *river* Bull's Run some three miles and ordered to *hold* itself as a reserve. I was in the rear with the medical wagons and my ambulance broke down so I was left in a bad fix. I was some time looking for my Reg. While we were waiting the battle had commenced some 1/2 miles from us in good earnest. At one time a shout rose

---

left U.S. Army Engineers to become brigadier general in CSA. He outmaneuvered a superior force at Harpers Ferry to escape capture and then did a superb job of bringing a large force by rail from the Valley to the aid of P.G.T. Beauregard in the piedmont at Manassas. During the battle, Johnston moved a large force by foot from right to left flank at a crucial time, likely saving the day for the Confederates in the maneuver. After this battle at Manassas, he was promoted to full general, retroactive to 4 July, but this promotion started unending tensions in CSA command, especially with Jefferson Davis, a West Point graduate, student of Napoleonic strategy, and often intrusive commander in chief. Kallman, *Historical Times*, s.v.

some distance beyond the hill and stretched from one Regiment to another. The courier said that the enemy had been repulsed and it made every soldier's heart leap for joy.

The Brigade was soon ordered up much to the gratification of many. As we were about to enter the field we heard that the enemy had taken some of our cannon. This produced an effect much to the contrary of what the others produced. On our boys went and took and took [sic] a position immediately behind our battery and in front of that of the enemy. The enemy opened upon us with shot and shell which flew so near our boys' heads that they immediately fell upon their faces. This was about 10 or 11 o'clock. Our boys lay there some 1 1/2 hours with shot cutting large trees entirely off within ten feet of their rear. My feelings at this juncture are not to be described by me. Dr. Black & myself took shelter behind some trees; but was soon obliged to leave.

The first man wounded in our Reg. was Lt. Owry of Co. D "Smy[th] Blues."[27] He was struck in the mouth by a fragment of a bomb. He came out and we commenced dressing the wound but before we had done anything others were brought out and being desperately hurt we left him to attend them. From this time on numbers were brought out. The fight in the meantime grew hotter and hotter. We found it very unsafe for us to remain there, so we fell back some distance in the rear. Shell after shell burst above us, ball after ball burst whizzing through the air and striking a hill some distance [behind] and made the dust fly. We attended some wounded at a house near the scene of action but were compelled to retire. We had the wounded conveyed to a creek near by and there did all that we could do for men in their fix. I witnessed an amputation and my ideas were not very far from right.

About 4 o'clock I rode back to the field in search of a case of instruments we left. I did not find the instruments but I witnessed the oft described horror of a battle field. Men lying in every nook and corner, wounded dying and dead. I found a wound[ed] Yankee sitting under a bush. My soul was sorrowful. I looked upon him not as an enemy. I could not realize it. I think he was mortally wounded. I gave him some physic[28] and filled a cup with water and left him to the mercy of those whose duty it was to look after him. I was too much engaged to do more. My fears were very much relieved to find some of the "Blues" out

---

[27] Apparently R.G. Owry, originally a captain who had helped organize a military police patrol before Virginia seceded. Wilson, *Smyth County History*, 235-39. He became a lieutenant in the Confederate company once war came.

[28] Physic was a general term, sometimes meaning a cathartic or purgative, other times a pain-killing dose of morphine or cocaine. The context suggests a pain-killing physic. *McGrew's*, s.v

there. One poor fellow—one with whom I was well acquainted was lying near where Sherman's Battery[29] was taken by our Reg. His name was E.H. McCready.[30] I doubt not but he was a brave boy and died in the full discharge of his duty as a soldier. He was shot through the heart.

I met the boys before I got to the body and got them to go back with me. We then carried him and laid him beside Capt. [H.] *Hall*, "Dare Devils" of our Reg. who was shot through the head [31] —Six other "Blues" were wounded — two dangerously. I found and did what I could for several other wounded soldiers and then returned to the creek where I had the pleasure of meeting with Major Kent [32] & Col. [James F.] Preston. I heard that Col. P had been killed.

The wounded were convoyed away, or all that could be[.] several were left in my charge which I had convoyed in litters up to a house in the vicinity; but here they were obliged to lay [sic] out of doors in the yard. The yard was covered with wounded from all most every state in the SCA [sic].

Oh War! Horrible, unrelenting work of Envy
who has imbued his hands in blood
And taught the sons of men to make a death
That nature never made.[33]

---

[29] The infamous William Tecumseh Sherman (1820-1883) enjoyed considerably more success later after transferring to the western theatre to serve under Ulysses S. Grant. In this engagement, Sherman commanded an infantry unit and not an artillery battery. The Federal artillery companies reported as lost to the Confederates in this engagement were those of Captain James Brewerton Ricketts (1817-1887), a New Yorker and West Point graduate noted for extreme bravery in both battles of Manassas, and Captain Richard Arnold (1828-1882), a Rhode Islander and West Point graduate who was that day acting assistant adjutant general with 2nd Bde and filed the official report of loss. Arnold, "Report No. 50," *Official Records*, ser. 1, vol. 2, 450-51; see also table of batteries, ibid., 328.

[30] Dr. T.L. Sexton, only Smyth County Blues veteran to survive into the twentieth century, confirmed that Edward H. McCready of the Blues Company D was the first resident of Smyth County to die in the war, falling on this day at Manassas. Wilson, *Smyth County History*, 239.

[31] Possibly H. Hall, as reported by Col. J.M. Heck, 25th Va. Infantry, *Official Records*, ser. 1, vol. 2, 254-56. Of the Dare Devils: "...a company of rough mountain boys from Grayson County. They entered the service bragging they could lick the Yankees with hickory sticks," notes, Glenn McMullen, shared with me.

[32] Possibly R.C. Kent of Wytheville, who corresponds with Judah P. Benjamin concerning mountain and valley campaigns, *Official Records*, ser. 1, vol. 4, 235, 240.

[33] Quoting a poem by by an unidentifiable author.

MONDAY, NEAR MANASSAS JULY 22ND

This morning after paying some attention to the sick in [my] charge I left for camp. Worn out almost entirely by the duties of the day and the watching of the night I barely could get to camp. After getting something to alleviate the gnawing of the stomach I felt very much refreshed. It rained all day. We had no shelter except what could be made with blankets. [34] I could find no dry place to stay and by the way of passing of time which seemed to pass very lazily along I went to the [Manassas] junction. I again saw sights—sights that were more heartrending if possible than those I witness [sic] the day previous. My heart bled to see men of our own nature, of my own standing, fighting in a common cause with myself and others all filed like so many precious brutes in porches, tents, houses & wherever they could be lain. Several were lying so that the rain blew upon them and they had not the power to protect themselves from the weather. Many wounded prisoners were there also. My reflections were sad when I looked upon them and contemplated their position and the cause that prompted them to do that which brought their present condition. I went back to camp a sad sick hearted boy.[35]

NEAR MANASSAS, VA TUESDAY JULY 23

All nature looks green and refreshed this morning but saddening sights are evident not far. O what a contrast! There is no occurence worth noting of to-day. I wrote several letters to my friends.

NEAR MANASSAS, VA. JULY 24; WEDNESDAY.

We had a regular sick call this morning—a good many sick—drilling commences to-day and a great many are always ready to take advantage of this part of the services.

---

[34] Soldiers called this camp near the battlefield Camp Maggot. The water was not fit to drink, and there was an infamous stench. See John Overton Casler, *Four Years in the Stonewall Brigade*, ed., James I. Robertson, Jr. (1904. Reprint ed.; Dayton, OH.: Morningside Bookshop, 1994) 40, 50.

[35] Casualties were actually low compared to later fights: Confederates, 1,982 (387 killed, 1,582 wounded, and 13 missing); Federals, 2,896 (460 killed, 1,124 wounded, and 1,312 missing). However, it was the first major conflict witnessed by the diarist and by most of the troops; and even the veterans of the Mexican War had seen nothing on this scale for more than a dozen years. Wert, "Bull Run," *Historical Times*, s.v.

I went to the junction to-day in order to mail some letters—there a good number of persons there who seem to be worse. Nothing more occured worth noting.

NEAR MANASSAS. JULY 25; THURSDAY.

After sick call this morning I went to the junction with Dr. B in order to assist him dress some wounds. I found he had a hospital and a goodly number of patients—all lying upon straw. I was very busy there until evening.

A great many Citizens of Montgomery, Wythe & Pulaski Counties came to see their friends. Many of them brought conveniences for the wounded soldier in shape of shirts, sheets, pillows &c. I returned to camp in the evening and found a recruit there for our company.

We are faring badly here—the water is very muddy and impure:

The food is bad.

NEAR MANASSAS, VA. FRIDAY JULY 26TH

Nothing of interest to-day. I have been very drowsy and dull to-day—felt very badly. Two of our boys came from Winchester to-day. I learn that A.J.S. [Alexander J. Sanders?] is very unwell[.] I wish he was here to get a discharge. I was fearful at first that he he [sic] could not stand the exposure to which we are exposed.

NEAR MANASSAS, VA. SATURDAY JULY 27

I was up at sunrise this morning. Nothing occurred outside of the usual exercises of the day until evening when the Reg. was ordered out. I had the ambulance made ready for marching and started after the Reg. but it had not left the field. We were then ordered to pack to leave which order was hailed with delight. We moved some 3/4 of mile in westerly direction. I don't think the situation is bettered a great deal—water being the greatest object now. I am tollerably [sic] well fixed now—having fixed up my tent again. I feel quite secure. All the companies have tents now.

I have just attended prayer meeting, being the first services I have attended for a long time. It is duty that we should not fail to attend. I felt as if I were sitting at home in some familiar church when the singing broke upon the evening air. Oh! it was so sweet! So refreshing to the mind! Many sweet thoughts of home and friends were brought fresh to my memory by simply hearing the music! How differently it sounded to what we hear from morning 'till night. The Chaplain is an old man, and to all appearances a very rough man.[36] I will try and make it convenient to attend every night.

We can hear nothing different from the movements of our enemy. I do really wish that some sort of peace would be declared.

NEAR MANASSAS, VA.

SUNDAY JULY 28TH, 1861

This morning 105 men were up to be examined, prescribed for and administered to. I am very busily engaged until about 10 o'clock. After that time I have some spare time. I found my clothes very dirty this morning and_______. [sic; his blank space] I went to the creek, washed and dressed in clean clothes. I felt some-what relieved. I went to the place appointed for preaching but could not stay 'till preaching commenced. I went back and attended some sick ones and then into my tent and wrote a letter to Mrs. (Mary) Tomlin.[37] I ate no dinner to-day. I went to sleep and slept a while and went to preaching at 4 o'clock. The sermon was the first I have heard since April, when we were in Richmond. I cannot say that the sermon was the best I ever heard or at least I do not think so.

The text was the 23rd Psalm and 4th verse:

Yea, though I walk through the valley
and [sic] shadow of death,
I will fear no evil;
for thou art with me;
thy rod and thy staff shall comfort me.[38]

---

[36] Apparently this chaplain was W. Gaines Miller (b. 1805) of Montgomery Co., VA; although older and, at least according to the diarist "very rough," Miller was noted for service to the troops, including medical assistance in hospital and in the make-shift field tents near the scenes of battle. Charles F. Pitts, *Chaplains in Gray: the Confederate Chaplains' Story* (Nashville, TN.: Broadman Press, 1957), 96. VA. Census, vol. 3, s.v.

[37] Mary Tomlin was a family friend of the Faris's. She took a maternal interest in the diarist. Born in 1810, she had a home in Marion Township in 1870, VA Census, 1870.

[38] Psalm 23:4. A Psalm of David. He has altered King James translation, which is the one he customarily used: "Yea, though I walk through the valley of the shadow of death, I will fear no evil: for thou art with me; thy rod and thy staff they comfort me."

The first of his discourse was devoted to logical reasoning on experience, it[s] uses & benefits. "Experience," says he, "is the only thing by which we may know really the nature of an object. We know religion only by experience. Without or aside from experience we can have only a vague idea of what is the true nature of things, but with experience we know positively." He spoke at some length of David the "sweet singer of Israel" and the sad experiences of his life. He knew things more positively than most men of his age because he had experienced more. His writings were pointed to us as the cravings of his soul and the longings of his heart. We were then pointed to David's life for a precedent to our difficulty. I came back to camp. A very hard rain fell this evening but I was kept perfectly dry in my tent.

Mr. E.W. Sanders came into camp this evening. How glad I was to see him. He brings news from home that all is sad and dreary—crops good &c. He also brought me some shirts from some lady—how kind is that—I hope to be able to repay them some day.

Dr. & Mrs. Faris wrote me a few lines—I am closely engaged taking an inventory of what medicines we have on hand and also make a request for more—I retire late to-night—after "Taps".

NEAR MANASSAS, VA.

MONDAY, JULY 29, 1861

This morning I was up somewhat earlier than usual making pills for "sick call". Over 130 were up this morning to be physicked [sic]. My berth is becoming harder & harder. Nothing occurred worth noting to-day. I commenced writing a letter to Dr. F. to-day. Mr. D.B. Snapp was in our camp this evening. A very heavy rain fell this afternoon—I am perfectly dry in my tent.

CAMP NEAR MANASSAS, VA.

TUESDAY 30TH, 1861

To-day Andy Sanders came from Winchester where he has been in hospital for some time. We intend making an effort to get a discharge for him. We made the effort but failed. I am sorry for this. I know he can never stand the duties of a soldier. I sympathise with him and his pain but the law of military are [sic] so rigid. I think Andy will have to go home yet.

Nothing of interest occurred to-day worthy of note. The weather is exceeding warm.

WEDNESDAY, JULY 31ST

CAMP NEAR MANASSAS

To-day nothing outside the usual routine of duties occurred 'till evening. After dinner Capt. A[bijah] Thomas from Smyth[39] came with a coffin to get the remains of E.H. McCready who was killed on the 21st inst[ant; that is, July]. We went out and disinterred the body and placed it in the coffin and sent it to the depot. Mr. E. W. Sanders will take charge of the corpse to-morrow morning. Thus the last sad office has had [sic] been filled by us and we consign him to the land of his birth there to rest until Heaven and Earth shall give up their dead and the sea its dead to be judged by the Father of Righteousness. It must be heartrending to his parents to see their son brought home a lifeless corpse but they have reasons to be proud of their son. He did his duty and fell in the thickest of the fight for a cause common to us all.

Nothing else occurred to-day worthy of note.

THURSDAY AUG 1ST, '61

CAMP NEAR MANASSAS, VA.

Every thing as usual [.] Mr. E. W. Sanders left for home this evening. He had the kindness to give me some change before he left. I needed it very much too.

Sickness seems to threaten a great many of our boys—many are becoming ill every day.

---

[39] Apparently Abijah Thomas, most prominent antebellum industrialist in Smyth County and son of Welsh immigrants. "His developments of the iron industry in mines, furnaces, and foundries along the South Fork [of the Holston River] and on Staley's Creek made him a wealthy man for his day, and if the Civil War had not destroyed these properties and involved him heavily he would in all probability have amassed one of the great fortunes of the state." At this time, Thomas was apparently an officer in one of the Home Guards that patrolled in Smyth County. Wilson, *Smyth County History*, 180-81.

[FRIDAY] AUGUST 2ND, 1861

We left our encampment to-day and went to a camp one mile east of Centreville [Fairfax County], Va. I had the pleasure to-day of seeing my brother C[harles]. I met with him on the road between Manassas and Centreville. I should not have known him if he had not spoken to me. We walked to-gether from there to his camp near Centreville. I had a good deal to talk about. I regret to see him somewhat addicted to drinking. I felt it was my duty to talk to him about it and will do so soon. I found on arriving at his camp that there were many there that I knew. Cousin Bill & "Eddy" Webb & my bro accompanied me near our camp. I found P.H. Ruffner & "Bud" Almond at Centreville. Bud knew me as soon as he saw me, Ruffner did not.[1]

Our encampment now is upon the same ground that the yankees [sic] occupied before the engagement on the 21st inst. I find scattered about many envelopes beautifully set off with drawings of the once glorious fallen stars and stripes. Some have the Goddess of Liberty supporting the flag staff in one hand and pointing to it with the other. The motto beneath is: "Your country's flag, defend it". The answer this motto got on the 21st is better known than described. It is said by the citizens of Centreville that when the Yankees went to Bull's Run that morning they were singing "Dixie" but when they came back, from some cause or other, they were singing "Get out of the Wilderness", and some said that all H—l couldn't take Bull Run. I hope they will remain of that opinion for surely I do not want to see another engagement . We slept out under the trees the following night.

CAMP NEAR CENTREVILLE

SATURDAY, AUG. 3RD, 1861

The weather is very oppressive now. I feel very much debilitated from the effect of the heat and exercise. Many of our boys are giving way also. I fear fever will commence its ravage in the army.

Nothing of any importance occurred to-day. I wrote two letters—one to Aunt A M.J. another to Capt. C.B. Beatie.

---

[1] Charles Apperson is listed with Co. C, 7th Va. Infantry; J.W. Almond is also listed, and it is noted that he was promoted to captain of Co. C. Roster for Co. C also lists Ruffner and Webb, as privates; there are two Edward Webbs in C Co., one Edward C. Webb and one Edward W. Webb. It seems likely that his visitors were with C Co. of 7th Va. Inf., and thus were J.W. Almond, P.H. Ruffner, and either Edward C. or Edward W. Webb., in addition to his brother Charles. Scott, *Orange County*, "Appendix—Confederate Soldiers."

Our water here is good but a long way off. I hope our men will soon now be relieved of diarrhea.

CAMP NEAR CENTREVILLE, VA.

SUNDAY, AUG. 4TH 1861

I attended preaching to-day[.] was not at the place appointed in time to hear the text—not much of a sermon though.

In the evening I went again to hear him. His text was Joel 1:19: "Unto thee o Lord will I cry in time of danger."[2] He said some good things but they seemed out of place somehow or other. His principal topic was that innate principle in man to cry to the Lord for help whenever danger seemed nigh. He [said] that principal was a principal fixed [,] firm and immovable in the very soul of man. Even the most confirmed infidels and unchristian have given the lie to their *doctrine* by this voice of the soul of man. Naturally an infidel when on the deck of his vessel in a storm denied the existence of a God and yet could not refrain from crying out for His protection. He then spoke of the propriety of it when sincerely and prayerfully offered. Thus we as a people should, in the midst of our dificulties cry unto God for assisance; and He would give us aid and power to wrest ourselves into deliverance from the hand of the subjugation.

Nothing else worthy of note transpired.

CAMP NEAR CENTREVILLE, VA.

MONDAY, AUG. 5TH 1861

To-day I have been very unwell. The oppressing effect of the sun seems almost too much for me. Headache, nauseated stomach, dullness of energy, drowsiness &c were my ailments. I took no medicine, however, and felt something better at night.

I am sure that I do no violence to truth when I say that I have never seen anything so abused in my life as medicine is here. Men take it entirely too much. Their laziness will cost them something of great value—health. An election came off to-day that I regret very much to be compelled to take part in. The Election for 3rd Lieut— J.M.T[homas] & D [avid W.] B[ear] are the candidates. I have allways [sic] looked upon both as good friends and hate very much to

---

[2] Joel 1:19: "O Lord, to thee will I cry; for the fire hath devoured the pastures of the wilderness, and the flame hath burned all the trees of the field."

vote but I had promised and so have to vote. D. B. was elected by a triple majority.[3]

CAMP NEAR CENTREVILLE, VA.

TUESDAY, AUG. 6TH, 1861

The paymaster commenced upon our Regiment to-day. The exclamation that, "he has come at last!" is often repeated. Nothing worthy of note occurred to-day—I heard that 13 regiments of our of our [sic] soldiers had crossed the Potomac above Relay House—I can not vouch for the truth of this however [;] I am very busy. I wrote a letter for Mr. E. H. Sanders to-day. I am something better in feeling than I was yesterday.

My Bro C[harles]. and two friends—J.W. Almond & P.H. Ruffner came down to see me and staid [sic] some three hours. I was overjoyedto see them. They are a wild set of boys. Ruffner doesn't seem to have changed any at all either in character or body.

CAMP NEAR C[ENTREVILLE]— VA.

WEDNESDAY AUG. 7, 1861

The paymaster commenced on the Blues and I among the rest got some of the monthly trash. We received $47.76 each for our time since we left home until the 30th June.

Several do not care now how it goes. We got a good deal of the Confederate States money—payable at any bank.

Nothing else worthy of note occurred to-day. I got a letter from Dr. Quisenberry to-day—He is well—says the militia has been ordered out in that county (Orange) and were at Mitchells Station [Culpeper] County two weeks but have been sent home again.

The Dr. does not seem to be much of a fighting man himself—he is exempt from military duty.

---

[3] David W. Bear (1840-1918) of Co. A, Jenkins Brigade., 4th Va., had enlisted at Wytheville. Joseph M. Thomas (b. 1838) served in Co. D, 4th Va. Inf., Va. Brigade., and eventually became captain. *Smyth County Families and History*, ed., Jim Presgraves (Wytheville: Private Printing, 1974)., hereinafter *Families and History*. See also Mack D. Sturgill and Kenneth L. Sturgill, *Smyth County Virginia Cemetaries*, vol. 2 (Marion, VA.: Dean Tucker, 1994)., hereinafter cited as Sturgill, *Cemetaries*.

CAMP NEAR CENTREVILLE VA.

THURSDAY AUG. 8TH 1861

Last night was an unusually warm night. I was up sooner than usual this morning. Business was plenty during the day. I spent the day at a monthly report for July. Slept some two hours after dinner.

The Brigade was order [sic] out this evening to see Prince of France who was said to be passing.[4] But before we could get to the road his honor had passed. Two carriages were all the traveling accomodations I saw for himself and cortege. He came from Washington City. What may be the intention of his visit here I know not. I have no doubt very public affairs brought him to our soil. He has seen the Despot, Lincoln, and I presume is going to see old Jef[5] . Would to God that our troubles may find a pacification in the Prince. And if not a peace maker a Layfayette.[6] The crowned Heads of Europe are not wholy [sic]

---

[4] The diarist may have confounded names and identities of the Bonaparte family in this era. The Prince Jerome Napoleon (1784-1860) died before the war. Apperson may be talking about an American Bonaparte, Jerome; or he may be talking about Joseph, the Prince or Plon-Plon. Louis Bonaparte, Emperor Napoleon III (1803-1873) recognized the Confederate States as belligerents in the war. He was involved in much diplomatic intrigue throughout the war, including the sponsorship of an invasion of Mexico. His cousin Joseph Charles Paul Bonaparte (1822-1891) was known as Plon-Plon or the Prince. Prince Jospeh at one time after the war was in line of succession to the imperial throne; not possessing much power during The Civil War, he may be the person here described as visiting, probably as a military observer. Another possibility is Jerome Napoleon (1805-1870), son of the American Elizabeth Patterson and Jerome Napoleon, King of Westphalia (1784-1860). Although Patterson's marriage to Jerome was not recognized by Napoleon III (Jerome's marriage to Catherine, Princess of Würtemberg, gave him his title and bona fides), the offspring Jerome Napoleon was eventually received by Napoleon III. Jerome was not a prince; he did found a distinguished American line of Bonapartes, generally known as the Bonapartes of Baltimore, one of whom became an important Progressive Era politician, protege of Theodore Roosevelt, and a cabinet member. The American Jerome may be the person described here. In any case, neither Joseph the Prince nor Jerome the American was living in Richmond, and neither possessed significant power at this time; there is no record of either man visiting President Lincoln or President Davis. Owen Connelly, *Napoleon's Satellite Kingdoms* (New York: Free Press, 1970). Most likely of all is that a French diplomat unrelated to the Bonaparte family was visiting in Richmond on official business; and that is whose carriage and cortege passed by the Stonewall Brigade's camp.

[5] Note that even this early Abraham Lincoln has become in the diarist's language "The Despot." By contrast, Jefferson Finis Davis (1808-1889), president of the Confederacy, is treated much more familiarly as "Old Jef." Although early in the diary Apperson claims profound respect for Davis's strategical acumen, there is no great deference at all—and Apperson will soon follow the lead of most Confederate citizens in disdaining their commander in chief.

[6] Apperson hopes that the Bonaparte family may play the same role as did the Marquis de LaFayette (1757-1834), who led French troops and provided other support for the cause of independence in the American Revolutionary War. Note that Apperson, like most Confederate

conversant with our difficulty and may have sent the Prince over to see into matters, or France may want cotton. If so the Great Blockade of Lincoln will soon drop to pieces—and the Armada of Philip of Spain[7] be squandered to the four winds of the earth. I am writing after Taps and must retire soon[.] Not very well in my bowels.

CAMP NEAR CENTREVILLE, VA

FRIDAY, AUG. 9TH, 1861

Prince Jerome Napoleon passed along to-day on his way back to Washington. Gen. [Joseph Eggleston] Johns[t]on's division was ordered out near Centreville for his majesty to review[.] He came along the line in a carriage with two other Gentlemen. I did not get a good look at him. He had on white pants and whiskers *a la militaire*. His visit to the country at this time is a matter of curiosity to many. He evidently wants peace or cotton. Whether he is for North or South I am unable to say. I have great confidence in France. Jerome has been Louis Napoleon's diplomat in many cases. I do hope that something will be done for our difficulties. According to the usage of nations a prince cannot visit a nation at times of war and not visit the other without great *insult* to the one not visited. Prince Jerome has come to see both sections of our warlike country—may it be a precursor of peace!

The weather is very warm indeed—a beautiful rain fell this evening. I wrote a letter to cousin James Apperson this evening. J[ospeh]. M. Thomas [of Stonewall Bde.]is very unwell which I am very sorry to see.

CAMP NEAR CENTREVILLE, VA.

SATURDAY, AUG. 10TH, 1861

Something unusual transpired to-day. There has been some new arrangement in relation to the posts of the guard. We cannot get to the spring

---

citizens, regards the CSA as the heir to the American Revolution and regards this war as a fight for independence.

[7] Holy Roman Emperor Philip II (1527-1598)of Spain sent the famed Armada against England in 1588, but was defeated in a great naval battle in the English Channel, followed by a terrible storm that further dissipated his huge fleet. Again, Apperson uses an image from Whiggish history in which the alleged despot, Philip, is compared to Lincoln; the Armada is compared to the US naval forces, and by extension the English naval heroes and English liberties are paralleled with Confederate forces and ideals.

now without a pass frpm our Capt. Several Regiments seem to be moving towards the Potomac. We may expect stormy times soon. No prospect for peace as yet. I should not be surprised if we move toward Alexandria soon.

I rec'd A [sic] letter from Mrs. Faris to-day—glad indeed was I to hear from home— to get such good letters from my friends. I love true friends.

CAMP NEAR CENTREVILLE, VA.

SUNDAY AUG. 11TH, 1861

Another Sabbath has found us here—we should be thankful to Divine Providence that we have been permitted to see the bright sunshine of this morning. I know we soldiers are too careless about our spiritual concerns and often am I brought to reflect upon my own manner of being. I know I am a sinful creature and deserve the wrath of a Sovereign God, but how wretched the thought. Estranged from God and Godly people, to live without the hope of eternal salvation and the dread of everlasting punishment is a distressing thought.

I attended the preaching of our chaplain to-day. He may have preached a good sermon but I did not think so. His text—"Choose ye this day whom ye will serve." His principal topic or the principal part of his discourse was upon that innate principle in the soul of man that prompts him to worship something. "Man" says he "must worship Moloch or Baal, Brahmin or [illegible]—we will worship God or Mammon—." He does this from a prompting that he knows not the source. And between God and Mammon there is no neutral ground—peace cannot take a ground of neutrality—we must worship one and dispose the other or else we will love the one and hate the other. Thus reasoning he went on to a close by appealing to his hearers to heed the calling of the Saviour of sinners & c.[8]

Many, very many sick are now being administered to. The distressing influence of the sun is too much for our men.

I was very sick several hours to-day— got a letter from Mrs. Tomlin—she seems to have heard something derogatory to the bravery of Capt. [A.G.] P[endleton] and Lieut. [W.G.] Fulton[.] ["W.G." after name Fulton] Whether the change is true or false I am unable to say. She wishes them to rid themselves of the charge. This I hope they may do. She says she is expecting to hear a good report of me and will be disappointed if she does not. So far as hearing a report

[8] The Rev. Gaines Miller from Montgomery County was chaplain for this brigade.

from me is concerned, I hope if she hears any it will be *good.* But where in discharge of the duties incumbent upon me I feel that I have endeavored to discharge them to the best of my feeble ability. And there my conscience is clear. I feel that my case is in the hands of a higher tribunal than mere man. Thus if I have or have not done my duty in the sight of man that a good report may come I am perfectly indifferent.

CAMP NEAR CENTREVILLE, VA.

MONDAY, AUG. 12TH 1861

Nothing of any importance has transpired to-day. Our sick list seems to be gradually growing. Several patients seem threatened with Bilious R[h]eumatic fever, and Rheumatism and catarrh[9] are the principal complaints.

I wrote a letter to Mrs. Tomlin this morning.

---

[9] Rheumatism in 19th century generally referred to painful conditions in muscles, joints, and bones. In modern medicine, much more specific terms are used. Originally confounded with gout ("a metabolic disease resulting in an excessive concentration of uric acid in the blood from improperly metabolized protein"; characterized by swelling and extreme pain in joints, but especially in feet and big toe), rheumatism by the middle of the 19th century was recognized as an ailment separate and distinct from other inflammations and pains in muscles, joints, and bones. Group A hemolytic streptococcus is the "activating agent" for rheumatic fever, which was especially dangerous at the time if it attacked the heart muscles. Bilious fever referred to fever and pain associated with the intestines, and was also called enteric fever and enteritic fever. Bile is a thick, viscous fluid that passes from the bile duct of the liver into the common bile duct and then into the duodenum as needed. Its function is to aid in digestion, especially of fats. Both an excess of bile and too little bile were called biliousness or bilious in this period. It is likely that the bilious fever reported was typhoid, an intestinal disease easily spread during periods of "social breakdown" such as crowded conditions during war; typhoid was beginning to be recognized as a separate disease from other problems more generally described as bilious fevers and pains. Its easy spread through the stools of the infected in crowded camp latrines was not well understood until after the war. Bilious rheumatic fever suggests rheumatic fever associated with a heavy discharge of bile; it is also likely that bilious rheumatic fever was typhoid. "Gout;" "Rheumatism;" "Typhoid," *McGrew.* Catarrh is from the Greek *katarrhein,* to flow down; and was applied in 19th century to inflammation of mucous membrane, especially of head and throat. Here it seems to mean any coughing up of mucous. Dry Catarrh, also mentioned, referred to severe coughing, usually associated with emphysema or asthma. "Catarrh," *Taber's.* Note that these respiratory and enteritic diseases associated with unsanitary conditions in crowded hospital tents are the ones most puzzling to stewards and physicians of the era, and also the kinds of diseases responsible for the majority of death and severe suffering among patients otherwise successfully treated or operated on for severe wounds.

CAMP NEAR CENTREVILLE, VA.

TUESDAY, AUG. 13TH, 1861

Things are going on as usual. J[oseph]. W. Thomas is very unwell to-day.

WEDNESDAY AUG. 14, 1861

To-day Dr. Black detailed Dr. Snidow of Tennessee to assist me. This is something very agreeable on my part. Snidow seems to be a very agreeable young man and I think will make a very good assistant. Dr. B. has also made arrangements that will mean more for us to do—all those who are able to get to the medicine tent are compelled to come there and get each dose—those who are unable to come we must go to and administer each dose as it is to be given.

I wrote a letter to Mrs. F. this evening—

During the day to-day heavy cannonading was heard in direction of Alexandria or Fairfax. Many conjectures were proposed as to what the cause was—News came in the evening that Stewart [sic; J.E.B. Stuart) had attacked the enemy and killed several—another report says that the Federals had crossed the Potomac near Leesburg (Loudon County) where we had a large force and the late rains had swollen the river so that it was impossible for the Yankees to get back so our forces attacked and took 1700 prisoners. This report may be groundless and false, however.

Jo[seph] Thomas left for the Hospital to-day.

CAMP NEAR CENTREVILLE, VA.

THURSDAY, AUG. 15TH, 1861

Nothing unusual to-day—We heard cannon firing in the east again to-day without being able to account for it. The sick are not better. Fever seems to be threatening our soldiers.

I promised Lieut. [James W.] Kennedy to-day to write for his paper. It is a task by no means to be desired but if I can do anything to promote the interests of the [Marion] *Visitor*,[10] I am willing to do it.

[10] On this newspaper, see 37ff.

CAMP NEAR CENTREVILLE

FRIDAY AUG. 16TH, 1861

There has been a great deal of rain lately. To-day has been a very wet disagreeable day. Our Hospt. [sic; Bde. field hospital] at Manassas is broken up. I do not know what arrangements will be made about our sick now.

I have spent some moments in writing to-day.

SATURDAY, AUG. 17TH, '61

CAMP NEAR CENTREVILLE VA.

This day passed as others have usually passed with the exception that Mr. [Edward S.] Watson from Marion[11] came down and brought some of the company clothes. Mine did not come. The cloth was sent out in the country to be made up and the garments had not been made up. I and others will get ours with B.F. Leonard & Thos. Owry.[12]

I finished communication to the *Visitor* this evening. Lieut. Kennedy is very unwell—he came in my tent and I did what I could to relieve him. Afterwards Capt. Pendleton came with violent spasms of the stomach. I bathed the epigastrium with Chloroform Liniment and gavc him Laud. & H Annodyne [sic].[13] He soon got better.

---

[11] Edward S. Watson ran a dry goods store in Marion where the Marion National Bank later stood. Active in the deliberations concerning secession, he campaigned for a "less southern" pronouncement of secession; when war came, he enlisted in and served as captain for the Marion Home Guards, who were generally too old or too young or otherwise disabled for combat service. "Edward S. Watson," Wilson, *Smyth County*.

[12] Smyth County merchants.

[13] The epigastrium is the region above the pit of the stomach. As noted earlier, chloroform was generally used in the first half of the 19th century to relieve pain, especially as an anesthetic prior to an operation, although there were already a number of chloroform deaths causing concern among practitioners by the 1840s. In this case, Apperson is making a liniment, or strictly external medicament, to spread chloroform over the outside of the stomach to relieve the pain of stomach ache. An anondyne was any pain-reliever, in this case laudanum [Laud.], which is morphine, and heroine (H. anodyne). *Taber's.*; *McGrew's.* As also noted, the steward here is curing nothing, but rather treating by relieving pain, albeit with dangerously addictive drugs.

SUNDAY AUG. 18TH 1861

Nothing of any interest occurred to-day. We are having a great many cases of cramp colic[14] now, and some of them serious. We have one case that seems to have symptoms of Laryngitis—Dr. Black thinks it to be *Peripneumonia nothe.*[15] I am unacquainted with the complaint. The patient is hoarse, almost speechless—suffers with tightness in the throat & slimy mucus seems constantly running from his mouth. There is a strange sound in his throat which seems to be occasioned by phlegm collecting in the wind pipe or at the bifurcation of the Trachea from a want of power to expell it. The patient is continually changing his position—not satisfide [sic] in any way long at a time. The countenance looks vacant and anxious. I was ordered to give him [illegible] 3 tes di [three teaspoons diluted]—but was no better at evening. First a sinapism then an epiplastic were ordered with Hoffman's anodyne and Tinc[ture] of opium were ordered[16] —Dr. B evidently thought that there was some spasm there. Nothing, however, seemed to do any good.

I wrote to B.F. Leonard to bring me some onions and pepper and wrote to Dr. Faris to send them. Raining very much.

MONDAY AUG. 19TH

Raining again to-day. The case spoken of yeaterday seems no better. He is evidently worse. We continue the antiphlogistic with emetics[17] to expell the mucus secretions—he seems to be throwing out large quantities of *purulent* matter[18]—I fear some organic lesion.[19]

---

[14] Colic is "spasm in any hollow or tubular soft organ accompanied by pain," although its Greek root specifies the colon as the source of the pain. *Taber's.* Cramp colic is descriptive rather than analytical, but likely refers to intestinal colic.

[15] Bacterial pneumonia was still generally called peripneumonia following Hippocrates' notes. The conception of a bacterial cause did not develop until the 1880s, and Apperson and his colleagues, still following Hippocrates, treated peripneumonia with bleeding, or venesection. *McGrew's.* Black's label seems a bit idiosyncratic; nothe was an obscure and very rarely used English term literally meaning "nought" or "nothing" and connoting "neglected." OED.

[16] Sinapism was a mustard plaster; placed on the upper abdomen, it produced a discharge by stimulating inflammation. Epiplastic was an agency to counteract inflammation and fever. Hoffman's anodyne was a compound of ether to relieve pain in the "plasma," or blood and fluids of body. *Taber's.*

[17] Antiphlogistic was an agent to reduce inflammation; emetics were agents the produced vomiting. *Taber's.*

[18] Matter containing pus. *Taber's.*

[19] The purulent matter makes Apperson fear a tear to an internal organ.

We are quite busy—Dr. Snidow who is helping me assists me a good deal. I rec'd. a note from Joseph [W.] Thomas this evening. He [sic] says he cant [sic] get from the junction. I am sorry for it. I also rec'd. a letter from Mrs. Faris things—things at home are going well.

CAMP NEAR CENTREVILLE, VA.

TUESDAY, AUG. 20, 1861

This morning Mr. Wright of "Dare Devils" died—I was fearful of his case from the first. Dr. Black thinks it a case of Perinpneumonia Notha. Nothing of any importance occurred to-day.

WEDNESDAY AUG. 21ST 1861

Today I am 23 years old. May I never see another birthday with my country in this conditon[.] We heard various rumors to-day—viz. that Gen. [Henry Alexander] Wise & [William Starke] Rosencranz [sic; Rosecrans] had met and fought [20] —Wise whipped Rosencrantz's forces and took him prisoner—that Alexandria was abandoned by the Federals. That France & England had acknowledged the S.C.-&c -&c. None reliable though.[21] I have been engaged writing nearly all day—am tollerably [sic] well—Capt. Pendleton is very unwell. Wrote a letter for Dr. Quisenbery to-night.

---

[20] Wise (1806-1876), from Drummondtown (Craige County) Virginia, was honors graduate from Washington College (now Washington and Jefferson College) in Pennsylvania, and a former ambassador to Brazil, member of congress, and governor. An eloquent and militant speaker, Wise defended slavery and as governor put down the John Brown slave rebellion at Harper's Ferry and had Brown hung. At the Virginia secession convention, Wise supported secession and was an early and prominent volunteer for the Confederate army. Bright with promise, he was still inexperienced in military tactics, and he performed poorly in the field, especially in these campaigns of the valley and the western mountains. Rosecrans (1819-1898), from Delaware County, Ohio, was a distinguished graduate of West Point. A Roman Catholic and registered Democrat, Rosecrans was something of a political appointment, someone to whom Republicans could point as proof of a broad based and nonpartisan war effort, since Catholics generally voted Democrat and immigrant Catholics would be needed in the army. In the field, especially at the recent battle of Rich Mountain near Beverly, West Virginia, Rosecrans proved brave and successful, and his bold charge up Rich Mountain had much to do with McClellan's successes in western Virginia. These rumors are not only untrue, but opposite reality, for Wise failed in the west and Rosecrans enjoyed grand success. Faust, ed., *Historical Times.*

[21] Alexandria was not evacuated by the Federals. Napoleon III, as noted, schemed considerably, and recognized the Confederacy as a belligerant—a step toward recognition as an independent nation, but it had nothing to do with this battle; England did not recognize the Confederacy.

CAMP NEAR CENTREVILLE, VA.

THURSDAY AUG 22ND, 1861

Nothing of interest occurred to-day until night, when about dark an order came from Head Quarters for the regiment to prepare for a fight or a march to have everything so arranged that they could bundle up immediately. This was something not very easy or quickly done on my part. Drugs[,] lint[,] [22] bandages[,] and Hospital stores of every kind were spread promiscuously over my tent. I went to work and with the help of Dr. Snidow I suppose it was 2 o'clock [when] every thing was ready to be moved .

We then lay down to rest a while.

CAMP NEAR CENTREVILLE, VA.

FRIDAY AUGUST 23RD, 1861

As has often been the case we are not ordered off yet and had to unpack my medicines. Sick call amounted to 140 in number this morning. Capt. Pendleton was sent to Gen. Hospital—I fear he will have an attack of fever—We were ordered of[f] this evening about 5 o'clock to Fairfax Court House. The report in circulation is that the enemy has been making some demonstrations towards us. The march to Fairfax was a pretty hard one. Dr. Bear has taken very ill on the way—had cramp colic. We gave laudanum & brandy which did not seem to relieve him. A bystander proposed salt water until vomiting was produced—We gave the brine and found it relieved him immediately but the paroxysm would return again. However he got better and we were compelled to leave him.

I walked [to] Faiffax CH [Courthouse] with Mr. Rhodes of Pendleton's Artillery Company. Found him a very sensible man. I stopped awhile at the Hotel at the CH; found some of our boys there—all of [them] went after the Regiment. The brigade was ordered back about 10 miles below the CH. The alarm had been a false one—several brigades were out—all came back—I hated very much the idea of having to walk back to camp that night and resolved not to do so. I walked ahead of the Regiment in company with D.W. Venable[23] and

---

[22] Lint is not here cotton lint. In 19th century, lint [from Latin, *linteum*, that is, made of linen] was "linen scraped until soft and wooly for dressing wounds. *Taber's.*

[23] Possibly Charles W. Venable (born 1843), an early volunteer with Smyth County patrols, then member of Brigade who survived war and apparently relocated in Prince Edward County. See Wilson, *Smyth County*, 236, and *Virginia 1870 Census Index*, vol. 4, ed., Bradley W. Steuart (Bountiful, UT: Precision Indexing, 1989)., hereinafter cited as *Va. 1870 Census Index.*

stopped at the house of Mr. Joseph Robinson where we had left Dr. Bear that evening. Mr. Robinson gave us some bread and milk to eat which was very much needed. Dr. Bear was better—I remained with him all night.

Mr. Robinson is one of those who have felt the smart of having northern troops about his house and on his premises. He told me that $500—would not repay him for the damages he received. His grain was taken, hay[;] feed and [sic; word omitted] wasted [;] a large and splendid potatoe [sic] field was ruined—all his poultry killed and he could not say a word—this was the spirit of the "Grand Army". I feel sorry to record such deeds but I am afraid they are too true to be left unrecorded. I slept on a bed for the first time since I left home

SATURDAY, AUG 24TH 1861

This morning I arose sometime after sunup and ate a hearty breakfast. Then I left for camp where I arrive [sic] about 9 o'clock. I rec'd. a letter from Miss Columbia Thomas asking information in regard to her brother Jos[eph M.] . I answered her immediately. I rec'd. another from Mrs. Faris this evening[.] all as usual at Home. Nothing else occurred to note.

CAMP, NEAR CENTREVILLE, VA

SUNDAY, AUG 25TH, 1861

We are spared to see another sabbath morn—bright and sunny as it is. The weather is becoming very pleasant indeed. I wished to go to preaching to-day but was not permitted to do so. I was in hearing of the preacher's voice but could hear nothing. I went to see a case of Cholera Morbis last night & treated it. Sinapism to the epigastrium Tinct[ure] of opium—Rx. Cal[omel] 1gr [am] powder of opium1/2 gr[am]—give one every two hours.[24] My patient was doing well. I commenced writing a letter to Dr. Faris this evening but had not more than half finished it before the regiment was called out and we were on a march towards Fairfax again. We did not go more than 2 miles before orders came for us to come back to camp. The boys raised a shout and came back. I am unable to give any reason for such movements. I think the enemy must be changing

[24] Cholera is bilious diarrhea in Latin; "an acute infection involving the entire small bowel, characterized by profuse watery diarrhea and vomiting, which produces severe loss of fluids and electrolytes, muscular cramps, oliguria, dehydration, and collapse." Not available in this period, there is now a cholera vaccine, which must be administered with generous replacement of the lost fluids. *Taber's.* Treatment of 1861 is a mustard plaster, or sinapism, accompanied by pain-killing opium.

positions and wavering about which fools our pickets. I finished my letter to Dr. and wrote one to Mrs. Faris. Then visited Jno [M.] Preston[25] and retired near midnight I suppose—The weather is very fine—pleasant too.

CAMP NEAR CENTREVILLE, VA.

MONDAY AUG. 26TH, 1861

This day passed as usual. I have had a disagreeable headache to-day. Went to the spring and washed my body all over and put on clean clothes—I felt much better afterwards. I recd. two letters this evening—one from Capt. C. W. Beatie[26] & one from Uncle Chas. Jones. I had thought that Uncle Charles did not like my coming to the war, but from his letter he seems as devoted as ever. I wrote a short letter to cousin Bettie to-night—I had not heard from her for some time.

CAMP NEAR CENTREVILLE, VA.

TUESDAY AUG. 27TH, 1861.

I was up early this morning attending Hospital Stores, such as bedding, towels etc. etc. Nothing of interest occurred to-day. My headache of yesterday has not entirely left me. Our sick list seems to be diminishing somewhat[.] I hope soon to see good, healthy weather.

CAMP NEAR CENTREVILLE, VA.

AUG. 28TH, 1861

This morning Dr. Black awakened me and said we were under marching orders again. I rose and prepared to go the rout [e]. The Ambulance being at

---

[25] John Montgomery Preston, born 1838 in Washington County, was then private in Co. B of 48th Va. Inf.; he would be promoted quickly into officer ranks, would survive wounds at Gettysburg, and return to Smyth County after the war as a prominent farmer and local leader. Presgraves, *Smyth County*.

[26] Claiborne Watkins Beattie (born 1828) of Chilhowie, son of Robert Beattie, one of the first settlers of that community. The Beattie family owned the Town House, where their large extended family lived; their house was a combination house and stage coach tavern "which acquired a reputation in its day." C.W. Beattie was one of the first men in Smyth County to organize a volunteer Confederate patrol before Virginia seceded, and his Town House became a "favorite place for militia musters." Later he joined the Stonewall Brigade. Wilson, *Smyth County*, 236, 283. *Va. 1870 Census*, 1.

camp I prepared to go int it. Very little attention was paid to "sick call" this morning. I bundled up and went with the Reg.

I had the pleasure of meeting Charles Payne an old acquaintance of mine to-day. I knew him as soon as I saw him. He seems as usual. He is Quartermaster of [Milledge Luke] Bonham's Brigade. [27] He promised to visit me before very long.

It rained some to-day and we had to march. We stopped a short distance this side of Fairfax C.H. and remained some two hours I suppose. This waiting has been the most disagreeable part of the service to me.

After awhile however the order came for us to retrace our steps. This vexed the soldiers very much being the 3rd time they had been ordered here and back. I think the cause of this is Col. [J.E.B.]Stuart has took [sic] an advance position and one that is very important for him to hold and the enemy is not very well satisfide [sic] with troops so close to them. I have no doubt this will bring on a general engagements [sic].

We returned to camp—I was very much troubled[.] After I lay down some fellow came for me to extract some teeth—I pulled two very well for him.

I took some physic. too which I hope will do me some good.

CAMP NEAR CENTREVILLE, VA.

THURSDAY AUG. 29TH, 1861

Nothing of any interest to-day—We had orders to prepare to march if necessary. I suppose [James] Longstreet[28] who has a position in front and is

---

[27] Milledge Luke Bonham (1813-1890) of Red Bank, S.C., was a bold and courageous infantry leader cited by P.G.T. Beauregard for holding the center of his line at Manassas. His First Brigade was largely composed of South Carolina infantrymen but included some Virginians and North Carolinians. Bonham was contentious in his relations with professional soldiers and politically ambitious and later resigned his commission to serve in Confederate S.C. politics, including as governor. Edward G. Longacre, "Bonham," *Historical Times.* Charles Payne was apparently from Orange Co., *Va. 1870 Census.*

[28] James Longstreet (1821-1904), a West Point graduate and wounded veteran of the Mexican War, was the son of a "middling farmer" and grew up near Augusta GA. before removing to Alabama. A career officer, Longstreet was called "Old Pete" by his troops and "My Old Warhorse" by Lee. Cautious and at his best on defense, Longstreet performed well at "counterpunching," that is, responding to an enemy's bold charge. Commended at Manassas and later at Williamsburg, he was faulted for slowness at Seven Pines. His role at Gettysburg remains object of great controversy, some of it fueled by his own vigorous defense of his tactics in writings after the war. The diarist's sarcasm about Longstreet's desire for "sound health" by retreating from the front is a typical comment in an army whose other leaders were generally focused on bold charges and quick strikes. John D. Kallman, "Longstreet," *Historical Times,* s.v Contrast Apperson's notes

determined to have sound health. I learned to day that J[oseph] M. Thomas] arrived Home—also that Sampson Wolf was dead—died of wounds received on the 21 [July]. He was a good companion—a brave and worthy young man—may we never forget him! I wrote a letter to Uncle Chas. Jones to-night.

FRIDAY AUG. 30TH, 1861

(CAMP HARMAN IS NEAR CENTREVILLE VA.)[29]

Nothing outside of the usual routine of duties occurred to-day. The sick list is something smaller than it was sometime back. They are preparing pay rolls for us again. The Southern Confederacy is doing a good business in keeping her soldiers so well paid off.

I am busy making off reports to-day and will be busy for several days.

CAMP HARMAN SATURDAY AUG. 31ST

The weather is something cooler. This morning is beautiful, clear, and sunny. Sick call over and went to work on reports again. The day passed away as usual. I received a letter from cousin Bettie this evening. News from other points are somewhat discouraging—the enemy has taken Fort Hatteras[30] with all its contents. But it would be folly for us to expect to win every time. I wrote a letter to R.H. Dungan to-night. I do not know that he will ever get it though.

---

about Longstreet with his notes of the previous day about then-Col. Stuart, whose bold push to the front seems likely to bring on "general engagements."

[29] Camp Harman in Fairfax Co. near Centreville was named for Maj. John Alexander Harman (1824-1874), quartermaster to Jackson. A very capable administrator, Harman was given to rough and even profane language, but the normally strict Jackson tolerated these vices without complaint. This camp, unlike others noted by the diarist, was set near a good source of clean water, and was generally a healthy environment. Jeffry Wert, "Major Harman the Wagonmaster: 'Old John'," *Civil War Times Illustrated*, 20 (1981):8-13; Alexander M. Garber, *Stonewall Jackson's Way* (Staunton: Spectator Job Print, 1876).

[30] Hatteras Inlet on the southeastern NC coastline was one of the state's busiest ports, "a haven for blockade runners, and a major supply conduit for Confederate forces." Confederates constructed two forts to guard the inlet, Fort Clark and Fort Hatteras. During battles of 27-29 August, Flag Officer Silas Stringham, commander of the Federal Atlantic Blockading Squadron, attacked the forts from the sea with effective artillery fire. Fort Clark fell first. Despite reinforcements under Confederate Flag Officer Samuel Barron (1809-1888), Fort Hatteras was also surrendered. The Federals' Maj. Gen. Benjamin Franklin Butler (1818-1893), disgraced earlier, had urged this action, and its success raised his prestige although marines under his command were unable to effect a landing to participate in the battles. The loss of the two forts "shook Southern confidence" and restored morale to Federal troops, as well as partially vindicating Butler. Edward G. Longacre, "Hatteras," *Historical Times*.

This is the last day of summer. O what a dark gloomy summer this has been to the American people. Her business stopped—Her fields laid waste, her interests devastated and her promising children engaged in deadly strife. O may another summer bloom upon our country with peace and harmony. All is sad and dreary now and will not the searing frosts of autumn make us more gloomy in feeling?

I enjoyed a an [sic] hour very pleasantly with Dr. Bear to-night.

Every thing is quiet in this section—

CAMP HARMAN, SUNDAY SEPT. 1ST '61

God in his mercy has permitted us sinful *mortals* to breathe the cool, refreshing air, and look upon the bright sunshine of another Sabbath morn. A more beautiful morning I have not seen lately. How thankful we should be to God for the gifts of health and strength He has bestowed upon us, and the success He has permitted our arms to gain. I feel my sinful nature needs regenerating—I know with sorrow that I am a very sinful creature and I pray God may spare me of doom that awaits sinful men.

"Sick Call" is over—health is improving. I attended the preaching of our Chaplain Mr. [Gaines] Miller to-day. He preached from Luke 12th chapter 4 & 5 verses. He exhorted and recomended Godly fear, sincerity and perseverance throughout this "short, flickering life." "To fear God" said he "is to love Him".[31]

This has been the most quiet, pleasant Sabbath we have spent since we left Home. Nature seemed to lavish her mellow sunlight on all around. The soldiers seem cheerful and happy. Squads and groups were congregated around indulging in conversation or writing letters. Others seem to stroll along the different paths almost unconscious that civil war was abroad in our land—How will we spend our next Sabbath is a problem solved only by the lapse of time. Many that are now cheerful may rest cold and silent in death ere another sabbath morn shall break upon us.

I wrote a letter to E. H. Sanders this evening. After night I attended programs at Capt. P's [A.G. Pendleton] tent. How much like home to hear the soul stirring notes of vocal praise ascending to the thrones of God. I have Newton

[31] Luke 12:4-5: "And I say unto you my friends, Be not afraid of them that kill the body, and after that have no more that they can do. But I will forewarn you whom you shall fear: Fear him, which after he hath killed hath power to cast into hell; yea, I say unto you, Fear him." Words ascribed to Jesus (KJV).

Umbarger in my tent to-night very sick with fever. I am writing at "Taps" —. No mail this evening.

CAMP HARMAN, VA.

MONDAY SEPT 2ND 1861

I have engaged the bigger part of to-day in unpacking medicines—nothing unusual is going on. The weather is very fine now.

CAMP HARMAN, VA.

TUESDAY SEPT. 3RD, 1861

This morning I was awakened about 1 or 2 o'clock by Dr. Black who stated a man had been shot in the neighborhood. We repaired to the place immediately and found Mr. J. L. Watters of Co. G with his hand badly injured. The bullet pass [sic] through the palm of the hand and carried away a part of and shattered the metacarpul bones of the middle and fore finger. He looked badly—Dr. Black assisted by Dr. [John] Leyburn of Pendleton's artillery[32] took away the two fingers that had lost all important connection with the body and dress [sic] the wound and brought the man to camp. I have a piece of bone taken from his finger.

We got to camp about day break—I attempted to sleep a while but could do no good.

Dr. [Joseph] Crockett came back to-night—having been away sick. He seemed rather wrathy [sic] because we occupy his tent.[33] I have had severe headache to-day.

WEDNESDAY SEPT. 4TH

I have been very busy to-day removing hospital stores out of Dr. Crockett's Tent and putting them into a new one—I have a very good tent now. Mr. W. S.

---

[32] Dr. John Leyburn of Rockbridge Co. was a graduate of Washington College. Bean, Notes.

[33] Dr. Joseph Crockett of Wytheville was assistant surgeon of 4th Va. Crockett is discussed in more detail in Apperson's memoirs, *Reminiscences.* Described here as "wrathy," that is in the diarist's and memoirist's language, filled with wrath over the trivial, Crockett initially struck Apperson as "an erratic sort of person." Later, the memoirist decided that Crockett was likable enough, as well as competent, but he noted that the doctor "did not have a popular turn." Crockett died after suffering wounds in the battle of Gaines Mill, 27 June 1862.

Strother [34] arrived in camp to-day—I got three letters to-day—one from Dr. F. another from Aunt M[atilda Apperson] and one from my friend Joseph M. Thomas. He is at home and his health improving.

I answered Dr. F's letter to-night and wrote some for the "Visitor".

The sick list is growing smaller.

CAMP HARMAN

THURSDAY SEPT. 5TH

To-day has been a cloudy, rainy day. I was engaged making of reports this evening. Mr. [Wade] Strother and Lieut. [James W.] Kennedy[35] were with me until a late hour. I wrote some and retired.

CAMP HARMAN

FRIDAY, SEPT. 6TH 1861

To-day passed off as usual. I am not having so much to do now. Sickness seems to be abating somewhat. I wrote 'till a late hour to-night.

CAMP HARMAN VA.

SATURDAY, SEPT. 7TH 1861

Everything is quiet in camp. Nothing outside of the ordinary routine of events is occurring. I wrote to Joe Thomas this evening. I am in hopes Joe will be with us soon again. We rec'd a large tent this evening and will keep it for sick men.

I retired earlier than usual this evening.

---

[34] Wade S. Strother, apparently related to the Strother family that built the Continental Hotel that was site of secession debates, was from Marion. After the war, he served as circuit court judge in Smyth Co., 1866-69. Wilson, *Smyth County*, 96.

[35] James W. Kennedy, lieutenant in 4th Va. and an early organizer of the Smyth Co. Blues, was also involved with the *Marion Visitor*; after the war, he established another newspaper. Wilson, *Smyth County*, 173, 237.

CAMP HARMAN VA.

SUNDAY, SEPTEMBER 8TH, '61

This is another pretty morning. Bishop Johns of Richmond[36] preached [at] "Head Quarters" to-day. I would have been glad to have heard the sermon but could not go.

Mr. [Gaines] Miller preached this evening. I can give nothing particular of his sermon He discoursed principally upon the conditions of the Jews—How they had degenerated and what God had put upon them & c. He also exhorted the soldiers to do the duty assigned them faithfully and avoid asking why this is done this way and that is done that way—"Go and do yours."

I rode down to near Fairfax C.H. this evening with Mr. Strother.

I am well.

I wrote a letter to cousin Bettie to-day and rec'd one from Mrs. Faris, Mrs. F's letter stated that Mr. [John] M. Preston was dangerously ill.

CAMP HARMAN

MONDAY SEPT. 9TH, 61

This has been a beautiful day—though this morning was cloudy. I heard to-day that Col. [J.E.B.] Stuart's men had captured the Steamer "Pawnee" somewhere below Washington City—The truth of this I cannot vouch for the truth of the statement.[37]

---

[36] John Johns (1796-1876), Episcopal Bishop of Virginia, was a native of New Castle, Delaware. He graduated from Princeton University in 1819 and was ordained a priest in the Episcopal Church. He served several parishes in Virginia, and became assistant to Bishop William Meade in 1839. He also served as president of the College of William & Mary between 1849 and 1854. He baptized and confirmed Jefferson Davis and he baptized Robert Edward Lee. When Meade died in 1861, Johns became bishop. During the war, he was "roving chaplain" in Lee's Army of Northern Virginia. John Sumner Wood, *The Virginia Bishop: A Yankee Hero of the Confederacy* (Richmond: Garrett & Massie, 1961).

[37] The steamer USS. *Pawnee* was commanded by Stephen Clegg Rowan (1808-1890). Rowan, born in Ireland, immigrated into the US in 1818 and grew up in Ohio. Joining the US Navy, he served in the Mexican War, and when the Civil War broke out, he was commander of the *Pawnee*, whose early duty was to defend the District of Columbia during Abraham Lincoln's inaugural 4 March 1861. Early in summer of 1861, Commander Rowan led the *Pawnee* in a successful siege of Alexandria, "first amphibious assault of the war." Still later, Rowan's *Pawnee* was successful in the assault on two forts in Hatteras Inlet in North Carolina. Apperson is wise to be skeptical of these rumors. Far from the *Pawnee* suffering capture in the federal capital on this day, Rowan's ship was destroying blockade runners in Hatteras. Norman C. Delaney, "Rowan," *Historical Times.*; E.M.

Nothing extraordinary occurred to-day. I had the pleasure of being introduced to Dr. Bear's Ma and Aunt—very nice ladies I wrote a letter to Mrs. Tomlin this evening.

CAMP HARMAN VA

TUESDAY SEPT 10TH, 1861.

This has been a good day. Nothing of of [sic] more than ordinary interest occurred—The report that the "Pawnee" was taken—this is false. [J.E.B.] Stuart had some skirmish lately, took some prisoners.

I am well supplied.

I wrote a letter to Aunt Malinda. I took a bath to-day and have since felt Rheumatism in my right knee.[38]

WEDNESDAY SEPT. 11TH

Evening passed quietly and undisturbed to-day—I wrote a letter to Mrs. P. Faris of Triford [39] to-day.

CAMP HARMAN

THURSDAY SEPT. 12TH

The routines of Camp life is [sic] transacted to-day as yesterday. Those men who are in Hospt. tent are very unwell. Typhoid fever. Mr. W.[Wade] D. Strother left our camp this morning—

CAMP HARMAN VA.

FRIDAY SEPT. 13TH, '61

I have been very unwell to-day. Dr. Snidow is also sick. My head has been in agony all day. I took a dose of Sulph. Morph.[40] and apparently it only tended to

---

Eller et al., *Civil War Naval Chronology* (Washington: USG.P.O., n.d. [1961]), 26, hereinafter *Naval Chronology.*

[38] This is a general term for soreness and inflammation of joints. *Taber's.*

[39] Triford was in Rockbridge Co. Ray O. Hummel, Jr. *A List of Places Included in Nineteenth Century Virginia Directories*, Virginia State Library Publications No. 11 (Richmond: Virginia State Library, 1960). We cannot identify this Mrs. Faris or her family.

[40] Sulfate morphine (now known as morphine sulfate). "The sulfate [that is, salt of sulfuric acid] of an alkaloid obtained from opium and occurring as feathery white crystals." Actions and uses are described as "hypnotic" and in twentieth century, literature on morphine sulfate carries strong caution that it "is used by drug addicts due to its action on the central nervous system."

increase the disagreeable feeling. Mr. L.W. Segus—(one of the sick) is very bad—

I wrote a letter to sister Mary E. Gen. [Joseph Eggleston] Johnston was out on a review to-day—staid [sic] on the field until Batallion Drill was over. What the object of his visit is unknown to me—Perhaps it betokens something (?).

I have had Rheumatism in my knee all day.

CAMP HARMAN, VA.

SEPT. 14TH, 1861

I am not much better this morning—a very disagreeable sensation courses over my limbs and back and seems to concentrate its force in my head. I was engaged part of to-day in unpacking some new medicines we rec'd last evening and repacking such as we do not need. The Southern Confederacy seems to be waking up a little. She furnished us a splendid medicine chest compared with what we before had. We have a good stock of medicine in hand at this time. Mr. L.W. Segus is very unwell[.] He has been treated with brandy, wine &c.

I fear I will be sick. I took a large B. Mass pill at bed time—My tongue is very much furried.[41] We received news to-day that Rosencrantz [sic] & Lee have met and Rosencrantz was badly whipped.[42]

Taber's. As noted, the extremely addictive nature of opium and the distillate morphine was insufficiently recognized during the Civil War.

[41] Blue mass pill was prescribed for headaches of undetermined cause. It was a compound containing mercury. See Stowe's comments concerning the colorful and almost literary descriptions of health providers in the era; the diarist describes his tongue not only as *furry*, but *furried.* Stowe, op. cit.

[42] William Starke Rosecrans (1819-1898) was victorious at Rich Mountain and generally fought successfully in western Virginia in summer of 1861. Cheat Mountain in Middlesex Co. controlled several mountain passes in central western Virginia, including the turnpike between Staunton and Parkersburg. Confederate General William Wing Loring (1818-1886) faced Rosecrans, but was slow to engage his forces, leading to a dispute with Stonewall Jackson. Robert Edward Lee intervened, taking command of Loring's forces in "his first operation of the Civil War." There was success for the Confederates on 10 September, but heavy rains and great confusion thereafter (some of it caused when Lee's reconnaissance officer John A. Kimball was killed before he could make a report) took away the element of surprise. Lee withdrew his troops in disgrace on 15 September, and was called in the southern newspapers "Granny Lee." Jefferson Davis withdrew Lee from the scene and sent him to South Carolina to inspect and supervise fortifications. Jeffrey D. Wert, *Historical Times.*

CAMP HARMAN

SUNDAY SEPT. 15TH, 1861

To-day passed as usual until near night when it was rumored that we would move next day.

I am no better in health—worse if anything. I fear I have had a spell of sickness.

NOTE [sic, diarist's note]

The following is remarks written all at once. I was taken with a spell of fever and did not write daily—in fact wrote none from the date of last day noticed until the 24th day of October, being then at my fathers.

On Monday Sept. 16th our Brigade was ordered to march. we marched near Fairfax Station and pitched our tents. I was very unwell. Every symptom was that of fever. I felt I was risking my life to-day with the Regiment though I have great confidence in Dr. B. as a surgeon, and I hated to leave very much. The medicine tent was pitched and Dr. Snidow and and [sic] another young man (Heankins of "Pulaski Guards") proceeded to put things in order. I was to [sic] unwell to assist. I lay down in the tent to rest and sleep for the night. On Tuesday morning I was worse—Dr. Black advised me to be sent away. I agreed to it. He sent a man over to Fairfax Station to see when the "sick train" left that point but the man did not report in time for me to get to the Station in time to take the train. Consequently no other alternative was left me but to take the ambulance to Manassas or wait the train next day. I determined to take the ambulance that night. A. T. Sanders accompanied me, another young man named Poole was also sent away. Our trip to Manassas was a rough disagreeable one. Arrived there about 9 o'clock and went into the "Black Hospital" for the night. Next morning A. T. S. [Sanders] got things ready for us to leave. We left about 7 o'clock as we thought & were told for Charlottesville. The car the sick ride in is a freight box—a horrid place for a sick person to be cooped in. The trip was tiresome enough. We arrived at Culpepper C. H. about 4 o'clock. There we were stopped by the surgeons and ordered to the Hospital. I sauntered along nearer dead than alive to what is termed the "Barracks Hospital"—a pittiful [sic] place for a sick man. This was Wednesday evening and I lay almost insensible as to my true conditions until Thursday evening without being examined by any M. D. although there seemed to be a whole Regiment of Doctors there. A. T. S. went and brought me a Physician who gave me a purgative. I asked for a furlough to go to the country which was recommended by the surgeon without any delay. A. T. S. took the recommendation and tried to get Dr. Houston to assent to my removal but he was refused. Andy's endeavours were strong and I shall never forget his kindness. I lay from Wednesday until Sunday with little or no attention, food, or medicine. On Sunday morning however Uncle Tommy came and succeeded in getting me from such a place. I hired a horse buggy & boy which cost me $3.50c: I have but a faint recollection of what occurred between the C. H. & Uncles [apparenty Thomas Apperson]—When I arrived there all seemed glad to see me.

As to my own feelings I am not aware of having any. I felt that I was ailing—I knew that disease had fastened upon me but I know not the nature or form of what my health or body was suffering. I was put in a good airy room by my kind relatives and on Monday Dr. Somerville came to see me. What passed during the next two week [sic] I recollect but little. Father and Mother and Sister all came to see me, my Uncle Joe Apperson also. I talked and conversed with them but with how much rationality I cannot presume to say. My father was to see me tollerably [sic] often but I do not remember it. Dr. Sommerville requested that Dr. Stringfellow be called in—he was sent for by my Uncle.

Of these two worthy sons of Aesculapius I am forced to note a few things having no idea that it will ever reach the ears of either.

Dr. Somerville is a man apparently some 55 or 60 years of age. He has been a devotee of pill & powder from a young man and seems fully to understand his profession. Not only does he seem to understand his calling but he has learned in his course of long experience to soothe the patient with kind words and fatherly admonitions. Being a pious man his conversation often turned in that direction. He came to see me often and after I became so that I could speak with some rationality he spent several hours with me each time he came. Medicine was often the topic or a difficult case was recited by him with some degree of pleasure to him especially if his reputation was elevated any thereby. He gave me some very good tracts one day— Presbyterian in his views he was of course a strong advocate of *Infant Baptism.* I found myself before I was aware of it liking the old Gent splendidly—was always delighted when he came.

Dr. Stringfellow a robust pompous man of some 40 years is rather cool and reserved. Has some backwoodsman-like ways—having lived in Kansas. He seems to understand what he intending [sic] doing but he has no such smooth, soft, fervent feelings as Dr. S[ommerville]. Dr. Stringfellow came to see me Regularly [sic] and I have no doubt did his duty well.

At night I was troubled with severe sweating, my clothes and the covering and cloths of the bed were often perfectly wet. This debilitated me very much and caused the Drs. to give any quantity of quinine and Arom[atic]. Sulph.[sulfuric] acid.[43] At night I lay with no covering save a sheet and kept my room cool and well ventilated. Finally those *horrid* sweats gradually lessened in power until I believe while I write they almost entirely left me.

At the end of the third week of my stay at Uncles I returned down stairs. It was a hard task though I had been eating a considerable quantity of food from the commencement of my illness, and indeed it seems as if I had an inclination for food during my whole illness.

I felt that I was mending and walked out occassionally. One evening I rode up to M. Station 1/2 miles distant. Dr. [Sommerville] came to see me that evening. I continued to improve and by the 20th of Octr. I was able to ride to my fathers in a carriage. I am indebted to my Uncle and his family for the life I enjoy now. If I had remained at the Hospt. I feel sure nothing but Divine Providence could have perpetuated my existence. At my Uncles I received every attention that a son could expect. Cous. B—was my regular attendant. As attentive as a sister and kind beyond description she administered to my wants hourly. Many nice roast potatoes did I receive at her hands. I shall ever remember her with the affection of a brother.

Indeed it may be wrong to signalise one—all were kind, attentive and affectionate. While thanking and writing of friends I should not forget the Great God of Heaven and Earth in whose power it lay to will my existence at an end and the taper of my life would have been extinguished while I lay upon a bed of sickness and the mind was left unrestrained to wander whithersoever it would I could but look upon my past life as one of sinfulness and the present as that of perfect dependance [sic] upon the goodness and mercy of a just and righteous God. I could but offer up thanks to Him that all was well with me as it was. I tried to read the New Testament daily and resolved to read it daily but through the sinfulness of the flesh that resolve has been broken.

I wrote several letters during my illness and some were written and I knew nothing of their contents afterwards. Dr. Faris and wife wrote me one in conjunction and Mrs. F wrote one wholly herself. Oh! how much good it did me to hear from such esteemed friends. They seem anxious that I should visit them but I cannot, my time is too precious and my presence and services as

---

[43] Sulfuric acid was a "colorless, odorless liquid of heavy, oily consistency" administered to attack a deficiency of acid in the stomach [hypoacidity], the symptoms of which were thought to be these "night sweats." It is highly corrosive and very dangerous, and was diluted in this case with a compound of benzene marked by its pleasant smell, and hence Aromatic Sulfuric Acid. "Sulfuric Acid," "hypoacidity," "Aromatic," *Taber's.*

demanded at the Regiment. But if the dispos[ition] of human events will ordain that I should live until my time is out then I shall make an effort to see once more the majestic hills of the South West and grasp once more the hand of those i have [been] taught to love. If peace is soon restored to our now distracted and warlike country I will perhaps settle myself.

Never since I left my fathers roof have I ever known what Home sickness was until I was sick. In thought I wandered over all the scenes I had before passed over. I longed to be at *Home*—its quiet eves around the social hearthstone or festive board a kind existence [,] daily employment were all remembered.

But to return. On Sunday the 20th Oct. I started Home—to my fathers—my brother and father were along (my brother being also sick). The road was very rough—the carriage jolted me considerably whenever it got among the rocks. Soon we came to a country the roads of which I was familiar—I saw no alteration in the situation of things. At Zoar Church [Chesterfield County] by which we had to pass it was church day and I felt constrained to stop. I entered the church and I believe everybody knew me—I knew nearly all I ever knew before. I did not remain indoors long. When I went out I had many hearty shakes. Dr. Row and myself had a long conversation. The wind was cool and I became chilly and thought it best to leave. We came on ahead of the concourse of people that were at church. When we arrived at the Grove[44] we took dinner with my esteemed friend Dr. Quisenberry. Every thing there presented the same appearance that they did in days gone by. The old Store House where I had lived and worked still stood though unoccupied. Near night we left for home—2 1/2 miles distant. At my father's domicile once more and little expected too. I had thought perhaps I might be afforded the opportunity of visiting my friends this fall but I never thought to visit them in the garb of a soldier and under the disagreeable position of *being sick*. I had fostered the hope to attend some school of medicine and if I came in direction of home then stop and see them. But our country's condition broke up all such arrangements and sank every such hope and in the place and name of a sick soldier I visited the home of my boyhood.

Monday I spent home looking around.

---

[44] "The Grove" means Locust Grove in Orange County, where he grew up.

TUESDAY 22ND—

It rained hard all day. I was engaged part of the day in writing—wrote letters to Dr. Faris[,] J.W. Kennedy[,] 1st Lieut, "Smyth Blues" & Uncle Charles Jones. The balance of the day was spent in sitting about.

WEDNESDAY 23RD

I rode out this morning in the bright sunshine. I went to the Grove and found nobody at Home. I then went to the tanyard of Thos. Johnson and from there to J.F. Almond's. He seemed glad to see me but did not recognize me at first. Things look about as they looked before. After dinner I rode over to Richard Webb's. His son has been with Gen. [Henry Alexander] Wise [in Kanawha Valley campaign] and now lays very ill—all knew me there. About sundown I went back to the Grove with the intention of staying there but Dr. had not returned and I went home at the rate of 2-40 [two miles in forty minutes]. I arrived at home a little after dark. The wind blew rather cool and I was suspicious that it would do me no good. I was very sore from my ride.

THURSDAY OCTR. 24TH

To-day myself and brother rode down to the old Wilderness to a store kept by a Mr. Sims. He was not at home and his better half acted the part of the *store boy* which was rather agreeable to me as she was rather good looking and talkative and brought a young lady along. I made several small purchases and started for home. At the store I met the Rev. M. Chancelly a very worthy Baptist preacher. He was coming up to the road consequently we had his pleasure of his company. On passing the road that leads to my fathers I invited him to turn in and dine with me—he accepted the invitation. We had a good deal of conversation—agreeing sometimes and sometimes disagreeing.

FRIDAY OCT. 25TH

To-day was spent at home. Nat & myself walked out in the fore noon and in the same capacity that Nimrod of[45] old lived and died I had the fortune to kill a

[45] Nimrod was a mythical symbol for hunters, but apparently was also a real person in early Hebraic history. In the line of Noah, his son Ham had a son Cush: "Cush became the father of Nimrod, who was the first potentate on earth. He was a mighty hunter in the eyes of Yahweh." Genesis 10:8-9. See also 1 Chronicles 1:10. *The Jerusalem Bible*, trans., Alexander Jones et al., 1966. Additional notes: Nimrod "is a character of popular story (verse 9 records a proverb) derived from a Mesopotamian mythical hero of uncertain identity." There is also a tradition that Nimrod founded the City of Babel and caused to be built the infamous Tower there whose use was

bird and a hare. When I returned to the house though I had walked scarcely a mile in all & could scarcely walk. The afternoon was spent at the house.

SATURDAY OCT. 26TH, 1861

This morning I was up very early. My father keeping up the practices of Nimrod, had been out the night previous and informed us that he had a "Coon" up an oak tree. We went and at the second shot I succeeded in bring the wiley animal from his leavy domain[46] —dead. The balance of the day was spent in doors.

My appetite is of such a voracious character that I eat so much that I am very stupid for some time after eating. I hope to be well enough by the last of next month to return to my Reg. I can hear no deffinite [sic] and reliable news here—.

SUNDAY, OCTR. 27TH 1861.

The forenoon of to-day was spent at Home reading, eating nuts, &c. After dinner I walked to a neighbours house some two miles distant. The walk was nearly as much as I could stand. The folks knew me and seemed glad to see me. I spent the evening there.

MONDAY, OCTR. 28TH, 1861.

This morning I started early to see my Grandmother. I went by the Grove and took dinner with Mrs. Robinson and Mrs. Quisenberry, then started to Grandfathers. I saw a good many things on my way that I had before been familiar with. I have seen but few changes in the country and but few of these were for the better.

I arrived at Grandfathers a short time before night—had an affectionate meeting with my aged Grandmother. She has lived the period allotted to man but looks but little different from what she [sic; did] nearly three years ago. I have a presentiment that I shall never see her more. It is not my intention, or rather I do not expect I shall visit this part of Virginia again for a long time unless I am taken sick again. My interests and feeling seem to be elsewhere. I

---

curtailed when the unbelieving people of Babel were caused by Yahweh not to be able to understand each other. Thomas Bulfinch, *Bulfinch's Mythology* (New York: Doubleday, 1947) 310.

[46] Leafy home. Archaic usage, *leavy bowls*, sometimes poetically repeated in 19th century. "Leavy." *OED.*

promised Mrs. Quisenberry to-day that I would be see [sic] them again Tuesday afternoon.

I was very much affected to-night by my aunt's husband (Wright) coming home under the influence of ardent spirit [alcohol]. He is a good workman—brick layer by trade—. Oh! the misery! The misery ardent spirit brings upon the human race.

TUESDAY, OCTOBER 29TH 1861

I walked out this morning. The weather is very fine now. Nothing but what might be expected passed to-day. Until evening—conversation &c. with my relatives.

I bid them adieu, perhaps for the last time and started for Locust Grove where I arrived only a short time before night.

Dr. Q. came home after dark but had to leave in a short time—such is the life of an M.D.—he requested that I should remain until he returned. I was entertained by his lady rehearsing the events that had transpired in their immediate neighborhood and with which they have had connection since I left the county.

Retired late.

WEDNESDAY OCTR. 30TH, '61

This morning I read some of Professor Watson's latest *edition* on the practice of Med.

Dr. [Quisenberrgy] came near noon—but a few moments at Home when called to leave. He requested me to ride with him as it seemed impossible for us to have a chat at home. I rode some 7 or 8 miles with him to see a lady affected with *tonsillitis* and then returned, passed home and went to see a *man* in another direction. The trip was made pleasant and short by interesting conversation—at home again about 8 o'clock.

THURSDAY, OCT. 31ST, '61

To-day I rode with Dr. again in his breakaway[47] , to see a young man some 11/2 miles distant. We stopped at Wilderness to purchase some articles—I was

[47] Also called *break* or *brake.* A large wagon or wagonette, mostly a frame and usually without sides, used for breaking in horses. By the 1870s, the term means a kind of large wagonette, but given the time and place, it seems Quisenberry is using a horse-training break to make some of his rounds. "Brake, Break." *OED.*

invited to take some domestic wine made by a lady in the neighborhood and it gave me a severe headache so I did not spend the remainder of the day pleasantly. Went home— took dinner and rode out again. I was very drowsy and tired—Retired early.

FRIDAY NOVR. 1ST, 1861

This morning rose with the sun. The headache of yesterday had left me. After breakfast I walked home and when I arrived at home I found myself very much fatigued. I had promised to visit a neighbor and asked sisters to go with me which they did. We found Mr. Webb and family at Home and family well—all knew me.

After supper Mr. Webb & myself got in conversation on the various doctrines of the different churches and the proper mode of administering water for the washing away of man's sins. He being a Missionary Baptist of course upheld immersion. During the conversation he advanced a good idea that strengthens a much disputed point. Those denominations that practice the different modes of baptism that the application of water is simply fulfilling a command and it matters not which of the three modes is practiced. Mr. Webb says that it is but fulfilling the command and it does seem that Christ was baptised in the river Jordan and probably immersed then immersion is the application of water and for fear that sprinkling or pouring might not do it is best to be immersed.

I retired late—Raining very hard.

SATURDAY NOVR 2ND 1861

Rain is still falling very fast. The day must be spent indoors I have become tired of the *smart children* there and came away though it was raining very hard. My feet and legs were wet. I am very sorry to see ...[entry to diary stopped here].

SUNDAY, NOVR. 3RD, 1861

This is a wet morning though the sun shines very beautiful. I concluded to go to church—New Hope. Myself and father were ready and started about 9 o'clock. I found many old acquaintances there but feeling such anxiety to return to my post at Manassas. I did enjoy much pleasure from seeing them. The minister's text was "if the trumpet give the wrong sound who shall prepare for battle." I considered the text as badly handled by the preacher. [48] His first subject was death—the common lot of all men—its uncertainty—its terror—the horrors of the grave and [illegible phrases of six words] for the universal tyrant. Next was an obligation to seek mediation between God and man, and repentance through faith, and baptism typical of the death of the Savior. Finally the much harassed point as to the validity of sprinkling and pouring [in baptism], the admission into the church of non-professors of religion and predestination and election or the "final perseverance of the saints.["] All this from a text that, to me, leads to not even one point refered to. The Sacrament was administered—Politics had their share of mens' attention outside.

We came home—I had anticipated to visit Mr. H. Roach but was too late in arriving Home. Should be able to leave for my Reg. on Thursday.

MONDAY NOV. 4TH, '61

This morning I rose with plans laid to visit some friends and do some business also. I went to the *Tanyard* after a pair of boots, called at "The Goodes", had [visit with] Mr. and Mrs. Robinson—Mr. R[obinson] gave me a pair of yarn socks—very very acceptable in "times of war". At home to dinner after which I started to visit Mr. H. Roach—found him at home and about to pay me a visit. Mrs. R[oach] seemed glad to see me as did all the children. The greater part of the evening was spent in social chat—when Mr. R[oach] & myself[.] [W]alked over to his brother's a short distance across the fields. He was not at home but his pious feeling would not allow us to leave until we had a little supper. After this was over Mrs. Reynolds & lady came in and we spent a pleasant evening. The old Squire came in however an hour or so before we left. He being all wit and humor much more was added to the pleasure of the evening. His daughter Ann is something like her father in wit and is a very handsome clever girl. Near two o'clock I left them with many good wishes for my welfare in future. From there to my father's I had a dark muddy lonesome walk.

---

[48] Specifically, sounds from two different trumpets signaled specific and different actions, viz., assembling, charging in battle, and disassembling. The signal from the wrong trumpet could lead forces to charge at the wrong time, or to disassemble when the charge was needed. The image is in Numbers, but St. Paul in particular uses the image to make certain points. See Numb. 10 : 1-10; Joel 2 : 1, 5; 1 Th. 4 : 16; 1 Cor. 15 : 52. See also notes, *Jerusalem Bible*, ed., Jones.

TUESDAY, NOVEMBER 5TH, '61

As I had before anticipated I started, in company with my father, to Uncle Tommy's from where I propose starting to my Regiment after a day or so. The [Rappannock] River had been very high in consequence of the rain on Saturday and we concluded it more safe to go by Germans bridge and go up the River. I found it a long tedious road.— Once we were lost and had to retrace our steps for some miles or so. Stopped at Mr. S. Stringfellow's at Raccoon Ford [49] and purchased some articles and then pursued our trip and arrived at Uncle's a short time before night—To-morrow I wish to spend at his house— Rec'd three letters Mrs. Tomlin, A. T. Sander's & J. W. Kennedy.

WEDNESDAY NOV. 6TH, 1861

To-day has been spent chiefly in the parlour with my cousins. I have been kindly treated by my Uncle's family & though I am too poor to do anything that would return the same in in [sic] the same spirit it was done; yet I have a memory that [I] will not forget—such kindness with me will [n]ever sleep in oblivion's tomb.

I have determined on to-morrow as my day for starting to the field hoping in the meantime that the God of our Universe will dispose events so that I shall be able to reach my Reg. in safety and stand the winter so that my service will benefit my country and our cause.

I hate parting from friends but to-morrow as yesterday I leave some that I may never be permitted again to see. I left the home of my boyhood amid the tears of mother, sisters & brother, but God's will be done. War news—or anything reliable is scarce with me. It is reported that the Southern Confederacy is sending troops to Kentucky—I hope it is so. I would like to go and be one in the ranks of our brave boys to break the fetters that now holds [sic] Virginia's first-born[50] the iron grasp of tyranny.

I am writing at 9 1/2 o'clock p.m.—will retire in a very short time.

---

[49] A town on a ford of the Rappahannock River in Culpeper Co. Hummel, *A List.*

[50] In order to allay fears of relatively small states and thus ratify the constitution in 1787-1789, large eastern states such as Virginia and Massachusetts relinquished claims on western territories; Virginia relinquished claim on a huge section of today's Upper South and Midwest, and the first state organized from that territory was Kentucky, settled mostly by Virginians and thus "Virginia's first born."

THURSDAY, NOVR. 7TH 1861

The weather is fine now. I arose about sunrise. The air is fine and healthy. I have anticipated starting for Manassas to-day and will if nothing occurs. Uncle's folks seem somewhat anxious for me to remain with them a day or so longer but duty forces me to leave.

It is one of the painful necessities to part with those who have acted the part of friends when we are in ill health or in distress. So it was with me. I left my cousin and matronly aunt in tears though not 'till I had embraced each with a kiss. Uncle accompanied me to the spot where I got on the train for Culpeper C. H. I reported at the Hospital and found all things right. I eat and slept in the Hospt. for the night.

FRIDAY, NOVR. 8TH 1861

This morning I procured a passport for Manassas and left Culpeper at 1/2 past 2. I was in company with a young Lieutenant from South Carolina—Jos. L Rarden 7th S.C Vol. Corp. [Milledge Luke] Bonham's Brig.[51] —he was quite a nice young man. When I got to the junction of the two roads I found the 5th & 27 and 2nd Regts. of our Brig. *en rout [e]* for the valley of Virginia and learned that the 4th and 33rd would be along next day. I procured through the Kindness of the guards stationed with our baggage lodging and food until the regt. arrived.

Manassas seems a Second Babylon[52] in regard to some—Splendid houses are being erected for the army that will winter at Manassas.

News from the south is very discouraging. Accounts have reached us that the Northern fleet has made a formidable attack upon Port Royal [S.C.]—evidently

---

[51] Bonham (1813-1890) of Red Bank, S.C., graduated from South Carolina College (today University of South Carolina), practiced law, entered politics, and was active in battles with the Seminoles and in the Mexican War. He was elected to state assembly and to US Congress. He served bravely at First Manassas, helping to hold the center of P.G.T. Beauregard's line, but later quarreled with professional soldiers and left the army to become war governor of S.C. In that capacity he subdued those in the hill counties who were opposed to the Confederacy. Leaving war governorship in 1864 he returned to the army as cavalry officer. Edward G. Longacre, "Bonham." *Historical Times.*

[52] The Biblical account of Jewish captivity and exile in Babylon (ca. 597-538 B.C.E., the so-styled "seventy years of exile," even though it was only about 60 years), a rich and powerful empire, was often used by nineteenth century Protestants in their imagery. There is a hint in Apperson's notation here that with such luxury and opulence inevitably come slavery and dissolution borne of disbelief, thus a Second Babylonian captivity for believers.

intending to land at Savannah. The yankee programme seems to be a winter campaign in the south.

The prevailing opinion among our boys is that we will attack the yankees at Romney [53] which is the cause of our Brigade moving to the [Shenandoah] valley.

SATURDAY, NOV. 9TH, '61

The 4th Regiment arrived this morning but no conveyance seems ready to convey the 4th away. I walked around among the soldiers establishments—great [illegible] and wrote two letters—one to Papa & one to cousin Bettie. Rain commenced falling before evening and fell nearly all day—I am afraid it will be bad for us—our boys have no shelter to protect them. Cars could not be furnished to take them away to-day, and consequently the men must content themselves as best they [can] without food or shelter.

Several of the company, myself included went to the Station and ordered an oyster supper. We returned to camp about 10 o'clock and found the soldiers lying like swine in a bed although the ground was soaked by the rain that had fallen during the day. A. O. S[anders], J.W. K[ennedy]—Bradley Willmore & myself went to a fence in the neighborhood and made a large fire and sat by it 'till morning—I took cold—.

SUNDAY NOV. 10TH, '61

This morning we expected to leave early but in this we were mistaken. A train of cars ran up but there was not room enough to take the whole Regt. and three companies were left behind and did not not get off until the middle of the after-noon—the "Blues" were one of the three. Our trip was an interesting one. Many fair ladies were along the road which gave new beauty to the inspiring mountain scenery. Several camps are situated among the hills of the Blue Ridge—mostly for convenience of Hospital purposes I believe. Night came on before we passed Piedmont in Faquier County, and the remainder of our trip to Strasburg was performed after night. But the moon shone beautiful and bright giving to the gigantic cliffs a silvered appearance to our attentive gaze. The hills looked like terrible monarchs of ages and the deep ravines and gorges looked dark and gloomy. We arrived at Strasburg about 9 o'clock. Here all was mud and confusion. Some went to cooking but I went in search of some place to rest my sleepy frame. I found a half filled freight car and spread my blankets for a

[53] Possibly Rodney, in Bedford Co. Hummel, *A List.* Romney is not in Valley.

nap, however uncomfortable I might find my lodging place. I was called up to supper—drank a cup of warm coffee and lay down again and had a good nights rest .

CAMP 2 1/2 S.E. OF WINCHESTER.

MONDAY NOV. 11TH, '61

This morning six months ago we left this place and travelled the same road to Winchester. Much has transpired in our nation's history since then. We have under went [sic] arduous duties, encountered difficulties of no small degree—But that is now in the past and is looked upon with no small degree of indifference while we look ahead for more prosperous and brighter days. We are upon the track we went before and have new energies and bright hopes: but how soon these energies may be crippled and wasted and these hopes cast to the ground by disappointment no mortal tongue can tell. All the men believe they are going to Romney [Rodney?] to attack the enemy.

The day was pleasant and although I had not fully recovered my strength since my illness I followed the regt. on foot for a walk of some 14 or 18 miles. Soon after leaving Middletown in company with some friends I turned aside to a farm house to get something for my digestive organs to work upon. We stopped at the house of a Mr. David Miller and found a splendid meal and something to stimulate for those who partake [.] as I never indulge I asked to be excused. I never saw the Regt. any more that day 'till I found it in camp near a village called Kernstown[54][.] weary and worn out I sought a place to rest. Many of our boys seemed not to care for the march for hours after I lay down the three monotonous note of Sambo's[55] favourite instrument mingled with the revelry of camp. Ardent spirit had shared in making merry this day. A blanket on the wet ground and a blanket above made me a bed. We camped in a wood.

TUESDAY NOV. 12TH 1861

This morning I found a good fire when I left my bed of blankets and reported for duty—to commence next morning—The usual routine of camp-life was all that transpired to-day. I wrote two letters—one to Dr. F. & one to Dr. Q.

---

[54] Frederick Co. Site of numerous skirmishes in the next three years.

[55] Sambo was contemporaneous slang for African American, and was a profound insult. The instrument was the banjo, then associated with African American music more so than southern white music.

I have good—comparatively—lodging now. I have a cold.

CAMP NEAR WINCHESTER

WEDNESDAY NOV. 13TH, '61

Up early for "sick call". The sick list is not very heavy now. Timothy Hawkins will help me in the surgery. Nothing unusual passed.

THURSDAY NOV 14TH, '61

Nothing worth noting to-day. I learned that Loring's Brigade was on the way to join us. If true I am glad—some good friends of mine are in his command. This evening shows badly in the weather department, an[d] about dark rain commenced falling in torrents. I wrote an article for the "Visitor" [Marion newspaper] this evening.

Received a letter from Cousin Bettie containing one from Mrs. F.—

FRIDAY NOV. 15TH, 1861

Still raining and cold. I purchased two coats to-day—intend keeping warm if possible. After "sick call" I was engaged posting books. My tent is very damp and we made a large fire in front and made a bed of live coals in the center—it is very confortable now. The rain is still falling while I write —. I will write Mrs. F a letter and retire

CAMP NEAR WINCHESTER VA

SATURDAY, NOV. 16TH 1861

Old Aolas [Aeolus] [56] seems to be spending his fury this morning with vengeance. Every thing is on wave. To all appearances tents will suffer. The wind continued to blow all day. Trees were filled on every side and all day burning fires glistened on every side. Nothing unusual occurred during the day.

---

[56] From Homer's *Odyssey*: "King of the Aeolian Islands, father of Halcyone; appointed by Jupiter [king of all the Greek gods] keeper of the winds and later considered to be the wind god. He receives Ulysses hospitably and gives him, tied up and made harmless in a leather bag, all the ill winds, which are later let out by his companions." *Bulfinch's. Aeolian winds* is a common image in the Romantic era poetry and fiction that Apperson favored.

CAMP 2 1/2 S.E. OF WINCHESTER

SUNDAY, NOV. 17TH, 1861

The Sabbath day but no difference here—the wind is still blow [sic]. I spent nearly all-day in conversation.

No preaching in camp that I know of.

CAMP 2 1/2 MILES N.E. OF WINCHESTER

MONDAY, NOV. 18TH, 1861

This morning after "sick call" I went to Winchester with some sick men. Our men are very much exposed here and the effect is very obvious at "sick call". Twelve were sent from our Reg this morning.

I remained in Winchester several hours making some few purchases. Many fair girls were promenading the streets[.] I arrived in camp near night. We move to-morrow. I wrote two letters to-night—one to Mrs. Tomlin and one to Mr. Jno [illegible; Ernells?] at the request of his son who is sick in Hospt.

CAMP 2 1/2 MILES N.E. OF WINCHESTER VA.

TUESDAY NOV. 19TH, '61

We did not move to [sic] was anticipated yesterday. The Brigade has but few wagons and all them were engaged moving other Regiments—perhaps we will move to-morrow. For my part I am very well satisfide [sic] where we are. We will be further from town. Nothing unusual occurred to-day. I wrote a letter to Uncle Charles after night.

CAMP 2 1/2 N.E. OF WINCHESTER VA.

WEDNESDAY, NOV. 20TH, 1861

This was a pretty morning. Things go on as ususal. I had some short words with Dr. C[rockett]. this morning about keeping the Report books—he seems "monarch of all he surveys[.]" I was engaged writing in register to-day. We did not move.

Our company as well as others in the regiment has some members that indulge too freely in the use of ardent spirit. I have seen and noticed that its use become more extended every day—lately, at times, half the company seemed drunk, but I hope a stop will be put to so disgraceful a habit. Ja[mes]. T[homas]. came to my tent to-night and seemed anxious to quit the habit—D.

W. Venable proposed to draw up a pledge for the benefit of the company—he said he would sign it without hesitancy and use his influence to get others to sign it. J. W. Kennedy and myself drew up and 30 signed their names and took it to get others to put down their names. Oh what a blessing if the damning use of alcohol could be stopped in our army.

CAMP 2 1/2 N.E. OF WINCHESTER, VA.

THURSDAY NOV. 21ST

Nothing unusual occurred to-day—. The dull routine of a camp-life is gone through each day alike.

We are still waiting for orders to move to another camp. Much anxiety is expressed by the soldiers in regard to winter quarters—they fear they will remain in tents the whole winter.

CAMP N.E. OF WIN VA.

FRIDAY NOV. 22ND, 61

We were ordered to pack up this morning and move to another camp. We marched out about 8 o'clock and took the road to Winchester. How desolate and lonesome a camp looks after being left by an army! While at the camp we left this morning the weather was very cool. The wind blew hard and keen prompting the men to cut down a great many trees for fuel. Piles of immense logs—whole trunks of trees—were constantly burning[.] And when we left, the grounds around presented quite a ragged appearance. The man that passes there will see our mark for years to come[.] And indeed will not such marks be visible throughout Virginia? Our feelings morally temporary and socially will also receive marks from the hand of the war.

Many "fair ones" crowded the doors and windows of the houses in Winchester to look at us. How sweet to the soldiers to see the smiling faces of ladies greeting with smiles and bidding them God speed on our mission. It brings to my mind the friends of home and their association.

It strengthens and tightens the bonds that bind me to those whom I have learned to love. How we ought to live in—in the army different to what we do really life [sic; his exact words; the sense is that the standards of good conduct at home are lost in the army for many of the men].

I know many fond parents and looking sisters are deceived in the walks [conduct or manner of living] of a son or brother, believing and hoping as they doubtless do that all is well when it is not—many are drinking to the dregs the sinful cup of pleasure. How many mothers would be made glad and sister's fears would be banished if they only knew that their sons and brothers were living a sober attentive life in camp!

I walked along with the Regiment 'till we arrived at Winchester. There I was detained a short time to make some purchases and I did not overtake it again 'till our new encampment.

We stretched our tent and I laid down early—We have a very good encampment here—water and wood convenient.

CAMP 4 MILES E. OF WINCHESTER, VA.

SATURDAY, NOV 23RD '61

This morning was dark and cloudy rained some during the night—after the morning wore away pretty well the clouds dispensed and the sun shone out bright and warm With the help of D. W. Venable, Hawkins[57] and myself built a flue or furnace in my tent. It operated finely.

I read some and gosipped some until late—I wrote a letter to Capt. C. W. Beatie and wrot [sic] up my journal. My tent is very comfortable now.

CAMP 4. E OF WINCHESTER VA.

SUNDAY, NOV. 24TH '61

This is sabbath at Home but here in the army no one knows it but in name. Our chaplain is sick and we have no religious services in camp now. The day has been spent with me as it [should] not be spent. Reading and talking with some transient visitor soon wore the day away. It is night now. A part of the Regiment is now resting in quiet, careless slumber while some linger yet around the fires as if loath to give up its inticing warmth. The cry of the "Sergeant of the guard" sometimes aroused the stillness of the night. How careless some men seem. From their joyful and gleeful manner one would think the thought of home never pervaded their breasts. Others again are morose and sullen—pining for home and ever cursing the fate that finds them here. How varied are the inclinations and dispositions of man.

---

[57] Probably James Hawkins of Smyth Co., one of the first men to join the Smyth Greys. Presgraves, ed., *Smyth Families*, 9. The Hawkins family lived in the Chatham Hill settlements on both sides of the North Fork of the Holston River as it came through Smyth Co. *Heritage*, 210.

I look back at home with a wistful eye, all its enjoyment—all its clustered sweets and its bounteous pleasures are fresh and vivid in my mind. The pleasant emotions of social and mutual privileges are still green in memory but I look again at my country's bleeding conditions and I am content. I am almost forced to believe that I will soon become [sic] to love the life of a soldier. Its varied changes of fortune and misfortune, the goings down and uprisings all have their sweets and bitters.

Should my time [of army hospital enlistment] expire & I am still a healthy man I think the next enlistment for me will be during the war & sink or swim live or die.

I have been reading in a copy of the "Southern Litany Messenger".[58] I am delighted with it—one piece on female education is finely written.

I wrote two letters to-day—one to Bro Nat and one to Cousin Bettie. I am writing in my journal late—I will read the above and retire.

MONDAY NOV 25TH, 61

Clear and beautiful. I was up early—the day wore away as do the most of our time—I have time to study some but I find it almost impossible—so many interrupting me every few minutes. Capt. [Alex G.] Pendleton [newspaper editor and organizer of the original Smyth Greys] drew money for our company to-day. Rec'd the "Marion Visitor" [Pendleton's newspaper] and hear good news from our side in the North west[that is, northwestern Virginia and southeastern West Virginia].

I do not know what to think of my friends—I get no letters. The health of the Regiment is not as good—Parotitis[59] is prevailing to a considerable extent.

---

[58] "Variety" magazine founded in Richmond in 1834 by Thomas W. White. The magazine originally featured a combination of short stories, poetry, feature articles, literary reviews, and opinion. The poet Edgar Allan Poe became editor in 1835 and brought national attention to the magazine with his own poems and with his sometimes sharp-tongued reviews of poetry. In 1840 Matthew Fontaine Maury, an oceanographer and naval officer and later important leader in Confederate navy, joined the editorial team and transformed the magazine into one more focused on southern political issues rather than a variety magazine. Although Maury was gone from the offices by 1850, the *Southern Literary Message* became increasingly political and increasingly sectional where once it was national and literary. It continued publishing until 1864, growing more strident in defense of southern politics as the war went along. Neil T. Storch, *Encyclopedia of Southern History*, eds., David C. Roller and Robert W. Twyman (Baton Rouge: Louisiana State University Press, 1979); hereafter, *Encyclopedia*.

[59] "Inflammation of the parotid gland [salivary gland that extends to a point near the ear, hence parotic], either simple or epidemic. Synonym, mumps." Taber's. This case was epidemic.

CAMP 4 [MILES] BELOW WINCHESTER VA.

TUESDAY NOV. 26 1861

To-day the reg. was given the privilege of going to Winchester to see the execution of a soldier according to the usages of war. They avowed that he had attempted to take the life of his captain. He had fired upon him and wounded him severely. For this he was tried [,] condemned [,] and to-day he dies. How sad to think. A wife made a widow [,] 4 helpless children made orphans [,] and a man doomed to die an ignominious death by one rash unmeditated step. And worse, Ardent spirit did the deed. Fried a brain and put into the heart of the man to do that for which he now pays the penalty with his life.

Many availed themselves of the opportunity of going to town. Lieut [James W.] Kennedy & myself walked up but the execution was over. The condemned man was then before his maker.

We returned to camp late. I drew 26$ of my wages this morning.

WEDNESDAY NOV. 27TH '61

I went to Winchester, to-day to assist Dr. B with some medicine stores—He turned some over to the proper authorities.

I returned to camp about night.

THURSDAY NOV. 28, '61

This evening is cold and frosty. I was engaged putting up a bed to-day. I heard to-night that [John B.] Floyd's men had retreated back towards the Va & Tennessee Railroad. I wrote a letter home to-night and one to Dr. Faris. Raining now.

FRIDAY, NOV 29 '61

This is to some extent a damp morning but the appearance of the cloud seemed to fashion a pretty day but it was not. Nothing unusual took place. I ate breakfast with Capt. Edmondson[.] [60] We eat only twice a day. To-night our orderly came to me with a subscription to raise money to present Maj. Gen. Jackson a fine sword. Our company had subscribed some sixty dollars but for my part I had none to give for that purpose. It is true Gen Jackson has led us

[60] Possibly William Edmondson of Smyth Co., Co. A, 23d Va. Inf. Bn, John Echol's Brigade. However, Edmondson was listed as sergeant. *Smyth Co. Families*, ed., Presgraves, 10.

bravely on the battle field and has proved himself worthy of any and every gift that we can bestow—he merits honor and esteem and his valor and magnanimity as a general demands admiration from every one. But I am poor—there are poor men among us whose families are at home depending upon charity for support and if I have [money] to spare let them have it. It is now late—I have just returned from a patient with Cramp Colic. I have been posting our Books to-day—Read Gross' Surgery to-night.

Raining now.

CAMP STEPHENSON VA.

SATURDAY NOV. 30TH, '61

Raining slightly this morning—mud is plenty in camp. Cramp colic seems to be almost an epidemic among our soldiers now. Owing perhaps to the dampness of the weather and exposure Parotitis is going the rounds now. I am well so far except the appearance of something growing upon my breast just below the left nipple. What it is I cannot imagine. The first knowledge I have of the presence of such a thing was during my illness at my Uncles [sic]. It first felt about the size of the end of my little finger and was very sensitive to the touch. It continued to grow and is now about as large as half an egg and seems to be either incorporated with the costal cartilage[61] or firmly adhered to the rib—being utterly immovable. I have been using Vol. Liniment [62] upon it. I have been engage [sic] upon the report of this month.

I received a letter from my friend Mrs. Tomlin—She is a good woman to write me—it is pleasure to me.

I have plenty of company each night in my tent.

I retired late.

CAMP STEPHENSON VA.

SUNDAY DECR. 1ST, '61

Again we are permitted to breath[e] the pure air of another Sabbath morning and I feel the cool fresh and healthy breezes. How thankful we should be to our heavenly father for his mercy. But we are careless and unconcerned. I

---

[61] Costa is Latin for rib. Costal cartilage is cartilage in the rib. "Costa." *Taber's.*

[62] Vol. stands for volar or vola, having to do with the palm of the hand. The liniment is spread by the palm of the hand, or may be applied to the palm of the hand or the sole of the foot. Later volar and vola are replaced by the terms palmus and palmar. "Vol." *Taber's.*

have been hard at work every hour to-day[.] But necessity compells [sic] me to [work instead of recognizing the Sabbath in worship, reflection, and thankful rest].

I recd. two letters to-day. One from my brother at Centreville, Va, and another from Dr. V. Q[uisenberry]. Dr. writes me that my youngest Brother is severely attacked by Erysipelas [skin inflammation]. I am sorry to hear this. To-night I have had a good many visitors—good fellows though.

I think there will be rain or snow before morning.

CAMP STEPHENSON VA

MONDAY DECEMBER 2ND

I have been engaged to-day in writing our monthly report. Nothing unusual occurred. Camp-life is becoming monotonous.

TUESDAY DEC. 3RD '61

To-day as yesterday all is the same. I heard to-day that the yankees had fared badly at 'Evansport Battery'. I do not put much faith in the report. But I do really fear that we will have some hard battles soon. The weather is quite cool. Among the visitors to our camp are some very pretty ladies who condescend to show their faces occassionally. I am not much acquainted with the ladies in this section.

I finished my report to-day and wrote a letter to-night to send Dr. Faris by Mr. Fudge[63]—Who is in our camp at this time.

Things go on tollerably [sic] smoothly in camp now.

CAMP STEPHENSON VA

WEDNESDAY DECEMBER 4TH 1861

Mr. Fudge left for home this morning, I gave him "25" to take to Dr. Faris. I have been engaged in making an inventory of all we have on hand at this time. I got a letter from cousin Bettie[.] Uncle and his employer have fallen out terribly. Uncle will not remain longer than this year. I am sorry for Uncle and family.

---

[63] Possibly Granville Henderson Fudge (born 1841) of Marion, 1st Lt., Co. D, 4th Va. Inf. After the war, Fudge returned to Marion, serving for 9 years as Commonwealth Attorney. Presgraves, ed., *Smyth County*, 30-31.

I loan [sic] Lieut. Kennedy $20 last night[.] He is on a detail [assignment] for baggage

CAMP STEPHENSON, VA

THURSDAY DEC. 5TH, 1861

This has been a lovely day. Nothing unusual has occurred in camp. I have been busy all day—nearly finished taking inventory. There is considerable sickness in camp now. Parotitis [probably mumps] has been going the rounds.

I wrote a letter to night to cousin Bettie. It is after 10 o'clock and I will retire soon.

CAMP STEPHENSON

FRIDAY, DECR. 6TH, '61

The weather is fine now—I was much joyed to see Capt. C. W. Beatie of Smyth[64] in camp to-day. He hails from Centreville and reports that there is a great probability of a fight there. [General William Wing] Loring's Brigade or a part of it is at Strasburg [Shenandoah Co.]— our wagons started over to transport Baggage but were turned back at Newtown [Frederick Co.] and to-night they march again on the same mission. I got a letter from sister Mary.

Diptheria has made its appearance among our men. We have 3 cases and I greatly fear we will have it badly.

CAMP STEPHENSON VA

SATURDAY, DECR. 7TH '61

I am not in possession of any important news to-day. I was engaged writing a communication for the "Visitor[.]" I feel stupid and inactive. I have before mentioned a growth on my left side. It continues to grow and is painful to me at night especially when I make a deep inspiration [breathe in deeply], sneeze or cough. Its presence bears heavily upon my mind. From all I can gather from my knowledge and thc books it must be a fibro cartileginous tumor or some disease of the bone.

I retired late.

---

[64] Probably Clairbone Watkins Beattie of Smyth Co., one of the first captains of a volunteer group from Marion who eventually were brought into the Stonewall Brigade. Wilson, *Smyth Co.*.

CAMP STEPHENSON VA

SUNDAY DECR. 8TH '61

This morning I arose and found myself very unwell[.] I rested very badly last night. I have parotitis —my jaws as swollen [sic]. I have some unpleasnt feeling in regard to my health.

I rec'd. a letter from Mrs. Faris to-day. She invites me to come home at Christmas but an attempt to go home would inevitably end in futility. It would be almost infinite pleasure for me to see my dear friends but I cannot.

Heavy firing was heard in direction of Harper's Ferry[.] We are ignorant of the cause.

Linclon's proclamation is out. I have not seen it.

CAMP STEPHENSON

MONDAY, DEC. 9TH, '61

I am worse this morning. My jaws are swollen very much and I slept but little during last night. The weather is good.

No news —

CAMP STEPHENSON, VA

TUESDAY, DEC. 10TH, 1861

No better to-day. I am suffering no little pain indeed. I am too ill to write on passing events now.

CAMP STEPHENSON VA.

WEDNESDAY, DEC. 11, '61

Not much change in my jaws, and little in our every day affairs.

CAMP STEPHENSON, VA.

THURSDAY, DEC. 12, 1861

I feel something better now. I hope soon to be well again and once well of mumps one is not likely to be attacked again soon. I wrote two letters to-day—one to Nat and one to Dr. Quisenberry, and rec'd. one from Dr. F.

I understand the Confederate congress offers a premium up to 12 months to volunteers if they will reenlist at the expiration of their time and form themselves into companies and regiments. They are to have 50$ in cash and 8 weeks furlough. I think it wise and liberal on the part of our congressman.

Our cavalry took 9 of the enemy one day this week. I understand yankees are pretty thick about Romney [West Virginia panhandle then claimed by CSA and by Virginia commonwealth] and along the Potomac.

CAMP STEPHENSON VA.

FRIDAY, DEC. 13TH, 61

I continue to grow better. News reached us to-day that Charleston S.C. was on fire and burning rapidly—If true it is greatly to be lamented by us. I hope however much of the report will be contradicted.

CAMP STEPHENSON

SATURDAY DEC 14TH

I do not feel as well this morning owing to indiscreet eating yesterday. Nothing new has transpired within my range. I rec'd a letter from Mrs. F. to-day[.] I wrote a letter to Mrs. Tomlin to-day.

CAMP STEPHENSON VA.

SUNDAY, DECEMBER 15 '61

Last night some suspicious orders were given in regard to supplies for the soldiers &c. Every thing predicted a march and sure enough this morning we are ordered to hold ourselves in readiness. Our medicines are packed and ready to be moved. Rev[e]ille sounded on the morrow morning at 3 o'clock. Where we will go I know not, it is presumed by some to Martinsburg and others are fancying a fight with the enemy at Romney. It is rumored that reinforcements have been sent the enemy at Romney and if we go there to fight then we will have a hard fight. However our boys will fight a good fight just at this time. they want winter quarters and think a hard fight will be the means of getting them. The operations of the enemy seem to be not very active at this time—only waiting perhaps for an opportunity to "steal a march".

We had preaching in camp to-day by a Mr. Shelburn from Montgomery. His sermon is energised very much. I had not the fortune to hear but little of it. What I did hear was good. He spoke of our dependance [sic] upon God both individually and nationally. Then of God ['s] power in assisting those who call upon Him and deserve help. He dwelt with some degree of eloquence upon the occasion of Gods sending the destroying angel into the assyrians [sic] camp and smiting those who we[re] about to oppress His people[.]

Then with many exhortations to the soldiers of our army—to do our whole duty as men—both in camp and in battle he closed [.] An aged blind man named James Sterrit arose and attempted to address the audience a short time[.] I did not remain to hear him conclude.

CAMP NEAR MARTINSBURG

MONDAY DEC. 16 '61

Rev[e]ille sounded this morning at 4 o'clock, the encampment was soon alive with voices. Breakfast over and tents struck and a short time before sunrise we marched of[f] in the direction of Martinsburg[.] The morning was clear and pleasant though cool. The 2nd Reg led the way and the 4th followed with the other regiments of the Brig following in their respective places. We marched to within 2 miles of Martinsburg and camped near the big Spring. Our tents were pitched on the oposite [sic] side of the road where we were about the 1st of July last. The wind blew so hard that our tents were nigh being upset. What the programme will be to-morrow I know not. We have a number of boats along, evidently for something.

POTOMAC RIVER

5 MS. ABOVE WILLIAMSPORT VA.

TUESDAY DECR 17, 1861

This morning the soldier was up early and preparing breakfast. The men were speculating as to where we were bound[.] About 10 o'clock we were ordered to march. All the shovels, spades, axes &c were taken along also the the [sic] bedding and cooking utensils. We marched off at noon and took our way through Martinsburg down the main road. It stood very evident then that we we[re] going as many had promised to destroy dam No. 5 on the [Potomac] river heretofore strongly guarded by the Enemy. A short distance below Haynesville [Richmond Co.] we came to the point where a skirmish took place in July. Many trees were shattered among the boughs. Some two miles below Haynesville we turned to the left and marched in direction of Little Georgetown. After marching some 3 or 4 miles in that direction we were halted and informed that we had taken the wrong road and therefore we had to retrace our steps. We then marched in an Easterly direction until we came to the house of Capt. [R.T.] Colston [of 2d Va]. We camped in the wood between his home and the river. Rigid silence was enjoined upon us by the General. Reports say that the enemy is in pretty large [force] just beyond the river. I lay down in the ambulance with J. D. Hawkins and napped—I was not well and did not rest easy.

POTOMAC RIVER

WEDNESDAY DECR. 18TH, 1861

Last night a detail was made to commence operations on the dam and the axes soon rang loudly through the woods. The enemy soon discovered what was transpiring and commenced pouring bullets down upon the workmen. The fire was kept up until near night at which time I am now writing and the firing is still progressing. We were ordered from our position to a mile in the rear where we cooked some provisions[.] A cannon was seen and heard firing in direction of Williamsport [on Maryland shore of Potomac].[65] The cause and result of which we are ignorant. The 4th Reg. goes on picket to-night. I am writing about 2 o'clock. We went on picket duty this evening[.] We marched in direction of the mill and halted behind a large hill. The firing continued on both sides till [sic] night though I think without [sic] but little damage to either party. I learned we had one man wounded in the shoulder. The object for destroying this dam is to render useless the canal. This dam is one of the most important on the river and when destroyed the canal is emptied some 25 or 30 miles. The enemy is among the hills on the Maryland side and in the canal using the bank as a breast work. Our men can only get down to and from the mill after night.

It is thought the work at the dam will be completed to-night[.] We are lying very composedly in the wood. A detail with pick axes and hand spikes passed on towards the dam.

They were halted by a sentinel and asked who they were when a wity Irishman said "Faith and this is the *dam* detail colonel"[.] A company (Rockbridge Rifles) from the 5th Reg are in the mill protecting the workmen. I slept in the ambulance

---

[65] Brigadier Gen. Samuel Gibbes French, then of state ordnance, Virginia, CSA, reported on this firing from Federal forces on Maryland shore, 15-17 Dec., *Official Records* 1, 5:469-70.

POTOMAC RIVER

THURSDAY DEC. 19TH, 1861

This morning before I was up the Yankees opened [fire] upon the Mil [sic] with a piece of artillery. Four balls passed through the mill house which routed the boys, one making his escape at a time and as he ran up the hill whole volleys were fired at him. We could tell when ever one would leave the mill. He would have to run the gauntlet for some distance. All escaped but one—he was shot before he got through. Several bombs were fired over us but none did any harm[.] Two pieces of "Pendleton Battery" (Capt. McLaughlin) were brought out but the Gen. [Stonewall Jackson] would not allow them to be fired.

We were relieved by the 5th Regiment about 12 o'clock and marched out in an open field some distance in the rear. Our men and the Yankees were exchanging shots almost every minute[.] We could see both parties as they fired. The Yankees seem to lurk in the neighborhood of a large barn on the Maryland side. Gen [sic] Jackson took a piece of artillery and gave the barn a few shot. We have been expecting the Yankees to fire into our camp as they could do it very easily from several points on their side. It is said that the enemy has a good force and is in command of Gen. Dix. [66]

I wrote to Dr. F. this evening and rec'd. a letter from Uncle Charles.

The Regiment an[d] baggage moved near the river again to-night. Our camp fires and the Yankees are in sight . The Yankees fired the mill and the light prevented our men from working on the dam. The hard working are Irishmen and Gen. Jackson furnishes them spirit—they are the men to do the work!

ON THE POTOMAC

FRIDAY DECR. 20TH

This morning we marched to our cooking place and spent the day. Gen Jackson is determined not to leave until his work is done. The day was very cold. The [Smyth] "Blues" go on picket to-night [.] [A]fter dark the regiment was ordered near the river again. Sharp firing took place between our artillery and

---

[66] John Adams Dix (1798-1879), from Boscawen, New Hampshire, served in the US Navy in the War of 1812 as a fourteen year old. After naval service, he entered New York politics, becoming prominent as a Jacksonian Democrat and filling an unexpired US Senate term by appointment to 1850. A railroad entrepreneur, Dix reentered politics in the James Buchanan administration and, when Lincoln was elected and Civil War began, he received commission as major general of army volunteers from the newly elected Republican. A large army installation in southern New Jersey is named for him. Russ A. Pritchard, "Dix," *Historical Times.*

the enemy. One of our artillery men was slightly wounded on the leg by a piece of bomb. The "dam detail" went to work again to-night.

Our boys have been firing at the Yankees to-day as they did yesterday. Someone remarked to Gen. Garnett [67] that his men were fighting the Yankees without orders[.] He said that was all right. He liked to see men willing to fight and he came down there to fight.

ON POTOMAC RIVER

SATURDAY DEC. 21 '61

This morning is really a cold one. We have orders to march at 6 this morning[.] The dam was finished last night. We marched off with a scanty breakfast. We moved toward the main road very rapidly. An instance is worthy of note just here. I was somewhat roused this morning. Yesterday Lieutenant Sayers of Co. A. [68] took a poor harmless prisoner and brought him to H. Q. He was sent to the guard house for the night and had it not been for the kindness of some of the "Blues' he would have suffered from cold. This morning he came trudging along under arrest[.] I was sorry for the poor man and more so when I knew him to be the warmest friend we have in this section. He is an humble miller at Little Georgetown and while we were there treated us kindly. He had never seen so many men together before and saw his first cannon. He looked on with some degree of interest and was seen by this Lieut. whose zeal is beyond his discretion and love of for [sic] humanity and was arrested. Capt. Pendleton vouched to Maj. Kent for the loyalty of the prisoner (Mr. Laprose) but it did no good. The Lieut who arrested him wished to do something notable but treated a friend badly—We gave him protection from the cold chilling night air. The prisoner seemed to regret that he had been taken by his friends but maintained good humor all the while. He was set at liberty this morning and left us by calling God's blessing down upon our heads.

---

[67] Richard Brooke Garnett (1817-1863), attended West Point and graduated with his cousin Robert Selden Garnett (the first general of either side to be killed in battle (July 1861). A veteran of Seminole Wars, Garnett did not fight in the Mexican War; he fought successfully as a brigadier general, but quarreled with Jackson during the Shenandoah Valley Campaign of 1862 when he felt compelled to retreat before a large Federal force. He was part of the famed Pickett's Charge at Gettysburg; although too sick to walk, he rode in the front of his troops and was killed near the stone wall at Cemetary Ridge. His body was never recovered. J. Tracy Power, "Garnett," *Historical Times.*

[68] Possibly John A. Sayers, an original member of Smyth Volunteers and Smyth Blues, Wilson, op. cit., 235.

We took the Mcadamized road through Martinsburg to the place [where we] left our tents. Here we remained all night[.]

News reached us to-day that Mason & Slidell[69] have been demanded by England[.] Every one is looking towards England with a hopeful eye. It remains yet to be seen what England will really do.

CAMP STEPHENSON VA

SUNDAY DECR. 22ND 61

This morning is one of the coldest we have had. We left our camp and came to the old encampment again. The chimneys had fallen down and lay about in heaps. The ground looked like the site of some town now covered in ruins. The air is very cold.

I had my tent stretched and repaired my chimney, and am once more ready to deal out pill or powder. The weather is very cold now but I do not expect anything better than tents this winter.

CAMP STEPHENSON VA

MONDAY DECR 23RD, 1861

This morning the wind rose so that I could have no fire in my tent on account of smoke. Last night it rained and hailed and every thing was covered in sleet. I was engaged making our monthly report for October the original being lost.

The wind rose higher and still higher until I thought our tents would certainly go, but they did not.

News reached us of a fight at Dranesville a few days ago[70]—the fight terminated somewhat disastrously to our side.

---

[69] James Murray Mason (1798-1871), a northern Virginia aristocrat and graduate of the College of William & Mary, served as ambassador to England, as did John Slidell (1793-1871), a New Yorker who moved to Louisiana and rose to prominence in politics there. The two were sailing to England and France on a diplomatic mission on the British registered *Trent*, when they were captured and removed by Federal naval forces. Many Confederate observers presumed that the incident, coupled with British popular anger over the blockade that deprived mills of southern cotton, would bring England into the war on the side of the CSA. However, the men were released and tensions eased. Slidell and Mason then continued on, to France, where they won great sympathy but failed to gain French assistance. Patricia L. Faust, "Mason" and "Slidell," *Historical Times.*

TUESDAY DEC 24TH '61

This morning the wind still blows hard. I wrote two letters to-day—one to Dr. F. and one to Father's family. I rec'd. one from R. H. Dungan. He was at Mt. Jackson on his way to Strasburg. I hope to see him soon. I predict something will be done in this section soon. A pretty good force is collecting here. Some rumors of a ma[r]ch [sic] is in camp.

Tomorrow is Christmas[.] How sad and [illegible] here in camp! I presume many will get on the *limber* order[71] before to-morrow night. I promise myself no extra pleasure[.] I shall remain in camp I think.

CAMP STEPHENSON VA

WEDNESDAY, DEC. 25TH, 1861

Another Christmas is here. The gay[,] the buoyant and the pleasure seeking are an empire within themselves and enjoy as much of lifes sweetmeats as if they know not that every Christnmas draws them a year nearer to "that bourn from which no traveller returns"[.] [72]

Things are much more quiet in camp than I supposed they would be. There is some suspicion that we will not tarry here many days longer. We are being reinforced by Lorings Brigade.

I rec'd. a letter from my brother at Centreville.

CAMP STEPHENSON VA

THURSDAY DECR 26TH 1861

I have been engaged at our monthly report again. I wrote to R H D this evening. I steal a few moments and devote them in the perusal of Watts

---

[70] Dranesville is in Fairfax Co.; there was an engagement there on 20 Dec. In late Nov., Union cavalry had made an "expedition" to Dranesville; but this late Dec. fight was of smaller scale and did not make as much of an official registration for Union or Confederate records as the diarist does here. *Official Records*, 1, 5:448-49; 1128-29.

[71] Apparently, he means to say, relax by getting very drunk, hence *limber* in a later day's sense of *loosened up*.

[72] Shakespeare: "The undiscouered Countrey, from whose Borne No Traveller returnes." *Hamlet*, III, i. More probably Borne means here 'the frontier or pale' of a country [where before Shakespeare it meant "destination"]. *OED*.

"Improvement of the mind".[73] So far I have examined the work and am capable of judging it a is [sic] most useful work. The truth it teaches and the various characters it presents are evidence of a work of no mean merit. The small differences of right and wrong are so nicely and explicitly arranged that to see error and observe justice is rendered comparatively easy. But I should remember the teachings of the work or book I commend. And Watts says we must be slow to [illegible; sense of phrase is *accept*; but that is not the illegible word] a work and not be positive until we have pursued it in all its ramifications and viewed it in every light.

CAMP STEPHENSON VA

FRIDAY, DECR. 27TH 1861

The wind rose last night and was blowing furiously this morning—the day promises to be a cold disagreeable one. I have been writing all day. The enlargement on my side of which I have before spoken seems to be coming to "a head"—suppuration is evidently taking place so I hope it will develop nothing serious. [74]

Our boys received a lot of boxes from home this evening. When they were opened every one was anxious to see what his dear friends at home had sent him. Many received excellent clothes, some apples, cakes &c. I was among the unfortunate—got nothing a coat from Francis Taifer in Marion. However I do not complain. My friends in Smyth have done me many favors.

The progress of the war is rather slow. The prevailing opinion is that we have to go to Romney soon. Gen. Loring's command is in camp on the road leading from Winchester to Romney. So far as I am concerned and so far as my feelings go I had as soon go to Romney as anywhere. It is hardly probable that we will

---

[73] Isaac Watts, *The Improvement of the Mind* (1674. Reprint ed.; Morgan, PA: Soli Deo Gloria Publications, 1998). Watts wrote this discussion of the mind from the perspective of the evangelical Christian interested in the humanities and in a faith-based reason. Each of the perspectives is important to the diarist.

[74] Suppuration is the forming of pus, usually from an abscess created by liquid formed around dying white blood cells. Apperson may have had erysipelas [Gr., red skin], "an acute febrile disease with localized inflammation and redness of skin and subcutaneous tissue accompanied by systemic disturbance." Now treated with penicillin to kill the infectious bacteria, magnesium sulfate solution compresses on the red and swollen skin, and aspirin for pain, erysipelas is seldom a great threat. However, before penicillin was developed, the treatment was to await the bursting of the abscess, a procedure that sometimes caused the pus to enter the blood stream and cause a much greater infection. "Suppuration; erysipelas," *Taber's*.

see much rest and as to going into winter quarters except in tents I can hardly hope it.

CAMP STEPHENSON VA

SATURDAY DEC 28TH, 1861

I am still writing and likely to be for several days yet. The monthly report, quarterly report, and yearly report are all to be made off and handed over to the proper authorities, also returns to send in of medicine on hand [,] condition & c and what has been used and unavoidably lost.

Cold to-day—. I got a letter from Mrs. Tomlin. She writes more familiar every time. She goads me some about being low spirited—I will answer in a few days. To-night I washed a shirt and two kerchiefs. I can wash very well I think.

SUNDAY, DECR. 29, 1861

This morning is a beautiful one. The weather has been remarkably good and I hope it will continue so during the winter.

This day I know many of our friends are at home quietly enjoying its luxuries. I know that many earnest prayers must be offered up from the Home Altar. Would to God that the wickedness of our persecuors would come to and [sic] end[;] that all those now isolated from home and friends would enter into domestic peace.

I spent the day sauntering around camp. I commenced writing letters about night and wrote 3.—one to Dr.[,] one to Mrs.Tomlin and one to cousin Bettie. I also got one from cousin Bettie. Our comrade in arms—B. F. Leonard came in camp from Winchester this evening. He has a furlough for 30 days and will leave for home to-morrow. He has been ill for a long time. I hope his trip will be pleasing and beneficial to him. He will take my letters to Dr. & Mrs. F. I propose sending 20$ to Dr. F.

D. W. Venable[75] offers to lend me the amt. 'till I draw.

We are daily expecting orders to march. Some conjencture that we will go to Romney. Some think to the "Hanging Rock" and others hope we may go into more comfortable quarters.

---

[75] The Venable family operated a dry goods store at the depot in Marion, and D.W. Venable may have been related to R.J. Venable, the patriarch of that family business; Marcellus P. Venable was a partner of Capt. Pendleton in the newspaper business, and D.W. Venable may have been related to him.

Wilson, *Smyth Co.*, 166-667.

MONDAY, DEC. 30, 1861

This morning is clear and cool. B. F. Leonard left us—I gave 20$ for Dr. F.

I also drew 20$ from Capt. P. and handed it to Drury [W.] V[enable]. I have been engaged the larger part of to-day in mending my overcoat.

The enlargement on my left side was opened to-day by Dr. Black. Very little pus escaped. I am glad to see a deposit of pus for I fear it might terminate in something serious. I poulticed it [76] and hope soon to find it well.

J. M. Thomas is making an effort to get up a company to man heavy artillery—the condition under which the men volunteer is that they receive the bounty and furlough offered by congress. He is progressing favourably and I hope he may succeed. For my part I hope the company will not be raised although I was on the roll.

The Mason & Stidell case seems to excite some of our "boys". I do hope England will speak out and let us know to what extent they are for or against us.

(Note)

(The following incidents up to Christmas were not [illegible] at the time of occurrence or daily as they should have been on account of marching steadily. A note was taken however as they occurred.)

TUESDAY DECR. 31, 1861

When the the [sic] hour of midnight was summoned by Time's [illegible] the Old Year departed and another came in. I was engaged all day on reports—quarterly & monthly. I made an effort to draw my pay for my stewardship to-day but the little caring pay master was too nice for me to be prepared for him.

We received an order to-night to be ready to march to-morrow morning at an early hour. The packing of medicines were left to J. D. Hawkins. I did not get through my work till near midnight I then retired to rise early.

---

[76] Poultice is from Latin for "thick paste." "A hot, moist mass of linseed, mustard, or soap and oil between two pieces of muslin applied ot the skin to relieve congestion or pain, to stimulate absorption of inflammatory products and to act as a counterirritant." *Taber's*.

WEDNESDAY JAN 1ST, 1862

[He speaks to the year of 1862, anthropomorphizing it.] Bright, beautiful New Year's morn[,] a bad state of affairs you find[.] [C]an it be that you will pass away and leave our country as you found it[?]

At 3 o'clock reveille sounded and we rose to prepare for the march. About 6 o'c. we marched off towards Winchester. [77] We had supposed we were going to Martinsburg but now we were at our wits end—about a mile from camp we turned abruptly to the right on a very rough road. "We are bound for Romney," said some but I could not believe it. I supposed we were going to another camp where fuel would be more plenty [sic]. In this I was mistaken. The road we traveled was a rough one and led us onto the pike across the Allegeheny some 4 or 5 ms [miles] from Winchester. The wagons were much retarded by hills. Some of them upset and some broke.

The road across the mountains is a good one. We passed through Pugh Town [Frederick Co.] to-day—It is a poor looking place, apparently every house is a century old—No improvements are there beyond what the simple wants of an unostentatious simple people need.

Soon after we left this village we found we were not going to Romney. Taking the road to the right we were told that it led to Bath. [78] Some 1400 of the enemy were in camp there.

We camped on a high hill on the land of a Mr. Collins. The wind blew hard.

THURSDAY, JAN. 2ND, '62

This morning we were detaned [sic] some time waiting for the wagons. Some of the Company's wagons did not get up 'till this morning, consequently they had no blankets to cover with and no *grub* for supper or breakfast. Two 24-pound guns were on the road and one was stuck fast in the mud all night which stopped the wagons.

---

[77] Historian E.B. Long notes that McClellan was ill and Lincoln himself was effectively in command of forces in the area of Federal northwestern Virginia [soon to be the State of West Virginia] and northern Virginia around the Federal capital. Long also says, "Stonewall Jackson was on the march despite winter weather...on what is often called the Romney Campaign." Everette Beach Long with Barbara Long, *The Civil War Day by Day; An Almanac, 1861-1865* (1971; paper reprint ed.; New York: Da Capo, 1985), 157, hereinafter Long, *Civil War Almanac*.

[78] Town in Sheanandoah Valley county of same name; Jackson aimed to destroy the rail lines of the Baltimore & Ohio Railroad and also dams on the canal operated by Chesapeake & Ohio Canal Co. Long, *Civil War Almanac*, 157.

Gen Loring's command came up to-day. I saw the "Smyth Rifle Grays". They boast of seeing hard service and I suppose have and indeed they look rough enough for it.

I had the pleasure of friend R. H. Dungan's company to-day for some 5 or 6 miles. He is a choice fellow.

We passed over some horrid roads again to-day. Near night I thought I would try some house for a meal. B. F. Sexton and I accordingly *flanked* on a house in the country and called for a snack. The old lady said "God bless your souls yes you shall have something to eat" snapping her eye and talking alternately. We thought for sure we would get some good eatables now; but surprise was great when the stingy old soul came to us with a cold dry loaf of bread and cut two thin slices for us and a little girl followed in the rear with two pieces of what people in this country call *pudding*—we minced a while and started [out again on their march]. We had not gotten far before we met a "Smyth Blue" and some others in company with the old man of the house. He wanted to know if we had had something to eat. I told him, yes a little. He said come back and we should have as much as we could eat. Hoping to see the other boys chagrined we went back. This time we got a pretty good meal. Mr. Dix, the gentleman of the house gave me many items of Yankee outrage. He had hid his most valuable property and was sleeping in the woods at night. We also saw Mr. Buck who had been a sufferer. Finding the Yankees and union men were after him he packed some trunks with clothing and valuable papers[.] [H]e started away but was overtaken and his goods taken, he barely saved himself by taking to the woods.

Our camp to-night is near Unger's store at the crossroads. His (Mr. Unger's) store had been robed [sic] , and he forced to run and leave his family. The 4th Reg camped upon the side of the mountain. The camp fires gleamed brightly on every side.

FRIDAY JANUARY 3RD, 1862

The troops started early this morning but the wagons were detained until Loring's command passed. The wagons traveled slow. The train was at least 5 miles long. I went into the country and got my dinner near Oakland [Louisa Co.] and the people in this country are poor and somewhat illiterate. The illiteration [sic; illiteracy] may somewhat account for the Union grounds they have taken. They have been led and duped by a politician such as [John]

Carlisle[79] and others until they are with difficulty made to believe anything. They begin to see the war strength of the South and perhaps will not have the same confidence in others that they have heretofore had. To show the ideas these people have of strength in an army I will note what a man said of our numbers. He said he certainly saw 75,000 men pass when realy [sic] we only had between 12,000 and 15,000 and he saw not more than half the amount.

We had to travel very late in order to overtake the troops. There was a large creek which crossed the road some 7 or 8 times and in order to give the drivers a chance to drive with safety—it being very dark—large fires had been kindled so near each other that the light of one reached that of the other. Indeed the quantity of fence destroyed was shameful.

About 8 o'clock snow commenced falling and fell rapidly for a while[;] then turned to hail and rain. I felt very unwell. Staid [sic] in Capt. Whitescarver's[80] tent with a good stove.

The 1st Tennessee Regiments and a part of the 48th Va. met with a party of Yankee scouts this evening and had quite a skirmish. We lost some three or four killed or wounded and took 8 prisoners. Gen Loring asked permission to go ahead in order to give his men a trial. The Ark. and Tenn. troops are hard looking customers. The 1st Tenn. is armed with rifles throughout.

SATURDAY JAN. 4TH, 1862

This morning an advance was made upon Bath[.]] Loring's command went straight forward[,] a body of malitia [sic] on the left and Ashby's cavalry on the right.[81] We had hoped to capture the whole command of the enemy but they eluded our grasp and escaped.

We marched into the village a short time before night. The village was soon hunted over and but little was found. Some overcoats shoes tents &c were taken, also two pieces of can[n]on. The library and paintings and drawing implements

---

[79] John Carlisle (b. 1815) of Augusta Co. issued petition protesting the secession convention, broadside, 15 January 1861, broadside coll. 4714, VA. St. Library, *Southeastern Broadsides Before 1877; a Bibliography*, Virginia State Library Publications No. 33, ed., Ray O. Hummel, Jr. (Richmond: Virginia State Library, 1971), 397; *Va. 1870 Census.*

[80] Possibly Charles T. Whitescarver (b. 1823) of Blacksburg Township, Montogomery Co. , VA. *1870 Census Index.*

[81] Turner Ashby (1828-1862) was a cavalry general from Rose Hill in Fauquier Co. A volunteer who raised a cavalry force, Ashby had little formal training, but performed well for Jackson in this Bath campaign and eventually was given command of his own force in the Shenandoah Valley, where he was mortally wounded in the spring of 1862. John E. Stanchak, "Ashby," *Hist. Times.*

of the author, "Porte Crayon" (Alias [David Hunter]Strother) were captured. He is now on the staff of Gen. [Nathaniel Prentiss] Banks at Williamsport, his father owns the property of the Berkeley Springs at Bath. [82]

The village, though on the border of one of the poorest countries I ever saw is nevertheless a handsome space. The streets walks and aisles are capacious. The Hotel is an excellent one—new and well arranged. The Springs seem warm, or at any rate warmer than any running water I ever saw.

The 4th and 2nd Regiments were quartered in the hotel for the night but it was not so comfortable as the wagons did not come up and we were without blankets and there were but few fireplaces. Provisions were scarce also. I had eaten no breakfast except a piece of cold bread and meat and drank a cup of coffee and no lunch and no supper but: "a contented mind is a continual feast." [source of quote unknown, possibly a bowdlerization of Proverbs]

I found books in an office once occupied by a Yankee. I took some of them.

SUNDAY JANY. 5TH, '62

This morning we were marched back some half mile to get breakfast. I felt badly having sat up all the night before. We marched toward Hancock in Md. and stopped in about a mile of the river. Some can[n]onading took place between ou[r] side and the other. Little or no damage was done us and I know nothing about the other. The enemy seems to be pretty numerous about there.

Alpine Depot was taken and a good many valuable stores found. It is generally supposed that Hancock will be bombarded by our forces.[83] I

---

[82] Strother wrote and drew caricatures under the pen name Porte Crayon. He was opposed to secession, and urged that Unionist counties of northwestern Virginia, especially in the eastern panhandle of West Virginia become part of the new state. An early volunteer, he served in the Department of West Virginia commanded by New Hampshire transplant and Wheeling, WVA railroad man Benjamin Franklin Kelley (1807-1891) in a unit whose main function was to guard the lines of the Baltimore & Ohio RR. Banks (1816-1894), who commanded all Union forces in this area of the Sheandoah, was a self-made businessman from Waltham, MA and a leader in the northern Democratic party. Lincoln supported him, despite poor generalship in skirmishes with the Stonewall Va. Brigade. He was later transfered west to serve successfully under Grant in Mississippi campaigns. Cecil D. Eby, Jr., "Porte Crayon's Quarrel with Virginia,"*West Virginia History*, 21 (1960): 65-75; idem, ed., *A Virginia Yankee in the Civil War: The Diaries of David Hunter Strother* (Chapel Hill: UNC Press, 1961); Michael T. Cochran, "Banks," *Hist. Times*.; Jeffrey D. Wert, "Kelley," *Hist. Times.*

[83] Jackson's Va. Brigade won skirmishes and took materiel from several sites near Bath: Slane's Cross Roads, Alpine Depot, Great Cacapon Bridge, and Sir John's Run. Jackson was then successfully driving toward Hancock, as diarist opines; but his final target was Romney. Banks's

understand the citizens [of Hancock] have had warning. We have two 24-pounders and can throw shells to some extent. I stayed in Cpt. W's [Whitescarver] tent again to-night. Snowing again.

MONDAY, JANUARY 6TH, '62

This morning something of a backward movement was commenced. The Regiment marched in some two miles of Bath and halted. I was with the ambulance. The road was so slippery and thickly crowded with ambulances wagons and artillery that I was about 1/2 day going some 2 m[ile]s. Pretty heavy can[n]onading from the other side was kept all day.

Some few days ago two bottles of whiskey were stolen from me and this morning more was gone. This caused an investigation of the wherabouts it went and two men were returned to ranks.

The enemy killed and wounded some two or three of our men to-day. Co. A 4 Reg. was detailed to-day to take charge of the battery of large guns.

TUESDAY JAN. 7TH 1862

This was one of the most trying days I have yet seen. The Reg. was held back in order that the train of wagons could be in front [.] I kept the ambulance back and regretted it afterwards. The road became so blocked up that we could not get along at all scarcely. Gen. Jackson was out in the road with the teamsters managing the horses and pushed at the wheel Jehu-like.[84]

I drove on in front of the Reg. 'till about 2 or 3 miles from town when the Reg. left me to come with the slow going teams. The horses were often down flat

---

troops were essentially operating under the orders of Lincoln himself, since McClellan was ill, apparently with typhoid fever. Long, *Civil War Almanac*, 157.

[84] There are several Jehus in the Bible, but the diarist is probably talking about the "son of Nimshi." The prophet Elijah selected this Jehu to replace Ahab as ruler of Israel because the son of Nimshi was "zealous for Yahweh," he "driveth furiously," and he was determined to eradicate the worship of Ba'al. He metaphorically "drove" and pushed the wheel himself, and he killed many who served Ba'al. Ruling around twenty years, he accomplished much in moving Israel to a kingdom dedicated to monotheism. However, the Biblical images are not wholly good ones; there is some suggestion that Jehu was zealous more for himself than for Yahweh, that he was too bloody in his assaults, knew nothing of mercy and less of common sense and may have overindulged bodily pleasures. The diarist is thus again somewhat ambivalent about T.J. Jackson, who here is compared to a ruler who "driveth furiously" but not necessarily on behalf of divine plan, perhaps only out of his own personal human vision. Jehu is described in both chapters of Kings, but especially 2 Kings 19:14, 17. See also Herbert Lockyear, *All the Men of the Bible* (Grand Rapids, MI.: Zondervan Press, 1958) 180.

on their sides—men could not march without falling on the icy road. Gen. Loring had his command [that is, his part of the army] rushed on and stopped the wagons of the Regiments. The road got wors[e] and worse. Mr. Snodgrass of Co. A let a 24-pound gun pass over his foot and I had to take him in charge and no surgeons to attend him[.] I traveled 'till after two o'clock and stopped at the house of a Mr. Miller.

His wife was a plain good woman. I dress[ed] the injured foot and sat a while before the fire. [some words crossed out by diarist.]

WEDNESDAY JAN. 8TH, 1862

I sat by the fire 'till day came and I begged the woman of the house to give us some breakfast which she did. I was sorry for one thing however. When the lady went to her meat house to get some meat she found the soldiers had stolen half she had. The 1st Va. Reg. was close by her house. I presume they took it. It is wrong for our men to do so.

We were up and of[f] early and got in front of the wagons and artillery. The roads were worse if possible than yesterday. Both horses would sometimes fall at once. We crossed one creek some 8 times and had to break the ice. We often turned out into the fields. We got to camp near night at the crossroads. Here I found the Reg. having marched that distance (17) [miles] the night before. I was on business seeing some sick off to Winchester and compounding some medicines. We are having a great many sick now. I think it would be beneficial to the service for the men to be put into winter quarters now. Many hope that we will bring the winter campaign to a close soon.

THURSDAY, JANUARY 9TH, 1862

This day was spent in camp. Nothing was done except to send off some sick. Our army is in a bad condition. This trip will not remunerate the C.S.A. in my opinion.

All seem to be expecting a move towards Romney now. We are here at a point where we can go either to Winchester, Martinsburg, Romney or Springfield. Some conjecture that the men will not follow old Jack to Romney but this is all gammon. [85]

I have no doubt but they would follow him wherever he might see fit to lead them.

---

[85] "humbug, rubbish, ridiculous nonsense 1805." *OED.*

I wrote a letter to Dr. F. to-day and rec'd. one from Mrs. F. also.

FRIDAY JAN. 10TH 1862

This morning we prepared to move our encampment. The place we have is a muddy wet place.

The appearance of further movements changes every day. We infer from certain things that we will soon stop for the winter. It is reported that the Colonels from this Brigade rec'd furloughs. If this be so could it be that we will continue to travel?

I hope we will soon leave this dreary looking country. Rain and mud. Every thing [sic] is racking with a cough—many of our men are down with pneumonia—our army is becoming crippled from sickness. We moved upon the Martinsburg Pike about 1/2 mile from Unger's Store.

SATURDAY JAN; 11TH 1862

We sent 14 men to Gen. Hospt. this morning. I heard that the 1st surgeon called for transportation for 250 sick and an Arkansas Reg. for about 150. How long can we stand this? Our army will soon be reduced to a meagre force.

The rumor is current to-day that Bath has been reoccupied by the enemy again. Furloughs have been granted to-day to two privates[,] one commissioned and one commissioned officer in each company for 12 days. Furloughs are selling for 20$ among the boys. A. T. Sanders, Mr. Parish, R. C. Vaughan and Lieut Gibson get furloughs from "S. B. Co" [Smyth County Blues]. Raining again this evening.

I wrote a letter to Dr. Q[uisenberry] to-day.

SUNDAY JAN 12TH, 1862

Nothing unusual took place to-day. We are expecting a move soon in some direction. I wrote to Uncle C[harles]. Jones in Miss[issippi]. and my Brother at Centreville [Fairfax Co.]. I rec'd a letter from Mrs. F. dated 16th Nov.

MONDAY JAN 13TH, 62

Last night I was up nearly all night seeing to such sick men as would probably have to go to Winchester. An order came for us to send them off to-night but we could get no transportation for them.

This morning at an early hour we made preparations to march. We learned that we were going to Bloomery Gap to-day. Where that is no one knows. We started through mud & c and took a westerly direction—towards Capon Mountain.[86] The road was in a horrid condition and we traveled slow. The 1st Brigade was in front. It is said that the Yankees have left Romney. Some think that we will go to Blommery Gap and then we can go either to Winchester or Romney. We travelled about 10 miles and camped on the creek near the furnace.

It is very cold. [A] great many of our men have gone to Winchester of their own accord.

TUESDAY JAN. 14TH 1862

Last night it snowed again and this morning the clouds look dark and glowering. We still march onward and that we are going to Romney is now a fixed fact. The wagons go ahead of the troops to-day. We crossed the Capon River and soon after North River. Leaving Capon Mountain in the rear we entered a country something better in appearance than what we had seen for the past few days. I think the most beautiful mountain scenery I ever saw was seen to-day. The snows lie on the ridges and in the ravines which added to the prominence of view. I could see every rise and fall along the whole [range?] as far as my eye could search.

At the "Cross roads" the teams waited some time for the troops to come up. At this place the Yankees burned a storehouse about a week ago. Hampshire Co. [West Virginia but still claimed by Confederates, and with a sizeable number of Confederate volunteers and sympathizers] is ruined by the vandals that overrun her. I hope they have left not to return again soon.

We camped for the night about a mile beyond the cross roads and about 14 miles from Romney.

---

[86] Capon Mountain and Bloomery Gap are in what became West Virginia; but much of Capon Valley and of the Capon River that runs through it is in Virginia. The Capon Depot Road on which the diarist traveled is in Shenandoah Co. Hummel, ed., *A List of Places.* Although those on the Mountain were loyal to the Union and generally fought in blue, a number of men in the Capon Valley formed Co. F in Imboden's Cavlary Brigade. commanded by John Daniel Imboden (1823-1895), Staunton native and graduate of Washington College who moved west after graduation and became active in land speculation and also secessionist politics. Imboden became well known for his bold and slashing attacks, especially on Baltimore & Ohio railroad lines in area. Maud Pugh, *Capon Valley, It's [sic] Pioneers and their Descendants, 1698-1940* (Capon Bridge, WVa.: private printing, n.d. [1946-48]); Emory M. Thomas, "Imboden," *Historical Times.*

It is very cold and the clouds threaten us with falling weather. I procured some roughness[87] and hay for a bed in Capt. W[hitescarver]'s tent.

I rec'd. letters from Cousin Bettie and Mrs. Tomlin.

WEDNESDAY JAN 15, '62

Such a time none of us have ever seen—rain hail and snow falling rapidly. Many of our boys are without tents and shoes. We will endeavour to make Romney to-day.

We started off early. The wagons went in front but the regiment soon overtook and passed them. The 4th Reg. was not more than one third its usual size and only 2 captains. The road is very wet and slippery.

We passed the ruin of many houses lately burned by the Yankees[.] One was a fine steam tannery about 6 mis. east of R[omney]. On making Romney we passed some fortifications of the enemy though they were trivial looking affairs—only erected for a feint I suppose.

Romney is a deserted looking place. Situated as it is among some picturesque mountains forming something like a triangle around it. The town seems to have had some aspirations before the war, the houses lately built are good ones. But of all places I have yet seen there is more filth here than any of them. Not a street, walk, aisle, hole or corner but some putrifying pile and stinking mass is visible. The houses used by the enemy are worse than can be described. The Court House was used as a sort of Commissariat and was filled with rotten meat & c. The citizens are generally of the Union stamp and some seem rather odd in expression.

THURSDAY JAN 16TH 1862

Our men were all quartered in houses yesterday. I got a tollerably [sic] good [illegible; house?]. In a room adjoining mine is one containing a quantity of medicines, tents, harnesses and Hospital furniture which was taken from the enemy. Nothing of interest occurred to-day. The enemy destroyed a large quantity of ammunition before they left. It is said that the Yankees are at the mouth of Patterson Creek and are unable to cross the river. Wrote to Dr. F. to-day.

---

[87] Cornshucks for bedding. "De Vere, *Americanisms*. Roughness in South Carolina denotes shucks or cornshucks, on account, probably, of the roughness of the serrated blades." *OED*.

FRIDAY JAN. 17TH, 1862

This morning I assisted Dr. McGuire med. director[88] to pack and lable [label] such stores as come under his charge. They were sent to Winchester. I have been busy giving out medicine. Being alone I am very much confined[.] [Illegible name] has been turned over to his Co. This evening orders came for the men to cook a days rations and be ready to march at any time.

SATURDAY JAN. 18TH, 1862

We did not move last night and this morning it is raining terribly. The weather is some what warmer than usual. I have a severe cold and cough. The growth in my side has suppurated[89] and is now almost well.

I wrote to Dr. Quisenberry this evening.

Some think we will be ordered back to Winchester soon and there remain 'till the winter is over. It is presumed also that Gen. Loring's command will remain here.

SUNDAY JAN. 19, '62

This morning rain is still falling. The streets are in a horrid condition—sloppy and slippery.

I have been writing to-day. Attended church in the evening. The Rev. Dr. Foote[90] preached this morning but I could not go to hear him. The gentleman that preached this evening was unknown to me. He was in uniform—quite a picture to see in the pulpit. He read and sang a hymn commencing "The promises of my father will evermore stand good."

---

[88] Hunter Holmes McGuire (1835-1900) was a native of Winchester and longtime friend of T. J. Jackson. Son of a prominent physician, he earned medical degrees at Jefferson Medical College of Philadelphia and at Medical College of Virginia in Richmond. Before he could begin his career, the war came, he enlisted, and Jackson chose him to be brigade surgeon. McGuire wrote several sketches of Jackson, and is one of those most responsible for the images that the public has of the general. John E. Stanchak, "McGuire," *Historical Times.*

[89] The abscess has burst and discharged most of the pus. As noted, in 19th century, such suppurations were allowed to occur with no intrusion; in 20th century medical world, such abscesses are aggressively lanced and drained and then the area is carefully cleaned and protected because of the danger of infection if suppuration does not take place at once. "suppuration," "abscess," *Taber's.*

[90] Possibly the Rev. William Henry Foot of Fairfax Co. (born 1800), *Va. Census Index*, i.; *Va. Historical Index*, ed., Swem..

He then preached from Heb. 2 ch. 3 v. "Why will you neglect so great salvation as this?" [91] He argued the greatness of this salvation tendered by God to man. God alone was capable of such a plan of salvation through the blood of his Son. He spoke the merits of Christ's blood and and [sic] how elaborate the way of salvation—how finished before the saviour yield up the Ghost. Then why neglect it—why neglect that for which such precious blood as Christ's was spilled for. The plan of salvation was one that man could never conceive of and yet how easy. Not like the heathen with their sacrifices of human blood to Moloch or Juggernaut. [92] "Then" said he "it is complete and easy and is now offered to every one, take it or perhaps the spirit may cease to strive the angel of mercy may plume her wings and leave thee alone. To-day is the time. All the past is in eternity for where are thy yesterdays? In eternity! Where are thy tomorrows? In eternity! So all that is left you for penance and prayer is the narrow space of to-day."

His sermon was an edifying one, and the first I have heard in church since Nov. How sweet the minister's voice sounds in the narrow limits of the church. It is musical as it strikes the walls around and is reflected back to the ears of the listeners. So like home and its quiet.

MONDAY JAN. 20TH, 1862

I have seen mud and rain but never in my recolection [sic] have I seen so much as here. The mud is every where above and below. Rain falls rapidly day and night. The streets are like muddy pool.

---

[91] "How shall we escape, if we neglect so great salvation; which at first began to be spoken by the Lord, and was confirmed unto us by them that heard him;" Hebrews 2:3 (KJV).

[92] Moloch was a god worshiped by Semitic people living in ancient Near East several hundred years BCE; Jewish and Christian tradition often uses Moloch as a very general symbol for any worship of gods other than the monotheistic Judeo-Christian conception. Judeo-Christian traditions usually connote blood–sacrifice and even torture ascribed to worshipers of Moloch. Juggernaut is a Hindu god worshiped on the Indian subcontinent, several hundred miles southwest of Calcutta. Authorities disagree whether the Hindu sect Siva or Vishnu worships Juggernaut. Of interest to southern Christians is this image of a ceremony:

"The idol is a carved block of wood, with a hideous face, painted black, and a distended blood-red mouth. On festival days the throne of the image is placed on a tower sixty feet high, moving on wheels....While the tower moves along numbers of the devout worshippers throw themselves on the ground, in order to be crushed by the wheels, and the multitude shout in approbation of the act, as a pleasing sacrifice to the idol." Thomas Bulfinch, *Bulfinch's Mythology* (1867, Rev. ed.; New York: Thomas Y. Crowell, n.d. [ca. 1950]).

We rec'd. orders this evening to prepare to march but it was countermanded—

I wrote to cousin Bettie this morning—. I am unwell with a cough and cold. It is generally thought that we will go towards Winchester but any direction we could take will not surprise me. The creeks are evidently too high for us to cross many.

TUESDAY JAN. 21ST, 62

Raining still. Nothing of any note occurred to-day. The number of sick sent to Gen Hospital in Winchester as shown by the proper book is 3200. Our Regiment numbers 249 men for duty. Ten commissioned officers in the Reg—2 Capts. 2 1st Lieuts and 6 2nd Lieuts. Several of these Lieuts. are in command of companies in absence of the Capts.

Orders came this evening for us to be ready to march to-morrow at dawn. Gen Garnett is sick—I do not see how we can get along for the mud.

WEDNESDAY JAN. 22ND, 62

We did not move this morning as was expected last night. I am ready to march at any time but packing and unpacking is some trouble to me. Nothing new transpired to-day.

Our men are becoming lost to all sense of rectitude. Card-playing, drinking, swearing and fun making occupy the whole time of the men[.] Between 30 and 50 may sometimes be seen playing cards at one time in one room. I hardly thought Co. D. would ever become so wicked.

I understand we leave to-morrow at light. It may turn out as other orders have.

THURSDAY JAN. 23, '62

This morning we marched off. Taking the road towards Winchester. The roads were much better than I expected to find them. We left the road we came at [sic] turned to the right at or near Fredericksburg. Our road passed Hanging Rock [93] 15 miles from Romney. We camped in one mile of Hanging Rock [Pass].

---

[93] It is actually Hanging Rock Pass in West Virginia. Long, *Civil War Almanac.*

All along the road as we traveled to-day the bare walls and naked chimnies [chimneys] stood marking the spot some poor mans house stood once but now is in ashes by Yankee brutality. Hogs[,] cows and poultry lay dead all along.

FRIDAY JAN. 24, '62

This morning we started from our camp early. The day was very cold. We passed the Point of Rocks from where the [Confederate-sympathizing] malitia [sic] ran some time since. They we[re] effectually surprised and utterly routed. And though the malitia [sic] were whipped here by one (the 5th Ohio) regiment it it [sic] to all appearance [was] the strongest place I ever saw. The mountain rises high on either hand leaving a narrow pass not more than 50 feet wide at bottom, the road leads along the pass. The whole length is some 2 or 300 yds boths [sic] sides guarded by rough overhanging rocks. After passing through on the Winchester side there is a considerable elevation on which if a canon [sic] were planted it would cover and [sic] the road the whole distance. The malitia [sic] we[re] posted here when the enemy came but their pickets were taken and they fled in utter confusion.

A Mr. Blue or Blues lived here and seems to have been well enough to do in the world but the Yankees spared none—his house was in ashes.

I was told to-day that a Mr Reed, living on this road at the time the enemy came down, was murdered and thrown into the flames of his house. At another place the Yankees found only a poor woman and her child at the house. After tantalizing her so long as they chose they set her house on fire. She put it out. They fired it again and again and a third time. She then thought to save some of her bed clothes. They permitted her to save them till her house fell then took them to the burning house and threw them in. Her son, a little fellow was crying bitterly, but the unfeeling Yankee was yet untouched. They seized his hat from his head and threw it into the fire. These are only a few of the many outrages they have committed.

We traveled fast to-day. Got our breakfast after marching on this side of the mountain. The Regiment camped about 14 miles of Winchester. Commenced snowing about night. Poor men that we are. Gen. Loring's men seem much insulted at being sent to Romney and we to Winchester; but this trip is not to be desired by any one. Loring's men called our malitia [sic] cowards and many other names as we passed. They think Gen. Jackson partial to his old Brigade

Some of our boys asked some of the Tennesseans something about Rich Mountain.[94] This raised them to a high pitch. At Rich Mountain they were defeated.

SATURDAY JAN. 25TH, 62

The snow was about 2 inches deep this morning. We left camp after sunrise. Some think we will go to Winchester and others think we will camp a few miles this side. The sun shone out prettily about noon.

We reached camp some two miles from Winchester a short time before sundown. Thus we have completed a trip of some severity through as poor a country as I have ever seen. The people are simple as children almost. One illustration will suffice to show —. I give it as it was told to me. Some of our boys called at a house and asked the lady of the house if they could get a snack[.] The old lady with all her dignity, polished airs and, plaited hair informed that it was impossible "for" said she "the *head captain* of you all is here with a whole crowd and wants dinner. I am trying to fix it for him now and cant [sic] tend to yours while he is here." The boys, much interested to know who was meant by *Head Captain* ventured to peep into the old lady's parlour—there sat Gen Jackson and his staff. The boys left without any courtesy leaving the head captain to revel for a while in Buckwheat cakes and sausage.

We camped about two [miles] west of Winchester out in an open field where Gen Loring's men camped some time back W. W. Sanders Co. D. died last night. His brother will take his body home. Col. [James F.] Preston is also dead [.] [W]e lost in him a good officer.[95]

---

[94] 10-13 July 1861, battles of Rich Mountain and Laurel Hill in this part of early western Virginia campaigns that established the independence and eventual statehood of West Virginia; these battles made McClellan's early reputation for the Federal forces, and the way that Gen. John Pegram (1832-1865) found his forces encircled and then overwhelmed gave the native of Petersburg a great embarrassment, aggravated by his own capture and brief imprisonment. In time, Pegram recovered his reputation and saved the name of his family; he was from a prominent Richmond family that contributed many illustrious military leaders to Virginia and the US and was himself a high-ranking graduate of West Point. E.B. Long, *Civil War Almanac*, 92-94; James I. Robertson, "Pegram," *Historical Times*. 190

[95] Apparently William Sanders of Smyth County, listed as "died in the war" by Joan Tracy Armstrong, *History of Smyth Co.*, Vol. 1, *Ante-bellum Years through the Civil War* (Marion: Smyth Co. Historical Society, 1986) 222; hereinafter, Armstrong, *History of Smyth*. Colonel James Francis Preston of "Smithfield," his plantation near Blacksburg, VA., was so beloved by the men of the 4th Regiment that they named their encampment after him, and the place was called Camp Preston for some years thereafter. Subsequent leaders were often compared unfavorably with the respected Preston, and his death caused confusion as well as sadness. Preston suffered from

SUNDAY JAN. 26 '1862

Last night the wind blew so rapidly that scarcely a tent was left standing. The tent I slept in tottered and flapped dreadfully. I thought many times it would break from its fastenings like a ship from its moorings and be at the mercy of the storm.

Our camp presents a hard looking picture this morning. Tents all wrecked—some of men whose tents fell last night still lay under them as they fell, others have crawled out and gathered the fragments of theirs and with the help of some rails have made a poor shelter.

We we[re] proud of being brought back to Winchester but predict that we will nil it. It is understood this morning that we will build huts to winter in[.] This is unjust and unfeeling. We have performed many long hard marches for the protection of the valley in Gen. [sic] and Winchester in particular. We have been in active service two thirds of the winter and now we must build winter quarters for one third of the winter and an uncertainty at that.

News reached us to-day of Gen. Crittenden's defeat at Somerset. [96] Dr. Black has leave of absence for 20 days. I am glad for him to go home but sorry that I am left to make off reports &c without help. He put some things in my charge. The report this month will be a hard one to keep correct.

MONDAY JAN 27 1862

This morning the weather seems to be better. I wrote a letter to Dr. F. Nothing took place till evening when an order came for us to move. I learned the Fair Ground at Winchester is where we are going. I started off soon in order to choose a suitable house for my drugs.

---

rheumatism, and resigned his commission and went back to Smithfield, where he died soon after arriving. Notes on Preston provided by Glenn McMullen. See also Bean, Notes.

[96] Important battle, 19 January 1862, won by Federal troops in Kentucky. Known variously as Mill Springs, Logans Cross Roads, Somerset, Beech Grove, and Fishing Creek, this battle was fought along the northern bank of the Cumberland River; "the moderately small but startegically important battle...presaged things to come in the West, showed the weakness of the Confederate line, and boosted the Federal cause among the people of Kentucky and eastern Tennessee....It was the first break in the Confederate Kentucky defense line, which ran from Cumberland Gap to Columbus on the Mississippi." George Bibb Crittenden (1812-1880) of Russellville, KY, was a West Point graduate who was fighting for the CSA while his brother Thomas and his father John were both staunch Unionists. Crittenden was "demoralized" by the defeat, even and especially though he was ordered to take an untenable position "not of his choosing." Long, *Civil War Almanac*, 162; Charles M. Spearman, "Crittenden," *Historical Times*.

I found a good cabin and took possession.

Capt. Whitescarver and others sleep with me.

TUESDAY JAN 28TH 62

Our sick has been prescribed except it was done promiscuously[.] A part of the men have tents here and a part are in huts. The mud is almost knee deep all over camp. A pretty place for men, gentlemen to lie down for a night's repose.

WEDNESDAY, JAN 29TH 62

The dull monotony of camp seems again to surround us. The weather continues to be bad. I understand that the 4 Reg. will be the Town Guard. I think it injustice to us to keep us out here in this awful place when we might find good quarters in town. There is evidently some imperiousness somewhere and with that imperiousness much unfeeling ungratefulness. It is understood that we will not stay here long but will move across the Rail Road to some shanties there.

I got a letter from Brother Nat to-day.

THURSDAY JAN 30TH, 1862

Snowing this morning. Lieut J[ames] W. Kennedy sent for me to-day to see him. He is in town sick. I visited him and found him suffering some. Several of our boys are sick. Cold and its effects being the principal complaints.

FRIDAY, JAN. 31ST 1862

We moved to-day across the Rail Road. Co. E. & G get the huts[.] The other companies are in tents and will remain in them 'till huts can be built[.] I have a very comfortable hut and have been engaged to-day fixing up[.] D. W. V[enable] has been assisting me—he will stay with me.

SATURDAY FEB1, 1862

It is reported this morning that Gen Loring has been ordered back to the vicinity of Winchester by the war department in Richmond. Gen. Jackson seems not to have been informed in regard to the order and the report is current that he has tendered his resignation. If this is true the effect will operate unfavourable towards the diffusion in this quarter. But if Gen. Loring has been ordered back without regards to Gen. Jackson's position as a ranking officer it is of course injustice to his honor as a man and officer. How Gen. Loring can expect Gen Garnett to take a position with 2000 men that he himself is unwilling to maintain with 8 or 10000 is a mystery to me. We have guarded the Shenandoah Valley from the Potomac to Strasburg, from Berkely to the foot of the ride, and now it would be unjust to throw us at Romney while others take the valley.

I fear that if Gen. Jackson does resign, this branch of our army will become disorganised.[97]

Our men on furlough are coming in now. I visited Lieut. Kennedy to-day. While I was walking through Winchester I met Chas. Payne an old school mate. He told me of the death of H.P. [P.H.?] Ruffner. [98] I staid [sic] with him some time.

SUNDAY FEB. 2 '62

Nothing worth noting came to light to-day. I have been busy working on monthly reports as I have but three more days to finish. The weather is bad. Snowed lightly last night.

"Sick call" is rather indefinite now. Dr. [Joseph] Crockett has no system in any thing he does.[99] He declares he will have sick at 7 o'clock but is never seen until some hours after. I do not feel that it would be proper for me to presume to prescribe for all the men that would allow me to.

---

[97] This "Loring-Jackson controversy" seems to have been a matter of bruised egos for two good officers. Each officer was offended by being placed near each other, and each officer considered that he had been unrecognized for successes in these brief winter campaigns. Loring believed with others that Jackson was often emotionally unstable, if not mentally deficient; Jackson was most offended because he thought that strategists did not appreciate the dangerous forced marches that he was executing during these winter storms. With regard to tactics, Loring considered that Jackson was not protecting his flank, while Jackson—as seen in these diary entries already the master of the quick "horseless cavalry" infantry march— said with some reason that he was easily within support distance of Loring. Judah P. Benjamin, CSA secretary of war, was able to placate both men by promoting Loring and reassigning him to southwestern Virginia, where he distinguished himself in subsequent battles. The Virginia troops once under Loring were reassigned to Jackson's army. Benjamin's diplomacy in this controversy is credited with saving the Confederacy "its best strategist," Jackson. Stanchak, *Hist. Times*, 447-48.

[98] Apparently B.C. Payne, corporal in Orange Co. battery commanded then by Capt. Thomas J. Peyton. Ruffner is apparently P.H. Ruffner of Co. C, 7th Va. Infantry, then commanded by Capt. John C. Porter of Culpeper; Apperson had two brothers serving in Co. C. with this Ruffner. W.W. Scott, *History of Orange County* (Dayton, VA.: Ruebush-Elkins, 1907) 271-72.

[99] Dr. Joseph Crockett of Wytheville, VA. was assistant surgeon of 4th Va. Bean, Notes.

MONDAY FEB 3RD, 62

Quite a sensation is afloat in our camp to-day. There was some inkling of it yesterday but the truth could not be found. Lieut. Col. [L.E.] Moore is placed at the head of the Reg. Maj. Kent is promoted to Lieut. Col. and Capt. A. G. Pendleton is made Major. None of the changes seem to give satisfaction. Many believe that Capt's Updyke and Ronald will resign on account of Pendleton's promotion—them being older officers. Maj. Kent will resign by basing the cause upon Col. Moore—Kent having had the regiment under his charge and supervision since Col. Preston went home [was killed] thinks it due him to be made Colonel as one who has been maimed for Life while struggling for his honor and wealth and country.[100]

So far as a captains resignation is concerned it will do no harm[.] [T]here are others who will take their places. I hate to have any dificulty in any part of the theatre that I act but it is unavoidable though.

I became very angry this morning but I [word or words omitted?] not to have done so though it was justifiable[.] I asked for a detail to chop wood, the day was a bad one it is true, but we are compelled to have fire. One man from Co. F. and one from Co. D. were activated and the Lieut. of Co. F. promised me that he should come. I waited some time for him to come but he came not so I enquired after him when I heard that no man had been detailed nor did they intend to detail one. At this I felt somewhat riled for I have waited on that company as much as any one could and now they won't return any good act at all. I went to the Major and told him that I wanted wood and if I got it not I would leave the Medical Department. He sent some men to cut me a load. He also made a detail for some himself but the men refused to cut it. This is wrong. The "Dare Devils" came near disbanding this morning . They marched down

---

[100] "Go home" was often used to describe death, and in this case the meaning is doubled, for Col. Preston went home to die. The diarist seems to favor L.E. Moore for colonel because that officer was already "maimed" in service. Moore had been wounded severely at Manassas, and he probably resigned because he had never recovered sufficiently to ride a horse, rather than over some dispute about rank. Kent refused the rank of lieutenant colonel because he did not want Albert Pendleton to succeed him as major of the regiment. Kent was reassigned and took command of reserves in Wythe and Carroll counties, figuring prominently in the battles around Saltville known as Stoneman's Raid in December of 1864. Pendleton did become major of the regiment, but Captain Charles Ronald took command as the officer directly in charge of the troops. Bean, Notes.

and took quarters in some tents at the fair grounds. It has snowed rapid since morning.

TUESDAY FEB 4TH 1862

Though yesterday was a stormy disagreeable day, to-day the sun shines beautifully. Nature has once more put on one of her smiles that gladdens the heart of man. Nothing outside of the dull monotony of camp life occurred. The duty incumbent upon the 4th Regiment falls very heavily up the men. Every man has to stand guard every other night. This [w]ith the exposure they are necessarily compelled to undergo, taxes too heavily the physical energies of men. And after all this heavy duty the citizens of Winchester are not grateful—rather will they play the part of famished vampires and will draw the last dime a soldier has, and then turn him out to the misery of Winter's storm. I do not impeach all the citizens of Winchester with this penurious, merciless principle: for there are some, I have no doubt that are soul and body engrossed in the welfare of our soldiers and the cause of our country.

I finished the report of the month past and forward it to Med: Director.

WEDNESDAY FEB 5TH 1862

The weather is bad to-day and indeed it has been for some time. I rec'd a letter from Cousin Bettie to-day. She is well. I was called to see S. M. Sexton[101] to-night after 8 o'clock—had to walk some two miles into town.

THURSDAY FEB. 6TH 1862

This morning the sun shone out pretty. I have been engaged consolidating inventory of medicines. Maj. Kent left for home this morning.

I had the luck to partake of some good things sent to J. M. Thomas from Smyth[.] He made a general treat—candidates will electioneer[.] [102] His treating to eatables is well enough and should be remembered but treating to drink is beyond all question to be condemned. I wrote a long letter to Mrs. Tomlin and rec'd. one from home. Many of the volunteers are enlisting for the war and are

---

[101] S.M.Sexton was private in Smyth Blues; he fought in the major engagements of the Stonewall Brigade. and was killed at Gettsyburg. Armstrong, *Hist. of Smyth*, 222.

[102] On "treating" and "toasting" and "swilling the planters with bumbo," all part of rural Virginia electioneering, see Charles Sackett Sydnor, *Gentlemen Freeholders; Political Practices in Washington's Virginia* (Chapel Hill: University of North Carolina Press and the Institute of Early American History and Culture at Williamsburg, VA., [1952]).

going home on 50 [sic] days furlough.[103] I am glad to see it. Loring's command has arrived from Romney and is at the camp west of Winchester. It is strang[e] that such movement belong to such a man as Loring. Fearlessness has doubtless been one of Gen. Loring's admired qualities and no one would suppose that anything like fear would prompt him to act as he has done. But when we look at everything and examine carefully into his operations we are almost persuaded to believe that he was afraid of the *Yanks*. We learn that a part of his force was ordered to prepare to march in a [sic] hour. Leaving Romney in a hurry they hurried towards Winchester as fast as their baggage would allow over the roads. When a wagon would stick fast in the mud the baggage was burned and in this was a large quantity [sic] was consumed as though the fiendish Yankees we[re] in full charge at their heels. After he left I understand that Romney was pretty soon occupied by the Yankees again. This is the worst feature in the case. Our men gave the true citizens of Romney and adjoining country that they be protected from the enemy—that his desolating tread should no more startle them from their homes and thus gave them occasion to boast of their southern principles—and now they are left again to the mercy of a relentless foe in an exposed condition without any means of protection except to flee from the home they cherish. Such is their condition[.] [L]et us look to the result.

FRIDAY FEBRUARY 7TH, 1862

No new thing to-day. Time is passing rapidly. Days fly like moments almost. Our tour of enlistment will soon be ended. We will then turn our steps homeward once more. How pleasing the thought—how [we] longed for the time. We can then talk with the friends we love, roam the fields we remember so well with its paths, each leading to some cherished spot, and view again with new delight the gradual ascent of the good mountain where it rises majestically and bathes its top in the variegated clouds of heaven. And Oh! Could we be so

[103] The diarist may be incorrect about the length of the furlough. Enlistment commitments for many of the volunteers were expiring by winter of 1861-1862, and new volunteers were not immediately forthcoming. The Confederate Congress on 11 December 1861 passed a law offering inducements for long-term re-enlistment: A three-year commitment (or for the duration of the war, whichever came first) was rewarded with a bounty of fifty dollars and a 60-day furlough. However, the timing of the furlough had to be at the discretion of the officers so as to be "compatible with the public service." In addition, every soldier re-enlisting could choose the branch of service; and the soldiers could elect their officers. Douglas Southall Freeman, *R.E. Lee: A Biography*, 4 vols. (New York: Scribner, 1934-1935) 2:26.

fortunately blessed as a nation and people to have peace, blissful peace in our land.

D. W. V[enable]. went to-day to help bring the baggage from wagon. A. J. Sealy staid last night. J. M. T[homas] is on a big spree. A goodly number of the 4 Reg is reenlisting. Maj. Gen. Jackson's resignation was not excepted [sic]—I think he will remain with us.

CAMP PRESTON, WINCHESTER VA

SATURDAY, FEB 8TH 1862

The sun shines beautiful this morning and the day promises to be fine. I wrote a letter to Mrs. Faris to-day.

The men are reenlisting rapidly and going home on the furlough granted by congress, they having received the bounty of 50$ also. I am somewhat confused about remaining longer in the service. I have been trying to decide for some time.

My duty would prompt me to join right away but my immediate interests, pecuniary especially would dictate to me to go home and prepare to do something for myself. I have written Dr. F. but he has not answered me yet. I was called to see Thos. Schwartz[104] this evening—I fear he will be very sick. The people with whom he is staying seem to be kind to him.

SUNDAY, FEB.9TH 1862

This morning, from some cause or other the boys took a notion [to] go home by availing themselves of the opportunity of reenlisting. Some 30 put their names down for two years or during [sic; duration of] the war. Some got their furloughs & bounty and started homeward. I am proud to see it and cannot reconcile my conscience to stay away. News from Europe seems to be good. [105] I passed the day in camp. All are eager about going home.

---

[104] We cannot locate Schwartz in either Smyth Co. or Orange Co. records for the Brigade.

[105] The diarist was responding to an optimistic hearing of a speech of 27 January 1862 in Paris. "Emperor Louis Napoleon of France told the French people that the American Civil War has seriously compromised our commercial interests, but that France would confine herself to hoping for termination of the war as long as the rights of neutrals were respected." Long, *Civil War Almanac*, 163-4.

CAMP PRESTON, VA.

MONDAY, FEB. 10TH, 1862

This morning we are informed of the loss of Fort Henry on the Tennessee River. Two victories [Somerset in KY. and this one] for the enemy have thus followed each other quickly. I fear the effects of these defeats. [106] The southern people have found it harder to reconcile a defeat than anything else. We have been victorious until we are almost ready to believe that we will not meet with any reverses—we become careless and unconcerned. Let us prepare our minds for defeat as well as victory, let us not look at a reverse as our death knell but look up, prepare for the worse and hope for better. I visited T Schwartz this evening and found him very ill with *pneumonia.* I prescribed for him and promised to see him next day.

The work of reenlistment is going gloriously on. 27 of Co. D. got their bounty and furloughs and started for home.

I am undecided whether to enlist or go home and spend the summer in study[,] attend a course of Lectures [at Medical College of Virginia in Richmond] in the fall & winter and take a Diploma. J. M. Thomas offered to send me money to-day. What prompted him to make the offer I know not.

CAMP PRESTON VA

TUESDAY FEB 11TH, 1862

The sun shines beautiful this morning. Dr. Crockett visited Schwartz with me but did not change the treatment.

This mornings papers brings us the doleful news of another heavy defeat at Roanoke Island on the Carolina coast which resulted in the loss of Gen. [Henry A.] Wise's entire command. O. Jennings Wise badly wounded. [107] Three battles

---

[106] These were part of Federal "rivers campaigns" to clear passages on Cumberland, Tennessee, and Mississippi rivers; Ft. Henry and nearby Ft. Donelson guarded the Tennessee River, which "was an important river highway, bypassing the Mississippi," and the Union victory was of profound strategic importance, although the diarist focuses on the emotional significance of a fickle public response to a series of defeats. Long, ibid., 165-67.

[107] O. Jennings Wise was the son of the former governor and wartime general Henry A. Wise. He commanded the Richmond Light Infantry Blues, formed before secession by sons of the most prominent Richmond families. They became Co. A, 46th VA., and O. Jennings Wise was elected its captain. The 46th was fighting in the west under Brig. Gen. Robert Selden Garnett (1819-1861), where their losses were especially heavy and their heavily criticized commanding general was killed. Henry Wise then took command, and the army fought more successfully, but in this

lost and the enemy threatening to pierce the very heart of our country. The Burnside Fleet [sic] of the North is strong and will make us suffer along the coast. Every day our sky becomes more and more clouded.[108]

CAMP PRESTON, VA

FEBRUARY 12TH, 1862

The papers of to-day verify the statement of yesterday. Our loss is 300 killed and about 3000 prisoners. [109] The effect on the men seems to be of a rousing character. I am decided I think to reenlist: Every man able to handle a gun will be needed in this conflict. We have work on our hands—hard, tedious work—fraugh[t] with dangers inummerable. The enemy is advancing towards Tuscumbia, Ala. and will perhaps get possesion [sic] of of [sic] the Great Southern R.R. Route. At Weldon the enemy may probably get possession of the Weldon & N.C. R Road. With these two roads in their possession we will be cut off from the southern state[s] almost entirely.[110]

---

engagement his son the captain of the Blues was mortally wounded. Jeffrey D. Wert, "Richmond Blues," *Hist. Times.*

[108] Ambrose Everett Burnside (1824-1881) was not in command of the fleet, but was in command of the army forces that made the amphibious landing from boats commanded by Flag Officer Louis Malesherbes Goldsborough (1805-1873). Burnside's men continued on, capturing Ft. Macon and NC coastal cities, including New Bern and Beaufort. John E. Stanchak emphasizes,as does the diarist, the "emotional impact" of the "small" battles for a northern public still embarrassed by the large-scale defeat at Manassas. Stanchak, "Roanoke Island," *Hist. Times.*; see also John D. Kallman, "Burnside," ibid.. Cf. E.B. Long, who notes that "[c]ontrol of Pamlico Sound gave the Federals a first-rate base on the Atlantic coast for operations against North Carolina...a back door to Richmond had been opened and a vital Southern state dangerously threatened." idem, loc. cit., 168.

[109] CSA forces killed were officially 23; Shaw did surrender at least 2,500 men. Naval History Commission, *Civil War Naval Chronology*, Pt. 2, 1862 (Washington, D.C.: US Government Printing Office, [1946]) 20-21, hereinafter *Naval Chronology.*

[110] At this moment, northern Alabama was not in jeopardy, although a naval force did come near Florence, AL. before turning back toward TN. The attack, coordinated by Federal navy (Andrew Hull Foote [1806-1863]) and army (Ulysses Simpson Grant [1822-1885]), was focused on Fort Donelson in TN. as part of the continuing campaign to "clear the channels" and "open up the river highway" of the Cumberland River. The goal in TN. was not railroads, but rivers whose control would open up the entire "bread basket" state of the central South. The N.C. coastal story was a different matter, and the rail lines there were damaged. Weldon, N.C. was an important shipbuilding and repair dock, and the railroad from Weldon to Wilmington was one of the South's first important lines; infantry actions following up the Roanoke Island amphibious assault were aimed at that rail line. Long, *Civil War Alamanac*, 166-73.

But in the midst of trouble like this, and in reverses like those lately transpired we have something to cheer us—England has recognised the South as fair France follows in her wake. [111] Lieut [James W.] Kennedy expects to be sent home as a recruiting officer and wishes me to go also. I will if I can.

Senate has passed an important bill for the reorganisation of the army. Those of the 12 months men who does not reenlist are subject to a draft and can be called into service in 40 days from the expiration of his present term.[112]

I rec'd a letter from Nat and wrote one home. Nat has reenlisted.[113]

CAMP PRESTON VA.

THURSDAY FEBRUARY 13TH, 1862

This morning the shun [sic - sun] shone soft and beautiful. The Earth took the advent of Spring. No news. The accounts from the field of action is [sic] no better than before. Rumour speaks of victories for us in Ky. & Missouri. God see it may be so! In the battle of Roanoke Island it is said that the "Richmond blues" commanded by O. Jennings Wise Capt. lost all but nine. This is sad news to us but we must resign ourselves to bear it.[114]

---

[111] The diarist is responding to rumors and to some speeches by Confederate sympathizers in Parliament. On 6 May 1861, Lord John Russell had proclaimed that Great Britain recognized the C.S.A. as a belligerant in a war, with diplomatic and other rights attaining to such status; but Russell was clear in stating that Great Britain did not then recognize the C.S.A. as a nation. On 31 January 1862 Queen Victoria announced that Great Britain intended to remain neutral, while recognizing the two sides as belligerants in a war and while insisting on British rights to trade with either side and British rights to move their goods on the high seas without interference from US or C.S.A. Despite some speeches in Parliament calling for recognition of the C.S.A., no such recognition came. Emperor Louis Napoleon subsequently offered to "mediate" some disputes and interfered often, even sponsoring an abortive invasion of Mexico, but he never officially recognized the C.S.A. Long, *Civil War Almanac*, 70-71; 165.

[112] Virginia general assembly passed an act providing for "general induction into the militia" of all VA. white males between the ages of 18 and 40. Those volunteers currently serving who refused to reenlist became members of the militia as soon as their term of volunteer service expired; from the militia, anyone could be "drafted" into regular army or navy service. Commissioned officers could resign at any time, subject to certain conditions. There were exemptions for slaveowners who held more than 20 slaves. VA. *Acts of Assembly*, 1862, Pt. 1.

[113] Nat and William Apperson were on the roster of Co. C., 7th VA. Inf. commanded by officers from Culpeper until J.W. Almond of the Appersons' native Orange Co. became commanding captain later in this year. Scott, *Hist. of Orange Co.*, 271.

[114] Skirmishes in KY. were actually part of northern victories; skirmishes in MO. were inconclusive. Long, Civil War Almanac, 170. O. Jennings Wise died from his wounds, and his Richmond Blues suffered losses, although not to the extent reported here. Following the defeat at Roanoke Island, the Blues were transfered back to Richmond, where they served as a kind of

I know of nothing that is transpiring now in our immediate neighborhood.

CAMP PRESTON VA

FRIDAY FEB. 14, 1862

This morning is comparatively warm. I was late in retiring las night and consequently not early in rising this morning. I visited my patient [Schwartz] in town and think he is improving. I visited the Medicine College to-day and saw some fine specimens of anatomy.

I took cold last night and feel badly this evening. I am almost out of patience waiting for a letter from home. Retired late—very late the air is very cold to-night.

CAMP PRESTON VA.

SATURDAY FEBRUARY 15TH, 1862

This morning it is reported that the enemy and a part of our malitia [sic] had a pretty sharp fight yesterday in Morgan Co.[115]

"Hurrah!" for the "milish." Reports say that the Yankees first whipped them and had surrounded them and captured a goodly number of them and all their baggage. The malitia [sic] made a charge upon them and retook their baggage and drove the enemy off. Our Brigade received orders to prepare for active field service but I presume it was only that they might be ready to move in case the enemy threatened us too strongly.

I wrote to Secretary of War [Judah P. Benjamin] a few days ago to ascertain whether an artillery company would be rec'd. by the government—He writes that it would and the greater part of our Company had joined such a company some time ago.

I am very unwell to-night—I was out night before last with a sick man and got very cold. My head and throat are very painful.

---

police force until the 1864 Petersburg campaign. They remained under command of Gen. Henry Wise. Wert, loc. cit..

[115] Skirmish in Bloomery near Morgan Co., WVA. Skirmish was inconclusive. There was an earlier skirmish, 2 Feb., in Morgan Co., TN., also inconclusive, and the diarist may be conflating rumors about skirmishes in Morgan Co. Long, *Civil War Almanac*, 171; Charles Shetler, *West Virginia Civil War Literature; an Annotated Bibliography* (Morgantown, WVA: West Virginia University Library, 1963)., hereinafter Shetler, *WVA Civil War.*

It is reported that a fight is progressing at Fort Donaldson [Donelson] Tenn. and that we had won a victory in Ky but Gen. Floyd was dangerously wounded.[116] I look for Dr. [Harvey] Black back to-night. No more furlough are to be granted till further orders.

CAMP PRESTON, VA.

SUNDAY FEB. 16TH, 1862

I feel better this morning but I fear I will have some infection of the lungs if I do not take care.

In company with Lieut. [Andrew E.] Gibson[117] I went to church this morning in town—the Old school Presbyterian Rev. Dr. Kay from England preached[.] [118] The church is a good one and the congregation is good.

---

[116] No victory, but rather crushing defeat. John Buchanan Floyd (1806-1863) graduated from South Carolina College, became a prominent landholder in southwestern VA., was VA. delegate and governor before Civil War. A politician with a promising future, Floyd was a failure in battle. He was not wounded in this attack on Fort Donelson; he made some miscalculations and failed to defend a fortification that might have withstood Grant's assault. When it was determined that the fort would have to be surrendered, Floyd worried about his political prominence, which might cause the Federals to punish him severely. Thus, he fled, and it fell to General Simon Bolivar Buckner (1823-1914) to surrender. When Buckner inquired about terms of surrender, Grant told him the only terms were "unconditional surrender," producing Grant's famous nickname. Floyd was reprimanded for his poor performance at Donelson. This battle concluded the winter rivers campaigns that sealed off KY. and much of TN. from C.S.A., gave the Federals easy travel over the western Upper South, and established a new American hero in US Unconditional Surrender Grant. Charles M. Spearman, "Floyd," *Hist. Times.*

[117] Andrew E. Gibson (1838-1862) of Smyth Co. was an early volunteer in the Smyth Blues, who immediately elected him 2d Lt. He was unanimously elected captain in the elections of midwinter 1861/1862. He was a devout Presbyterian and apparently discussed religion with the always curious and inquisitive diarist. Armstrong, *Hist. of Smyth*, vol. 2, 126-28; Wilson, *Smyth Co. Hist.*, 237.

[118] We cannot identify this visiting British minister. Old School and Old Light refer to kinds of Presbyterianism in the antebellum US South. These Presbyterians emphasized predestination and election and a "rational" approach to questions of faith and salvation, borrowing heavily from John Calvin's reinterpretations of Protestantism after Martin Luther's heavy emphasis on salvation by grace and individual free will. New School and New Light Presbyterians in the middle of the eighteenth century emhasized grace and free will and especially used the technique of the massed-crowd outdoor Revival to *awaken* putatively dormant religious spiritualism in a movement generally called the Great Awakening. A Second Great Awakening began to occur immediately before the Civil War and it was still going on as the War broke. Apperson is very aware of the different appoaches to religion, and he seems to be interested in both Old Light and New Light sects of Protestantism. For concise descriptions of these movements in southern Protestants, see John H. Leith's essay on "Calvinism" in *Encyclopedia of Southern Culture*, eds., Charles Reagan Wilson and William Ferris (Chapel Hill: University of North Carolina Press for

The text is in Romans 8 ch. & 28 v. "All things work together for good to them that love God." [119] His argument was clear and forcible; but his English accent seemed a little affected. He preached of the special Providence of the Creator, how it worked many things for our good. Yet, we being shortsighted we see it not. Said he: "The world is filled with little machines all working to-gether for the benefit of man. The sun, the brilliant orb that sheds its renovating, verifying, and vitalising rays on the evil as well as the good operates in the morn—the moon on the ocean, the ocean on the earth, the earth on the atmosphere and the atmosphere on health, and health on wealth.["] And so in the affairs of state all have their sheriffs & magistrates legislators and governors, presidents or princes—all operating to-gether for the same object—all have their armies and navi[e]s and forces: It is so also spiritually and morally. Tribulation worketh patience, patience[,] experiences and experience[,] hopes, which shed abroad in the heart of man maketh not ashamed! [120] Physiologically it is the same working. The mind devises, the heart perceives, the will resolves and the hands act!" Man he said was the special object of God's Providence. He sendeth the rain to fertilize the earth, the sun to warm and give life and beauty to vegetation. He then showed some instances of God's watchfulness over his creatures. Daniel in the Lion's den—the fiery furnace, David's victory over Goliath and the crossing of the Red Sea by Moses and his people. Of this last he said—"High walls of stone were on both sides of them which it were impossible to scale—a terrible and bloodthirsty foe behind and the rolling waves of the Red Sea in front. But with trust in God Moses rais[ed] his staff and smote the liquid wave and it rolled high on either side, the children of Israel passed over[,] Pharaohs hosts followed, but followed to perish." He spoke at large of the power of Prayer. When Sennacherib threatened Hezekiah with a fatal siege, he sent for

---

the Center for the Study of Southern Culture, 1986). Note that Apperson's wartime mentor Harvey Black is very much a traditional Calvinist, as are their military commanders of the Brigade, Thomas J. Jackson and of the Army of Northern Virginia Robert Edward Lee (although Lee did worship as an Episcopalian, his basic beliefs and assumptions are very much Old School Calvinism, as they were for most Episcopalians of the era).

[119] For an Old School Calvinist, the remainder of the verse may be most important of all: "to them who are the called according to the *will of God.*" Romans 8:28 [ital. in King James version then used.].

[120] Romans 5:3-5: "[3] And not only *so*, but we glory in tribulations also: knowing that tribulation worketh patience; [4] And patience, experience; and experience, hope: [5] And hope maketh not ashamed; because the love of God is shed abroad in our hearts by the Holy Ghost, which is given unto us."

good old Isaiah and they two went to prayer and the destroying angel smote Sennacherib.[121]

At 4 o'clock I went to the the Northern Methodist church and heard him preach again[.] [122] This is a splendid church capable of seating 1000 persons. The sermon was not so good as this morning. The text was "There's more joy in Heaven over one sinner that repenteth &c."[123] The hymn sung by a splendid quior [sic; apparently, choir] was "All hail the power of Jesus' name." After preaching I visited my patient, took supper at "Randal Evans" and returned to camp. It snowed last night—cold to-night.

CAMP PRESTON, VA

MONDAY, FEBRUARY 17TH 1862

The air is cold and the earth is covered with icy sleet.

I saw a letter from Dr. B[lack] this morning to Dr. C[rockett] stating that he will not be here till the last of the week. I am getting exceeding anxious for him to return and keep the sick list straight I do not like prescribing and taking the responsibility of so many men. I am very unwell to-day. Nothing new —

---

[121] Second Chronciles 31:1-19. Hezekiah, successful ruler of a restored Judah, faced four crises in his very long rule, the first of which was the Assyrian invasion by Sennacherib. Sennacherib is also the name of the Assyrian Moon-god and the name as used in 2 Chr. is both a symbol of sin and the name of a threatening invader. According to Chr., Hezekiah's great faith caused Yahweh to send one angel who destroyed an army of more than 180,000.

[122] The Methodist Church had split into northern and southern divisions over the issue of slavery in 1845 after an especially divisive national session of the general conference in 1844; however, conferences in KY. and MO., and the Holston Conference of the mountains in VA., GA., and TN. formally attempted some reconciliation with the conferences of Northern Methodists, and some Northern Methodist churches were still functioning in this part of the Shenandoah Valley in northwesternVirginia and the Union territory about to become West Virginia. Note that Apperson attended Methodist church services in Smyth Co. and had friends at Emory & Henry College in neighboring Washington Co., and both of these counties are in the Holston Conference. Despite efforts at reconciliation by Holston Conference Methodists, the ministers and their congregations supported slavery and specifically supported the bishop of the Holston Conf., James Osgood Andrews, whose wife's ownership of slaves had produced the effort in the 1844 conference by northern Methodists to expel him and any other slaveowning minister. See Donald Gene Mathews, *Slavery and Methodism; a Chapter in American Morality, 1780-1845* (Princeton: Princeton University Press, 1965), 246-82. Holston Conference Minutes, 1845, Archives of EHC.

[123] Jesus' words quoted between parables, Luke 15:7: "I say unto you, that likewise joy shall be in heaven over one sinner that repenteth, more than over ninety and nine just persons, which need no repentance." And: Luke 15:10: "Likewise, I say unto you, there is joy in the presence of the angels of God over one sinner that repenteth."

CAMP PRESTON, VA.

TUESDAY, FEB, 18TH, 1862

I feel something better this morning. I hope soon to be well.

News by this morning's paper states that the Federals are making considerable headway down the [Cumberland] river and gives an account of two days fighting at Fort Donaldson [Donelson] and our men are truly victorious. While this report made our hearts impulsively heave with delight news came from Staunton that Nashville had been taken from us, this latter we will not believe until it is fully confirmed. [124]

I visited Thos. Schwartz this evening—found him decidedly better I think. I went also to the Hospital to see some of our boys. After I returned I pened [sic] a letter to Cousin Bettie.

CAMP PRESTON VIRGINIA

WEDNESDAY FEB. 19TH, 1862

Rain is falling this morning—more bad weather on us[.] News this morning does not confirm the taking of Nashville but gives some account of several of our steamers being burnt and destroyed to prevent the enemy from capturing them. Indeed our cause is getting dark and doubtful. The martial hosts of Yankees are swarming around us rapidly. We look forward to a day not far distant when we will be attacked hard. If the enemy gets the R. Road in Tennessee it will be a hard blow on us.

I have been in house nearly the whole day. Cold rainy and hailing. I have been reading Shakespeare's Othello—a very affecting thing.

CAMP PRESTON VA

THURSDAY FEB 20TH, 1862

All is excitement this morning. Fort Donaldson [Donelson] in Tenn. is undergoing a storm of shot & shell. Our men had fought bravely but by the dint of superior numbers they have been successful in capturing Ft. Donaldson.

---

[124] As noted, Ft. Donelson and Ft. Henry were both lost, and these "delight"-producing rumors thus are completely incorrect. The disbelieved rumor about Nashville was true, and TN. Confederate leaders led by Gov. Isham Harris removed to Memphis for their political capital. Note that this day of bad military news was also the occasion of the first session of the new Confederate Congress in its capital Richmond. Long, *Civil War Almanac*, 172-74.

Rumor states that Nashville is now in the hands of the enemy. We do not, and will not believe the reports until [it] is confirmed. Our cause is loosing [sic] ground now but we should not despair the least; but we can not bear adversity as we should. Our men have not been taught to bear them. Too much has been said by our papers and speakers about bearing ills and hardships. We have seen no hardships yet, we have no ills nor suffered any from inconveniences. Our pathway since the commencement of the war has been as far from thorns and snares as we could expect. But when the enemy has thrown himself around us like a mighty serpent availing himself of every opportunity to seize some weak and unprotected spot, and in this manner weakened our forces by piece meal, and robbed us of many arms and much ammunition provision stores &c while he got hold on our shores we may look for an era of hardships soon to cloud our sky darker and darker still, then we may look forward for a time that will try the souls of men.

I learn that the malitia[sic] is called out in the country. I hope to see them standing in one extended line. I know it will go hard with many of them but it went hard with us, we had to dry up soon and take it in good earnest.

I wrote a letter to Dr. F.

B. F. Sexton slept with me.

The nights are cold and disagreeable.

CAMP PRESTON, VA

FRIDAY, 21, 1862

This morning's paper states the fall of Ft. Donaldson [sic] but not of Nashville. Gen [Gideon Johnson] Pillow, [125] [Simon Bolivar] Buckner[,] [John Buchanan] Floyd are safe at Nashville. [Albert] Sydney[sic] Johns[t]on had arrived with 25000 men—a good reinforcement.

I got a letter from Ms. Tomlin to-day Mrs Faris is sick or so I learn from Mrs. T's letter. Nothing new.

---

[125] Gideon Johnson Pillow (1806-1878) was from Williamson City, TN. A successful attorney, he established a partnership with future president James Knox Polk, and became prominent in TN. Democratic politics. A veteran of Mexican War, he was undistinguished there and often quarreled with commanding general Winfield Scott; but he was protected by his benefactor, President Polk. In the Civil War, he received a political appointment as senior major general in TN. provisional army and he served poorly and ineptly. He, along with Floyd, was ineffective in the rivers campaigns that cost the CSA Forts Henry and Donelson. Like Floyd, he worried about special punishment because of his polticial prominence, and thus he slipped away and arranged for Buckner to accept the responsibility for surrendering. Edwin C. Bearss, "Pillow," *Hist. Times.*

CAMP PRESTON VA

SATURDAY, FEB. 22ND, 1862

This morning Dr. Black came in—I was quite glad to see him. Things will soon assume some regularity in the medical department I presume. I visited some patients in town to-day. Had the pleasure of being introduced to two daughters of Rev. Wm. Wilson[126]—two nice ladies. I saw Jas V Dungan in town—a part of Loring's troops left for Manassas to-day.

It will not surprise me if we have a fight here early this spring. A large body of wood oposite [sic] and in front of Ft. Alabama [Frederick Co.] was ordered to be cut down. Not much was done to it however.

CAMP PRESTON VA

SUNDAY FEB: 23RD 1862

Nothing unusual occurred to day. I spent the day in camp reading Shakespeare's "Rape of Lucerne". After sundown Jas. Meek and myself went to town with the intention of hearing a sermon but the crowd was too large to hold the crowd so we came back to camp.

I wrote to Mrs. Tomlin to-day.

MONDAY FEB: 24TH, 1862

This morning looked like a May morning but after sunrise a short time the wind commenced blowing rapidly and continued all day capsizing every tent and blowing away things away[sic]

Jeff Davis' inaugural was rec'd here this morning.[127]

---

[126] Possibly the Rev. William V. Wilson (b. 1819), who also lived in Marion Township, Smyth Co., and was sometime chaplain with Army of Northern Virginia. Charles F. Pitts, *Chaplains in Gray; the Confederate Chaplains' Story* (Nashville, TN.: Broadman Press, 1957), 157. VA. Census 1870.

[127] Inauguration was 22 February 1862. Davis stood in a "pouring rain" to deliver his first speech as president of the CSA, which had a bicameral legislature that replaced the earlier unicameral secession conference. The new political capital was Richmond. Davis called for divine guidance and intervention and invoked the constitution as gurantor of state rights in a federal system. He decried "unbridled majority" voting as the "most odious and least responsible form of despotism," and he said, "Civil War there cannot be between States held together by their volition only." Quoted, E.B. Long, *Civil War Almanac*, 174.

I spend a good deal of my time foolishly—gaming but not to bet. It is reported that our forces have evacuated Nashville—I hope not though.

CAMP PRESTON VA

TUESDAY FEB 25TH 1862

This morning the news from the battlefield in Tennessee almost strikes us dumb with astonishment and wrings our hearts to acknowledge it. Fort Donaldson [sic] capitulated with 12000 of our men after four days fighting. Nashville is abandoned to the Federals—the enemy is pouring his thousands down upon the Southern states—our Generals are retreating before him like sheep before the dog.

We have two horrid defeats to follow each other in rapid succession. Why is it? Has the chivalry of the South died away? or is our cause less important than it was a few months ago? Do we feel less patriotic than we did when we first rushed to the field to secure our rights, our honor and our all? I hope not! Something must be wrong when 12000 men [128]—fighting men are given over to an army not more than twice or thrice its size perhaps.

While our hearts sink within us we have something to cheer us. Gov. [Isham] Harris has called out the whole force of malitia [sic] of Tennessee. Our men seem to [be] stimulated to action by our late defeats and are now re-enlisting fast. The malitia of Va. are trembling now for their fate. They know there is but one alternative and that is for them to come out. We must present one solid front, one determined will to resist to the "bitter end" all efforts to subjugate us.

Reports came in to-day of the movements of the Federal troops towards this place by Harpers Ferry. Active movements are going on in Winchester moving commissary quarter master's and ordnance stoves. The evacuation of Winchester I think is not all improbable.

I rec'd a letter from Dr. F. to-day. He refuses to give me advice in regard to re-enlisting but intimates that it would be better for me to remain in the army.

---

[128] There is no agreement on the size of the force surrendered, with estimates running from no more than 500 to more than 15,000. The diarist's figure of 12,000 is accepted as a fair estimate by E.B. Long, op. cit., 172. The "twice" and "thrice" estimates refer to the strategic assumption of the day that an assaulting force needed a huge majority, perhaps ten times the number of troops to be successful against an entrenched position in an established fort on a river. Long estimates Grant's force to be 27,000.

He is correct but I have decided to remain before I heard from him. Mrs. F. is very sick which I am sorry to hear.

WEDNESDAY, FEB:26TH, 1862

Some orders came to-day for the Regiment to practice skirmish drill every day—the surplus guns are being cleaned and sent to the ordnance department. This looks something like preparing to battle. No papers came to-day. The condition of the Railroad rendered so by the recent rains retards our mails.

An election was held in Co. D. to-day for Capt. since [Albert Galatin] Pendleton [was] promoted, and 2nd Lieut. to fill the vacancy occassioned by the election of Captain. A. E. Gibson 2nd Lieut. was elected unanimously by those present and J. M.Thomas to 2nd Lieut. 1st Sergeant Bishop ran and came in one vote of tying the election. [129] I voted for Thomas according to army regulations on elections.

THURSDAY, FEB 27TH 1862

Nothing transpired to-day more than is usual. The wind blew hard. They are still moving stores from Winchester. The sick was moved from Shenandoah [Alum] Springs [Shenandoah Co.] to-day. I have been engaged in making off monthly reports.

---

[129] With reenlistment, troops reorganized their companies and voted for their officers. Results for Co. D, 4th VA. Inf. of Virginia Stonewall Brigade—still basically the original Smyth Blues—were Albert Gallatin Pendleton (1836-1901), captain; Andrew E. Gibson (1838-1862), 1st Lt.; James M. Thomas, 2d Lt. A.R. Bishop was barely defeated by Thomas for 2d Lt. and remained as lst Sgt., a noncommissioned and unelected position, but one of great power in terms of actually running Co. D in its day to day details. Pendleton was a prominent attorney with business interests in the *Marion Visitor*, the newspaper for Smyth Co.; he appears to have been unpopular with his men, but a powerful leader. Gibson was a well-respected lay leader among Presbyterians who had established no career before the war. Although very young, Gibson was described as a "beloved" patriarchal figure among the troops. Armstrong, *Hist. of Smyth*, 115, 126, 128-30 and appendix. Thomas, who offered to do the diarist some favors before this election, was apparently related to two prominent families, the Thomases and the Coles, and a maternal ancestor, Freelove Cole Thomas "suggested that the new court town of Smyth County be called 'Marion' for General Francis Marion" of Revolutionary War renown, Wilson, *Smyth Co. Hist.*, 320-26. The drinking sprees paid for by the candidates in the elections mentioned by the diarist earlier were occasioned by this feature of reenlistment and election of officers.

FRIDAY 28TH, 1862

Last night was a cold night. The wind continued to blow [.] The sick was being sent from Winchester to-day—hands are at work on the embankments. 5 days rations are drawn.

The enemy is reported in the neighborhood of Harper's Ferry. I presume an attempt will be made by him to reconstruct the Balt. & Ohio R.R. but that cannot be done while we are here.

I wrote to Dr. F. to-night.

SATURDAY MCH 1ST, 1862

I finished my monthly report to-day and handed it over. The prospect for some move grows more prominent [.] I think we will vacate Winchester soon—perhaps in less than 5 days. Two prisoners wer[e] brought in this morning with 14 horses. Gen Banks & McLeland [McClellan][130] are reported to have been at Charles Town last night. I do not believe it. The heavy ordnance is being sent away from this place. We will soon follow. I got a letter from Dr. Quisenberry and one from Cousin Bettie—answered both.

SUNDAY, MCH. 2ND, 62

Commenced snowing this morning and snow rapidly for a while. Preparations for moving are still in progress. Some very important moves are evidently on hand, but what they are none of us can see. Reports say that Commissary & Quartermaster stores have been removed from Manassas back to the interior. This impresses us with something like the opinion that our policy will be in accordance with the views of President Davis that is: to concentrate our forces somewhere from the coast so as to have them in bodies sufficiently strong to repel the attack of the enemy. The attempt to defend the entire coast has been a failure fraught with much harm to us. The enemy's intention may be to draw forces from Manassas here with the sole intention of attacking that point as he did in July last.

---

[130] Nathaniel Prentiss Banks (1816-1894), identified earlier, was indeed moving his forces toward Jackson's VA. Brigade., but he was not coming from Charles Town WVA.; instead, Banks was marching toward Winchester from Harpers Ferry. George Brinton McClellan (1826-1885), also identified earlier, was recuperated from illness, and was again active with his Army of the Potomac, but he was not in West Virginia. McClellan was about to undertake the Peninsula Campaign via Aquia Creek moving southeast of Richmond. Long, op. cit., 324-27. 210

I had an interview with Dr Black this morning in regard to my course for the next two years. He advises me to remain in the medical department and then finish my course [that is, curriculum at Medical College of Virginia]. He promises me also to aid in giving me a through ticket from the District at the University of Va if it can be done. And after consideration I think it will be best for me. If I were to go into any other department I would loose [sic] what medical knowledge I have acquired and would probably never again turn my attention to-wards it. I wish to go home if I can but the prospect is rather dull now. Dr. says he wanted for me to be here when the regiment is organised again. He will assist me in getting an appointment by the Secretary of War [Judah P. Benjamin].

MONDAY MARCH 3RD, 1862

This morning is cold and rainy. A part of the regiment goes on picket. Prospects for a move still seem evident to take place to-day or to-morrow. Dr. Black wrote me a note advising me to pack up but I did not receive it in time. He also sent me a letter of recommendation to the Surgeon General and advising me to mail off my application and show it to him. I did not do it because I had no idea of what form an application should be._ . [his punctuation showing something omitted on purpose]

TUESDAY, MARCH 4TH, 1862

This morning Dr. B. sketched a form for me and told me that it would be best for me to get the signature of Dr. [Hunter Holmes] McGuire Med. Director. I obtained the signatures of Col: [Charles A.] Ronald[131] and Maj [Andrew Galatin] Pendelton[.] [B]oth seemed perfectly willing to sign the recommendations. I then went to the office of Dr. McGuire and asked him to do me the kindness to sign it. His manner was such that I did not feel that he cared anything about accommodating a Hospital Steward and I felt somewhat abashed. I ventured to ask him. He took the paper and glanced it over and says: I am too busy this morning—come in this evening and I will look at it ." Thinks I, very good I'll not trouble you again. One moment proved as ample time [as] a thousand years to [illegible; sense is demonstrate or attest] to that [.] However I

---

[131] Charles A. Ronald (1827-1898) was an attorney and a veteran of Mexican War. Originally Capt. in Co. E, 4th VA., he was elected Col. in command of entire Stonewall [Virginia] Brigade. once Jackson was elevated to corps commander. James I. Robertson, Jr., *The Stonewall Brigade* (Baton Rouge: Louisiana State University Press, 1991).

suppose such rebuffs are such as all of us may expect as we go on through life. I don't like to trouble big men though.

I sealed up the papers and put them in care of the post master.

I was called to see D. Trucks of Co. "A." He has nearly run his race by drinking. What a lamentable thing to see so promising a young man become a victim to so defaming a vice. It is to [be] hoped that we will not be troubled so much as heretofore by the use of ardent spirit. President Davis enjoins many penalties on the liquor makers.

It will be a blessed thing in this time of trial to see all of the liquor manufactories closed and its vendors out of employment. Prospects for leaving here in a day or two are not so good as a day or so ago. Rations are being brought back from Strasburg.

WEDNESDAY, MARCH 5, 62

Every thing is quiet in camp. The men are as unconcerned about the enemy as if they were in Maryland. It is reported that an engagement at Leesburg [Loudon Co.] [132]—but like other reports I expect there is not much truth in it. Lieut Jas. W. Kennedy has resigned his commission as 1st Lieut to Co. D. There will be another election now. I feel sometimes like I would like to be an officer but upon consideration it will be best for me to continue in the Medical Department as I hope to continue the practice of medicine hereafter. There is one thing however I ought to do: that is study more. I waste many hours that are precious, and, if the[y were] properly improved would in the course of time, render good account.

I put my name down for reenlistment to-day.

THURSDAY MCH 6TH, 1862

Moving seems fresh again to-day. I have packed up to get all things ready to move. It is hard from any idea what will be done. The malitias [sic] are working on the fortifications that are in the neighborhood.

FRIDAY, MARCH 7TH, 1862

To-day firing of canon were distinctly heard in the direction of Bunker Hill [Bedford Co]. Col: [Turner] Ashby is down on the enemy. About 3 o'clock

---

[132] Banks's forces were advancing against a much smaller force commanded by Jackson, and the Federals successfully occupied Leesburg on 8 March. *Official Reports*, 1, 21:22-28, 550.

orders came for us to pack up and be ready to march immediately. In less than 1/2 an hour all were ready. We moved down the road something like a half a mile. Fences were immediately thrown down and the troops took position.

The wind blew cold and raw. We remained on the field and made fence Rails \ suffer. The enemy is reported to be in 8 miles of us. Ashby drove him back to-day! A rumor is afloat that 135 Yankees were captured at "hanging rock" [133]—It needs confirmation.

The soldiers seem in fine spirits. Whenever Gen. Jackson came along the [word missing] he was applauded most enthusiastically.

There is a much larger force here than I had anticipated on. I have no doubt the enemy will be surprised to find Winchester harder to get than they expected.

The people of Winchester are very much excited. Women & children were walking the streets and crying rapidly.

SATURDAY MCH 8, 1862

Every thing is quiet this morning—no enemy in sight—We marched upon the hill on which Fort Alabama is situated. From this hill a most splendid view of the country on the east can be obtained. The canon [sic]—one 42-ponder and one 24-pounder could wake the enemy for a long distance. But it is not expected that these guns will not be used as there is no ammunition with them. On the west the Pugh Town [Frederick Co.] road commands the hill i.e. there seems to be a higher point on it than the hill fortified.

A detail was made to fall [sic] some timber near in order that a clearer range might be obtained and perhaps also with the intention of forming an *abatis.* [134] . We returned to the field and remained 'till near night when we went to our quarters again.

Some things have occurred to-day that may be worthy of notice. For some weeks past the men of the 4th Reg. seem to care nothing about the position they hold as men fighting for Liberty and Rights. Co. D. Has [sic] been foremost I ought say. A part stays in town a part in the country, a part in the fair grounds and a few at camp, not with standing repeated orders for every man to be at his post. Some are doubtless under the entire control of the little archer Cupid and

---

[133] Hanging Rocks in Hampshire Co., WVA. 22nd Federal cavalry co. organized in Washington, PA. and known as Old Ringgold Cavalry; it was based in WVA most of the War.

[134] Abatis is "a defence constructed by placing felled trees lengthwise one over the other with their branches towards the enemy's line, and piling them up until a shelter for workmen is obtained." *OED.*

"Strong indeed must be the heart
In which love can find no tender part."

hence rules are violated, the law to which we are subject is set at variance and exhortations are unheeded. To-day and yesterday it became imperatively necessary for every man to take his place and I believe most of them but some few were missing. So soon as the Regiment stopped and prepared to make a stand several wanted to go to town some for bread some for clothes, some for one thing and some for another and of course were refused by Col: Ronald; but some went anyhow and were sent for and brought in at the point of the bayonet.

To-day one came and asked the Col: to allow him to go for clothes[.] [T]he Colonel's tender heart gave him permission with the injunction to return immediately. The boy (Jno. N. H.)[135] started and took a friend with him saying to the Captain [Pendleton] that the Col: gave both permission. He [Ronald] saw it and was very much fretted—The consequence was that Hall goes into the guard House.

It is to be regretted that there seems to be a want of interest among us. The enthusiasm that prompted many to leave home has faded and left in its stead a dont-care feeling. Our men must rouse up. The time is rapidly approaching when we must take the field for a summer campaign that promises to be active and bloody, & he that shuns the duties impressed upon him as a soldier is unworthy of the rich boon of Freedom.

SUNDAY, MCH: 9, 1862

This is a lovely morning—clear and sunny. There is but little of interest to-day. Col. Ashby had a skirmish to-day [and] brought in one prisoner. The large canon from Fort Alabama are being moved to-day. These are all the heavy pieces here.—The wagoners were ordered to harness their horses to-night—we may leave to-morrow. Mt. Jackson [Shenandoah Co.] is thought by some to be the point that we will go. We will doubtless fall back to some strong point. Manassas is also being evacuated. Guns &c are taken to Gordonsville [Orange Co.].

I wrote to Dr. F. to-day.

---

[135] John N. Hall, of Smyth Co.

MONDAY MARCH 10, 1862

We expected to have left here this morning but it rained hard and I presume prevented our movements. The news is of no importance to-day. The probability is that we will move to-morrow. Gen. Jackson with a part of his staff were viewing the grounds this evening. What his intentions are is a mystery.

I read part of the History of Poland to-day—There seems to me to be some analogy between our struggle and that of the aspiring Polanders but I hope our fall will not be like that of that fallen nations [sic; poss.]. I have been reading Johnston's Chemistry of Human Life—a very instructive work.

TUESDAY, MARCH 11TH, 1862

This morning we were ordered to pack up. After packing up and lying round for some hours, or until about 2 o'clock we were summoned to take the field. Reports came that the Yankees were marching upon us very rapidly. Cannon were heard in direction of Berryville [Clark Co.]. [136] Our lines were thrown out across the valley below Winchester so as to guard the road to Martinsburg [Martinsville in Henry Co.] road. Soon however the 4th Regt was ordered upon the hill crest of the road where a battery stood. [F]rom this place we could see very plainly all that passed below. The maneuvers of our men just below us and the shifts and changes of our cavalry at the edge of the wood. [J]ust before night the enemy made his appearance about two miles from us. The pickets could be seen advancing and ours falling back, two regts were seen to enter the wood on our left and I presume went into camp, as the smoke soon ushered [sic] out. Farther on our left in a field the enemy's bayonets were seen glistening in the evening sun. The attempt to attack our left was very evident. Far toward Millwood [Clarke Co.] we could [see] Taliaferro's [137] command in a long line

---

[136] Jackson was taking most of his VA. Brigade., some 4,600 men, on a rapid retreat up the Shenandoah Valley southward. He was preparing for a major engagement elsewhere. There was a skirmish at Stephenson's Station (Depot) in Frederick Co., apparently what Apperson heard. Federal forces commanded by Banks were in process of recapturing Winchester and pursuing Jackson. *Official Records*, 5:4.

[137] William Booth Taliaferro (1822-1898) of Gloucester City in tidewater graduated from The College of William & Mary and read law at Harvard University. An officer in Mexican War, he later served in VA. gen. assembly. Originally commissioned to command VA. militia in east, he was a strict disciplinarian and extremely unpopular with his men. Reassigned, he joined Jackson's VA. Brigade, but he could not get along with Jackson. Although he conspired against Jackson in Richmond among poiticians weeks before this action, Taliaferro fought with distinction, especially in this Shenadoah campaign of 1862. Edward G. Longacre, "Taliaferro," *Hist. Times*.

coming forward. This was encouraging to us. It came near the encampment we had left and halted.

Night came on. Two premises were made by us. One that we would remain 'till morning and give battle, the other, that a retreat would be effected beneath the cover of night. The latter was correct. About dusk we left the field. Taking the road we passed through Winchester but not through the main part of the town. Loud shouts were heard in Main and Market streets. The soldiers seemed some-what animated rather than depressed. This animation was from the effect of the excitement of the evening and of the present moment of moving. I know many fe[l]t sad at heart to leave a place where we had been protecting for the last 12 mos. and now looked upon as home almost. Some had ties that bound them to the place, the ties of love had fastened upon them. But it was of no avail. They had but to bid their sweet hearts good by [sic] take one last kiss and leave them to the fates. This was sad indeed. Many exp[r]essed themselves that they would sooner fight than leave those endearments behind.

I did not from the first think that Gen. Jackson would give fight with his small force. But after leaving Winchester I thought it probable that we might return next morning and have a round or two.

Gen. Jackson commanded his Colonels to meet him in council that night. They did so. He told them the chances for and against them. And said that one of the best opportunities was now offered for a brilliant victory that had been offered during the War, and then asked the opinions of the officers assembled with him. All opposed fighting I think but one perhaps.

This may be a matter of some discussion whether he ought to have fought or not. If he fought he did it on his own responsibility as he had been ordered by a higher power to evacuate the place. He had moved all his stores away, and nothing was now left to do but march his command wherever it was ordered. If now he had fought a superior force and won a victory his fame would have been complete but on the other hand if he had fought a superior force contrary to orders and had been whipped the whole South would have been rife with a condemnation of the act. But looking at the thing as it was I think we ought to have fought. They will construe it into a victory any how; and could have done no more any way. The force of the enemy here on hand was estimated at 16000 ours did not exceed 5000—10 Regts one batallion and some malitia[sic]. We had a good proportion of artillery with Col: Ashby's cavalry. Great victories have been won with greater odds than that. In Poland 10,000 fought 100,000 and was victorious. A force of the enemy is reported to be advancing from towards Millwood and if true a retreat is wiser that it would otherwise would seem to be.

We marched with in two miles of Newton [Newton Stephensburg in Frederick Co.] and camped at the house of a Mr. Barton. The farm and improvements were equal if not superior to any on the road. Plank fences[,] stake fences and stone fences all laying out his farm in good lots; but when [the] enemy comes his plank and stone fences will be in ashes. Capt. [A.E.] Gibson and myself went into the kitchen and got a bite of vi[c]tuals. I was proud to get some sour milk of which I drank about a quart. I laid down in the wagon to sleep.

WEDNESDAY, MCH 12TH, 1862

This morning we were roused early and took a snack and started towards Strasburg [Shenandoah Co.]. As I traveled along I could not help reflecting upon the distressing necessities of war. We are now leaving the most beautiful part of Virginia's soil—this the garden spot of, I might say, the whole south. The inhabitants are to some extent those who think more of money and land than they do of politics and country. We are evidently in a country now where we will not be so much exposed to the doings of disloyal men.

We marched within two miles of Strasburg and camped on a hill above the creek.

The sun shines warm and the men seem to enjoy it very much.

THURSDAY, MARCH 13, 1862

To-day passed in lying round. We rec'd news that a fight had come off at Norfolk between the Virginia and some of the Yankee boats. The Virginia sank two and disabled another. This is news to us. [138]

---

[138] The *Virginia* was the former USN. *Merrimack*, which was rebuilt by the Confederate navy into the world's first "ironclad" fighting ship. The initial fighting in Hampton Roads did bring terror to Federal forces, with even President Lincoln in "dread that the *Merrimack* [sic] would sally forth to destroy the fleet and appear off Washington or New York." However, by 12 March, the Federal's ironclad *Monitor*, a quick boat with a turret gun that could revolve rapidly and fire accurately, had fought the *Virginia* to a draw. The slower, less powerful, and more awkward *Virginia* could not be deployed as once hoped, and soon was destroyed to prevent the Federals from capturing it. When Apperson heard reports of 12 March, he was not hearing about the fighting that day between *Virginia* and *Monitor*, but rather the first fighting in which wooden vessels of the Federal blockade were rammed by the *Virginia*. Apperson was thus hearing what citizens of Washington, D.C. were hearing, to wit, a terrible new ironclad monster was destroying the Federal fleet in Hampton Roads and was ready to come up the Potomac or even out to sea and

I wrote to Dr. W. Faris.

FRIDAY, MARCH 14, 1862

This morning some appearance of rain.

It is reported that some 60 of our brigade remained in Winchester and were taken prisoners. I have not the least doubt that some did; and should they be taken again by us death should pay the penalty.

It is said that a large body of the enemy has been as far up as Newtown. Orders came this evening for us to be ready to march to-morrow at 4'o A.M.

I have been engaged all day assisting Dr. Black make off property returns.

SATURDAY MARCH 15 1862

This morning according to orders all were up. Soon after sunrise we started taking the McAdamized road[139] through Strasburg up the valley. Rains poured down. We pass some three or four villages—some with 20 or 30 houses. About 4 o'clock we got to Woodstock [Shenandoah Co.]. This is a very respectful village. Larger than I expected to see it. Here a good many malitia seem to be on the [illegible] for the war. Some had old rifles but most of them were unarmed. We marched some two miles further and camped on the road side.

News of a victory in Arkansas to-day but reports[140] vary very much.

SUNDAY MARCH 16 1862

Some expected and others hoped to remain in camp to-day but and [sic] order came for us to pull out which we did about 11 0'clock. The road was very muddy. We passed through Edinburg which is a very nice village—nice too by having for its inhabitants some fair ones of beauty.

---

then into New York harbor. Long, *Civil War Almanac*, 180-83. Eller, ed., *Civil War Naval Chronology*, Pt. 2, March 1862, 30-32.

[139] The most advanced kind of overland roadway in the era. "Macadamize, verb, trans., to make or repair (a road) according to J[ohn] L[oudon] McAdam's system, which consists in laying down successive layers of stone broken into pieces of nearly uniform size, each layer being allowed to consolidate under the pressure of ordinary wheel traffic before the next is laid upon it." *OED*.

[140] The campaigns along the Tennessee and Mississippi Rivers continued, and these would all result eventually in Federal victories. There was fighting on 13 March at Spring River, Arkansas, but it was inconsequential and not a victory or a loss for either side. Long, *Civil War Almanac*, 182.

Dr. [George] Bean[,] Mr. [A.E.] Gibson & myself flanked for some dinner. At the home of a Mr. Bowman we got a fine meal. Dr. Hay & Maj: Mercer[141] were there. Brandy was handed round pretty freely.

When we reached our brigade again it had gone into camp. Col [Charles A.] Ronald met us. Talked to us about the impropriety of leaving ranks to get dinner.

We are camped in the wood near a Mr. Ripley.

Several Rifle Companies were sent to Col: Ashby who is said to be at the camp we left on Saturday. This is certainly a very fine country here. Our camp is a good situation. I loade[d] out of the wagon as much medicine as I thought I would need and pitched my tent. Francisco & C.G. McLemore will sleep with me a few nights.

MONDAY MARCH 17TH, 1862

We had regular sick call this morning. There is always more sickness when we are in camp than when we are marching. The list is crowded this morning. Many of our boys are trying to play off.

I am sorry to see some few of the 4th Regt declaring that they will go home. If the mass of people do not do better I fear our case will yet prove a hard one. Every man must put his shoulder to the wheel and aid. They must not turn their whole attention to who will be in service and who will not.

I wrote two letters to-day—one to cousin Bettie and one to Dr V Quisenberry[.] Have been working in property returns to-day.

TUESDAY MARCH 18 1862

Nothing to-day but a report that our forces have been whipped again at Newbern N.C. The day has been fine.

We have gotten no letters for some two weeks.

WEDNESDAY, MARCH 19TH 1862

The day has been spent in camp[.] [N]othing worthy of particular notice occurred. The malitia is slow in their manifestations of patriotism. Some have

---

[141] Possibly Thomas H. Mercer, *Official Records*, 12:779, 780-799; also possibly George W. Mercer, apparently from Rural Retreat, Armstrong, *Antebellum Years*, 227; the more famous Hugh Weedon Mercer (1808-1877), a native of VA. and West Point graduate, was already a colonel commanding 21st GA. and serving with Jackson in the Valley at this time. Edward G. Longacre, "Mercer," *Hist. Times*.

responded to the call of the Governor [John Letcher] but not as many as in the spirit that they should have done. The camp we occupy is in a tollerably [sic] nice place for a camp. We are in sight of a village called Hawkinsville [Sussex Co]. In the surrounding country there are some very pretty farm houses in the neighborhood. The Shanandoah [sic] runs along at the foot and between our camp and the Blue Ridge.

THURSDAY, MARCH 20TH, 1862

CAMP 2 MI. ABOVE EDINBURG

This morning during "sick call" it was announced that a march was on hand. And when we found our wagons gone, having been sent away yesterday to carry stores from Mt. Jackson to New Market [Shenandoah Co.], every thing was thrown into confusion. Companies were crowding the few wagons with knapsacks and bedding[.] Some were breaking up boxes and trunks and heaping together all the baggage likely to be left so that it could be readily destroyed when the regiment started off. I was troubled more than any one. The enemy was reported to be in four miles of us and no wagon to take my medicines. I unpacked some boxes and selected the most valuable medicines and put them together with the determination of leaving nothing valuable if I could carry it. Finally a part of my things were put in different wagons wherever I could find room enough to put anything until I had the pleasure of seeing all on. We had barely gotten our things loaded up before our wagons came but we had nothing much to put in them. The wagons moved off and we remained until about 2 o'clock when we marched off toward Mt. Jackson. We passed the 37 & 21st Va Reg near our camp.

At Mt. Jackson the streets were crowded with wagons conveying stores away. Some excellent Hospitals have been erected here—the best I have seen—but they are being vacated now. Nearly all the medicines have been taken away but an order was sent in[:] the surgeon to keep the [words missing, page torn] space for more sick.

I went into the kitchen and got a snack of vi[c]tuals.

The provost guard are stationed here. They had lost a prisoner—a Union man. This guard is deficient as well as the remainder of our army—too much liquor is drank [sic] for the good of the service. Some of them will walk up and down the streets and talk and look big but when the time comes for action they are not there.

We marched two miles west of Mount Jackson and camped. I found my baggage all right—my tent up and a good fire in my stove. Mr. Francisco had things comfortable.

It seems that the enemy is pushing on us, which renders activity necessary. When we get past New Market we are comparatively safe. As we are now the enemy could flank us by way of Warrenton [Fauquier] & Louray [?] from Manassas. From Culpeper C.H. to New Market is a good McAdamized road and should the enemy push us past New Market and follow us up [Joseph Eggleston] Johnston can throw his force to New Market and attack them in his rear. This seems to be the plan.

It is a sad matter indeed to give up this the finest country we've seen. We passed the celebrated Stirnberger farm to-day. It belongs to Brigadier Gen. Weems of the malitia. It is an excellent farm indeed [on the north fork of the Shenandoah River where it crosses the Valley pike]. Lovely plains surrounded by a slight elevation around it and further off the [B]lue Ridge on one side and the Allegheny on the other. If our men would just step forward now in this emergency and make and [sic] demonstration towards the enemy, though they had not an arm the effect would be great. But we leave a section and the enemy comes in and fares as well as we. This will not do. Some sacrifice of life, property and time must be undergone before we shall win for what we now struggle.

It is reported that Maryland is rousing.

Ed. Note: At this point, portions of the diary are missing, either lost or never recorded. He picks up a brief set of entries in May, after which there is another blank space until October. Unrecorded is the springtime reorganization of the old Virginia Bde., with Charles A. Ronald becoming regimental commander; Confederate losses of manpower and territory as McClellan moved inexorably toward Richmond; stunning successes for Jackson's Bde. in the Shenandoah Valley, from which his legendary status emerged because of the ability of his infantry to move almost as fast as cavalry —which must have been an incredible challenge for Apperson and the medical corps, who were having considerable difficulties with Jackson's earlier, much more slow moving marches; the wild "ride around McClellan" (12-15 June) that the westerner J.E.B. Stuart accomplished by bringing his cavalry completely around the brilliantly directed but very orthodox, even stately, march of the Union general's huge force (estimated at more than one hundred thousand men, with some eighty thousand available at any give time for a major assault on the Confederate capital); and then the so-styled Seven Days Campaign, from 25 June to 2 July, when Robert Edward Lee coordinated feints and skirmishes successfully with Jackson to drive the Federals from Richmond. It should be noted that the Seven Days Campaign cost the Federals around 16,000 casualties, but it also cost the Confederates at least 20,000 casualties. It should also be noted that Lee's bloody and not particularly successful assault at Malvern Hill [Henrico], which concluded the Seven Days Campaign, was as much a tactical victory for the much-maligned McClellan as it was a tactical blunder of over-aggressiveness for the justly celebrated Lee. As E.B. Long notes, "The guns fell silent on Virginia's peninsula, but the Federal army was still there, and not too far from Richmond at that." [142]

THURSDAY, MAY 1, 1862

DR. SHELBY'S [ROCKINGHAM CO.]

Owing to the active movement of our army, and the inconvenience of obtaining nothing as well as perhaps the want of time, I have left a space—a blank between this date and the date furnished in my diary some two months ago.

Since then more has transpired than I am able to write on or even note. The battle of Kernstown [Frederick Co.] has been fought and the Valley almost entirely given up to the enemy. [143]

---

[142] Long, op. cit., 235.

[143] Again "the fog of war" makes the diarist record a defeat with long-term consequences for the loss of the Valley, when military historians now record a tactical victory for Jackson with long-term consequences for the protection of the Valley as Jackson's enclave. Jackson acted on poorly gathered information from Ashby that Gen. James Shields commanded a small Federal force at Kernstown, a little south of Winchester. Attacking on 23 March, Jackson brought his force of 3,500 against Shields's strongly entrenched force of 9,000. West Point guidebooks of the era indicated that an entrenched force could protect itself against an attacking force three times its size, and thus the poor intelligence sent Jackson "against the book," with a hopelessly inadequate ratio for a serious attack. Casualties were high for a brief engagement, more than seven hundred for Jackson and almost six hundred for Shields. Long remarks, "Kernstown marked the opening of what would become the famous Shenandoah Valley Campaign. Furthermore, it had its effect: Gen. J.E. Johnston had directed Jackson to divert Federal attention from his main army and keep troops from the gathering Army of the Potomac [McClellan]. Jackson did so by attacking. Washington, fearing a threat on Harper's Ferry and Washington, ordered Banks and his Federal troops to return to the valley and others that had been heading for the Peninsula were withdrawn from McClellan's command. The threat also influenced Lincoln to keep Irwin McDowell's large corps south of Washington, instead of sending it by sea to the Peninsula....Thus, what became the First Battle of Kernstown was a small battle large in results. For the remainder of March, Jackson withdrew up the Shenandoah, protected by Ashby's cavalry, while Banks and his Federals slowly pursued as far as Strasburg." Long, op. cit., 188.

In that engagement our loss in killed, wounded, and missing, falls not short of 600 [sic]. The 4th Reg't lost 76—Co. "D" lost one killed, and three wounded.

The Conscript Bill has been passed. I have been to Richmond and assigned to duty to the 4th Reg't as hospital steward since I left off my diary.

To-day we are in Rockingham County near Dr. Shelby's on the road marching towards Port Republic. Last night rain fell rapidly and the ground was wet and the roads were almost impassible, but now the ground is thoroughly saturated with water and the condition of the roads indescribable.

We are detained to allow the train of wagons to pass. A team is stalled opposite our last night's camp. The poor horses are cruelly beaten by the drivers impatient to pass. Some wagons have been upset in the hurry of the drivers to pass. Some got in front of other teams. Col. Jesse S. Burks' command[144] is in front of us, but fortunately our teams are in front. Some of the regiments have had nothing to eat this morning. By noon the trains had passed and we were allowed to go forward, but often we were called to a halt to allow the wagons in front to get forward.

Orders from Headquarters require the roll to be called every hour and absentees marked. The further we go the worse the roads get. After traveling some two or three miles from 1 o'clock to 6 o'clock, we were orderd to press forward to our wagons. From this time till 9 o'clock, I walked through mud and water. Regiments became broken into fragments of companies and every man seemed to be thrown upon his own exertion and choice in regard to reaching camp. Dr. Snidow and I walked briskly until about 7 o'clock and kept tolerable free from mud, but then night set in and our fate was settled so far as our being plastered with mud. Turning off the road at various places in order to avoid the ponds of water that collected in the road, we would frequently go down knee-deep in mud in the open fields. Camp after camp was passed but no tidings from the 4th Reg't. No one could tell us where it was. Coming at last to the camp of the Commissary of our Brigade, we were told which light came from our camps. In our course to reach them, I went through thickets, over plowed fields and deep creeks and down steep rugged banks. Finally we did arrive and were among the first in camp. Others came in with a shout. The camp fire at night to a very poor weary weather-beaten soldier is like home to the evening shepherd or husbandman.

---

[144] Col. Jesse S. Burks, who graduated from Virginia Military Institute, commanded a brigade. in Jackson's valley campaign.

FRIDAY, MAY 2, 1862

NEAR PORT REPUBLIC, ROCKINGHAM CO., VA.[145]

Many of our boys remained behind last night and came in this morning. Gen. Jackson met them and told them to hurry to camp. He thinks, I suppose, they should have come up last night, which they should have done. Gen. Jackson has much to bear from men when they are worn down. I am told he worked manfully yesterday in getting wagons safe across the marshes, and while the men complained it was not without a cause. Many sank into the mud last night and when they pulled out of it, they were barefooted, having lost their shoes in the mud. Today no shoes can be obtained from the Quarter Master and consequently they must remain barefooted.

The Commissary Stores are being curtailed—wheat for coffee and nothing for sugar.

To-day we have been at the same place. Various orders have come and we are ready to move. At five o'clock Taliaferro's and Burk's commands are passing. I suppose they will take the advance which belongs to them now. The enemy is reported to be in cannon shot of us—movements are active.

I rec'd three letters to-day, one from my sister and one from other friends. What a pleasing thing it is to correspond with friends. How I do love a good letter. It fills my memory with all the pleasing associations of other days and all the friendly connections I have formed and love to cherish. My breast is filled with emotion with hope for the peace of home.

I hoped we would move to-night; we did not.

SATURDAY, MAY 3, 1862

TOP BLUE RIDGE, BROWN'S GAP

This morning at half past seven we marched off. Taking the road towards the mountains we entered Brown's Gap and pursued our way up to the mountains.[146] The scenery was good considering the season. The barren hills look sad and the rocks stand out badly. . . . [illegible section] This is evidently a good place to ambush the enemy. From the jutting ledges men could do terrible execution without endangering themselves. After winding around many ravines and hills, we are at the top about one o'clock and ready to descend the

[145] Port Republic is southeast of Harrisonburg and near Brown's Gap. Hummel, *List.*

[146] A pig iron furnace; there were a number in the Blue Ridge.

mountain. Where we are going is not known by any. It may be that we will be held ready to reinforce our forces at any place in the eastern portion of the state or perhaps anywhere else.

I might make suppositions, viz., Jackson will either make the railroad, ostensibly leaving the Valley as if on retreat, and when he reaches the railroad he will push for Stanton; or he will go towards Culpeper and cut across the country to New Market and then cut the supplies of the enemy; or he is going to reinforce Gen. Johnston's forces at either Yorktown or Fredericksburg. [T]his first seems more probable.

We are camped out at a hotel at the foot of the Blue Ridge miles from Charlottesville. The march to-day was brisk and continuous one. We traveled 9 hours.

[T]he sick list is always large on a march. Larger in the 4th Reg't than in any other from what I learn. Orders from Gen. [Charles Sidney] Winder[147] put all those complaining in the rear of their respective regiments in charge of the Assistant Surgeon. Some 38 of our reg't had to march in that way and a delapidated set they were. Rheumatic patients, and those affected with bronchial diseases, diarrhea, dysentery, and all other diseases almost had some victims. While some are really sick, there are others who are too lazy to live and try to dupe the service at every opportunity and cheat the service out of their time.

Our camp is on a stream. I washed and took off some winter clothes. The weather is warm.

SUNDAY, MAY 4, 1862

ALBEMARLE CO., VA.

This morning at 8 o'clock we moved off. Gen. Winder issued orders in regard to the troops carrying their knapsack and some discontent prevailed. For

[147] Charles Sidney Winder (1829-1862) from Talbot City MD., was a West Point graduate noted for heroism on frontier duty in the antebellum West. In 1854, he was promoted to captain, possibly being the youngest man so promoted in US army before the war. He resigned his Federal commission to join the CSA as a major of artillery and participated in the bombardment of Ft. Sumter. Promoted to Brig. Gen., he was selected by Jackson to command the Stonewall Brigade. He was noted for very strict discipline and great personal bravery. "He led them into battle for the first time during Jackson's 1862 Shenandoah Valley campaign. Though his conduct did not gain the brigade's affection, it earned their grudging respect. On one occasion, when he stood up to Jackson, the brigade cheered him. During the Seven Days Campaign, he directed his men with gallantry." Jeffrey D. Wert, "Winder," *Hist. Times.*

my part I can but support my commander's orders and he that does not is remiss in duty.

Our troops have had their own funds and are too stubborn to be governed by any authority. I expect to render mysefl unpopular with the men but I cannot help it. When I see a man destroying himself out of honor, I cannot but tell him of it.

We passed White Hall [Albemarle Co.] about noon. Several fair ones were there which animated our boys not a little. I had the pleasure of conversing with one a short time. She seemed inclined to ridicule us for retreating as she called it.

We were at Mechum River Depot [148] [Albemarle Co.] on the Virginia R.R. about 5 o'clock p.m., having been very much retarded in our march. Here those of men, who were barefooted, sorefooted, sick and otherwise incapable of marching, were left at the Depot to be sent on the railroad cars. We then proceeded to camp half mile up the road [to] Staunton.

It was very evident now that we were going [to] Staunton and probably before many days we will witness a conflict.

Our sick moved tolerably off well though the company increased rapidly. It is termed Co. "X" or "Crockett's Battalion." [149] Orders are to be up a half past three [A.M.] tomorrow.

MONDAY, MAY 5, 1862

NEAR MECHUM'S RIVER DEPOT, ALBEMARLE CO.

This morning we were up early to fulfill the order of last night. For a time we had some hopes of getting a ride on the cars, but when we started off we took as the boys say, "The gravel train"—we took the dirt road on foot.

This part of the country looks better, I think, than that we passed over day before yesterday. Several good farms, elegant houses, with beautiful yards in front and a large number of nappy hedges were on our road. And to add a finish

[148] The town is Mechum's River, sometimes spelled Mecham's River. The Virgina Railroad had a depot at the town. Humel, *A List.*

[149] Joseph Crockett (1833-1862) from Wythe Co. was physician attached to Co. A, with rank of Assistant Surgeon to regiment from 4 May 1861; this was apparently the Crockett about whom the diarist was critical and even sarcastic in earlier entries. During this march, Dr. Crockett seems to gain considerable respect from the diarist steward. James I. Robertson, *4th Virginia Infantry,* Virginia Regimental Historical Series (Lynchburg: H.E. Howard, 1982), 46.

to all that is beautiful in nature, there were some pretty girls. The people showed real Old Virginia hospitality here. One of the most elegant yards I have seen was at a Mr. Farrow's.[150] Nothing seemed to be expensive, but taste and care were plainly shown. Gravel walks in different directions leading to the front door, on each of which were beautiful spring flowers just blooming. The squares or peats were green. Upon each side of the walks leading to the main entrance sat a spaniel of mink color save a few dark spots on his ears and sides. We got to Greenwood Depot [Albemarle Co.; on the same VA. RR. trunk] about one o'clock and found that the troops would be conveyed on the cars and the baggage wagons could cross the mountain. I felt a desire to cross it on horseback. I left the depot at 1 o'clock and started after the wagon while we [Co. A or "Co. X Crockett's"] were in front. When I reached the summit of the mountain I turned to view the scene below. And of all that I have ever seen in the way of beauty, magnificence, and glory, the panorama before me surpasses anything I ever saw.

On my left was a Valley which seemed to run up against a mountain, perhaps 15 miles distant; below in the direction from which we came was one broad expanse as far as the eye could reach.

In the Valley were houses and hills, meadows and lawns, upland and lowland ponds, streamlets, plowed lands and wheat fields. I looked upon this great handiwork of Creation and wondered if an atheist could look upon this and say there is no God—no Supreme Ruler to create all this beautiful scenery we traveled on. This gap is where the Central R.R. runs over the mountain.[151]

The western side of the mountain is not as fine as the eastern. I passed Waynesboro [Augusta Co.] about 4 o'clock. It is a small village of about 200 people. Myself and G. Hale, wagon master,[152] went to a house and procured dinner and overtook the wagons at camp two miles from Staunton.

---

[150] Possibly A.S. Farrow (born 1835), whose widow still maintained a residence at Miller's Township in Ablemarle Co. in 1870. *VA. Census.*

[151] Apparently Afton Mountain, the most prominent natural site near Waynesboro.

[152] Possibly Gideon Hale (born 1832), a farmer of Co. F "detailed as regimental wagonmaster" for Stonewall Brigade on this Valley campaign. Robertson, op. cit., 52.

TUESDAY, MAY 6, 1862

[AUGUSTA CO.] NEAR STAUNTON

This morning we moved into a wood where we remained all day. I finished the monthly report for April and handed it in. The enemy has fallen back down [northward] the Valley. [153] My first opinion of Gen. Jackson's movement is only partially correct, though it may have been otherwise had the enemy stood his ground. We leave tomorrow morning at dawn.

WEDNESDAY, MAY 7, 1862

BUFFALO GAP [AUGUSTA CO.]

This morning we left camp entirely ignorant of where we were going. We passed through Staunton and took the road to Westview [Goochland Co.]. At Staunton the Battalion of cadets [from Virginia Military Institute] joined us. [154] There were all young men hardly out of their teens. With the C.S.A. uniforms they will look fine, but with dust and sweat they will look no better than we do.

At night we went into camp almost 13 1/2 miles from Staunton. I borrowed ten dollars from Dr. Snidow to buy some shirting and it cost seventy-five cents per yard. I will be compelled to have them made by some lady.

We have a new ambulance and the sick increases. We are in a hard-looking county [Highland Co.] now. The enemy is not far off.

THURSDAY, MAY 8, 1862

[HIGHLAND CO. NEAR MCDOWELL BATTLEFIELD]

This morning we left camp early and proceeded towards Shenandoah Mountain. In the gap of the mountain, near "Mountain House," we passed the baggage of the troops before us. Here were some dead horses, the result of a skirmish yesterday in which our men killed 3, took two and killed five horses. It seems that there was some mistake or we would have taken a larger number of

---

[153] The Valley's elevation climbs as one moves southward on the Valley roads; thus Jackson goes "up the Valley" in a southward direction while Banks's forces on this day move "down the Valley" in a northward direction.

[154] V.M.I. Keydets, led by superintendent Gen. Francis H. Smith joined Jackson as the former instructor prepared a bold and risky maneuver to force Banks's troops into retreat down the Valley. The Keydets stayed with Gen. Jackson, even during the dangerous battle of McDowell, but they did not take part in this fighting. Bean, Notes.

prisoners. A flanking party was sent out with instructions to go to a certain Valley and intercept the enemy while retreating; but instead they went to the wrong one and found that they had come out immediately upon them. The enemy escaped with the loss [of] of great deal of their baggage. We reached a valley east of McDowell and heard cannon in front of us. Immediately a horseman came along and told us that we were skirmishing with the enemy but there was no prospect of a fight that evening. Soon we were ordered to return to where we had left our knapsacks and blankets. We returned but had been there but a short time when we heard cannon firing in the direction of the enemy. The long roll beat in two regiments, nad we were soon called to the ranks. Gen. Jackson's dispatch to Gen. Winder was, "Hurry up, I am pressed." Some confusion followed but soon all was right and we were on the way to the battlefield.

I was on horseback and when we got to the foot of the mountain [Bull Pasture Mountain], I found it impossible to get up. The wounded were being brought down in stretchers made of guns and blankets. The groans and cries were distressing in the uttermost. The assistant surgeon of each regiment in our Brigade was directed by the Medical Director to repair to the sick depot and assist in dressing wounds. Myself and Dr. Black went up front with the 4th Reg't.

After seeing the battlefield by the moonshine, we saw the regiment in position and went back to the Valley to render some assistance to the unfortunate. The wounded were lying all around and their suffering seemed severe. I do not know where the surgeons belonging to [Gen. Edward] Johnson's army[155] were—their men were suffering from want of attention.

About 1 o'clock the Reg't was ordered back to camp and we went. I was never so sleepy and tired. We got to camp a while after 2 o'clock. The result of the battle was that we were attacked by the enemy and fought them two hours.

The 12th Georgia Reg't was first to be in the battle and that with the 25th Virginia suffered at least half the losses. The 10th Va. suffered much and fought well.

---

[155] Edward Johnson (1816-1873) of Salisbury, VA., was nicknamed "Allegheny Ed" for his prowess for and fondness of mountain fighting. A West Point graduate, Johnson had served with distinction in Seminole Wars and in Mexican War, and counted Lee, George Pickett, and James Longsteet good friends before the war. Serving with 12 GA. Inf., he coordinated maneuvers with Jacson's VA. Brigade. Trusted by Jackson, Johnson fought successfully in this bloody battle of McDowell, and his wound, whick kept him out of the fighting for a full year, caused problems for the CSA command, and especially for Jackson. John E. Stanchak, "Johnson," *Hist. Times.*

Col. Gibbons was killed. The 37th, 21st, 48th, the Irish Battalion, 58th, 52nd and 44th Virginia Regiments were also engaged. We won the field. Gen. [Edward] Johnson was wounded in the ankle. [156]

FRIDAY, MAY 9, 1862

[MCDOWELL, HIGHLANDS CO.]

This morning we were expecting a fight. I met the Va. 48th Reg't and found none of Capt. [Robert H.] Dungan's company[157] hurt. We marched out towards the field. I counted the wounded at the sick depot and made out 160. When near the battlefield we found the killed lying at the foot of the [Bull Pasture] mountain, 31 in all. I obtained permission to go upon the battlefield and I went in company with Captains [Alexander M.] Hamilton and Laughlin.[158] From all I could see of the different positions occupied by both sides, I am forced to the conclusion that the loss on our side was much larger than theirs.[159] The hills and grounds showed marks of bullets near our position but on their side there were but few. I saw where one Yankee had sat behind a tree and shot several times. The cartridge papers were thickly strewn but he paid for it with his life, I expect, as there was a large pool of blood near.

We marched past McDowell, a small village[.] [T]en dead Yankees were lying near some houses. At their camp were knapsacks, tents, cooking utensils and all the necessities of war. Several of the tents were still standing. At the creek several boxes of ammunition had been thrown into the water. All along the road were crackers strewn. The Quartermaster's Depot was burning. We passed to a

---

[156] Jackson won this engagement, known as the Battle of McDowell or Bull Pasture Mountain, and his rapid march there and bold maneuvering added to this legendary status. However, historians Stanchak, Robertson, and Long all note the heavy costs of this engagement: 256 casualties for Federals, of whom 26 were killed; but 498 casualties for Jackson, of whom 75 were killed. Also, the loss of Edward Johnson for a full year hurt the Confederates. *Offiical Records*, 8 May 1862. Long, op. cit., 208-209.

[157] Robert H. Dungan from Smyth Co. joined the original Smyth Rifle Grays as their 1st Sgt. He quickly became captain during reorganization of that co. into a part of 48th VA. Rgt. Armstrong, *Ante-bellum Years*, 162.

[158] Alexander M. Hamilton (1830-1863) was apparently a Presbyterian from Rockbridge Co. A successful farmer, he joined 4th VA. Inf. at beginning of War and had just been elected captain 6 April during Jackson's Valley Campaign. Robertson, *4th VA. Inf.*, 54. We cannot identify a Capt. Laughlin.

[159] Correct. See 227 ff. It was a costly victory for Jackson.

point a short distance from McDowell and camped. We passes [sic] a wounded Yankee on the road. News reaches us to-day that fight was going on at Willliamsburg with some success to our side.[160]

Many Yankee letters fell into our hands and strange to say I have not read a really intelligent letter yet. All are vulgar and illiterate. From the letters in our hands and other things, all the troops we fought at McDowell were Africans. [161]

SATURDAY, MAY 10, 1862

[MONTEREY, HIGHLAND CO.]

This morning we left the camp early and marched all night, leaving Monterey to our left . Near night we were told that the enemy was in ambush. This not far from us. When near the place designated the ambulances and ordnance wagons were stopped and the regiments led the way, but no enemy was found. Gen. Jackson in a daring way took the lead at the head of a cavalry company and went through the narrow defile between the mountains. [162]

We went into camp about 1/2 mile below a Mr. Fletcher's. He had a fine meadow and I took advantage of the opportunity and gave my horse a good grazing.

---

[160] Rumors were incorrect. In sharp fighting on 6 and 7 May during McClellan's Peninsular Campaign, Federal generals Joseph Hooker (1814-1879) and Philip Kearney (1815-1862) defeated rearguard units of Joseph Eggleston Johnston's retreating force commanded by James Longstreet (1821-1904) and Daniel Harvey Hill (1821-1889). On 6 May Federal forces occupied the old VA. capital. Long, op. cit., 206-08.

[161] The diarist is declaring his racism herewith. Likely no black troops fought in blue under Banks in this Valley Campaign, although in fact there were two black soldiers James Cooley and John Ross, both from Marion and *both literate*, fighting voluntarily in grey for the Virginia Brigade. He particularizes the racist insult by saying *African*, assuming that the continent produced no literate people at all. In the racist mentality of that era, he is saying that these white northern soldiers write as if they were no better educated than Africans. On the racism of the era, most useful on this point are two books, George Milton Fredrickson, *Black Images in the White Mind; the Debate on Afro American Character and Destiny, 1817-1914* (1971. Reprint paper ed.; Scranton, PA.: Wesleyan University Press, 1987) and Winthrop D. Jordan, *White Over Black; American Attitudes toward the Negro, 1550-1812* (Chapel Hill: University of North Carolina Press for the Institute of Early American History and Culture at Williamsburg, 1965). On Cooley and Ross, see Wilson, *Smyth Co. Hist.*, 261-65.

[162] Jackson pursued Banks down the valley northward toward Franklin [in WVA.] as Federal general John Charles Fremont (1813-1890) rushed to Franklin to reinforce Banks's troops. On 13 May, Jackson turned his troops again up the valley southward, hoping to find Banks at Strasburg [Shenandoah Co.] and fight in the main valley. Long, op. cit., 208-13.

SUNDAY, MAY 11, 1862

[NEAR FRANKLIN, WVA.]

This morning we were up and off bright and early. The 4th Reg't. lead [sic] the way. All along we could hear the enemy. We got within four or five miles of Franklin and learned that the enemy had made a stand and probably had received reinforcements [from Fremont]. Opposite the house of a Mr. [name illegible] one of Co. "A" [David Findley][163] was accidentally shot through the knee joint. The bullet severed the capillary artery and shattered the lower end of the femur thighbone. Amputation was found to be necessay, chloroform was administered and Dr. [Harvey] Black performed the amputation. Varicose hemorrhage was so excessive that all the veins were tied, rend[er]ing the operating very protracted and tedious. Findley bore it well and the anesthesia acted fine. [164]

In the meantime, skirmishing was going on actively between our forces and the enemy. Cannonading from the enemy's side was kept up without much effect. Co. "C" of this Reg't lost one man, mortally wounded in the abdomen. He was conveyed to the house of a Mr. [name illegible] and left with a nurse.

I did not go to the 4th Reg't for two or three reasons. I did not know where to find it, and it was dark before I finished with the wounded on hand. The regiment came at 2 o'clock in the morning. We expected a general engagement next day. We can get no position for our artillery. The mountains are filled with so much smoke that you could not see our men 200 yards in the distance. Our boys charged the enemy and they fled, throwing away their knapsacks which we got. [165]

---

[163] David Findley (born 1827 in Smyth Co.) was a day laborer in Marion and a private in Co. A. Tall for that era [5' 11"] with blue eyes and light hair, he was not released from duty until the following December. Robertson, *4th VA. Inf.*, 50.

[164] Apperson apparently witnessed an amputation before this operation; this is the first time that we find him assisting with an amputation. Harvey Black was a serious student of surgery and an excellent practitioner and teacher. However, he had his limits, as did all surgeons of this era. Chloroform was a dangerous anesthetic and by this date in 1862 was already responsible for at least fifty deaths on the operating tables; indeed, the fifty recorded deaths "was only the tip of the iceberg." It would be the 20th century before there was "the systematic and highly professional field" of anesthesiology. "Those dangers were neither understood nor appreciated in the early days [1848-1890] of anesthetic practice, and even had there been, liberation from pain was so welcome an achievement that the attendant dangers could be disregarded." *McGrew's*, 15-18.

[165] Robertson reports that the smoke was so thick and acrid that it contributed to Jackson's decision to return to the main valley to seek a fight rather than continue pursuing Banks. Idem, *Stonewall Brigade.*

MONDAY, MAY 12, 1862

[POSSIBLY FRANKLIN, WVA; POSSIBLY SHENANDOAH CO., VA.]

This morning our baggage was sent back. Notice was given that preaching would be at 11 o'clock. During the morning several regiments had been sent out.

Only the 4th and 27th of the Brigade were left in camp. Cannons were firing at intervals. We lay around, mostly sleeping, especially the 4th Regiment, as it had no rest the previous night.

TUESDAY, MAY 13, 1862

[NEAR MCDOWELL, HIGHLAND CO.]

We are up and going early. Our mail bag was found and brought to us. I suppose the carrier lost it. The marches are as tedious as ever owing to so many wanting to ride. I carry knapsacks and overcoats as much as I can. To-night we camp at the same place we did on Saturday night [near Monterey, Highland Co.]. A cloud came up and rain fell rapidly all night. I could not keep dry in a wagon. We are yet ignorant of our destination. Perhaps we will go to northern Virginia or back to the wagons.

WEDNESDAY, MAY 14, 1862

[AT FORMER FEDERAL CAMP NEAR MCDOWELL]

This morning the roads were terrible and it was still raining. The boys had to take the mud and it is just as deep as the dust was yesterday. Not far from camp I found our company wagon broken down and all our cooking utensils and provisions in the mud. Our camp is near McDowell which we reached about sundown. I had orders for the surgeons of the different Regiments of the Brigade and by the time I delivered them, it was night. No supper in the camp, so I went to the "Dare Devils" [166] and got some grub. All our ambulances are

---

[166] Capt. Peyton N. Hale commanded the Grayson Co. Dare Devils, a county unit that joined 4th VA. Inf. Robertson reports, "[t]he most flamboyant of these county units was the 'Grayson Dare Devils.' Ninety-four of its 97 members were farmers living near the North Carolina border. Gaudily attired, this company took immense pride in its marksmanship. When 135 recruits responded to the first call for the 100-man unit, the captain [Hale] eliminated the 35 excess

ordered to report to Wilson's Tavern, I suppose to carry the sick and wounded away. I think this finishes this country. It is a waste now—people and all are gone.

Our camp is near McDowell on the same ground as the Yankee army encamped upon. The air smells bad from the carcasses of dead horses and putrefied meat left on the butcher's ground—There was a great many dead horses on the road. What may cause it we cannot tell unless it is from want of forage. We have not gotten more than 72 rations for man or beast for some time.

THURSDAY, MAY 15, 1862

[FORMER FEDERAL CAMP NEAR MCDOWELL]

Still raining this morning. We have many cases to sent [sic] to General Hospital at Staunton. [167] News from Richmond, Williamsburg and the Northwest is startling to us. Norfolk and Williamsburg have been evacuated and our troops are moving towards Richmond. [168]

---

applicants by staging an unorthodox shooting match. Each man had to fire at a target while on a dead run. Those widest of the mark were dropped from consideration." idem, *4th VA. Inf.*, 1.

[167] The CSA established field hospitals near major battlefields, and Apperson generally worked at these hospitals. There, surgeons conducted triage, deciding which cases had to be taken on at once and which could be postponed until transportation to permanent general hospitals, such as the fine one in Staunton. Those with minor illness or injury were also treated at the field hospitals, or even in the campsites. Apperson visited the general hospitals, often complaining of the privileged, and in his view even pampered, physicians working there. Medical historians rate the general hospitals as being good for the era, and perhaps surprisingly, even as late as 1864, well stocked and well supplied. Surgeon Lafayette Guild (based in Richmond) reported, "even after the bloody battles of the Wilderness and Spotsylvania (May 1864), that there was no suffering among the men from the lack of medical supplies or surgical attention." There was, however, a grave problem with transportation, for ambulance wagons were in short supply. Each regiment was to have at least two, but apparently that was only a "paper list"; and of course two wagons was hardly sufficient for some of the more bloody engagements that a regiment fought. There was an ambulance manufactory in Richmond, but it failed to produce the numbers of wagons needed. H.H. Cunningham, *Doctors in Gray; the Confederate Mecial Service* (Baton Rouge: Louisiana State University Press, 1958) 118-20.

[168] The ports of Norfolk and New Orleans were officially reopened to commerce by President Lincoln on 12 May 1862; and the Federal rivers campaign continued apace in what Apperson calls the northwest, with major successes at Memphis. Meanwhile, Nashville not only remained Federal, but a pro-Union rally was held there. There were northern successes in northern Alabama and northern Mississippi and in Arkansas this week, and Apperson may be calling that territory northwest. Long, op. cit., 209-15.

At Williamsburg I understand General [Jubal] Early was killed.[169] The 7th Va. Reg't is with that Brigade. I am anxious to hear from brother Nathan and others engaged there.[170]

We got to camp at sundown. Crossing the Shenandoah Mountain was a pretty tiresome job to us. I cannot see how an army could ever take such a place, no assailing party could ever get up the mountain. Raining very rapidly. I loaned my horse and have been walking through the mud.

FRIDAY, MAY 16, 1862

[SHENANDOAH CO.]

This morning rain is still falling. To-day is Thanksgiving day, and we will remain in camp to observe it, I suppose.[171] As to fasting, we have been at that for

---

[169] Jubal Anderson Early (1816-1894) was wounded by a minie ball in the shoulder in the Peninsula Campaign at Williamsburg, and he was evacuated to a general hospital; but he recovered quickly. Early, "with his abrasive and sloppy image, emerged from the Civil War as one of its great characters. Hard-drinking and sharp-tongued," he cultivated this image for himself, especially in memoirs after the war. Actually, he was from a prominent family in Franklin Co. and was well-educated, graduating from West Point, serving with distinction in the Seminole War and then practicing law successfully in Lynchburg. A courageous general, he bounced back from his shoulder wound and joined Apperson's own VA. Brigade. with a brigade command under Jackson for this Valley Campaign. Fred L. Schultz, "Early," *Hist. Times.*

[170] Nathan apparently survived this engagement, although he is not listed in 7th VA. Inf. William, apparently a cousin born in 1835, survived the Williamsburg fighting, but perished in the successful defense of Richmond variously called White Oak Swamp, Frayer's Farm, Nelson's Crossing, and five other names. David Riggs, *7th Virgina Infantry*, Virgina Regimental Histories Series (Lynchburg, VA.: H.E. Howard, 1982), 61. Long, op. cit., 211-34.

[171] Thanksgiving as we know it was a Civil War, and northern, creation in 1864. The Confederate Thanksgiving was proclaimed on 28 July 1861 as a praise to God for the successful defending of southern territory to that date. Other Confederate Thanksgiving days included this one, 16 May 1862. Federal Thanksgiving was proclaimed on 28 November 1861; another Federal Thanksgiving date was 6 August 1863. On 20 October 1864, Lincoln set the fourth Thursday as a national day of Thanksgiving to God, and that date was gradually accepted by southerners some years after the war. Long after the war, associations with the pilgrims of New England from preexisting in-gathering harvest celebrations in the northeast were gradually melded with this official Civil War commemoration. During the war itself, southerners kept their Thanksgiving observances completely separate from Federal ones, and of course did not talk about or celebrate pilgrims of New England; the Confederate Thanksgiving was very much a product of Protestant churches. As Apperson notes here, the Confederate faithful in their observances, far from establishing a feast at a harvest in-gathering, practiced fasting in the late spring planting season, although the diarist is obviously sarcastic in noting that they had all been "fasting" during the Valley Campaign. At the same time, the pietistic Apperson obviously wants serious prayer and

some time, but praying is not engaged in enough for the good of our cause. I fear our men are in awful condition to rest. No shelter from falling rain and no protection from the wet ground. All day we lay in a swamp exposed . . . . [illegible sentence] At 11 o'clock that night I was called to see a patient from Richmond with cramp colic. After relieving him, I went to bed. The news from Richmond is of an exciting character, the enemy is still moving upon the city. I understand that we will march towards Harrisonburg [Rockingham Co. in Valley] by taking the left hand road to-day. This looks like going into the Valley again.

SATURDAY, MAY 17, 1862

[BATH CO.]

This morning we were off early. We sent 15 men to General Hospital [Staunton], some with measles and other fever cases. We traveled down the Warm Springs Road and passed Lebanon Springs. We passed through Jenkins Gap and then we had a splendid country [Augusta Co.].

I went ahead and at a house of a Mr. Hogshead [172] I got a good dinner and a snack for Dr. [Joseph] Crockett. At the Stribling Springs [Augusta Co.], once the Augusta Springs, the improvements are good and will accommodate a good number of visitors. I do not admire the cottages very much. The water is a combinaton of sulphur and alum. The sulphur is not so strong as to be unpleasant. The first Brigade camped at the Springs and was ordered to fire off and clean their guns. News from Richmond is uncertain. The Yankees make an attack ere long.

---

reflection during this time of crisis in the "northwest" and in the Peninsula Campaign and in his own Brigade's Valley Campaign. See dates, Long, op. cit.. On Confederate religious observations, Pitts notes that Jackson and Lee were unusual in making sure that every unit actually was assigned a paid chaplain, in addition to three other categories of missionaries and other unpaid ministers. Most CSA units were more haphazard and random in their assignments. Note that one Tennesse unit demanded and was granted the nation's first "colored chaplain," Uncle Lewis after the Battle of Shiloh and until the end of the War. He was noted for stirring revivals and large-scale conversions; deeply revered, he was yet a slave, and thus had no recognized surname during his chaplaincy of more than two years. Pitts, *Chaplains in Gray*, passim and esp. 49.

[172] Possibly George Hogshead (born 1824), who had a farm in Rockingham Co. near Augusta Co.

SUNDAY, MAY 18, 1862

[STRIBLING SPRINGS, AUGUSTA CO.]

The day was fine. Mr. [L.C.] Vass preached to us at 10 o'clock. [173] His text was the poor publican's prayer: "God be merciful to me a vile sinner." [174] His sermon was short and pointed. The whole service occupied only one hour. A slight shower of rain fell during the evening. Myself and [Robert] Francisco [175] visited the [Stribling] Springs and tasted the water. We saw also a large tame bear.

---

[173] Lachlan Cumming Vass (1831-1896) was chaplain of 27th VA. Inf. A native of Fredericksburg, he attained baccalaureate and graduate degrees from Princeton and became a Presbyterian minister. He also attained divinity degrees, from Danville [VA.]Seminary and Union Theological Seminary of Richmond. He was serving a congregation in Amherst, VA when he left to join 27th Inf. as chaplain. Traveling with the fighting men, he was present at major conflicts, and was captured at Frederick, MD on 10 July 1864; after a month's confinement at a hospital in Baltimore, he was exchanged for a Federal soldier held by CSA and became chaplain at a post in Petersburg. Following the war, he served as chaplain at UVA. Lowell Reidenbaugh, *27th VA. Inf.*, Virginia Regimental Histories Series (Lynchburg, VA.: H.E. Howard, 1993), 181. See also Pitts, *Chaplains in Gray*, 156.

[174] The actual words from the KJV, "And the publican, standing afar off, would not lift up so much as his eyes unto heaven, but smote upon his breast, saying, God be merciful to me a sinner." Lk 18:13. Publicans were tax-collectors, and in the Roman Empire they were paid poorly, but were permitted to keep part of what they collected, as long as the Empire got its share, an arrangement that laid open opportunities for serious abuses. Ronald Brownwig notes, "Luke brings out very clearly Jesus' application of the word 'lost' to the publicans, as though their livelihood made them inevitably 'sinners.' Idem, "Tax Collectors," *Who's Who in the Bible*, vol. 2, *The New Testament* (New York: Holt, Rhinehart, and Winston, 1971). Soldiers by the nature of their task in war are often similarly "lost" and almost inevitably "sin," and Christ's forgiveness could be applied here to humble sinners among the soldiery. According to Pitts, it is unlikely that the Rev. Vass considering fighting itself sinful, and he also likely regarded the CSA cause as justified in the eyes of God; but "justified" and "righteous" soldiers could still do sinful things, such as gambling, whoring, drinking, stealing from each other and from local citizens; and these sins sprang from their "lost" state during stressful war. Pitts, op. cit., passim.

[175] Robert Lafayette Francisco (born 1825) was a cabinetmaker from Smyth Co. Detailed as Quartermaster Sergeant with Co. E of 4th VA. Inf., he became Capt. QM in June. Robertson, *4th VA. inf.*, 50.

MONDAY, MAY 19, 1862

[STRIBLING SPRINGS, AUGUSTA CO.]

This morning we were off at 1/2 past 5 o'clock. The 5th Reg't is from this country principally, and the people who had friends and relatives in the Reg't came flocking to the road to see them.

At many places were crowds, and their meeting was most affectionate. At Mt. Zion the crowd was larger than any place before. One instance I noticed particularly. A soldier apparently 33 years old stood talking very animatedly to a group of children among who [sic] was a woman holding a baby in her arms. The Reg't move[d] on, the band struck up, and the soldier started to take his place in the ranks. He seized his wife's hand and bade her goodbye and started but there was a little duty yet to perform—and to remind him of it the dear wife caught hold of his arm and said: "kiss the baby first." The soldier turned and kissed his offspring and then joined his file and we were soon away down [northward] the Valley. This man had a patriotic heart—a love of country that stimulated him to great and honorable deeds. He had something to sacrifice, something to lose—that dear woman may never see her husband again, that baby may have taken its last fatherly kiss and these little boys and girls may not be administered to by that parent again.

The roads are bad. We reached Mount Solon [Augusta Co.] at noon. Here the young and fair girls congregated; with many colored frocks they looked like a flower bed. At this place a large spring flows up and furnishes water for several flour mills.

We passed through a beautiful country. [W]ent in search of something to eat. We visited four or five houses before we could find one with any of its folks home. When we did it was the house of the kind and hospitable Mrs. Davis [his sentence structure and punctuation] gave us an excellent dinner and sent a snack to Col. [Ronald]. We got to Bridgewater [176] in advance of the Brigade. The bridge across the South Fork of the Shenandoah River had been burned and the river was bridged by placing wagons across and laying planks on them.

Bridgewater is a very nice place—larger than I expected. The enemy occupied it a very short time and persuaded a great many of the slaves to leave their masters in this neighborhood.

---

[176] Bridgewater is in Rockingham Co. and lies just beyond the North River and a few miles north of the county line separating Rockingham Co. from Augusta Co. Jackson's men are now going down the valley northward, almost circling back from the route they took a few days before.

We camped 1/2 [mile] outside this village. I am unwell to-day. the weather is fine. We will go to the Lower Valley, I now am sure.

TUESDAY, MAY 20, 1862

[BRIDGEWATER, ROCKINGHAM CO.]

This morning the men were ordered to stack their knapsacks and leave them under a guard and take their blankets for a tramp [march]. We passed through Dayton about 9 o'clock and reached Harrisonburg before noon. We did not stop to enquire the Yankees who had burned a great deal of fencing. We marched to Big Spring and camped. Part of [Richard Stoddert] Ewell's division[177] joined us this evening[.] Brigade in which are the notorious Louisiana Tigers[.] I saw some of them. I went to the house of a Mrs. Brock to get something to eat. The cooks [slaves] were at home but none of the whites. I got a good meal for a quarter. After I ate the old top [Mr. Brock] came. I went into his house and apologized for being in the kitchen during his absence, but he said it was all right. He gave me an awful tale of Yankee outrage—the Yankees circulated some gold and silver and United States notes. Mr. Brock lost one Negro by them. He is a wealthy old codger. [178] I got to camp near night.

For a few days I have been riding a horse picked up by S. H. [179] and supposed at first that he bought him, but I understand he did not and I found out that the horse [came from] this neighborhood [Bridgewater]. I told S.H. if any one could produce the proper credentials, I would have to give up the horse. I have heard that the Yankees have gone to Western Virginia. If this is so I presume that Gen. Jackson will follow immediately.

---

[177] Richard Stoddert Ewell (1817-1872) was born in D.C. but grew up in Prince William City. He graduated from West Point in 1840, served in Mexican War and was breveted Capt. in conflict. He served in Southwest thereafter and was on sick leave in VA. when the war broke out. Joining CSA army as Lt. Col., he quickly advanced to Maj. Gen. by time of Valley Campaign. "Old Bald Head" was a fine horseman and shrewd tactician and distinguished himself in this Valley Campaign and in Seven Days defense of Richmond. Some of his command included the famous or infamous Louisiana Tigers. Dale E. Floyd, "Ewell," *Hist. Times.*

[178] Possibly Archibald and Sarah Brock, he born in 1791 and she in 1793 of Linville Township in Rockingham Co. VA. Census, 1870.

[179] Possibilities are Samuel Hymon, Samuel Howe, Samuel Hicock, Samuel Houston, and Stephen Hackler. Robertson, *4th VA. Inf.*; Presgraves, ed., *Smyth Co.*. Since the young soldier apparently stole the horse, the diarist seems to be protecting his identity, even here in the confines of a private entry.

WEDNESDAY, MAY 21, 1862

[MASSANUTTON, PAGE CO.] [180]

We were in expectation of going forward down the Valley [north into WVA] but when we got to New Market [Shenandoah Co.] we turned in a southerly direction [up the Valley] towards Page County and encamped in the gap in the [Massanutton] mountain. Some one started the report that we have been ordered to Richmond and we are going straight to Gordonsville [Orange Co. near his birthplace]. I do not see the cause for, or the policy in, such a move.

We have many northern papers and of all the inconsistent lies I have ever seen are contained in them [his sentence structure]. To listen to them we have never won a victory and never fought without a superior force—when we fight at all and when we are not fighting we scarcely have no [sic] men—and half our army has to be kept in the service by the other half. The rebellion is quashed and the Southern Confederacy is played out. Nothing to do now but close the war when Abe [Lincoln] and his [cabinet?] shall think proper. This is well enough to be read by northern people who know no better.

When the rebellion is crushed many now living will be in dust. In some of our boys the spirit of these papers do [sic] no good. We have some prisoners in a farm on this road—some union men too. Many of those, who have deserted from our army because of such frivolous scribblers, will be captured.

THURSDAY, MAY 22, 1862

MASSANUTTON, PAGE CO.

This morning when the time came for starting we moved across a mountain gap called Massanutton. From this height a most beautiful picture of nature is a broad and extended plain. New Market and Mount Jackson both could be seen very plainly. The Valley [Macadamized] road looks like a gray line made through the Valley—not a fence appeared on the road. Very little corn will be cultivated in the Valley except against the mountains in the north. The land seems to be plowed.

We soon passed the road that led to Gordonsville. Passing by Hamburg [Shenandoah Co.] we saw Dr. [Harvey] Black's man [slave] Abe—sick. I gave him some medicine. 3 miles further and we were at Luray [Page Co.] This is a better village that I expected to find it. Many ladies were on the porch of the

---

[180] Massanutton Mountain separates Rockingham Co. from Page Co. The Gap in the mountain where Apperson camps may be in either county; the town is in Page Co. Humel, *A List.*

hotel. I saw a young lady—a Miss Brown—with whom I traveled when coming from Richmond. Page County can at least boast of some good-looking and many homely [181] girls.

We went into camp near Springfield and Dr. [Joseph] Crockett and myself put our horses into a field to feed awhile. Mr. Chadock, the proprietor,[182] invited us to partake of supper at his house, which we did. I prepared some bandages and some instruments.

FRIDAY, MAY 23, 1862

[SPRINGFIELD, PAGE CO.]

This morning we started from camp after 4 and went down the Front Royal Road. Our wagons were left at camp—about noon we were marching very rapidly and the sun shone almost warm. The men began falling out of rank in squads. The 4th Regiment was soon reduced to a mere skeleton. It does seem to me that the men have become lazy and careless—I know they can do better if they will. [183] After several rests the ranks became fuller. At 3 o'clock we heard cannon, indication that the fight had commenced. We were then 8 mi[les] distant from Front Royal. [184] In about 5 mi[les] of Front Royal we found the road was blocked by the enemy and we were obliged to go across the country to

---

[181] Almost illegible. He may say *comely*, but the contrast between *some pretty* and *many homely girls* seems to fit his style of writing and to express his meaning.

[182] Possibly Chadduck. A Catherine Chadduck (born 1801) still maintained a place in Springfield in 1870, and was the widow of a Chadduck who owned a good-sized farm there. VA. Census, 1870.

[183] Fascinating observation because this is exactly the moment when Jackson's entire VA. Brigade. was gaining its reputation as the "horseless cavalry" who could "gallop" anywhere on foot. For perspective on the "inside" and "outside" view of the Brigade., see Roberton, *The Stonewall Brigade*, passim.

[184] The VA. Brigade., plus CSA MD units defeated a force under Col. John Reese Kenly (1818-1891). Federal forces suffered more than 800 casualties, including Kenly, who was wounded and captured. This relatively small victory gave Jackson a good place from which to cut off Banks's march toward Winchester. Moreover, as Long notes, "Jackson's rapid movement and victory at Front Royal caused fear in Washington of a major northward move by the Confederates, possibly even toward the capital. This distracting diversion took attention form McClellan's efforts on the Peninsula near Richmond." Long, op. cit., 215. Kenly, originally from Baltimore, recuperated and was exchanged for a CSA soldier; he was promoted to Brig. Gen. and given command over MD forces. He would fight again in the Valley,but he also distinguished himself in fighting in the east. At war's end, the City of Baltimore awarded him a commemorative sword, and the State of Maryland commended him. Jeffrey D. Wert, "Kenly," *Hist. Times.*

the road at the foot of the mountain. Prisoners commenced passing. I saw one meet an acquaintance—both from the first Maryland Reg'ts [that is, one from CSA 1st MD and one from USA 1st MD]. One of the reg'ts is from our side and the other on the side of the Federals. Batches of prisoners commenced coming faster. We marched on until we reached Front Royal. When a short distance from there we heard the shouting of men and the car whistle. When we got to the place we passed through with the bands playing gaily. The citizens crowded the streets. Much excitement prevailed. When we got into Front Royal we found that the 1st Maryland Regiment on our side met the 1st Maryland Regiment on the Federal's side, and they settled the question they both ardently wanted to settle.

Our side nearly captured the whole regiment. When we got to Front Royal the car whistle sounding and the men cheering very rapidly [sic]. We were told that the "Louisiana Tigers", "Wheat Battalion", had charged and taken the train of cars heavily loaded. [185]

Everything was exultation in the village. We passed through and turned into a field to rest for the night. We learned that Cap't [George F.] Sheetz was killed in a charge to-day. He was a brave and gallant man and was just upon the eve of promotion. How sad it is to see the flower of chivalry of our land thus be sacrificed. The report is that 300 prisoners are taken. [186]

---

[185] Chatham Roberdeau Wheat (1826-1862) was son of an Episcopal clergyman from MD but preaching in Alexandria. A college graduate, from University of Nashville, he studied law, but left law school to fight in Mexican War. After that war, he practiced law briefly in New Orleans and served in LA. general assebmly, but he "filibustered" in Caribbean fighting and he also fought alongside English volunteers in Guiseppe Garibald's revolutionary forces in Italy. When Civil War broke out, he returned to LA and took command of the notorious Tiger Rifles, former convicts and other "unsavory characters." Apparently only Wheat could control these courageous but undisciplined and almost criminal men. Successful at 1st Manassas, where Wheat was nearly killed, the Tigers fought well in Valley Campaign, as here noted, and in Seven Days Campaign defense of Richmond. "Wheat was mortally wounded at Gaines' Mill 27 June 1862, and without his leadership the battalion was ineffective. In August 1862 [Wheat's Tigers] was broken up and the men transferred to other LA. commands. Although they carried a banner depicting a lamb, with the motto [from William Blake] As Gentle As, the Tigers had a well-deserved reputation as fierce fighters and troublemakers." Richard M. McMurry, "Wheat's Tigers' and Jeffrey D. Wert, "Wheat," *Hist. Times.*

[186] T.J. Jackson's official report, # 59, commends Sheetz and notes that his commander Turner Ashby "met with a body of the enemy posted as a guard at Buckton in a strong position, protected by the railroad embankment. Ashby drove back and dispersed the enemy, but with the loss of the most valuable of his followers, among them Captains Sheetz and [John]Fletcher." Jackson reports the capture of 700 prisoners on one day of fighting and 200 on a second day, for a total of 900,

SATURDAY, MAY 24, 1862

[FRONT ROYAL, WARREN CO.]

Last night I was roused from my novel couch [sleeping under the stars] by the rain falling on my face. I got shelter and went to sleep again.

I visited the village this morning and am agreeable [sic] surprised to see the large amount of store captured. The depot is filled with boxes containing clothing, arms and ammunition and accoutrements. Several other houses are filled also. The cars have several hundred sacks of salt and barrels of flour. The court house is filled with prisoners.

We moved off after our rations came up. The bridges across the Shenandoah [River's south fork] and Cedar Creek are saved. The Yankees attempted to burn them but failed. We met several small batches of prisoners and one very large squad, perhaps between 300 and 400. Though I felt exultant at our success, I could but feel sorry for the sufferings of humanity. About 3 mi[les] from Front Royal we were detained in the road some three or four hours. We were then ordered to take the Chapel Road which leads out into the pike at Middleton [Frederick Co.] Three wagons passed us which were taken near Winchester early that morning. Gen. [Richard S.] Ewell is behind us. Our army is divided into two divisions. General Ewell has command of the right, while Gen. Jackson is with the left. The left is composed of Taylor's Brigade, Taliafero's, Campbell's and the 1st Stonewall Brigade. Soon we heard cannon in the direction of the Valley road. We moved on more rapidly. Prisoners commenced passing all covered with dirt and blood.

In one batch was a woman dressed in a riding habit. She had a very unconcerned air. Many horses were taken alive. One of our cavalry said they were avenging Capt. [George F.] Sheetz who had fallen the day. When we got to Middletown [Frederick Co.] I rode down to Main Street and rode up it. Things showed that strange scenes had been transacted here to-day.

General Jackson and staff were riding down the street very hurriedly. Soon the column was about-faced and commenced a hasty pursuit just above Newtown [Newtown Stephensburg, Frederick Co.] The column was halted by the Yankees endeavoring to make a stand at a point near the village. Soon they

---

although Long estimates the number to be 800, Long, op. cit., 215-16. Thomas Jonathan Jackson, #59, *Official Records*, Ser. I, 12:700-12, esp. 703.

gave ground before our parrot guns and we entered the village just at dark. The citizens were jubilant. All the windows were lighted up. We pushed on amid the rolls of shouts of the men, cheers of women and blast of bugles. At Barton's Mill we came upon their pickets. I had found a demi-john of turpentine and wished to save it and was going across a field to a house with it when a ball whistled past me. I sat my load down and returned to the reg't. The firing became pretty heavy. The 33rd Reg't was in front. It gave way and the 5th Va. went in and then the 27th Va. under Col. [Andrew Jackson] Grigsby. We moved on slowly and cautiously.

We came near having a serious matter here. While the pickets were fighting, something in a burning wagon began to burst and make considerable noise. My first thought was that bombs were in the fire and were bursting and I advised the men to look out. Some left the road and went into the field. One of the regiments behind, supposing the enemy had managed to flank us, commenced firing on our own men in the field. This produced some confusion for a short time, but all was again restored to order. We moved on slowly to Kernstown [Frederick Co.] where the Yankees made another stand. A few skirmishers drove them back. Our regiment had diminished to three companies. Many had fallen down in the road and gone to sleep. General Jackson ordered us to rest till daylight. I do not remember to [have] ever had a sweeter sleep for an hour. My horse was worn out. I gave him a feed of oats, and I went to sleep and slept for several hours.

SUNDAY, MAY 25, 1862

[KERNSTOWN, FREDERICK CO.]

This morning as soon as it was light enough to ensure safety, we moved on. Beyond the [grinding] mill near Winchester, on a high hill, I could see a body of Yankees. From this hill if they had a battery they could have racked us along the road. Two regiments, the 2nd Virginia and the 5th Va. were sent forward to support the 27th which had to take the hill. Gen. Jackson stood in the road and watched the movements till the hill was taken and then ordered the Rockbridge Artillery up. the cannonading commenced at 5 o'clock and was kept up for some time. The 4th Regiment was also sent out on our right to guard the batteries. Troops came down the road very rapidly. The cannon balls flew high. About 7 o'clock the sounds of Ewell's guns were heard on our right. The enemy then gave way and commenced a retreat, and we followed in pursuit. Dr.

[Joseph] Crockett and myself mounted horses and left the wounded to join our Reg't, which had not been engaged. We overtook it just as it was going into Winchester. This was by far the most exciting scene I have ever witnessed.

The pavement was crowded with old men and children, old ladies and beautiful girls. They were busily handing out bread and meat and fresh water. Many were crying. The name of Jackson was lauded to the skies. Shouts for Jeff Davis and the Confederacy were rising high above the tumult. The artillery went along the street west of Main Street, part of the infantry along Main St., and Ewell's forces along Market Street. Many a brawny soldier shed tears as he pushed along to do the work before him. I rode along as rapidly as my horse could carry me. Soldiers were appropriating the contents of knapsacks to their convenience as the article suited. Now and then we passed dead Yankees and a broken gun—both alike emblematical of what will be the result of the attempt of the North to subjugate the South. We pursued the fugitives for 4 mi[les] north of Winchester and the cavalry went in.

Bunches of prisoners were being sent in till night and very many negro [sic] women were with them—one prisoner had a negro babe on his shoulder.[187] Opposite Camp Stephenson [at depot in Frederick Co.] we halted and some cavalry with General Jackson in the lead went down upon the enemy. The infantry stopped, and I went to sleep for several hours. When I awoke I found the Reg. had gone into camp. Dr. [Joseph] Crockett and myself went to Winchester to assist dressing the wounded.

Ed. Note With the second victory at Kernstown and the recapture of Winchester, the steward closed this diary section. He rested on a high note of optimism, but one modified by his sense of sadness for the mounting losses, such as George F. Sheetz and even a dawning sympathy for the Federal troops killed.

187 Some slaves had been encouraged to flee their captivity when Federal troops were victorious in Winchester ealier, although there was yet no official US policy to free the slaves.

Part Three

"The Sad, Blighting March of Mars"

8 October 1862–15 April 1865

From Sharpsburg to Appomattox Court House

FROM SHARPSBURG TO APPOMATTOX COURT HOUSE

During some of the most hectic fighting of the Civil War, the steward abandoned his diary. As he notes on 8 October 1862, in the aftermath of the Battle of Sharpsburg (or Antietam) on 17-18 September 1862, the fortunes of war had certainly changed dramatically. The first section of this third part of the diary is less a diary than a brief history catching up the reader on what has happened between the second battle of Kernstown in the Valley Campaign and the invasion of Maryland at Sharpsburg. As an historian, the steward functions well, accurately noting how much had changed once President Lincoln issued the Emancipation Proclamation and how utterly that document changed the nature of war and political history. Apperson of course went into The War primarily because of pride in his region and resentment over criticism from northerners. For him, this fight was definitely about place *in a geographic sense, about the land and the rivers that he loved. His identification with Virginia was in that sense very concrete and particular, the farming boy's traditional loyalty to the land he farmed. Yet he also went into The War because of* place *in another sense. Slavery gave a white man a* place *in society in economic terms, in class terms, and in social terms. He fully intended to buy his own slaves some day. When Lincoln declared that the slaves of those in rebellion would be freed on 1 January 1863, he was affirming what Apperson had long suspected, viz., that Lincoln really was an abolitionist who intended to work radical change in the social structure and the political economy of Virginia and the entire South.*

At the personal level, some other interesting things emerge. Dr. Harvey Black has become the benefactor of the young steward, functioning in wartime much as had Dr. Faris in the antebellum days. Dr. Black was largely uninterested in defending slavery and almost as "agnostic" about the theory of state rights as was Robert Edward Lee. He was a devout "Old Light" Presbyterian, fully dedicated to the most traditional interpretation of John Calvin; that is, Harvey Black believed that a select or elected few had been chosen by God to produce as much justice as was possible on this earth, and thus the primary loyalties of a man (and he certainly was gender-specific on this point) was to place, station, and duty. Dr.

Black therefore worked as a physician for the Confederate army because that was the duty that grew naturally, almost organically, from his station as a trained physician in Virginia. Apperson was occasionally mortified and always disappointed to see how unenthusiastic his mentor and benefactor Dr. Black was about the Confederacy, its generals and politicians, and about State Rights and its political institutions. Indeed, in some ways Black was unenthusiastic about the basic fact of Virginia land in that geographic sense of place. No, Dr. Black worked to help boys who had been shot because he was a physician. He was not working on behalf of any mortal cause. As the diary progresses in this third part, note that the course of the Confederacy begins to flag and falter, and as it does, the diarist steward begins to flag and falter in his loyalties. Indeed, after Gettysburg, he perceives the end of the various causes attaching to the Confederacy, and he begs Dr. Black to let him leave the field hospitals in order to study medicine in Richmond for service in a postbellum world.

This last request—denied emphatically by Harvey Black—introduces the most interesting aspect of their friendship in the enormity of the Civil War. Dr. Black is not even interested in the idea of a mission as a physician; even that much is too un-Calvinist and too "modern" and too "earthly" for him. He is devoted to duty according to his assigned station in place, and that is why he keeps serving the Confederacy. He will do so until there is no Confederacy, and then he will serve the mission as redefined, presumably by God Himself, in a postwar world. He refuses to bless Apperson's plan to leave, and effectively blocks his leavetaking. Thereafter, Apperson, once so fervid, almost rabid in his pro-Confederacy, grows listless and gloomy, while Dr. Black, never passionate in his Confederate loyalties, remains exactly as before, a sturdy and unbending Calvinist determined to do his job as God has laid it out for him.

Finally, the diarist and young benefactor seems to accept Dr. Black's own set of values, finishes his duties because he should and not because he wants to, and then makes his peace with the postbellum world where he will himself emerge as a peacetime leader in his region pioneering in the treatment of the insane while building educational institutions and trying to develop a truly New South economy of industrialism and commerce in the Virginia highlands.

[WEDNESDAY] OCT. 8TH, 1862

BUNKER HILL BERKELEY CO VA [WEST VIRGINIA]

A space of nearly seven months lay between the date that the pen was laid down to the date on which I now write. Vast and important have been the changes, mighty the work and glorious the accomplishment thereof. The time noted by me was a trying time. Hardly a ray of light could be seen to cheer the despondancy of our hearts. The power of the enemy seemed to have encompassed us on every side, and encircled us in a deadly, anaconda-like fold.[1] But the present date can be marked by the historian as one of light and hopefulness. A time that our soldiers can look back with the feeling that the husbandmen can look back at this season when he sees the work of his hand in a plentiful, abundant harvest. We see the fruits of the harvest under Mars in the battle of McDowell, Winchester[,] Port Republic[,] all the fights before Richmond, Cedar Mountain, the battle of Manassas the 2 times, surrender of Harper's Ferry and the fight at Sharpsburg Md. All these have occurred with the army of Northern Va. and all victories to us except the Sharpsburg fight which was not a defeat. [2]

In other parts of the South victory has crowned the efforts of our gallant troops—and now there is only a small [sic] part of the Southern domain in the hand of the enemy. Memphis is yet in his hands and the water courses of the Mississippi and the Carolina Coast also. N[ew] Orleans suffers under the rule of [Benjamin Franklin] Butler. [3] Andy Johnson is Military Governor of East Tenn. and is in Nashville.[4]

---

[1] In fact, General Winfield Scott (1786-1866) at the beginning of the war had proclaimed an "anaconda" policy of strangling the Confederacy by capturing the rivers and the coastline and then squeezing the CSA much as would an anaconda snake one of its victims. In the second section of the diary, Apperson seems very aware of the fact that Federal successes in the river campaigns and on the coast are significant, but now he seems to forget those problems, and he uses the anaconda imagery only as one more negative image of the northern opposition. Scott, a septuagenarian native of Petersburg with "small army" experiences made largely irrelevant in this huge new war, had to leave active duty, but he lived to see vindication of the anaconda policy by War's end, which he witnessed in retirement at West Point, where he had studied and taught with distinction. Patricia L. Faust, "Scott," *Hist. Times.*

[2] True enough, but R.E. Lee did feel compelled to abandon the field and thus abandon the strategy of "taking the fight to the North." Lincoln considered the result good enough for the Federal cause to mark the occasion with the Emancipation Proclamation. Note that Confederates again call a battle by the name of the town nearby, Sharpsburg, while Federals call it by the name of the physical feature, Antietam Creek. In this case, because Lincoln attached the significant Emancipation Proclamation to the results of the battle, most historians now call it Antietam.

[3] Benjamin Franklin Butler (1818-1893) of New Hampshire began political life as a moderate Democrat who hoped to avert Civil War. Indeed, he even nominated Jefferson Davis for US President in Charleston, S.C. convention of 1860. When the War came, Butler served with US forces, and emerged as a surprisingly radical force, issuing a famous "contraband" order that freed slaves of those in rebellion as northern forces conquered land, an order that Lincoln remanded, but that did serve as a basis for Lincoln's own Emancipation Proclamation. In May 1862, Butler

Our armies have been into Maryland under Lee & Jackson and into Ky. under [Edmund] Kirby Smith & [Braxton] Bragg. [5]

It is to be regretted very much that I have been compelled to allow such a breach in my memoranda but it was unavoidable. I now commence again while the army is quiet—gain strength & recuperating after the many hard fought battles of the summer.

---

was sent to New Orleans to serve as military governor, and he dealt effectively, if harshly, with southern white dissidents there. His "Women's Order" declared that white women who insulted Federal occupation troops would be treated as prostitutes. He thereby "created a national controversy....His enemies contemptuously dubbed him 'Spoons' Butler [claiming that he stole silverware and was otherwise corrupt], and Confederate Pres. Jefferson Davis went so far as to declare him an outlaw." Southerners also called him "Beast," and the politic Lincoln removed him from this post in December of 1862, returning him to military duty, where he "mismanaged" several assignments, angering US Grant and Lincoln. He was later important as a Republican congressman from Mass., and was active in impeachment of Andrew Johnson. John D. Kallman, "Butler," *Hist Times.*

[4] Andrew Johnson (1808-1875), the future vice president (1865) and president (1865-1869) of the US, was then war governor of Tennessee. A loyalist Democrat originally from N.C., Johnson, who was seldom called *Andy*, was a self-educated but very intelligent man with considerable political experience at the local and state levels in Tennessee. Very much "plain folk," he was opposed to slavery, but also deeply racist, he was very effective in organizing and running loyalist Tennessee during the remainder of the war. His papers are collected at University of Tennessee and have been edited for easy use by LeRoy Graf et al.

[5] Of course, Lee was not long in Maryland, but Smith did have some successes in an attack into Kentucky. After Sharpsburg, the CSA reorganized its army and promoted James Longstreet to Lt. Gen. in charge of a First Army Corps; T.J. Jackson was promoted to Lt. Gen. and placed in charge of Second Army Corps. Apperson and the soldiers from both his birthplace in Orange Co. and his adoptive home in Smyth Co. remained with Jackson in the new Second Corps. Edmund Kirby Smith (1824-1893) was raised and educated in Alexandria and then graduated from West Point (1845) and was shortly thereafter cited for bravery in the Battle of Cerro Gordo in the Mexican War. Afterward he became a warm friend with future CSA generals Lee, Albert Sidney Johnston, John Bell Hood, and Fitzhugh Lee. In this reorganization, he was promoted to Lt. Gen. and placed in command of the trans-Mississippi forces. This assignment was almost doomed to failure by fall of 1862, for the Rivers Campaign and the brilliance of Ulysses S. Grant were both in full force; however, it was Smith's force that held out longest in the fighting in the trans-Mississippi. David K. Snider, "Smith," *Hist. Times.* Braxton Bragg (1817-1872) was a native of Warrenton, N.C. who became a prominent planter in Louisiana. A graduate of West Point and a veteran of Mexican War, Bragg was a competent strategist but unpopular with his men. Promoted to full Gen. he became commander of the Army of Tennessee. He did fight effectively in this period, and had remarkable successes in Tennessee in spring and summer of 1862; he even invaded Kentucky, as diarist predicts, but he was forced back by superior Federal forces. Albert Castel, "Bragg," ibid..

[Apperson inserted eleven asterisks to show the end of his reminiscences and the beginning of the diary entry for 8 October 1862]

****

The enemy is at Harper's Ferry, and on the Maryland side of the river opposite Shepherdstown [WVA]. He seems to be easy as much so as do we.[6]

Dr B has been called to the post of chf surg of Division and I am still with him. Col. [Charles] Ronald is commander of the Brigade and Gen [John Robert] Jones of the Division. Gen Jackson is commanding a Corps [2d Corps] of J.R. Jones' and A.P. Hill's Hills Division.[7] Capt [Andrew E.] Gibson was killed at Manassas[8] and Lt. [Joseph M.] Thomas is Capt of Co D now.[9] Lt. [John J.] Bishop[10] was wounded at Manassas and J M Williams at Sharpsburg.[11]

---

[6] Indeed McClellan was so "easy" that he angered Lincoln, who wanted vigorous pursuit of Lee's forces into VA . As Lincoln feared, Lee took this respite after Sharpsburg [Antietam] to reorganize and regroup and then attack aggressively again. Long, 272-73.

[7] John Robert Jones (1827-1901) was a native of Harrisonburg and graduate of VMI in 1848; he instructed in military schoosl in FL and MD, but returned to VA when the war came, joining 33rd VA Inf. and commanding a company. Praised by Jackson for his bravery and effectiveness at Manassas and in the Valley Campaign, he was promoted to Lt.Col. Jackson personally brevetted Jones Brigadier Gen., but the Confederate Senate never officially confirmed promotion. Although wounded, he performed briliantly again, at Harper's Ferry and at Sharpsburg, "where on the 17th his men held Lee's far left against an artillery barrage, then repulsed an enemy advance." Another wound, plus an ulcerated leg, eventually removed him from duty at Chancellorsville, where of course he lost his champion Jackson. Berated by superiors for cowardice, he never received his promotion and was driven from the eastern army; in TN, as a civilian but still pro-Confederate, he was captured and imprisoned for two years by the Federals. He fought effectively for Jackson and military historians now regard his slide into disgrace as a tragic miscalculation by CSA superiors and politicians. Edward G. Longacre, "Jones," *Hist. Times.* Ambrose Powell HIll (1825-1865) from Culpeper, VA, was distinguished graduate of West Point, successful in Mexican War, and brilliant as Col. with 13th VA. Inf. in Valley Campaign and in Seven Days Campaign defending Richmond. Joining Jackson at Rapidan River his 13th Inf. "teamed with him...to [earn] a deserved reputation as one of American's great fighting units at Cedar Mountain, 2d Manassas, and Sharpsburg." Like Jones, A.P. Hill suffered after Jackson's death at Chancellorsville and was never effective again without the cooperation of his slain friend and sponsor. Edwin C. Bearss, "Hill."

[8] Andrew E. Gibson (1837-1862), a merchant of Smyth Co. was an early officer in Smyth Blues, had been QM. and then became Capt. before 2d Manassas. He was mortally wounded at Groveton on 28 August1862, part of the Battle of 2d Manassas and died on 30 Aug. Armstrong, *Ante-bellum Years*, 126-28.

[9] Joseph M.Thomas (1834-1912) was a farmer from Smyth Co. As a judge in a squire's court case concerning a freed "woman of color" Tabitha, Thomas was instrumental in allowing her to stay in Smyth Co. as a freed person despite Commonwealth law to the contrary. Originally a Sgt. in Smyth Blues, he was elected to officer ranks, becoming Capt. of Co. D by election on 29 August

The newspapers are full of European intervention again, a thing of no importance to us as I do not believe such will be the case for a long time to come. Our army is very much decimated in numbers but all who are subject to the Conscription act are being called out and put into the ranks.[12]

Abraham Lincoln has lately [22 September 1862 after Lee's forces abandoned the battlefield at Sharpsburg and left MD] issued a proclamation declaring the slaves of all rebel masters free after the 1st day of next January [1863] and promises to protect and uphold them in any act they may do in order to maintain their alleged freedom. This has aroused all the slumbering ire that South possesses and strong grounds are being taken in [Confederate] Congress to raise the black flag.[13]

1862. He served another year, and then resigned his commission because of "insipient pthosis[sic],' apparently ptosis, a drooping, in the 19th century usually describing an uncontrollable drooping of an eyelid, more rarely then an uncontrollable dropping of a visceral organ in the abdomen. He eventually farmed in WVA and lived until 1912 in St. Albin's, WVA. Armstrong, *Ante-bellum Years*, 16; also Robertson, *4th VA. Inf.*, 76; and "ptosis," *Taber's*, s.v

[10] John J. Bishop (1837-1862) was a cooper in Smyth Co. and originally a Sgt. of Ordnance in Smyth Blues, Co. D. Elected 1st Lt., he was wounded and captured at 2d Manassas, exchanged for a Federal prisoner on this very day [although the diarist does not mention that fact], he never recovered from his wounds and died on 30 October. Robertson, *4th VA. Inf.*, 40.

[11] John M. Williams (born1839) ran a grain mill in Smyth Co. on eve of the war. An original Smyth Blue, he was appointed 2d Lt. on June 1862 and then 1st Lt. during 2d Manassas in late August 1862. He was cited for bravery, but wounded at Sharpsburg and was brevetted Capt., appointment confirmed officially in spring of 1863. However, his wound, to right leg and groin, caused disability, and he resigned his commission in January of 1864 with permanent disability. Note that Co. D included a namesake, born in 1841, who was a day laborer whose arm was shattered by a minie ball at 1st Manassas and then served as an ambulance driver, apparentely at least part of the time for Apperson. However, after one month of service as an ambulance driver for Harvey Black's field hospital in Stonewall Bde, this other Williams was released from service because of his own disability. Although Apperson knew and served with both, he is clearly talking about the officer. Robertson, ibid., 80.

[12] The Confederate Conscription Act, as noted earlier, caused great controversy in some states, but in VA compliance was sufficient that there were generally enough forces available to Lee at least in 1862 and 1863. One point of controversy and resentment was the exemption of those who owned more than 20 slaves [because of fear of slave rebellion if the masters went into service], which occasioned class resentment among the majority of "plain folk" who owned no slaves or very few slaves. Another source of resentment, common also for the Federals, was the system that allowed a wealthy draftee or conscriptee to pay a "bounty" to another man to serve in his place, thus allowing the wealthy to "buy their way out" of fighting in the War. See Freeman, *R.E.Lee.*

[13] The Proclamation, besides redefining the Federal war aim as one of Freedom instead of Union, was popular with Labor and other workingclass groups in England who earlier had been sympathetic with the CSA because of their need for southern cotton for their textile mills. The Proclamation was also popular with the middle class of England and France, who were increasingly antislavery. Perhaps more to the point, Lee's inability to invade and stay in MD and

The season is dry—very dry—no rain has fallen since 1st of August of any consequence. The dust in our camp is shoe mouth deep and every puff of wind sends it in your face and eyes.

I have some opportunities for reading now and have been reading Surgery in "Neille [sic] & Smith's Compendium"[14]—Small pox is said to have broken out in Winchester—orders issued this morning for all recruits and conscripts to be vaccinated.

I have not heard from any of my Uncle's since February—I saw yesterday that Prentiss in Mississippi had been burnt by the enemy. My Chas. suffered in the force [or face?] of the fight , I fear.[15]

I have been reading but little to-day. Orders and blanks for quarterlies [quarterly reports], monthlies [monthly reports] and registers for surgical cases [an official listing of the surgeries performed] were sent over by Med. Dir. [Dr. Hunter McGuire] and distributed by us to Brigade surgeons. This evening is almost disagreeably warm.

McClellan's success in driving southern forces from Federal territory in MD convinced British and French diplomats and policy makers that US forces bid fair to win the war despite the reverses of summer 1862. As the diarist shows, Lincoln's Proclamation also redefined and repositioned the competing and contending armies and "belligerant states," for it suggested that Confederates were fighting on behalf of slavery, something clearly not the case for many southern soldiers before the fall of 1862. Apperson is among those who always defined slavery as a part of the way of life of southerners and abolitionism as a threat to the identity of his region. It should be noted that there remained many southerners, not least R.E. Lee, T.J. Jackson and Harvey Black of Apperson's immediate acquaintance, who resented this new identification since they were not supporters of slavery—or of states' rights. The black flag imagery was common to the era and suggested that one was fighting against pirates or other outlaw and unprincipled foes; the connotation is that one does not fight with gentleman's rules of war under a black flag.

[14] John Neill and Francis Gurney Smith, *An Analytical Compendium of the Various Branches of Medicine*, 2 vols. (1850. 2d rev. ed.; Philadelphia: Blanchard & Lea, 1852). Smith (1818-1878) and Neill (1819-1880) were teaching physicians who produced this basic medical-college textbook in several editions in this era.

[15] Charles Jones was the brother of Apperson's mother Matilda Jones Apperson, and he was one of the two uncles who sent him money and encouraged him to move "west" into either Georgia or Mississippi. In September, CSA forces attacked US Grant's forces in northern Mississippi in an attempt to distract Don Carlos Buell from his fight in KY during Braxton Bragg's invasion. It was assumed that Grant was heading to KY to reinforce Buell in his fight against Bragg. Grant and federal forces won the various engagements in and around Corinth, MS, and Prentiss was scene of a skirmish in which part of the village was burnt; Charles Jones had a plantation in vicinity of Prentiss. Grant was slowed in his advance to help Buell, and the strategy was partially successful, but Federal forces won the engagements and brought great damage to Northern Mississippi. Long, 269-273.

THURSDAY, OCT. 9TH, 1862

CAMP BUNKER HILL VA. [WVA]

The weather continues unpleasantly warm and everything is parched with thirst. The dust in all the roads is several inches deep and the wagons and teams in passing to & from stir it up and the air is filled with the dust. It is evidently jeopardizing the health of men and beasts. I have felt some symptoms of a dry cough, occassoned I infer from inhalation of dust. We have some hope that our camp will be moved. In fact the Brigade did move it [sic; its] camp a short distance.

I moved my trunk and our books down to-day. Dr. B. procured a 2-horse wagon from the QM. and tent for our use.

Near bed time orders were sent for the infantry pickets to be strengthened and the Regiments were sent out. What it means none of us can divine. The enemy is either advancing or the order is for precautionary purposes.

Dr. B. paid me $5.25c—& $3.60 for sugar & coffee $1.50 for horse feed and for one stamp.

Rec'd a letter from Laura F.—.

FRIDAY, OCT. 10, 1862

BUNKER HILL [WVA]

Everything is quiet this morning. The orders of yesterday evening could have been for nothing more than to make the pickets vigilant. Jas. Cooly[16] came over in the morning to commence working for Dr. B & myself. I have been somewhat inconvenienced by having to go to the Brigade for meals. His charge is heavy—20$ per month, I am fearful it will be a loosing [sic] matter to me—10$ from my small wages will leave but a small sum for other necessities. However I must have something to eat if I do not make a cent.

Rain commenced falling slowly and steadily and continued during the day. It is hailed with delight—no more dust to choke us at every turn.

---

[16] "Jas. Cooly" was James Cooley, a free African-American resident of Marion, VA. All of the Cooleyes were skilled bricklayers who had their own contracting firm in Smyth County. James Cooley enlisted in the Confederate Army as did another African-American, John Ross. Wilson, *Smyth County History*, 262-63. Note that Apperson complains of Cooley's charge for his services as cook, but does not doubt the quality of the services, nor does he make racist remarks as he often did with black people whom he did not know well.

Business with us is dull. I have considerable time for reading. Have a tent and books also. If we remain at this post during the winter I promise myself some instruction. Dr. [Lafayette Hall] Jordan sent a note and afterwards came for me to glance over and give him some ideas about quarterly reports. I promised him to assist him to-morrow if the weather will permit. [17]

I presume that the weather will be cold now in a few days. Wrote to Mrs. F & Laura.

SATURDAY OCT. 11TH, 1862

BUNKER HILL VA. [WVA]

As anticipated last evening the air is cool and refreshing this morning—rain having fallen slowly during the night. Arrangements were made this mornig for me to mess[18] with Dr. B. , Maj. [Douglas] Mercer, [19] Col. [Andrew Jackson] Grigsby[20] & Capt. Hunter[21].—after breakfast I went over to the Brigade and finished quarterly report for Dr. [Lafayette Hall] Jordan . 3 o'clock to dinner with Col. [Charles Andrew] Ronald and returned to my quarter and afterwards rode over again on business.

My attention was attracted his evening at Dress Parade by the reading of orders—the decision of the Courts Martial now in session. Heavy penalties are imposed on men absent without leave, desertion, cowardice, insubordination, and various misdemeanor. One man was trotting up and down the line while on

---

[17] Lafayette Hall Jordan (born 1838) became Asst. Surg. of Reg. on 6 May 1862; he was transferred to general hospital at Petersburg on 10 February 1863. Robertson, *VA. 4th Inf.*, 58. He was living in Mt. Jackson (Shenandoah Co.) in 1870. VA *Census*. 1870.

[18] Mess was traditional military term for the place of eating and the act of eating. *OED*. Generally officers messed with other officers, and in this case officers of the medical corps are messing with noncommissioned members of the medical corps such as Apperson.

[19] Douglas Mercer is identified as QM for Bde. with rank of Major. Robertson, *Stonewall Brigade*, 86.

[20] Andrew Jackson Grigsby (1819-1895) was from Rockbridge Co., VA; after attending Washington Col. [now Washington & Lee Univ.] in Lexington, VA., he moved to MO.; he fought in Mexican War and afterward taught in Lexington, VA. A resident of Giles Co. when War came, he was appointed Maj. of 27th VA. Inf. and was promoted through combat up to full Col. He was brevetted Brig. Gen. and so served, but was apparently never confirmed. In 1863, he resigned commission and served in CSA House of Rep., in KY delegation. "A bluff soldier much given to swearing." Reidenbaugh, *VA. 27th Inf.*, 147.

[21] John A. Hunter was a surgeon with rank of Capt. He generally served field hospitals and became Medical Director of Army of No. VA. and Army of SW VA. Reidenbaugh, *VA. 27th Inf.*, 153. He was born in 1825 and was living in Chatham (Pittsylvania Co.) in 1870. VA. *Census*, 1870.

dress parade but I did not learn his name or offence and when he stopped and was marched away the band struck up "Jordan is a hard Road to travel."[22]

I went to see Maj. Sexton[23] this evening in regard to commutation for rations. He is of the opinion that I am only entitled to 25c per day which is not enough.

SUNDAY OCT: 12TH, 1862

BUNKER HILL VA. [WVA]

The air is cool this morning and remained so during the day with showers. At evening every prospect for a raining season. Col. Charles Lee Jones[24] of Washington D.C. is a visitor to our Headquarters. He has been a prisoner but lately released.

Col. Grigsby arrived late last night from Winchester—An accident happened to him in which his horse by falling hurt one of his legs very much—He is *Hors de combat* [a "work" or "product" of combat, that is, temporarily out of action due to combat injury]. [25]

---

[22] Possibly Richard A. Jordan (1842-1864), Pvt., Co. H of 27th VA. Inf. Native of Lexington, VA., he was often sick, with long stay in gen. hospital. He is listed as "arrested" and held until Battle of Chancellorsville, where he was wounded (3 May 1863); recovering, he was captured at Gettysburg (3 July 1863), and died in prison at Ft. Delaware. Reidenbaugh, *VA. 27th Inf.*, 154. Jackson made displays of punishment for men court martialled, esp. for "cowardice" and "desertion." Indeed, he once executed several convicted deserters in front of open graves with the full Division assembled in "three-sided" formation. An execution squad of a dozen men shot each of the convicted, who fell into his appointed grave. "Officers then marched their regiments past the graves, to impress indelibly upon them the awful consequences of desertion." Robertson, *Stonewall Brigade,* 141, citing two eyewitnesses.

[23] Probably Joseph Carpenter Sexton . Born in 1833, he was a mechanic who joined Co. A of VA. 4th Inf. He was appointed Asst. Commissary for Reg. and would have been in charge of such rations. Robertson, *4th VA. Inf.*, 72. He was living in Black Lick Township in Wythe Co. in 1870. VA. *Census.* Sexton's clerk was a mechanic, John McAllister Sexton (1843-1864), of Co. A, apparently no relation. Still another Sexton involved in Commissary was Charles McDonald Sexton (1839-1915), a farmer in Co. A. Apperson would have to deal with all of these Sextons concerning rations, but only Joseph Carpenter Sexton was the officer in charge.

[24] Possibly Charles Lee Jones, who was born in 1834 in New York to Virginian Charles Lee Jones who then moved to D.C. Father and son C.L. Joneses were residing in Richmond in 1870. VA. *Census.*

[25] Grigsby was often wounded or otherwise injured, and it took much to put him out of action, even briefly, as here. Surviving soldier and memoirist John O. Casler reports that during the Peninsula Campaign Grigsby was wounded and lost his horse and had to limp over to a spring to ask some soldiers to pour cold water on his wound. One asked if the wound hurt, to which

We have sad news for our cause from the Western Dist. Gen's. [Earl] Van Dorn and [Sterling] Price made an attack on Rosencrantz [sic; Rosencrans] at Corinth[26] and was badly whipped and driven back 25 miles. No heart should quail but meet the reverse with the same magnanimity we have regarded our victories.[27]

Early this morning I rode over to the Brigade for some articles of medicine and met Captain Dungan[28] who had just arrived from home. (he was wounded in the foot at Cedar Run [9-10 August 1862].)[29] and gives me very disturbing

---

Grigsby is said to have replied, "Yes, Damn it!....It was put there to hurt." John O. Casler, *Four Years in the Stonewall Brigade* (Guthrie, OK: private printing, 1893), cited by Robertson, *Stonewall Brigade*, 122.

[26] See earlier note on efforts to take the pressure off Braxton Bragg in KY by preventing reinforcements to Don Carlos Buell. On 5 October 1862, William Starke Rosencrans [biography earlier] drove Confederates from Corinth into Chewalla, ten miles to the northwest during very bloody fighting, that is, 2520 casualties out of some 23,000 effectives. Long notes, "The Southerners succeeded in taking the pressure off Bragg in Kentucky by preventing reinforcements to Buell, but they failed to capture the important rail and road center of Corinth, or to wreck Rosencrans' force and thus make Grant pull back toward the Ohio. Long, 274-76. Sterling Price (1809-1867) was from Prince Edward Co., VA., but migrated with his family in 1830 to Missouri, where he became a prominent planter and "the embodiment of Missouri rural aristocracy." Dean E. Smith says that Price "launched his Civil War career fighting to hold Missouri for the Confederacy, and he never stopped pursuing that elusive goal throughout the conflict. In the process he alienated Southern leaders, including Jefferson Davis." Long, "Price," *Hist. Times.* Earl Van Dorn (1820-1863) was from gulf coast of Mississippi and graduated, low in his class, from West Point, 1842. He gained fame as a cavalry leader in Mexican War and considerable national recognition for combat with Comanches in western territories thereafter. Promoted to Brig. Gen. with CSA, Van Dorn "never lived up to his country's early expectations." Phillip R. Rutherford and other military historians put much of the blame for the defeat at Corinth on "poor staff work and his inability to handle details." Colorful and controversial, Van Dorn "was killed by an irate husband at his headquarters in Spring Hill, Tenn., 7 May 1863." Rutherford, "Van Dorn," *Hist. Times.*

[27] A formulation, "great souledness" or "bigheartedness" very loosely translated, from Aristotle, *Nicomachean Ethics*, Bk. 3., trans. with commentary, H.H. Joachim (1951. Rev. ed.; Oxford: At the Clarendon Press, 1966), ed., D.A. Rees.

[28] "Captain Dungan" is Apperson's friend Robert Henry Dungan who had left his educational pursuits at Emory & Henry College in Emory, Virginia in order to join the Confederate Army. Dungan was a1st Lieutenant in Company B of the 48th Virginia Regiment, which was organized at Seven Mile Ford, Virginia and known as "Jackson's Old Division." Wilson, *Smyth County.*

[29] Engagement in Culpeper Co.; also called Battle of Cedar Mountain and Battle of Slaughter Mountain, and Battle of Southwestern Mountain. Nathaniel Banks's corps of John Pope's large army attacked A.P. Hill's two corps of T.J. Jackson's large force; although Banks withdrew, casualties were high for this brief fight—2,729 according to Official Records and to E.B. Long. Moreover, the engagement demonstrated what a huge force was marching with Pope. Long, *Civil War Almanac*, 249-50; *Official Records*, 10 August 1862. Besides periodic bouts of influenza and

news as regards to the sickness of the citizens of Smyth. I rode over to Maj. Ballards[30] quarters—Chf Commissary—to consult him about commutation of rations &c. He was not at his office—I rode over again in the evening and saw him. He says 25c per day is all the commutation allowed in camp but when men are on detached service as I may be at times they are entitled to 75c per day. He also refers me to Maj. [Joseph Carpenter] Sexton to make arrangements about rations. I saw him and will draw for one week at a time. When I am not present where I can draw in kind I must keep account and rec'd commutation for it. I propose making Cooly go over every week and draw my weekly ration.

I have been introduced to Col. Peck and Maj. Williamsof the Louisiana Brigade. A portion of the day that I was not engaged I sat round the fire in conversation with Col. G[rigsby] who was nursing his leg. After night I read some of the first chapters of 1 Kings. Rain falling at bed time.

Horsefeed is scarce & my horse is falling off daily. The Flour is gitting [sic] very scarce in the Commissary Department also.

MONDAY, OCT: 13TH, 1862

BUNKER HILL, VA. [WVA]

The day has been partially busy. Commenced drawing rations—drew for 7 days—Went with orders to Dr [J.A.] Straith[31] for sending sick of Brigade to Hospt. & for drawing stimulants for the use of the different Brigades in Division D.

News from [Sterling] Price and [Earl] Van Dorn ameliorated smartly—rumors of a success by [Braxton] Bragg over [Don Carlos] Buell [in KY]. Dr. Gibson of Aldie [Loudon Co.] called to-day. Lt. [John J.] Bishop[32]

---

other diseases, Smyth Co. suffered economically, esp. with cost of salt (although produced in Saltville of Co.) and other food and dry goods. By this time, more than 800 famililes of Confederate soldiers were supported by government relief funds, called the levy. Armstrong, *Ante-bellum Years*, 128-29.

[30] Major Ballard was chief commissary and had authority over Maj. J.C. Sexton.

[31] J.A. Straith was chief surgeon in Bde., replacing Harvey Black after he was promoted to divisional surgeon. Bean, Notes.

[32] John J. Bishop(1838-1862), a cooper of Co. D, 4th VA. Inf., was originally an ordnance Sgt. but was promoted through ranks of Lt.; wounded and captured at 2d Manassas, 30 August 1862; exchanged for Federal prisoner, 8 October Robertson, *4th VA. Inf.*, 40; The femoral artery "begins at the external iliac artery and terminates behind the knee as the popliteal artery on the inner side of the [thigh bone]." "Femoral Artery," *Taber's*. Ligature is a "thread or wire for tying a blood

doing very well—femoral artery has been ligatured. Dr. Burton's report for August was returned for correction.

Have been reading Don Juan[33] to-day—not much interested.

TUESDAY, OCT 14, 1862

BUNKER HILL, VA. [WVA]

On last Thursday Gen [J.E.B.] Stuart[34] with 1500 picket men started on a tour through a part of Md. and extended his trip as far as Chambersburg, Penn. He returned last evening crowned with success in every particular. On reaching Penn. he commenced pressing horses—at Chambersburg the Homeguard hid themselves. He destroyed a machine shop and it is said exported from the haul is a large amount of specie [money in gold or silver instead of paper money or notes]—. Instead of returning by the same route he went he made a circuit around by Leesburg [Loudon Co.] entirely encircling [George B.] McClellan's whole army. On his route he came upon a quantity of ammunition lost by Gen. [James] Longstreet and destroyed the whole lot. At Leesburg a force attempted to stop him but Virginia's shore was before him and he was bent to make it. Throwing a few shot and the way was clear—. He brought some 800 horses. The

vessel or other structure in order to constrict or fasten it." "Ligature," ibid.. In fact, Bishop did not survive after all, succumbing on 30 October in the town of Aldie

[33] *Don Juan; Cantos* (1824) is a mock-epic poem in heroic couplets by George Gordon, Lord Byron (1788-1824). The cantos use the form and structure of high romantic epic poetry to tell a story of a great lover and soldier, but the tone is ironic, witty, and ultimately sad. Given Apperson's high-romantic, even naive, taste, and his approach both to lovemaking and to principled war, this style of complex and fey comedy would not appeal to him. American editions were produced by C. Wiley publishers in New York in 1824 and kept in print. Another likely edition available to Apperson is that published by W.A. Leary publishers of Philadelphia in 1848.

[34] General James Ewell Brown Stuart (1830?-1864) was the most romantic of the Confederate cavalry leaders; a man of plain folk origins in the Virginia highlands, Stuart attended Emory & Henry College and West Point. After some two decades of frontier battles with Indians, esp. in Kansas, Stuart resigned his commission and joined the CSA army when War came; a wild-riding and dashing cavalry officer, Stuart was not of Lee's class or status, and sometimes was resentful of the aristocracy in CSA army, as some of the officers from old families were distrustful and disdainful of him. He did commit a fatal error once, in losing communication with his superiors during Gettysburg (3-4 July 1963), but generally Stuart rode hard, observed closely, and as Lee reported, "He never brought me a piece of false information." In this instant, Stuart effected a bold raid, attempting to destroy an iron bridge over the Conococheague Creek near Chambersburg, PA. Although the ride was typically romantic, he failed in this effort. John D. Kallman, "Stuart," *Hist. Times.* Stuart Papers, Emory & Henry College Archives. William G. Bean reports that Stuart did not secure any money in specie or otherwise as the banks, forewarned, hid it. Bean, Notes.

Old Dutch farmers of Pennsylvania have felt that there was very little protection in their government and that it was hard that they had to furnish horses for an army of rebels. By way of a joke or otherwise it [sic] said that Gen. Stuart told them that Gen. Mclelland [sic] had ordered it and would no doubt settle the bill—some were told that the South would have war and they were now called upon to contribute something to its support.

The feat itself is one of the grandest of the war, or even of history, and reflects great credit on the commander.

Many speculations are advanced on the prospects of peace. Some of the will-be-prophetic [sic] seems to think that it is not far distant. Some are basing their hope and argument upon the tyranny of the Northern Government, upon its own subjects.

I have been reading Don Juan to-day—quit before finishing it for want of interests—"read" Neille & Smith" —. [Neill and Smith, *An Analytical Compendium*]

Wrote a letter to my Father's folks and one to Dr. F: also rec'd one from Dr. F:—Capt [Robert H.] Dungan called on me to-day and had a prolonged chat. I had some information of matters and things from Home in Smyth [Co]. How I have been disappointed in somethings! How many wolves are in sheep clothing!

Read a chapter in Kings [of *Bible*] and retired.

The weather is cloudy, pleasant, agreeable.

BUNKER HILL, VA. [WVA]

WEDNESDAY OCT: 15, '62

Rose early this morning, more from necessity perhaps than otherwise as I was suffering slightly with cold. The day was spent principally in reading. I went with some orders to the Brigade—It had been moved towards Smithfield [Albemarle Co.] this evening for some purpose. I suppose it is merely to protect some details [assigned combat units] that are destroying the Rail Roads. The track is being taken up and laid across timbers and burnt so as to warp railing which renders it useless.

I rec'd a letter from Cousin Bettie to-day. W.A. Bell [35] paid me 10$ which I loan [sic] him some time ago.—Jas Cooly ["freeman of color" and successful

[35] William Anderson Bell (1836-1930) was a farmer in Smyth Co. who joined Co. E and served first as an infantryman and then as an ambulance driver, beginning those duties on 13 October 1962. Soon, on 23 October 1862, Bell would be wounded in a fight with another CSA ambulance driver; confined at a Warrenton [Fauquier] CSA holding facility, he was captured by Federals in

bricklayer of Marion who joined Stonewall Bde.] went to Winchester to-day and bought some mess [kitchen and dining] furniture [really utensils] at an unreasonable rate. $2.50c for a coffee pot.

Dr. Straith was in our tent to-night and in course of conversation remarked how all the social connexions [19th cent. usage] of his neighborhood were broken up since the beginning of the War. The [illegible] will cause any of us to have serious & sorrowful reflections. Virginia has scarcely a neighborhood but what some breach has been made in it in the last year. Some noble citizens gone whose family is now separating never again to to [sic] be bound to-gether by the same ties that held them before. There is not a young man in the army that will ever find the same condition of things at home when he returns. O what a change there will be to those who live to see it.

BUNKER HILL, VA. [WVA]

THURSDAY, OCT: 16TH, 1862

D[rury] W. Venable was at my tent this morning before I got up. He is driving an ambulance, hauling wounded from Shepardstown [apprently Sheppards or Shepherds in Buckingham Co]. Loan Him 10$[36]

I traded horses to-day with Maj. [Douglas] Mercer [Bde. QM]. I expect I made a bad exchange. The horse I had got from Mr. Hutchinson in Loudon Co.[37]—a large horse that travelled very finely, but the number of his years were too many for me, or too many for him to see many more. The horse I got is a small sorrel 7 or 8 years old low in flesh and lame, he travels only tollerably [sic] well. I hope by attention to improve him in flesh as well as gait.

Made a requisition for stationery to-day.

March of 1863; exchanged, he was captured again and exchanged again, and then sent to Richmond general hospital "suffering from debility at war's end." However, he flourished in peace time, making his home in Blacksburg and living to be 94 years old. Robertson, *4th VA Inf.*, 39.

[36] Drury W. Venable (born 1848) was a carpenter from Smyth Co. detailed as an ambulance driver in Co. D of 4th VA. Inf. He was captured by Federals at Spotsylvania (1864), but later exchanged. Robertson, ibid., 78.

[37] Possibly George H. Hutchinson, b. 1826; or Henry B. Hutchinson, b. 1822. VA. Census, 1870.

The enemy is reported to be in Charlestown [then Charles Town, WVA] in force, and the 1 Brigade is on the left of Charlestown on the R.R.—some cannonading has been heard.[38]

I have not read much to-day. About 9 o'clock orders came in informing us that the Division was under marching orders. Dr. Straith was in our tent, He has been assigned to a board to consist of two med: officers for the examination of applicants for discharge or leave or certificate of disabillity. He does not seem well pleased with his new position. The order came to-night with direction for the board to procede [sic] at once. This may or may not have the desired influence over the particular evil that is intended to operate on [viz., soldiers pretending to be sick or otherwise disabled]. That too many are discharged and furloughed our General [T.J. Jackson] sees plain, and has appointed the board to remedy the wrong, if any wrong there be.

While I was writing copies of the orders rec'd I heard Parson Tibbs voice outside. He enquired for Dr B[lack]'s quarters. Thinking that he had left the command because of the hard shower that had fallen a short time before I felt like running a joke on him and said in a disguised tone that Dr B. was not at these quarters. Dr B. had gone out in this time and commenced telling him that Col. [Charles A.] Ronald was wounded and the Brigade was used up. No joking now. He went out found Col: R badly wounded in left thigh by a fragment of shell—it passed by the side but on the outer side of the femeral artery and perhaps imbeded itself the substance of some of the muscles of the thigh. Some of Carpenter's Battery[39] was wounded also and in the same ambulance. Finished dressing the wound and returned to our tent and lay down to sleep. If a move is made to morrow I am hard up for a horse.

BUNKER HILL, VA. [WVA]

FRIDAY, OCT: 17TH, 1862

This morning we were up early, breakfasted and packed up to leave. I went over to see Col. R[onald]. Doing very well—two others of Co. "D" came in and

---

[38] On 16 October 1862, McClellan sent out two "major Federal reconnaissances," one from Harper's Ferry toward Charles Town. This is a small town in WV panhandle, not the capital city. Long, 279.

[39] Capt. Joseph Hannah Carpenter , born in Covington, VA. in 1834, graduated from VMI in 1856 and became deputy clerk of court, a political stepping stone in VA., in Allegheny Co. Elected captain in VA. 27th Inf., he was tranfered to his own battery; later elected LT. COL., but declined. Wounded in head, he never really recovered and died in faciltity in Bath Co. in February 1863. Reidenbaugh, *27th VA. Inf.*, 134.

their wounds were dressed. I rode on to the Regt. to have my horse shod—got one shoe put on him. He travelled better. Saw the boys—"Smyth Blues" has J[ames] Wilburn[40] killed and [Albert] Lambert[41] slightly wounded. The Reg't. has suffered considerably. Lt. [Preston E.] Stamper[42] "Dare Devils" killed and several of the same Co. [F} wounded, among them Lt. [Troy C.] Cornett[43] badly in shoulder by an exploding ball. I have doubted the explosive quality of these balls, having not seen the effect where they bursted but in this case I think it true that they do explode. We found a fragment of one in his shoulder, and the flesh was very much blackened with powder. The ball is intended principally for igniting caisons. Lt. Cornett had the head of the scapulae[44] shattered, the acromion process[45] broken and the joint badly injured every way. Excision[46] was performed by Dr. [John P.] Walls[47]—I have the acromion process.

The troops are cooking and preparing for another trial I expect. The Regiments are pretty full now and ought to stand a hard fight.

Gen. Lee & Gen. Jackson went down this morning. Our wagons were "packed" and stood 'till late when they were "unpacked" and dinner cooked. Just as the sun went down the Old Brigade[48] marched past my quarters and took

---

[40] James H. Wilburn of Smyth Blues Co. D died from wounds received at Kearneysville, WVA. on 16 October. Unknown age or occupation. Robertson, *4th VA. Inf.*, 80.

[41] Albert Lambert enlisted in Smyth Blues in 1861 and was in Co D. *Smyth Co.*, ed., Presgraves. Age and occupation unknown; Lambert deserted on 19 November 1862, was arrested, court-martialed, and jailed in Richmond, February to June 1863; released on 2 June 1863, he deserted again on 24 January 1864. Robertson, *4th VA. Inf.*, 60.

[42] Preston E. Stamper (1836-1862) of Co. F was farmer from Smyh Co.; elected 2d Lt. on 6 April 1862, he was killed at Kearneysville, WVA on 16 October 1862. Robertson, ibid., 74.

[43] Troy C. Cornett (1839-1915) of Co. F "Dare Devils" was a farmer and Cpl. at muster in 1861. Elected 2d Lt. on 24 April 1862, he was promoted to 1st Lt. on 17 September 1862. Shoulder fractured by this wound at Kearneysville, WVA on 16 October 1862, he never recovered fully, and was permitted to resign his commission because of disability on 18 December 1863. He then farmed in Cromer's Rock. Robertson, *4th VA. Inf.*, 46.

[44] Scapulae are shoulder blades, that is "large, flat, triangular bones that form the posterior part of the shoulder." *Taber's* s.v.

[45] Acromion Process is "the lateral triangular projection of the spine of the scapula that forms the point of the shoulder and articulates with the clavicle." *Taber's.*

[46] Excision is to cut away or take out; in this case not only the bullet, but also the bones of the Acromion Process were removed. The next note indicates that our Steward kept the latter as a souvenir.

[47]John Perry Walls, age unknown, was assistant surgeon in the Stonewall Bde. A native of FLA, he graduated from The College of Charleston, SC. Bean, Notes.

[48] "Old Brigade" is possibly Co. B , 48th Virginia Regiment originally organized at Seven Mile Ford, Virginia by James Greever, Capt., and known as Jackson's Old Division. Apperson's friend

the road leading to Martinsburg [WVA]. As it strucke [sic] the village the band of the 5 Regt. struck it up and cast a lively air upon breeze—Col: [Andrew Jackson] Grigsby, commanding, dashed by with a large cavalry escort. The Brigade was full and in fine spirits. Looking at I felt some emotions of pride that I am a member of it. Only yesterday it seemed almost annihilated, really it was scattered, and now it has thrown itself together and marches out for some deed of nobleness while other Brigades lie here and look on with wonder and amazement. An officer remarked to me to-day that it did seem as if that Brigade could never be sent on any expedition without getting into an engagement of some kind.

We lay out in the open air under a tree —. Orders came for the division to move at 6 to-morrow[.] [M]edical wagons except one to each Brig: and Ordnance of the Div, will remain at camp.

I got letters from Cousin B. & Sister Mary E. Aunt M. sende [sic] me a message to write her—I shall not comply —.

NEAR MARTINSBURG VA [WVA]

SATURDAY. OCT: 18, 1862

Up early this morning—Breakfasted before sunrise. After making some arrangements about sending Lt [Troy C.] Cornett & another man to G.H [General Hospital; this one at Winchester] Dr B[lack] & myself moved off after the Div. which took the road to Martinsburg[.] Overtook Dr. Suphers of La. and rode nearly all the way with him. On reaching Martinsburg the division [turned] to the left towards Hedgesville [Berkeley Co., WVA] and camped in the first woods near the town. The first Brigade is destroying Rail Road.

The citizens of Martinsburg are the most unsound and bitter enemies we have travelled among—the citizens of Maryland not excepted. Not a handkerchief waves to us here but after a curl of the lip from some Yankee love striken woman. The stores are all closed and nothing can be had for C.S scrip [Confederate money]. There are perhaps a few who are sound noble hearted southern men—the Hunters, Faulkners, and Joneses. [49] A Mr. Robinson living

---

Robert H. Dungan was an officer in Co. B 48th Virginia Regiment. Wilson, *Smyth County History*, p.237.

[49] Edmund Pendleton Hunter was prominent attorney in Martinsburg, and was also patriarch of a large family of "ardent rebels." Charles James Faulkner was former congressperson and minister to France during administration of James Buchanan. Faulkner returned to US when the War came, and was seized by the Abraham Lincoln administration and thrown into prison at Fort

within a hundred yards from camp is a good secesh [supporter of secession]. Our bands enliven the air and I hear the troops shouting as they pass through the village. I presume they do it to annoy some of the citizens. Our government ought by all means to cause the doors of those Union merchants to be opened.

The air is very cool to-night—the chills of winter are fast approaching.

I wrote some orders to-night and will retire early because of the coldness of the tent without fire.

CAMP NEAR MARTINSBURG, VA

SUNDAY OCT. 19, '62

There is dense fog hanging over the earth this morning—I washed and dressed after breakfast. The command repaired to the R. Road and commenced its work of destruction. About noon the machine shops, hotel & depot was fired by the 1 Brigade [First VA Bde, or Stonewall Bde].

I rode down late in the afternoon and found large crowds of females near the fires evidently trying to show their contempt for the "rebels" who were going the "Whole hog[.]" One woman said she could stand a shower of grape [shot] as thick as ever hail fell if her people (the Yankees) would come. I found some of the boys had stoves and I made a rush to get one too. I rode past a large building that was burning and found some in a cellar. I got one. When I came back I found Dr B[lack] had gotten one also. I took them before me and returned to camp. I got two letters. One from Dr. F. and one from Mrs. Tomlin. Dr's letter informed me that he could not get the cloth I wrote him for some time ago at a less price [sic] than 3$ for an inferior article of paltry cotton and by waiting a while [he could] send a little better at 4$. The [illegible; refers to "paltry cotton"] cant [sic] be gotten. I wrote him not to get any. I wrote to Cousin Bettie —

Our stove has been put up and the tent is quite comfortable.

We have news from Ky that Bragg has given Buell a most terrible thrashing—9000 prisoners 42 pr of cannon &c. I hope it will be confirmed. Days of peace seem to be in the future—Factions are springing up at the North

---

Warren in Boston harbor. He was eventually exchanged for a northern congressman who had been captured at 1st Manassas, and from spring of 1863 served on T.J. Jackson's staff. Notes, William G. Bean. Jones may be Lt. Roger Jones, who helped capture John Brown at Harper's Ferry and then joined the CSA. Shetler, *WVA Civil War Literature*, 516-17.

and the administration is suffering. The democratic gains are largely in the ascendency.[50]

I wrote Dr. F. a letter and instructed him not to buy at the prices. The seared leaves of Autumn are now visible to us from the Blue Ridge on the east and North Mountain—a range of the Allegheny [crossing Craig, Botetourt, Allegheny, Rockbridge, and Augusta counties] on the west. The sun has lost its force and the mornings are hazy and frosty. We may soon expect fierce winter to compell [sic] these two belligerant powers to lay down their arms at least for a while.

NEAR MARTINSBURG VA [WVA]

MONDAY, OCT: 20TH, 1862

No new incident has transpired to-day for me to chronicle, amd I am to[o] stupid to make comment on any passing subject and too much limited in knowledge itself to do justice to any topic in times like these. I have been read[ing] anatomy closely to-day and really believe with some pains would form an improving taste for that branch.

I rod[e] to town this morning and spent a short time eying the ruins of the splendid workshops there. That which cost thousands and thousands of money now stand a mass of blackened ruins. The Balt. & Ohio [Railroad] Company has a contract with the Northern Government for indemnification for all the loss sustained to the R Road. Hence the destruction of these shops, while it may for a time inconvenience the Co. will not be to it a loss, but to The Federal Government a direct taxation to replace *in status quo*. Tearing up the R Road track is a heavier job than one at first thought would suppose.

Dr. [Hunter] McGuire Med: Dir: Va came by this evening and said that we had left our sick at Bunker Hill [Berkeley Co., WVA] to starve—they were

---

[50] As the diarist suspected, rumors exaggerated Bragg's successes. Bragg, along with Kirby Smith, did enjoy some initial success invading KY. However, at Perryville, or Chaplin Hills, on 8 October 1862, Buell's forces stopped Bragg's and Smith's advances and drove them out of KY and back into TN. Buell lost some 845 killed and 2851 wounded in that day's fight, and more than 500 were missing, but few were prisoners, so the 9000 figure is hopelessly inaccurate. Bragg's losses were heavy, making more than a fourth of his invading force. On his retreat, however, Bragg did move in an orderly way and captured much ordnance and quite a great deal of grain and other foodstuffs. Buell's slowness in following up his victory at Perryville angered Lincoln, and on 24 October he removed Buell from command. On the other hand, Jefferson Davis was equally unhappy with Bragg, and the CSA president removed Bragg from his command, reassigning him to be chief of staff. Long, 275-81; John E. Stanchak, "Perryville," *Hist. Times*. Lincoln did experience some political difficulties, as the War became more unpopular.

running over the country to obtain something to eat and that the blame was thrown on us—I replied that I knew the men were left there but I did not know what we could do. Dr. B[lack] had gone over to his Headquarters and he [Black] would perhaps see him. I am sure it is not the duty of the Division Surgeon to say what will be done with inefficient men when the orders from the commanding general [T.J. Jackson] orders them [to remain] in camp at his own discretion. If the sick were to be left there and the command did not expect to return for a lengthy period it was the duty *of the* General [Jackson] to issue our orders to the Surgeon of Division instructing him what to do—we are not commissaries [the officers in charge of supply, in particular foodstuffs].

NEAR MARTINSBURG VA. [WVA]

TUESDAY, OCT 21ST, 1862

Dr B & Maj. [Douglas] Mercer took an ambulance and went to Winchester this morning. The Division moved in direction of Shepardstown [Sheppards in Buckingham Co.]—We did not move our quarters. I have been reading a book entitled "The Diary of a Physician," a work of some interest and perhaps instruction I have a very high appreciation of the trials that meet the young and ambitious [doctors and medical personnel] who are limited in their means, having known what it is to want myself.

I have not been outside the limits of the camp to-day. Camp has some charms like those of home itself to me. I have nearly every convenience that I wish and hence am contented[.] I fear when Dr. [R.T.] Coleman[51] returns from Richmond that he will take the place of Division surg: and Dr B. will return to the regiment.

BUNKER HILL, VA. [WVA]

WEDNESDAY OCT 22, 1862

I write from Bunker Hill again[.] [T]hough I write from this place we did not come here until Thursday 25 inst.— Owing to the movements I have not had an opportunity to continue my diary sooner. We moved down on the R

---

[51] R.T. Coleman was more highly thought of by military superiors than by the diarist steward. Originally surgeon with 2d Bde, he was assigned to general hospital in Richmond. See commendation and assignment, William B. Taliaferro to A.S. Pendleton, 13 August 1862, Report No. 30, *Official Records*, Ser. I, 12:191. Actually, he is not complaining about R.T. Coleman in particular; he is anxious to continue working directly with Dr. Harvey Black, Dr. B, who by now is a mentor and benefactor.

Road some 2 mi. below Martinsburg [WVA]. The Road is entirely destroyed. The track taken up and the ties laid in piles with the Railing crossing these piles and then set on fire so warping and twisting the iron as to render it useless.

In passing along I could but have very unpleasant reflections. The wealth and pride of our country are wasting before the the [sic] sad blighting march of Mars. Here for instance the most excellent and elaborately constructed road in the South is now a worthless mass, a wreck of what men call "something splendid"—money, labor, and all the fruit of invention's genius expended [.] [T]he hope of the lovers of public improvements all reduced to ashes—worthless cinders. How men seem content to undo what others have done to gratify the thirst for waste & ruin. It is indeed an inherited prosperity which grows as the human family progresses in age and greatness.

I was Gen. [John Robert] Jones' head nurse nearly all day and amused myself reading "Physicians Diary". The first Brigade returned towards Bunker Hill at the leave of Gen. Jackson while the remainder of the division staid to finish the Road.

Near night Dr B & myself rode to our quarters which were on the bank of the creek below the sillhouse[52] and mill. We found Maj [Douglas] Mercer and two friends about sitting down to dinner.— Maj. [James Williams] Green [53] Q.M. [quartermaster] an[d] ____ Q.M. of [Gen. Jubal Anderson] Early's Brigade. All Drinking.—James Cooley[54] pitched our tent and we hoped for a good night's rest. About 8 o'clock Maj Mercer sent word for his teams to be brought away. Whether or not he intended it as a[n] insinuation to us that he would like to be rid of our Company and wished to leave us I am sure I cannot tell; but at all events Dr. [Black] did not think proper to follow. We remained.

Maj Mercer is a fine looking gentleman of commanding appearance and I expect fills his appointment as Maj & Q.M. as well as anyone. He has seen much of this world['] s ups and downs, having lived in Texas, New Mexico & Arizona, took part in the Mexican War and was in the Regular service in an expedition to

---

[52] Sillhouse, or sillary, gradually became the word sellery and then cellery. Generally, all these words refered to a building where wine was aged and then stored. Occasionally it refers to any kind of storage for liquid, and sometimes any kind of storage for anything. *OED*.

[53] James Williams Green (1824-1884) was attorney and commissioner of courts in Culpeper Co. Enlisted as Lt. in 7th VA Inf., became Regt. QM; and then on 1 November 1861 became Maj. and Asst. Commissary of Supply for 7th VA Inf. under Gen. [James Lawton] Kemper. Riggs, *7th VA. Inf.*, 76

[54] "Freeman of color," see notes. This is the first instance in which Cooley seems to be performing menial, almost servant-like, work. Unlike other chores, errands, and work, there is no mention of any payment to the black soldier for this work.

Utah. He seems conversant with the manners and customs of all among whom he has travelled and is an entertaining conversationalist. His life has evidently been spent where this world['[']s pleasures were most desirable to him—fast women[,] fast horses and fine liquors and he is at home.

Dr. B has resolved to mess to himself. We have some news from Ky. of a not cheering kind. The report of the fights there are all false. Some vile miscreant has started the lie to answer [Don Carlos] Buell caring nothing about the value of truth and the sacredness of of [sic] its character.

[BUNKER HILL, WVA; ON ROAD TO MARTINSBURG, WVA]

THURSDAY OCT. 23, '62

This morning we were up and had our wagon on the road at 6 A.M. Ordered it to join Gen. [John Robert] Jones' train and we rode on to Martinsburg. I got my breakfast at a house on the suburbs. The citizens seem to be exulting in themselves —The rebels are doubtless leaving town. I would be willing to see this part of the State [WVA] cut off and banished forever.

We moved on with the Division reaching Bunker Hill a little after noon. Camps are changed somewhat. Gen. Jones's camps is near the Stone Mill on the Smithfield Road. Dr B's tent is near. Maj. Mercer is west of us some 1/2 mile. He seems to shun us. We have made arrangements to mess alone. It is with much difficulty that we can get started. Our culinary furniture [silverware and flatware] is scarce and no provisions on hand— Jim [James Cooley] is a good cook though and will make things clean. He made out a tolerable meal.

The weather is getting very cool, in fact uncomfortably so without fire.

We shall miss the horse feed that we have been getting heretofore—it will not be so plenty and regular I fear.

BUNKER HILL, VA [WVA]

FRIDAY. OCT: 24, 1862

To-day has been one pretty full of business. Orders to copy & issue and distribute. I rode this morning to Gen. [John Robert] J's [Jones] Head Quarters and handed in a report of killed and wounded of the 1st Brig. near Kearney's ville [Kerneysville, Berkeley Co., WVA] Then went to see Dr. Whitehead's staff serving Gen. [Richard Stoddert] Ewell's[55] Div. to obtain some vaccine virus. I failed in the main—I think S[mall] Pox is being distributed very rapidly in the valley.[56]

Maj. [William] Terry [commander of Co. A, 4th VA. Inf.], who was wounded at Manassas, returned to-day.[57]

Troops are moving, I understand, towards Culpeper [Culpeper Co]. Two days rations are cooked.

BUNKER HILL, VA. [WVA]

SATURDAY OCT. 25, '62

The sun shone warm to-day until evening when the wind commenced blowing quite cool. Clouds were gathering and seem to threaten a shower before morning.

I walked over to the Reg't this evening and remained an hour or so. After dinner some orders came for the examination of all employees in the Medical Department that they may be disposed of as to allow the weakly conscripts to take the places of able bodied men. I copied [the orders and took them] and went to each Brigade—Serg[eant] C.C. Hinkle 37th Va Regt 3 Brig is the appointed officer to examine the men.

Gen. D.H. Hill's[58] Division has moved in direction of Smithfield—Gen Jackson has moved his quarters also. Some move seems evident. Can it be that

---

[55] Ewell (1817-1872), see earlier notes; by now, Ewell had lost his leg and had not yet returned to official duty; although by 23 May 1863, he would again ride horses and fight effectively in the field. Dale E. Floyd, "Ewell," *Hist. Times.*

[56] There was a terrible epidemic of small pox, and it hit the Army of Northern Virginia, and especially the Stonewall Brigade, very hard. One epidemic dated from the Sharpsburg [Antietam] battle of October 1862, and persisted until early winter of 1863; a second one immediately developed in mid-winter of 1863 and persisted until 31 January 1864. CSA medical authorities, especially surgeon and prolific writer Joseph Jones, were upset because they already understood that vaccination could prevent the spread of the scourge. Medical officials were ordered to collect vaccine crusts from patients but also from the arms of children; and these crusts were used to prepare vaccine. Things improved in the final months of the War. Cunningham, *Doctors in Gray*, 194-98.

[57] William Terry [1824-1888] was from Amherst Co. Joining 4th VA. Inf. as Lt., he was promoted to Capt. early, and then Maj. on 22 April 1862. Sustained wounds in left arm and side, 28 August 1862 at Groveton [Prince William Co.]. Robertson, *4th VA. Inf.*, 76.

[58] Daniel Harvey Hill (1821-1889), a native of York, SC, he chose a military career when still a child. Graduating from West Point in 1842, he studied with a group of 15 cadets who eventually became generals in the War. Decorated in Mexican War, he later taught at Washington College

we will attack McClelland [sic] again! O how my heart revolts at the thought of seeing the bloody scene of another battle field! Has not blood enough been already spilt to to [sic] appease the war demon that rages in our land?

Surgeons Straith[,] [John Perry] Walls & [Malcolm N.] Fleming[59] were with us 'till late. These are three men of differences in character. [John Perry] Walls is a sound[,] sensible[,] social man. Quiet spoken an[d] decisive[,] not very precise about matters generally. Is a good physician, has been a professor of anatomy. [Malcolm N.] Fleming is one whose cast of countenance has something solemn and stern[,] a mingling of destiny and determination while behind all this can be seen wit and humor which turns nearly everything into jest. Careless perhaps in all matters of domestic arrangement—kind and gentlemanly. Straith is vastly different from either[.] [S]ensible and minute in his conversation. Well read and has a good understanding of manners, & is quite precise in their use. His writings are prolix, aye, profuse with every point explained until former explanation itself becomes confused. No error escapes him, and his own works are done in strict accorndance with his Conscience. He will make his mark in the world and do humanity a vast amount of good. Popular at home and easily becoming so abroad & he labors to maintain that popularity and is ambitious for an enviable standpoint in his profession[.] which I doubt not he will yet reach. He is constantly engaged—losing no time from his duty. Whether or not from his competency he was lately placed on a board to examine applicants for furlough or discharge which place he fills with honor to himself and the Government.

The wind blew cool near night and some indication of a cloudy spell.

BUNKER HILL, VA. [WVA]

SUNDAY OCT; 26TH, 1862

This morning the sky was obscured by clouds and a light drizzly rain was falling which increased during the day 'till near night when the rain had set in[,] in good earnest, cool too—wind N.E.

(now Washington & Lee University) and Davidson College. Historian Hall Bridges labels Hill "Lee's maverick general," and Robert D. Hoffsommer says, "possessed of bravery that approached recklessness, he earned respect and affection from his men. He was also abrasive and outspoken toward his fellow officers, and his relations with them suffered." Hoffsommer, "Hill," *Hist. Times.*

[59]William G. Bean supplies the full names. See Bean's notes on Walls.

Dr. [Joseph C.] Stiles[60] has been holding a series of meetings in Ewels [sic; Gen. Richard Stoddert Ewell's] Div: which resulted in much good. He commenced last night in ours Friday [24 October] but I expect the weather will break him up. I have not been able to hear him though I learn he is an excellent man. Indeed I have not heard a sermon for a long time. Preaching is so seldom and irregular in camp that I greatly fear all of us will loose [sic] all the taste we ever had for serious, solemn discourses.

The truth is very obvious that we are becoming depraved. The character of our fallen nature is such that the life we are now leading meets no rebuffs as we go down down [sic] in the mire of sin and folly. And there is scarcely a soldier in our ranks who will not admit but that of all men and all classes of men a soldier in this struggle should strive harder to gain the aid and approbation of Divine Control.

Gen DH Hill's Div: I heard Gen [John Robert] Jones say while in our tent to-day was engaged in destroying the Winchester & Harper's Ferry road. He also stated he had heard that Harper's Ferry had been evacuated by the enemy. This needs but little reliance till further confirmed. If such is the case can it be that the enemy is going to change operations anywhere[?] It seems that the best policy that can be adopted by us would be to fall back and allow the enemy to proceed into the country and then fight him. It [sic] scarcely to be doubted that a large fleet of iron cased boats are now in course of erection for the purpose of a conquest along the southern shores. But woe be unto the man that leave the boats.

Capt: J[ospeh]. M. Thomas took dinner with us and spent nearly the whole day. He is one of my good friends.

I got a letter from Mrs. Tomlin to-day dated May 29th. I wrote her this evening. The old lady is in Wythe [Co.] now so I directed it to her there.

I have been reading Physic some to-day—finished anatomy. Read several chapters of 1 Kings.

---

[60] The Rev. Joseph Clay Stiles (1795-1875) was a Georgia Presbyterian minister who made a pre-war career in pulpits in New Haven and New York; relatively Old Light and conservative, he engaged in debate in broadsides and letters with Alexander Campbell, founder of the dissenting Campbellite sect. According to William G. Bean, "With the coming of the war, he returned to the South and was a popular, roving chaplain in Lee's army. His son Major Robert Stiles, was an artillery officer in the Army of Northern Virginia and was the author of *Four Years Under Marse Robert* (Washington, D.C: Neale Publishing Co., 1903)." Bean, Notes.

BUNKER HILL VA [WVA]

MONDAY OCT: 27TH 1862

The sun rose clear and the day was fine though cool. No business of any importance.

I drew rations for 4 days. This ends with the month [of October]. Dr. Stevens of the La. Brigade was in our tent at least half the day. The order taking away ward masters &c seems to operate badly with him [change in policy concerning junior staff assigned as ward masters and reporting to senior surgeons; in the case of Stevens, his staff was significantly reduced by the new policy.] He has some young Dr's detailed in his department that he is not willing to part with. I think with him that the Med: Dept. is almost imposed upon.

I attended the preaching of Dr. Stiles to-night at the camp of the 1 Brigade. His sermon was simple, plain, and practicable. His remarks were based upon the first clause of Isaiah 5th chapter. [61] A vineyard was planted by a prince and he worked it after planting the choicest of plants and looked forward to a fine crop but when he went to gather it the grapes were evil and poisonous. Now this vinegrower had done all he could—all that was in his power to make the vineyards yield a lucrative, healthy crop but alas! it would not. And so said the minister it is with you. God has created you for a wise and good purpose, he has placed you in a world formed by his own hands and all that is contained therein has been for [man's] convenience; he has given man a Bible of truths and wisdom to be governed by—containing laws for individuals & nations—He has even given his Only Son to die that man might be saved yet he is in upon rebellion against all of God's works.

The minister traced a long line of analogies between God[']s love towards his people and a father's love for his children. God has done all that he can do, both by warning and encouragement as a creator, father, and benefactor. He shows man to a sinner and God his only refuge, the one being to whom he can appeal for justice which as he said would scarcely come. While God is kind, benevolent, and holy; he is sure with justice; for when he cried Mt. Sanai's [sic] Top : "That I am the Lord thy God, thou shalt have no other gods before me", The

[61] Isaiah 5:1. "Now will I sing to my wellbeloved a song of my beloved touching his vineyard. My wellbeloved hath a vineyard in a very fruitful hill." (KJV) The prophet quotes God throughout all 30 verses of the chapter.

mountain was rent and the clouds were smote by his power.[62] This is in substance a part of his sermon. Space will not allow more—There was appointments made for next day & night. I returned to camp and retired after reading awhile.

CAMP NEAR WIDOW ALLEN'S [CLARKE CO.]

TUESDAY OCT 28TH, 1862

Last night sometime the Gen [John Robert Jones] got orders [from Gen. T.J. Jackson] to move. We were up early. The whole army will move together. I am much dismayed to-day. This morning my horse was loose minus halter. Some man needed one I suppose. We moved in direction of Smithfield. The 1st Div. in front and A.P. Hill[']s following—just as we struck the pike below Berryville [Clarke Co.] D.H. Hill was passing. I stopped at the house of a Mr. Whiting in this (Clarke) County and asked for dinner. I came in at the back of the house and sent one of the servants in to acquire if I could get a snack. I rec'd an affirmative answer with the message that it would be brought out to me. This I did not like—'twas the cold shoulder. The waiter came with a plate filled with good vi[c]tuals and I took it into a small dining room and ate it at my leisure. I was determined to let them know that I was not as they seem[ed] to suppose, an outside beggar, so I sent in a 5$ bill and asked the lady to take her change—she came to the window and seem[ed] reluctant to take anything—I insisted however and she took 70 cents for two of us. I was as polite as I possibly could be to the lady. Our camp is near the residence of the widow Allen. A magnificent country all around.

This is indeed one of the most desirable countries I have ever seen. The fertility of the land is excellent; the view of the Blue Ridge on the S.E. is fine; the Shenandoah winds its way along the base of the mountain. [T]he society claims, with merit too, to be as pure as any in Virginia. Here live the descent of many of the old families of English origin. [63] The relics and manners of some of superb

[62] Exodus 20:1-3: "And God spoke all these words, saying, I *am* the Lord thy God, which have brought thee out of the land of Egypt, out of the house of bondage. Thou shalt have no other gods before me." (KJV) Ex 19 describes the scenes on Mt. Sinai.

[63] Clarke Co. was claimed early by large planters of the First Families, who established claims in 1730, and then sent sons, or sometimes went themselves soon thereafter, making Clarke somewhat different from the other Mountain and Valley counties, where a landed elite formed from Scots Irish migrants some two decades later. "With men such as Robert Carter and William Beverly leading them, the large planters of the East, bearing such prominent names as Fairfax, Burwell, Page, Washington, and Lee" became the almost mythical elite "Tuckahoe" to the equally

old Virginia gentlemen still linger around many of the families and mansions. We see here all that is substantial, elegant amd polished. The farms seem to have rec'd. more attention than is usual in so extensive a section for husbandry. Every farm seems to have an ample supply of woodland attached to the farmhouses to be useful.

I rode out with the hope of procuring some butter, eggs, or something that might be relished by our mess and went to the Widow Allen's. [64] I did not expect to procure much from her but thought I would try by way of experiment. I rode up and sent in a negro [sic] to make the inquiry. He failed to return with an answer as soon as I thought necessary. I went in myself and found the Old Lady and young lady, her daughter I suppose, surrounded by a dozen or more soldiers to whom she was distributing fruit and talking at the same time. I addressed and made inquiry—no indeed she had no butter[,] and chickens and eggs she never sold—I remarked that people had done many things lately that they had never done before—while I was talking to her she was thrusting apples into my hand—I took them to satisfy the goodness of her heart.

I failed to procure any "forage" [sic] and returned to camp

CAMP NEAR MRS. ALLEN[']S CLARKE CO.

WEDNESDAY OCT. 29TH, 1862

I hardly expected to remain here to-day, but I believe the move was made principally to change camps. We are now in an excellent camp, and this country has not been over run by the army much.

I thought yesterday that a movement might be made with a view to attack and destroy the forces of [Franz] Sigel [65] which is somewhere between Culpeper

---

storied "Cohee" of the plain folk Scots Irish. Willard F. Bliss, "The Tuckahoe in New Virginia," *VA Mag. of Hist. and Biog.*, 59 (1951):388-96. By traditional understanding, the Cohees raised livestock [husbandry] and the Tuckahoes tobacco, but here the elite are found raising livestock with the use of slaves on large and well-tended holdings.

[64] Possibly Nancy Allen (born 1792), who was then more than 70 yrs. old and who owned a farm in Long Marsh Township of Clarke Co. VA. Census. 1870.

[65] Franz Sigel (1824-1902) was born in Baden, Germany and graduated from Karlsruhe Military Academy; politically liberal, he fought against Prussia in the unsuccessful revolution of 1848, fled, and eventually came to St. Louis, where he was teaching school at outbreak of the war. Lincoln appointed him Brigadier Gen. as part of a plan to attract antislavery, Unionist immigrants. Rapidly promoted to Maj. Gen., Sigel fought brilliantly at Pea Ridge (8 March 1862) in western campaigns and was then transfered to the Valley. He became commander of the Dept. of WVA, but never again enjoyed success, and indeed was disgraced by defeat at the Battle of New Market (15 May 1864). "Sigel was an odd combination of ineptitude and ability. On the record

& Manassas but as yet I see no further chances. Orders came of different kinds for the government of the Med Dept. I was at the Brigade this evening —

I rec'd. a letter from sister Mary this evening bring[ing] me the sad news that sister Bettie is very low with typhoid fever and Mother is also down with an absess. They are earnest in entreaties for me to come home for a short time. This is impossible while it would be the most desirable to me. I might be as they said useful in "giving medicine"[.] I wrote a letter to them promising to come home as soon as I can. As we are now there does not seem to be much probability of any of us getting home soon. Many are dying and those that survive will be worn out in constitution and energy. Some dry wag remarked the other day that many a woman would be fooled after the breaking up of this war. They would marry some young man that had been in service under Jackson and think she had a prize but it would be nothing but a worn out specimen of a man—no use at all—on her hands to nurse and perhaps to support.

CAMP NEAR MRS. ALLEN'S CLARKE CO.

THURSDAY OCT 30TH, 1862

This is a beautiful day—I rose before sunrise as I do usually and after breakfast went to the creek not far distant and bathed and changed my underclothes. I walked over to the Brigade took dinner with Capt [Robert LaFayette] Francisco [QM]—had a chat with Maj [William]Terry[66] , and returned to quarters. Nothing worth recording is transpiring now.

I was engaged during the evening making envelopes. Capt [James W.] Shields[67] paid me 6$ in full of [sic] commutatuion of rations when I went to Richmond last spring.

---

his military performance, aside from Pea Ridge, was little better than mediocre. But he unquestionably helped the Union cause by rallying German-Americans to the flag, and he held their loyalty to the end." Robert D. Hoffsommer, "Sigel," *Hist. Times.*

[66]William Terry (1824 1888), was from Amherst Co., but moved to Smyth Co. and joined Co. A of 4th VA. Inf. Lt. at muster, he was rapidly promoted, eventually to Brig. Gen. Often wounded, he survived War but drowned at his home in Wythe Co. long after the war. Robertson, *4th VA. Inf.*, 76.

[67] James W. Shields , age unknown, entered service 1 May 1862 as field and staff officer in charge of commissary for 4th VA. Inf. Promoted to Capt. in Dec. of 1862, but apparently breveted Capt. in this month. Re earlier remarks by diarist complaining of commissary and reimbursements. Suspected of wrong doing, Capt. Shields was "dropped from the rolls July 31, 1863, by order of the Inspector General's office. Ibid., 72.

CAMP NEAR MRS. ALLEN'S [CLARKE CO.]

FRIDAY OCT. 31ST, 1862

Another lovely morning—I have never seen such weather.

I went to Brigade with some vaccine virus. Dr. [Joseph Clay] Stiles was preaching when I went over. I heard the larger part of his sermon but did not hear what text he based his argument upon. He seemed to be solely bent upon stirring up the spirit of the members—made some beautiful appeals to them saying that wherever they were then God be also. He said that it fell upon individuals to pray for God to help them and bring the sinner to a right sense of his case. What said he one man might do and what the sins of one might prevent. He spoke of the defeat of whole people of Israel because one man had sinned. "Oh," said he "what more encouragement do you need than the words of God himself,—a whole bible full of promises!" "If there had not been a single individual converted for 20 years by all the preaching that might take place during that time and all the truths of the Bible have fallen unheeded to the ground then you would have encouragement enough in the one promise that wherever ye be there will I be also." The power of God to save all that called upon him for safety was fully proven from scripture.

And I might give in this scattering[,] promiscuous way nearly all his fruits and most prominent remarks but it is needless. The lecture looked upon here is one indeed that would do better for fancy's work than real fact. The minister in a slight depression in the land with perhaps a hundred lying & sitting around him listening to his teaching—some holding their arms in their hands. A short distance beyond and in fair view of where I sat were a parcel of careless men trying to have sport out of a squirrel—and fired some 7 or 8 shots at it—a thing contrary to all military law. Men & officers on duty marched back and forth around, the smoke from the camp fire seem[ed] to settle in the wood and was of considerable annoyance.

I returned to Hd. Qer's. Dr. B. for some cause or other commenced quizzing me on auscultation[68]. I had never done more than give that a glance and was

[68]Auscultation is "process of listening for sounds within the body, usually to sounds of thoracic or abdominal viscera, in order to detect some abnormal condition, or to detect fetal heart sounds." *Taber's.*

rather verdant [69]—or so I felt; but to acknowledge that I had not studied it when the book was before I consider equally as criminal as not to know after studying with proportionate pains.

His first question was "What is the difference between the Bronchial sound and the viscular murmur?" I was somewhat confused and answered with some incorrectness. From that he continued his quizzing—He proposed that if I would glance [at] the article in "Wood's Practica" [70] he would see how much I knew when to-morrow comes. This I must cheerfully accede to. I believe unless I have a stimuli I will never learn medicine. As I go on viewing the the [sic] different branches and their numerous ramifications, learning just enough to see the endless amount I have left unlearned my spirit sinks within me—the future days of my pupilage look dark and dreary, while I plunge deeper and deeper in the complex labyrinth of that oc[c]ult study. To-night I have been trying to get my brain settled on auscultation but my sleeping energy has such a powerful grasp up[on] my body that I have to lay down the works and go to bed.

I wrote to Nat to-day; giving him information about home difficulties. Gen Lee's Adj[utant] G[eneral] [Robert Hall] Chilton [71] has been promoted and A.P.

---

[69] The diarist has picked up a Byronic usage, despite his dislike for the mock-epic *Don Juan.* From the *OED*: "Verdant...[fig.] Of persons, Green, inexperienced, gullible. *Juan XV, 93*: Because my business is to dress society and stuff with *sage* that very verdant goose."

[70] George Bacon Wood, *Treatise on the Practice of Medicine* (Philadelphia: Griggs & Elliott, 1847; 1866). Wood(1797-1879) provided this treatise, usually called in shorthand *Wood's Practica* for medical students, and it was widely used, especially at the Mecial College of Virginia. Wood earned the M.A. and the M.D. from the University of Pennsylvania, and between 1835 and 1859 established a flourishing private practice as well as serving as attending physician at Philadelphia's Pennsylvania Hospital. Renowned for his eloquence as much as for his technical expertise, especially on auscultation and percussion, he delivered addresses to physicians and he delivered clinical lectures. Much published, the classically trained Wood often wrote verse and essays as well as technical medical treatises; and he helped in organizing physicians in the US into a professional force with high standards of training. He also published a widely used translation and updated revision of Dioscorides' *Materia Medica* (rev. ed.; Philadelphia: Griggs & Elliott, ca. 1860), and it is likely Wood's edition of *Materia Medica* that the diarist was studying—and using for filling prescriptions as pharmacist

[71] Robert Hall Chilton (1815-1879) was from Loudon Co., and graduated from West Point in 1837. He served in Indian territory with distinction before Mexican War, and during it "he won the brevet of major at Buena Vista, where he carried to safety the wounded Jefferson Davis." After Mexican War, he was paymaster in US army for 16 years, resigning in 1861 to become adjutant general with rank of Lt. Col. in CSA. From May 1861 to October 1862, Chilton served as chief of staff to R.E. Lee. This appointment to Brig. Gen. was never confirmed by CSA Senate. He moved to Richmond to serve as Inspector General of Lee's ANV. He did serve briefly in a tactical setting in battle in May 1864 defense of Richmond, acquitting himself brililantly with infantry and

Mason acting. I heard to-day that D.H. Hill has been taken from Jackson[']s Corps.

I drew rations to-day commencing Nov: 1.

CAMP ALLEN, CLARKE CO.

NOV. 1, 1862

This morning Dr. B rode to Cablestown village—monthly reports of sick and wounded from the 3 & 4 Brigades were brought in. It is to be regretted that so little care[,] interest and taste is manifested in making reports for the sick & wounded; out of reports of 10 Regt's besides Batteries only two of the reports are correct. Some are ridiculously erroneous—errors that one who had never seen a report before might discover forthwith. Yet these regiments are in charge and the reports are made under the supervision of full surgeons [trained physicians duly licensed as surgeons; not stewards such as Apperson]. Dr. [LaFayette Hall] Jordan [Asst. Surgeon of Reg.] sent a message for me to come over. I infered he wished some instructions about the reports—I went in the evening and found my inference correct. He had nearly finished the report—and done it correctly too—we'll furnish a handsome return.

Three ladies visited the Gen. [John Robert Jones] to-day—his wife and two Misses Schultz of Winchester.

I read auscultation part of to-day. When I went over to the Regt I concluded to attend preaching having been invited over by parson Newman. I went and heard Dr. [Joseph Clay] Stiles preach an excellent sermon. Prayer by Mr [Abner Crump] Hopkins chaplain of the 2d VA[72] and a hymn commencing

"Life is the time to serve the lord"

Dr Stiles rose and the first words out of his mouth were, "God made this world in six days, and could have made it just as easy in six seconds". "And he can convert every soul here to-night just as easy as he can convert one." Giving as his text, or rather as a groundwork for his sermon the 6 verse of the 1 chapter Jonah reading thus: "What meanest thou Oh sleeper? arise, call upon thy God, if

---

attached cavalry in driving out an invading Federal force, the Army of the James. After that engagement, he returned to Inspector General's post. Edward G. Longacre, "Chilton," *Hist. Times.*

[72] Abner Crump Hopkins (1835-1911) of Powhatan Co. graduated from Hampden Sydney College and Union Theological Seminary in Richmond; minister of Martinsburg Presbyterian Church at outbreak of War. Chaplain of ANV 2d Army Corps. After War, pastor of First Presbyterian Church of Charles Town, Charleston, WVA for 45 years. Dennis E. Frye, *2nd VA Inf.*, Virginia Regimental Histories Series (Lynchburg, VA: H.E. Howard, 1984), 107.

so be that God will think upon us, that we perish not."[73] Dwelling only a short time on what might seem the principal thought presented in the text, that to rouse sinners to a sense of their danger as the shipman [shipmaster] aroused Jonah: he threw a few hints to the members to throw of[f] the coldness of their hearts in the cause of God, and pray earnestly to Him to save the the [sic] thousands of souls that were being wrecked in the storm that was waged by sin, and then commenced a sermon on the character of sin. This is the third time I have heard him preach and each time the terror and miseries and influences of sin seemed to be the most prominent feature in his sermon.[74]

Deviating first to the law of God as emanating from the God-head for the exclusive Government of his creatures that it was just, benevolent, wise, and inevitable—dealing fairly and squar[e]ly with sovereign and subject; thus the arrogant, presumptive, nature of sin as proceeding in direct conflict with this great and good law—had laid the axe at the very root of the great shelter that had its being for the protection of Mankind and was striving to cheat God and rush the whole universe into irretrievable ruin.

Said he "I will not try to show you the enormity of your sins, nor will I attempt to classify your sins, nor will I attempt to enumerate your sins, for the smallest sin you ever committed, and which you commit every day, hour, minute and second you live, and upon every foot of ground you tread will be sufficient to bring you up to the flaming bar of God; your sins are far too varied and diversified—too many of God's beautiful benign laws are trodden under foot to be classified, the sands on the sea shore and the leaves in the forest will far [sic] be a number beneath the number of your transgressions. Then O what a thought! What a chilling, blasting, thought that the smallest of all these will bring you before that God of justice! I am a sinner, my body is full of sin, and I would not for ten thousand worlds look at that awful book wherein they are recorded! No I would not!

"I know myself for all this: for I would be stricken down—the cannon has not been forged nor the ball cast that would kill me as dead as to behold the enormity of my sins."

He gave to sin several systematic classes viz—Arbitrariness. Incorrigibility. Progress and Fruitfullness. Wherever it has entered, wherever it has sway it is

---

[73] Words of the shipmaster to Jonah, Jonah 1:6b (KJV).

[74] Such a sermon would be more New Light and evangelical than Stiles may have been in peacetime; such evangelical fervor was very much in keeping with what Pitts finds in the CSA army chaplains generally (Pitts, *Chaplains*, esp. 111).

content with nothing but supremacy. It turns out law and order, crushes benevolence and truth, laughs at holiness and virtue, rejects immutability and denies the authority of immutable laws, mocks at the warnings of God's holy words, and scoffs at all His divine attributes. It brings God's [word missing] down on the [illegible; sense is *sinners*] often in a summary way or the whole universe would be transformed into hell. Sin entered Heaven and aspired to thrust God and holiness out and reign, God saw it and cast angels into outer darkness. It entered the world, destroyed the family of the Garden of Eden, overturned the intentions of the Creator of Man, brought defilement and misery on all generations to come. Hence again, did it cause God to visit the the [sic] world with retributive justice—for forty days and forty nights was all that which the Creator had promised "good and very good" deluged[;] "every living thing was swept from the face thereof"—the elements poured forth fire & brimstone and swept cities from the face of the earth that no man afterward knew where they stood. Then a sinner in your breast this minute lives! Your breast harbors a dream that will turn heaven and earth into hell and thrust your soul into damnation and darkness forever!

That it is *incorigible* is equally plain. Persuade it and do what you will it still tends the same course. God warns you of that. No expression in the Bible is so often used as that sin is *against God*. It is at enmity against God and His ways of Holiness. The Creature may be reformed to sin never. The Creature may turn away from sin, may cease to be drawn by it and take up Christ & his virtues; but sin is still the same lawbreaker, the same enemy to all the virtues of man and attributes of God that it was at first.

It lures the men of earth into the belief that God is a liar and his book a fable, that virtue is comely [sic], truth oppressive and the ways of holiness sad and weary. God, knowing that sin could never be reformed thrust it into hell—banished where it could be restrained—where his mercy could never reach.

That sin is progressive is manifest in every act whether good or evil a man does. One sin gives room for another. Every sin committed gives less compunction than the one before. Conscience speaks up and the mind banishes it easier, until finally, it has entire control. If we do a good act sin is impertinent and seems to laugh at our credulity, which when spoken, destroys faith. From the fall of angels till now it has roamed over the world, and but for the check given it by God would have cheated Him out of the enire universe every [sic] since.

Now look at the fruits of sin. All through the Old and New Testaments we see its fruits—fallen angels, destroyed worlds, kings destroyed, wars waged, and deeds of horror and misery committed in all ages and by all classes. God's chosen people after having given up to the abandonements of sin suffered defeat, disgrace, [illegible] and death, and finally lost favor with their Divine Protector. Solomon once a favorite of Heaven to whom was entusted the building of the temple to contain the ark incurred the displeasure of Heaven that generations afterwards felt the chastisement [illegible] upon him for transgressions.

Having proved that sin is arbitrary and incorrigible and progressive and that it fastens upon many with a defying hold—a hold it claims, having transformed the very nature of man and made him prone to sin. What no[w] must be done to protect the body from this awful being? Go to God. Seize upon his divine attributes, acknowledge his power and claim protection. He alone has proven to make sin loose his hold and through the plan of salvation through Christ you may be saved. But stay where you are and vengeance will reach you. Sinner you are on the track. God is rolling along with all His heavenly thought. His goodness, love, mercy, Holiness [illegible] the high estate of the God be altered not a hair's breath will turn not to the right or left, He is on the [track] and you are a sinner, sin and God moves in the other direction, therefore He strikes you [illegible] you beneath all this [illegible] justice. He is not a car that can leave the road and [illegible] still. If a car leaves the road it would be a car still, but with God, if he moves right or left He would be not God; therefore He keeps straight [and immutable] and if you will [move away from Him] what terrible consequences. It is your fault not His —.

This is in substance his sermon—I was compelled to leave before he closed. He was commencing an appeal to the members in [sic] to flee to Christ and be saved—I regarded it a fine [illegible], well illustrated discourse.

I returned to Hd Qtrs.—Dr. B. got me on auscultation—I am a dunce in it—

CAMP ALLEN, CLARKE CO.

SUNDAY, NOV. 2, 1862

This morning we were expecting a general review. I rode over to the Brigade and borrowed a sword from Dr. B. The review was postponed 'till to-morrow.

I spent the afternoon in writing in my diary and reading in my Bible of the wicked kings [illegible names of three kings, possibly Abijah, Baasha, and Elah] and about good Elijah proving to the heathen that his God of Spirit was the true God.

Early this morning we heard cannon firing in the direction of Paris in Ashby's Gap [Fauquier Co.] and it continued all day. No account has reached us yet. It is reported that on yesterday afternoon that one of [James] Longstreet's Divisions and a portion of [J.E.B.] Stuart's cavalry had an engagement with the enemy near Aldie, Loudon Co., and took 70 prisoners. [75] No orders have been rec'd. I learned Andy Sanders [76] returned this evening. I am anxious to see him. I went to Capt. [Robert H.] Dungan's camp this afternoon—had loose chat and rigermarole. Dr. B has gone to the preaching. I wish I could have gone too.

About 8 o'clock orders came for 1 day's rations to be cooked, wagons packed and to hold the troops in readiness to march. The firing over the mountain continued until a later hour.

[CAMP ALLEN, CLARKE CO.; THEN ON THE ROAD TO WINCHESTER, CLARKE CO.]

MONDAY, NOV. 3, 1862

This morning we were up at sunrise and breakfasted. I rode down to Cabletown [Clarke Co.] to exchange a pair of gloves for Dr. B. Had a very good ride and when I got back the Division's wagons were just moving out. After laying around Hd. Qtrs. for some two or three hours, the Division moved up [southward] the Winchester Pike, and camped about 5 miles from Winchester. The country is a very pretty one.

---

[75] There were "operations" in Loudon Co. on 26 October, but no real skirmish and no prisoners taken. There had been a Federal reconaissance on 8 October to Aldie, but no skirmishes there. J.E.B. Stuart had by this date completed his "ride around McClellan," cutting wires and taking provisions and generally demonstrating that McClellan's forces could not stop him. The diarist may have confounded rumors of Federal actions at Aldie with Stuart's completed ride. On 2 November there was skirmishing in Philomot and Snicker's Gap (Loudon Co.], and the cannonading and gunfire there could be what the diarist heard. McClellan was moving in the Warrenton area, and James Longstreet's corps positioned themselves in his way by establishing a line at Culpeper Court House in Culpeper Co. There was no fighting then, and Longstreet was not wounded. Long, 280-85.

[76] Andrew Tate Sanders (1837-1877), a friend from Smyth Co. who was a clerk in civilian life. Sanders was often sick, but his sicknesses were not always believed to be legitimate illnesses by other authorities. Apperson hoped that Sanders could be excused from further active duty, but then his friend was captured at Kernstown (23 March 1862) and imprisoned until August. The diarist hoped to go see him and talk with him about his many troubles.

It is rumored that Gen. [James] Longstreet was killed yesterday, though the report is not much credited. Some firing was heard to-day. All accounts we get from the North through the papers say that McClelland [sic] is advancing.

The wind blows very cool this evening. Truly has bleak November come and many of our poor soldiers poorly clad. But they seem to be buoyant. Nothing can dispirit them.

[CLARKE CO.; ON ROAD TO WINCHESTER]

TUESDAY, NOV. 4, 1862

The air is cool this morning. I went to the regiment and had a long chat with Andy Sanders. Some things that have transpired have made me almost distrust my own nature.

How can it be that some women profess so much sanctity, so much rectitude, even venture to give others a code of morals by which to be governed and yet stoop to base, ungrateful acts themselves? I do not wonder at the fall of one who once I thought did me an injustice. And while I reflect upon it as due to so haughty a nature, I can but regard her with sorrow and pity. [77]

I gave Andy Sanders all the accounts that I have been keeping for him since he was taken prisoner [23 March 1862].

At night I felt lonesome and sad—my reflections seemed to lead into a melancholy channel. My future walks would seem to be crowded by disappointments. I have a continual dread upon my mind that some misfortune awaits me somewhere. To drive away this dull monster, I wrote a letter to Cousin Bettie. She is a good girl, a firm friend, and will make a worthy wife. I hope she will get some good husband who will do well.

[ON ROAD TO BERRYVILLE, CLARKE CO.]

WEDNESDAY, NOV. 5, 1862

Very suddenly this morning, we have orders to pack up and leave. The wagons moved immediately and troops moved about noon. Taking a direction midway between Berryville and Winchester, we proceeded to a point near Mr. Spitzer's on the pike leading from Berryville via Millwood. We arrived at our

---

[77] While he went to talk with Sanders about his friend's health, imprisonment, and other misfortunes, Sanders brought the diarist news of Apperon's former Smyth Co. girlfriend, identity not revealed in diary or "Reminiscences" memoirs.

camp which is on the south side of the Pike. In looking back at the troops it can plainly be seen that the Regiments have increased largely. Good must be the enemy's division that meets this one now.

I rode to Capt. [Robert LaFayette] Francisco's [QM] quarters and borrowed some candles. Finished auscultation [in Wood's *Treatise*] to-night.

CAMP NEAR MR. PAGE'S,[78] *CLARKE CO.*

THURSDAY, NOV: 6, 1862

This [diary book or notebook] book was given me to-day by Dr. B. It was found in an old English pannier [basket] captured at Harper's Ferry at the surrender of the Federal forces at that place. I intend to appropriate it to a continuation of my diary—my last book being filled.

No news of importance to-day. Surg[eon] [Hunter] McGuire was at our tent also surg[eons]. Hinkle, Burdette and [W.S.] Love—all on business. Dr. McGuire says the enemy is taking possession of all the Gaps in the Eastern side of the Blue Ridge, and that Gen. [T.J.] Jackson expected the enemy in Front Royal [Warren Co]. He (Gn J.) moved his Hd. Qurs up to Ninevah [Warren Co.] below Front Royal. Why it is that the enemy is being allowed to proceed up [southward] the mountains in that way I cannot see.[79]

Monthly reports of the 1 & 3 Brig. were handed in to-day—The 1 Brigade reports do very well but the others are pretty hard lot. Dr B rebuked me to-night, and very justly too, for speaking disparagingly of the reports before surgeons. I am wrong in doing so; but no presumptuous or arrogant spirit prompted me to do so. There is one thing sure, the reports are wrong, and in many cases ridiculously so, and if I laugh it is justified but courtesy discountenances it. I am very glad Dr B did so. It will make me more cautious and courteous.

---

[78] Several Page families of Clarke Co. were "Tuckahoes," that is, descendants of elite easterners who had come to the co. in the 1730s. This particular Tuckahoe may have been Eliza Page (born 1800), a widower who operated a farm in Millwood. VA. Census, 1870.

[79] Actually McClellan was hardly moving, proceeding at what E.B. Long labels a "snail-like pace." Republicans had maintained a majority in Congress in the elections of 4 November 1862, despite losses in the Northeast, and Lincoln may have felt emboldened to move against "Little Mac," with whom he had been patient despite long ago losing confidence in the general. He removed McClellan from command of the Army of Potomac and replaced him with Ambrose Everett Burnside (1824-1881). Long, 285.

Had a lesson on percussion[80] and pointed out one on coryza[81] for to-morrow night. The air is getting very cool.

CAMP NEAR MR PAGES [CLARKE CO.]

FRIDAY NOV. 7TH 1862

Slight sprinkles of rain fell last night and this morning by 8 o'clock it was snowing.

Have been at work on reports all day—been busy—I had to go round to all the Brigades to get some points. Capt Earhart [paymaster] has money to pay off the troops. Some have drawn and others are making preparations to draw. It is a question where I should draw—Med. Regulations seems to throw it upon the senior surg[eon] of the Reg't and some new plan of making out the field and staff is afoot—I shall try that first. I learn that many of the boys who are absent without leave are being deducted largely in the payroll by the Pay Master—This is all right. Good soldiers have done their duty and worthless men have run over the country shirking duty and shunning battles. Now they have their reward.

From a letter from Dr. Coleman to Dr. Fleming to-day we learn that he will be back in a few days. Then Dr. B. will return to the reg't.

The snow has fallen nearly all day but slowly. M[oses]. Gibson[82] came for names of the new officers of 14 La. Infantry—Return for Med. Off. is nearly ready—we will have the whole concern ready to-morrow.

Drew rations for 7 days to-day.

CAMP NEAR MR. PAGES [CLARKE CO.]

SATURDAY NOV. 8TH, 1862

Commenced early this morning to write on reports—finished and took them up to Gen Jackson's Hd. qurs. His head quarters are on the Front Royal pike about 8 miles from that place. It [sic] worthy of notice that his head quarters is the least attractable place I ever saw of the kind—no display, no

---

[80] Percussion is "use of the fingertips [not an instrument] to tap the body lightly but sharply to determine position, size, and consistency of an underlying structure and the presence of fluid or pus in a cavity." *Taber's.*

[81] Coryza, from Greek for catarrh, is "an acute catarrhal inflammation of the nasal mucous membrane accompanied by profuse nasal discharge." *Taber's.*

[82] Moses Gibson, age unknown, occupation unknown. Served 2d VA. until 31 October 1862; detailed as clerk to Surgeon Hunter McGuire in Nov.; later promoted to hospital steward. Robertson, *4th VA. Inf.*, 52.

ostentation, and none of that unnecessary military etiquette that can be found at many places. Two or three wagons[,] three or four tents and a few horses tied near comprise all that may be seen about his camp. Couriers coming and going, but no guard around his encampment.

I had a very pleasant ride. Having gone towards Millwood when I started by direction, I went several miles out of my way. I went by White Post, which is a village of about a dozen houses. I do not know its history or anything about it. I met with a Mr Meade[83] living at that place who seemed to be a knowing man—or seemed to think I did not know what I was inclined to hold or that I did. He said that D. H. Hill had a corps of troops in his command and that he ranked [outranked] Jackson. I tried to convince him that he was wrong, and told him the true position as regards corps that our army stood. He was invincible and was not convinced 'till he met a Major and asked him. He then acknowledged the *corn*,[84] and said he was informed so by Dr Ward and some other gentleman from Richmond. [85]

I note this merely to show how some men will hold on to any idea because it came from a distinguished person.

The country about here never fails to arouse the purest admiration whenever I ride over it. Fine farms enclosed by stone fences and splendid country houses scattered all over the neighborhood. Very little stock was seen though. The mountain gorges were very plainly seen as I rode along. The snow bringing out the crests and depressions more plainly to view. As might be supposed one would, I thought of the trerrible scenes that might be enacted here in a few more days. Not more than two centuries and a half ago the red savage roamed at large here. Those cultivated fields were then covered in one unbroken forest; the Delawares & Tuscaroras followed the deer and bear along the base of the ridge, the banks of the Shenandoah and the coves of the mountains.

Nature indeed was supreme in all her workings and governings. And until the pale face came and drove the red man back to the forests of the west the country knew no change in perhaps a thousand years. But now the picture for reflection is a sad and dreary one. It may be said that my musings are always

---

[83] Possibly Francis B. Meade (born 1816), of Chapel Township, Clarke Co. VA. Census, 1870.

[84] Apperson's italics. Usage in context is *nonsense*, with connotations of humor, even a joke or gag.

[85] Possibly William Ward, born 1827, of Richmond, who may have traced his ancestry to the Seth Ward family of 17th cent. prominence. VA. Census. 1870. "Ward," *Encyclopedia of Virginia Biography*, ed., Lyon Gardiner Tyler (5 vols.; New York: Lewis Historical Pub. Co., 1915), vol. 1. Hereinafter, *VA. BIOG.*

sad, pensive, melancholic, but how can they be other wise[?]. The terrible hand of civil war is devastating this fair land. I see houses standing alone, tenements vacated, and improvements of every kind falling to ruin. Can it be that as time rolls round that all these things will as gradually return to the state from which it was brought? Can it be that the thunder of heaven will roll alone along above the top of the mountain?—That no fiery mouthed monster in the hands of men of angry hearts will again wake the sleeping echoes of those hills?

In this neighborhood the brave Gen. Daniel Morgan[86] used to live. His dwelling yet stands and still is know[n] as Saratoga. Mrs Page lives there at this time. The old chieftain lies tranquil in his tent while thousands of cannon reverbrate around his resting place. There are many interesting incidents connected with this country in the life of Morgan. An old mill stands [at] Millwood that was erected by his supervisor.

I returned to camp about 3 P. M., collected 35$ of Lt. [Conway] Newman[87] , and 10$ of [Robert C.] Fulwider, [88] for I[saac]. Brown,[89] and 10$ of Capt. [Joseph M.] Thomas for [Samuel Rush]Sayers.[90] Traded shoes to-day an old pr for a new pr. Paid Capt. [Joseph M.] T[homas] 20$ for [James] Cooley.[91]

---

[86] Daniel Morgan (1736-1802), was born in Hunterdon country, N.J. colony and moved to VA. colony in 1750s, becoming captain in colonial army during French & Indian (7 Years) War; captured and imprisoned in Quebec, 1755. Released after war, Morgan became military leader in Revolutionary War, serving as Brig. Gen. in Continental Army. He was awarded gold medal and congressional citation, 17 January 1782, for Battle of Cowpens, S.C., a battle generally regarded as a turning point in Cornwallis's British Army final and unsuccessful march through Carolinas and to Yorktown. He built Saratoga in Winchester (Clarke Co.), led VA. militia against PA. insurgents during Whiskey Rebellion, 1794; became Federalist and served as Member of US House of Rep., 1797-1799. "Morgan," *VA. Biog.*, vol. 2.

[87] Conway Newman (1837-1917) was farmer educ. at UVA who joined 13th VA. Inf. as pvt. but was elected 1 LT. 23 April 1862; and later Capt. Wounded at Gaines Mill (27th June 1862), he survived to surrender at Appomattox C.H. Later Postmaster in Orange Co. Riggs, *13th VA. Inf.*, 131.

[88] Robert C. Fulwider (born 1841) was cabinet-maker who joined 4th VA. Inf. as drummer. In 1864 he was detailed as a nurse and served in Winchester General Hosp., where he was captured in May 1864 and later exchanged and transfered to 51st VA. Robertson, *4th VA. Inf.*, 51. There is no record of him in 51st, James A. Davis, *51st VA. Inf.*, Virigina Regimental Histories Series (Lynchburg, VA.: H.E. Howard, 1984); and no record of his life after May 1864.

[89] Isaac Brown (?-1863), unknown age and occupation unknown; joined Co. D of 4th VA. Inf. and was wounded at Gaines Mill (27 June 1862) and at 2d Manassas (30 August 1862). Fulwider apparently borrowed the supplies on behalf of the incapacitated Brown, with whom he served. Brown was captured at Gettysburg (3 July 1863), imprisoned at Point Lookout Prison MD, where he died and was buried. Robertson, 41.

[90] Samuel Rush Sayers (1833-1914) was from Wytheville. Surgeon at muster, 4th VA. Inf., he was transfered to 27th VA. Inf. Robertson, 71. With 27th he was wounded and captured,

Capt [Robert LaFayette] Francisco [QM] did not draw money for us to-day.—The order appointing a Board for the examining candidates for discharge or furlough has been rescinded and that board dissolved and one ordered from each division to meet and conduct business under the same rules and regulations of the other one. Surg. [John Alexander] Straith 2 Va Infy; [92] and surg Hinkle 37 Va Inf.[93] are appointed to officiate. Some dissatisfaction arises among the surgeons of other Brigades because they think this board a thing of indignity, though [such dissatisfaction is] uncalled for, I think.

CAMP, NEAR MR. PAGE'S [CLARKE CO.]

SUNDAY, NOV: 9, 1862

This morning before we were up orders were given for rations to be cooked and be ready to move at 9 A.M. Preparations wer[e] made accordingly but by the hour appointed for us to move orders came for more rations to be cooked. From some cause or other we did not move at all. The sick were to be sent in stage wagons—The sound of canon has been heard in direction of Front Royal all day. I wrote to cousin Bettie. Have spent the day in reading, sleeping and laying round generally. Read *Miltons Poems* some—the wind blows cold indeed and the weather promises to be wintry early.

Gettysburg (4 July 1863); imprisoned in Baltimore, he was later exchanged and returned to 27th until transfer to 4th VA. Inf. Reidenbaugh, 173. He survived to surrender at Appomattox and lived in Wytheville. Capt. Thomas borrowed money or supplies on behalf of surgeon who then worked under him.

[91] Cooley was a free person of color, already identified. This record shows that Apperson paid him for his nonsoldier services, such as cooking and setting up tent headquarters. Apperson apparently borrowed from his captain, Joseph M. Thomas, in order to pay Cooley.

[92] John Alexander Straith (1835-1872) was physician appointed Asst. Surg., 2d VA. Inf. However, no official records show him serving after 1862, although he clearly is serving on this date. After War he moved to Charleston, WVA, where he developed a medical practice. Frey, *2d VA. Inf.*, 131.

[93] There is no Hinkle recorded for 37th VA. Inf. Thomas M. Rankin, *37th VA. Inf.*, Virginia Regimental Histories Series (Lynchburg, VA.: H.E. Howard, 1982), nor in Cunningham, *Doctors in Gray*, though he obviously appears in diary several times in capacity of surgeon of some authority.

CAMP NEAR WINCHESTER [CLARKE CO.]

MONDAY, NOV. 10, 1862

Five oclock was the hour appointed for the troops to move this morning. We were up and had breakfast and were ready to march at that hour. The sun shone clear and warm. I learned that we would not move very far. The troops and wagon trains preceded Gen. [John Robert] Jones wagons. I remained behind to come with them.

We arrived in Winchester about noon and pitched our tents immediately under the hill on which are the fortifications thrown up by the enemy—or commenced by us [early in 1862 at beginning of T.J. Jackson's Valley Campaign] and finished by the enemy. Here both wood and water are scarce. Owing to a want of honesty in some body our head quarters can't furnish an axe at all.

To-day we got the "Richmond Daily Dispatch" and "Whig". It is too much for my narrow mind to draw any but erroneous conclusion from the news. As regards "recognition" [as an autonomous nation state] by England [it] seems to [be] more doubtful than it has been for a long time. It has ever been a dangerous reliance. The Democrats have carried the day in N. York and several other states. [Horatio] Seymour is elected Governor of the State. [94] Excitement is represented as very great. Tammany Hall [center of NY City Democratic politics] was crowded by enthusiastic northerners. The Dem. and abolitionists seem to be growing more jealous every day. An issue is growing up between them which I do hope may cause them to stop and reflect awhile ever they do anything. I have looked with intense interest to the feuds of the two parties and the factions likely to spring up among them. It is possible that that day is not far

[94] Horatio Seymour (1810-1886) was Democrat elected governor of NY in 1862 along with "sizable gains" for Democrats in NY state and congressional elections. Seymour, a War Democrat, was fervently for Union, but opposed the Emancipation Proclamation and generally opposed Radical Republicans. He defeated the Radical Republican nominee James Wadsworth in this election. However, Seymour, a conservative businessman who operated a bank and helped build and maintain the Erie Canal, was only somewhat reluctantly a politician, and he was particularly uncomfortable as a national spokesman for antiwar feelings. Indeed, Seymour was indefatigable in filling NY's large "muster roll" of troops and he worked tirelessly on behalf of the war efforts. Stewart Mitchell, "Seymour," *Dictionary of American Biography* , ed. Dumas Malone et allii (New York: Charles Scribner's Sons for American Council of Learned Societies, 1935), vol. 17. There were also Democratic gains in NJ, IL, and WI, but as noted earlier, Republicans retained control of both houses of US Congress. Long speaks for mainstream political historians in noting, "[u]ndoubtedly war weariness accounted for many of the Democratic victories." Long, 284.

distant when we can stand and look on calmly while they wear themselves out and have to give in. Not that I think that the Democrats will offer anything more acceptable to the peace of the Country than their brothers the abolitionists have done, or will give up their mistaken veneration for the "Old Flag"; but the result will be with these dissentions [sic] will ripen into a war among themselves—a contradiction in the management of the war.

The movements of our army here in the valley are singular. The division is guarding three roads, viz. 2 Brigade on the Romney [WVA] Road, 3rd Brigade on Pughtown [Frederick Co.] Road and first Brigade and 4 Brigade are on the Martinsburg [WVA] Pike.

WINCHESTER, VA.

TUESDAY NOV. 11, 1862

This morning early I mounted my horse and rode down to the Brigade which is in camp a few hundred yards in rear of widow Carter's house. I went down to get a muster and pay roll for myself. My horse is very lame. There seems to be an epidemic of sore feet among the horses of the army. I see numbers limping about wherever I go. It makes its appearance nearly like the scratches, only below the usual seat—the postern point—on the "heels" of the foot. It is of a cracked condition with a puslike discharge very tender and seems very painful. I heard some horses are losing their hoofs [sic].[95]

When I got back to the point where I left the camp I found preparations were being made to move. Gen. Jones had obtained a house in town and was about to take up quarters there.

The house we occupy is a large house in the suburbs near Mr. Shouttz's.[96] The building is a good one and commodius [sic]. The room Dr. B. occupies is on the 2nd floor on the corner. I can't say that I am pleased with the move. Dr.

---

[95]William G. Bean describes the disease as striking just above the horse's hoof, and sometimes causing the hoof to fall off. If it was an "epidemic," it did not attract the attention of the close student of Jackson's life and career (Robertson, *Stonewall Brigade*). Bean does note a similar epidemic among the horses in the northern Army of the Potomac, at this time, shortly after Ambrose E. Burnsides replaced George B. McClellan, Notes, William G. Bean. Bean's observation is corroborated in the diary of Col. Charles Shiels Wainwright, *A Diary of Battle; the Personal Journal of Colonel Charles S. Wainwright, 1861-1865*, ed., Allan Nevins (1962; reprint ed.; New York: Da Capo, 1998), 124.

[96] Writing almost illegible. Clarke Co. census lists no one named Shoultz, Schoultz, or Schultz, or any variation of the name. VA. Census. 1870.

Coleman will be here soon and we will move out to take the air, which on the whole is healthier than indoors for a soldier any how. Here we are under the necessity of putting our horses at a distance from us, in charge of the *drivers.*

I was very sleepy at night and retired early after reading Wood [*Treatise*] on *angor animi.* [97]

WINCHESTER, VA.

WEDNESDAY, NOV. 12TH, 1862

This morning I took the rolls and walked down to see the paymaster Capt. Earhart to raise my sallary [sic]. My horse being lame I arrived there about 10, and found the house crowded, so much so that I did not get in until sometime after noon. My rolls were not finished entirely but the P[ay].master seemed to be an elegant gentle man and accomodating he fixed them for me. I drew pay for six months including Bounty, amounting in all to \$178.00 without clothing. The stoppages [deductions from pay] were for 1 pr. pants 4\$, 2 pr drawers at 75c = \$1.50, 2 woolen shirts at \$3.75 = \$7.50. Total \$16.50 c. leaving me a ballance [sic] of \$159.50 c. This with amt. on hand is a very snug amt. of cash on hand; but how long will it last here where prices are almost fabulous for everything[?]

While being compelled almost to spend a considerable amount I ought by all means to make as far an advance as I could [that is, to save as much money as possible despite high expenses; by *advance*, he means to say *savings*].

Maj. [Elisha Franklin] Paxton of Gen. Jackson's staff (A.A.A.G.), is, I learn, to be our Brigadier General. This will be a source of much unsatisfaction. Many of the officers talk of resigning. Col: [Andrew Jackson] Grigsby will I am sure. While Paxton may be a man suited to the place and may prove himself worthy of such a charge, I think it [sic] making some discrepancy with older officers in the Brigade.[98]

---

[97] "Feeling of dying." *Taber's.* Writing is barely legible.

[98] Elisha Franklin Paxton (1828-1863) was from Rockbridge Co., VA., and attended Washington College and Yale University, taking degrees at each school. He also earned a law degree from the University of Virginia. After practicing law in Ohio, he came to Lexington in 1854, where he became friends with T.J. Jackson; on the eve of the War he retired from the legal profession because of poor eyesight. When the War came, he joined Rockbridge Rifles of the Virginia 27th, whom he served as lieutenant. Eventually this unit became part of Jackson's brigade, and Paxton was elected major. Performing well at Manassas, Paxton became known as "Bull" and was praised by Jackson. However, his men hated him, and he was "diselected" as major. Jackson then appointed Paxton to his staff as assistant adjutant general ["AAAG" above]

I walked downtown this evening and saw Jno Hull [99] who has just arrived from home.

Rain has been falling to-day.

I have read to-night "Acute Laryngitis" and its mucous, submucous, and pseudo-membranous forms.[100]

WINCHESTER, VA.

THURSDAY, NOV. 13, 1862

Dr. Coleman arrived to-day and will take charge to-morrow. We will return to the Reg't. He is an insinuating man and one of the most loquaciouis I ever saw. Really I think from appearance [that] talking is part of his being. A nice gentleman though he is, and one whose energy and pleasing qualifications fit him well for the part he fills. He is anxious for a clerk and asked me to recommend one to him. Mr. Sexton has asked me to recommend one to him. This I would do but the man that I would recommend I fear will not suit him. C.M. Sexton[101] has asked me to get him a position several times but I am afraid that the requirements of this place will not suit him and I would not like to be instrumental in placing a man in the place whom Dr. Coleman would be likely to find unable to his work.

---

with rank of major. As Apperson notes, protest was led by Colonel Andrew Jackson Grigsby, commander of the 27th. Grigsby did indeed resign in protest. The final verdict on Paxton's eventual performance remains unclear: His forces were in reserve at the victory in Fredericksburg and again at Chancellorsville. On 3 May 1863 at Chancellorsville, as Frank "Bull" Paxton prepared to attack under Jackson's orders, he was killed by a minie ball. He is buried very near his sponsor and fellow townsman Jackson in the Lexington cemetary. Jeffrey D. Wert, "Paxton," *Historical Times.*

[99] John N. Hull , age and occupation unknown, enlisted 31 July 1861 in Smyth Co. Blues, which became Co. D, 4th VA Inf. Subsequently he was captured at Spotsylvania (12 May 1864), imprisoned at Elmira Prison NY, and then paroled. Robertson, *4th VA. Inf.*, 57.

[100] Laryngitis, a scarring of the throat, is often a complication of measles morbilli, and can be mitigated by diet, cleanliness, and effective nursing care; it can sometimes be prevented by vaccines developed in the 1960s. In 1862, it was not connected with measles morbilli ['morbilli' meant 'little disease,' to distinguish it from 'il morbo,' ('plague')], and instead doctors looked at the mucous membrane as a possible site for the onset of the disease. "Measles Morbilli," *McGrew's.*

[101] Charles McDonald Sexton (1839-1915) was a Smyth Co. farmer who enlisted in Co. D, 4th VA Inf. On 29 June 1863 he was detailed to CSA Commissary Dept.; surrendered at Appomattox C.H. Robertson, *4th VA Inf.*, 72. Buried at Old Bethel Cemetary, Smyth Co., Sturgill and Sturgill, *Smyth Co. Cemetaries*, vol. 2:150.

I was at the Post Commissary this morning and obtained cotton, sugar, and molasses at big prices though. The fore noon was spent in looking over some papers & c. and this evening Dr. B proposed that we ride to the battlefield of Kernstown [23 March 1862]. My horse was very lame and ought not to have been used, but I have been anxious to see that ever to be remembered field, and this visit would perhaps be my best opportunity, as I contemplate it, to go. We first obtained a pass which is required to leave town and went on the Strasburg Pike as as far as Kernstown. Leaving the Pike there to the left passing an old church and entering a wood we came to the point where the first shot came so near us. Following the track of the army until we reached the field. We noticed some change in the appearance of distance—things seemed nearer. The trees were marked and scarred by hundreds of bullets, the most of which have been chopped after, I suppose by visitors [seeking souvenirs]. Furthermore where the two armies met in full force the bushes, trees, fences, and every prominent thing shows plainly that the truth has been told about the desperateness of the conflict. In a clump of undergrowth trees and bushes scarcely a single one is left untouched. The most of the shots from our side seem to have been aimed nearly correct, neither too high nor too low, while from the other side nearly all seem too high. The stone fence behind which the 23d and 37th Reg'ts. protected themselves before the advance of a column of the enemy pouring a perfect volley, was well marked. At one spot a large walnut [tree] stood that had been purged by a cannonball and the tree had been noticed by a great many as they passed. We found to our mortification that some ignorant, insensate man had cut the tree down and split it up to make firewood. Had the tree been mine nothing would ever have caused me to allow it to be destroyed. It would have been a relic for a number of years. I took some specimens from it and propose to send them home in some shape.

It is now pleasing to visit the field of our former strife and will be more so hereafter. Here on this field as noble set of patriots marched into the conflict as ever honored a Spartan's ranks. Many of those who went in never came out, but now lie covered by the Mother Earth. Poor Sam Neff[102] fought his last fight here and now rests from his labors. I could not find the graves.

We returned to town by a back way very well pleased with our trip. To-night I have been writing but will retire soon I think.

---

[102] Samuel Neff (1838-1862) was a miller from Smyth Co. who joined Co. D, 4th VA Inf. and was killed at Kernstown in Valley Campaign, 23 March 1862. Robertson describes him as "5'7", dark eyes, dark hair, dark complexion." Idem, *4th VA Inf.*, 65.

CAMP NEAR MRS. CARTER'S[103] *[CLARKE CO.]*

FRIDAY, NOV. 14TH 1862

This morning Dr. Coleman took charge of the affairs of the Division and we moved down to the Reg't. While the place we occupied at the Headquarters of the Div: is very pleasant I was not so well satisfied. My expenses were heavy and our place seemed issolated [sic]. Dr. B turned over the wagon and team to Dr. C[oleman] and took a receipt therefor [sic]. The papers were handed over also.

When we got to camp the 4th Reg't. was just starting out on picket at Bunker's Hill [Bedford Co.]—a distance of 8 hrs. This is very well. The trouble of a trip on picket is saved us which is one by no means to be wished.

My horse so lame this morning that I forbare [sic] to move him. I fear the disease among our horses will be something of more infection than we may now suppose. The first I have noticed of the disease is that it breaks out very suddenly,—in cracks & fisures [sic] on the heels of the horses['] hind feet first and afterward extends upwards to a point of the junction of the two latteral [sic] and middle line of the foot. Above the hoof large cracks open and a thin yellowish pus escapes. The whole covering of that part of the foot seems inclined to separate from flesh leaving it in a white ulcerous condition. There does not seem to be much fever, really. The system is to some extent affected, as may be seen by a loss of flesh and spirit of the animal. On moving the horse these fisures [sic] open; the tendons are stretched which seems very painfull [sic]. The infection is extending to nearly the whole number of the horses we have, both wagon and riding. I have been undecided about applying *a poultice* [104] to the place as that is what would be done were it human. This evening after washing the place and trimming the hair off as well as I could, I applied a strong solution of *Caustic Potash and Turacin Cerate* and bandaged the parts. [105]

Col. [Andrew Jackson] Grigsby took leave of his regt. (27th) this evening. He leaves to-morrow—having resigned his comm[ission]. and obtained leave of absence for 20 days. I am sorry to see him leave. He is a gallant officer—has

---

[103] Possibly farm of Emily S. Carter (born 1810) in Greenway Township, Clarke Co. VA. Census. 1870. She may have claimed descent from the "Tuckahoe" family the Carters, re Bliss, "The Tuckahoes of New Virginia."

[104] "(L. *pultes*, thick paste). A hot, moist mass of linseed, mustard, or soap and oil between two pieces of muslin applied to the skin to relieve congestion or pain, to stimulate absorption of inflammatory products, and to act as a counterirritant." *Taber's.*

[105] William G. Bean says, "a plaster containing a small amount of copper." Bean, notes.

made himself conspicuous for acts of bravery in every conflict, and now leaves us under circumstances not very pleasant. His mind is one of those unbiased minds, that will give the Devil his due.

To-day after we came down one of the "Dare Devils" came to see Dr. B about an *eruption* on his body. At first glance at Dr. B. I saw that he regarded the case with some suspicion. The eruption too presented an appearance that would excite suspicion in anyone. On his limbs were small *papular* [106] eruptions, some had gone further in their course than others. Those that had gone seemingly for a longer time presented the different shapes of *variola.* The history of the case too was sufficient to support the conclusion. He had been a prisoner and returned within just a short time. One of his mess mates who had been sleeping together was sent to [Winchester General Hosp't. day before with an infection. He is sent away to be examined next morning.

CAMP NEAR MRS. CANTERS [CLARKE CO.]

SATURDAY, NOV 15, 1862

If Old Nick had paid us a visit this morning there could have been but little more of a stir than was. The variola case has been examined by Drs. Black, Walls and [Samuel Rush] Sayers—all pronounce it genuine. The Brigade will be separated from the Regt, and that company [Grayson Dare Devils from Co. F, 4th VA Inf.] from the Regt, and this case - from the [F] Co. Water has been procured and I have vaccinated all that were present, not before vaccinated. Dr. B. asked me if I were willing to remain with this part of the camp. I of course am willing to do anything that will be of any benefit to the men. It would be cowardly for me to leave now, though I might not risk anything if I were to leave.

My horse's ~~hoofs~~ feet are no better. Dr. B. is using Bichloride of Mercury on his in strong solution.

D[rury].W. Venable [ambulance driver of Smyth Co. in 4th Inf.] sent me by [George Washington] Barger[107] a bag of smoking tobacco—I have but little use for it.

---

[106] Of the papule, Latin for pimple. "Red elevated area on the skin, solid and circumscribed." "Papule," *Taber's.* Often related to variola ("acute, contagious, systemic, viral disease…." *Taber's*), as Dr. Black and the diarist surmise.

[107] George Washington Barger (born 1839), was Smyth Co. farmer born in Montgomery Co. who joined Co. E of 4th VA Inf.; wounded at 1st Manassas (21 July 1861), he was detailed as a

I sent him 20$ as he has no money and the Company [E of 4th VA Inf.] is out on picket and Capt [Joseph M.] *Thomas* can't send it to him. He is Driving an ambulanse[sic] between Winchester [Clarke Co.] and Staunton [Augusta Co.]

I have not been doing much to-day. When the boys came in to-night they were very much surprised to find things so changed. I expect we will go into quarantine if this Disease shows itself any further.

CAMP NEAR MRS. CARTER[']S [CLARKE CO.],

SUNDAY NOV: 16, 1862

The case of variola is quite plain this morning. Dr. Coleman came to see it and seemed confident that it was small pox. He advanced considerable argument on the susceptibility of the disease. It would be an effort of vanity were I to attempt to follow his prolix[,] fluent and sometimes eloquent tongue, but some of his ideas would do to keep if they could be found and applied in after days. He relies firmly on vaccination as a preventive and advances a theory on the effects of vaccine and the susceptibility of ~~the disease~~ variola afterward. That some are infected after vaccination, and some worse than others, and some not at all is accounted for in this way. Suppose the susceptibility in one case be 8 and in another be 6. another 4. The strength of the *virous* [sic] is 4 and operates on the system to its full amount. In the case where it is 8 the grade of disease [its severity] would be 4 - the remainder after taking away the effect of vaccination, which was 4 - in the case of 6 - the disease would be two and in the last would be nothing and so on. [108] This theory to one listening at his descriptions is very

---

nurse, Winchester General Hospital, December 1861; detailed as ambulance driver, 28 September 1862, where Apperson worked with him. Robertson, *4th VA Inf.*, 38. Transfered to Co. F, 4th VA Cav., 13 August 1863, wounded in action and captured, Woodstock (22 October 1864). No further military records. Lived and married and farmed in Montgomery Co. in 1868. Robert J. Driver, *14th VA Cavalry*, Virginia Regimental Histories Series (Lynchburg, VA: H.E. Howard, 1988) 99.

[108] William G. Bean notes, "Dr. Coleman's theory was that the effects of vaccination depend upon several factors—upon the individual, his or her immunization, and also upon the potency of the vaccine." The hypothesis never bore up under testing. Instead, this phenomenon of ineffective (even disease-producing) vaccination is now called Spurious Vaccinia, and it was a problem for both Federal and Confederate forces, but especially so for the Virginia Brigade in this campaign and again, even more strikingly, during and after Chancellorsville (May 1863). According to H.H. Cunningham, "Spurious Vaccinia" refered to "large, repulsive-looking ulcers supposedly caused by impure vaccine virus" that "began to appear at the place of vaccination." Joseph Jones, CSA surgeon and a medical writer much respected during and after the war, opined

nice and perhaps plausible, but in looking over the chances against it, it faces [disproof]. Many men are known to have been vaccinated without effect after the 1 time for several times—there the insertion of matter [virus crusts] produced the same result. He said if one case could be found where after vaccination for several attempts it failed and there was infection he would give up the theory; though this may be I don't think there would be any reason to give up any theory even after repeated experiments to the contrary. By considering the changes in the *constitution*, the manner of insertion, and all the peculiarities of the system, it will naturally be infered that no theory will prove strictly correct.[109]

I was very much interested in his conversations. He asked Dr. B. how many of his boys he intended to make Dr's—Doctor said none of these unless they wished to be for he did not believe any one would become proficient in medicine if they were compelled to adopt it against their will. Dr. B spoke of the little incidents that change a man's feelings. How a very insignificant occurance [sic] might cause a child to determine his course, and follow it with diligence, or on the other hand, when a child's antipathies are once set against a profession an attempt to make him follow would be ruinous to him in future life. Coleman said that as a general thing the parent was inclined to make his smartest child a lawyer, and that it is generally looked upon as the 2nd grade of men who make followers of Hippocrates. How few men there are who have studied medicine

---

that "constitutional syphilis could be transmitted by the vaccine lymph." Some Federal doctors made a similar diagnosis, and according to Cunningham, smallpox was often confounded with syphilis, but these authorities were simply wrong, for no one could catch either from the vaccine for the other. Some vaccine may have been impure, but a more likely explanation came from surgeon O. Kratz at a February 1864 conference of army and navy surgeons of the CSA to discuss the problem: "[T]he principal cause of the deterioration of the vaccine virus [was] the indiscriminate vaccination and re-vaccination from arm to arm." Cunningham believes that Kratz's explanation could be valid, "since soldiers often vaccinated each other with almost any sharp instrument that came to hand." Still later, Jones offered the very plausible hypothesis, independently offered by Federal doctors, that "incipient scurvy" caused the "untoward effect," because "the same vaccine which produced grave effects upon those men suffering from the results of poor diet, exposure, and fatigue produced no ill effects among those who were healthy and well-fed." Cunningham, *Doctors in Gray*, 200-01.

[109] Although his terms are in his own words "prolix," the diarist suggests that the question must be approached by a more careful "scientific method" in which one variable is tested at a time in an hypothesis that is quantifiable, refutable, and above all susceptible to repeatable tests. As Cunningham notes elsewhere, the surgeons and physicians of the CSA and the US army and navy were meticulous in keeping records, and attempted inductive reasoning after careful observation, but seldom proceeded with controlled experiments grounded in the reasoning of scientific methods. Cunningham, 5, 112.

that were proficient in the literary branches of knowledge. It has been remarked that a certain man has taken the degree of A.M. at college and is now going to study medicine. "He ought to have studied law. Yes, he has thrown away all that polished talent by entering the field of medicine." He said as a class of men the medicine students were generally those who are notorious for smoking, carousing, and recklessness. At every Med: College midnight was made hideous with carousal of students. But, said he after going into the world they are made better men. No class ever reformed so effectual [sic] as the young Dr. and his seasons. He sees the last moments of all ages, sexes, classes, and every denomination—the evil and the good. The mother by the bed-side of her dying infant is a scene that will touch the heart of the most dissolute. She breathes the poisonous contagion of the most deadly disease, offers herself up a willing sacrifice to her affections while the physician must stand by and behold the work of nature. In society his place requires him to hold himself in dignified position, and nothing is as much respected by the world as is a dignified physician. He said he knew he was a better man than he was when he started in life—he was a lover of human nature and the more he saw and felt of the suffering of mankind the more he came to be aroused by the best of God. "Whenever I am brought to the bedside of the sufferer, my feelings seem touched by that Ithuriel wand that causes the waters of humanity to gush forth."[110] Part of his conversation I endorse as true, but a part I disdain.

The case of variola was sent off to-day. His mess mate is confined to narrow limits, and how he will pass his time is yet to be seen. No communication with others is allowed. His food is cooked and brought in about 50 yds of his bunk and set down and then he goes and gets it. He was seen sending papers from his knapsack to-day but was stopped. This seems hard. He wishes to write to his mother but is not allowed to use his own paper. When he was stopped he said "O Shuw!" [O Pshaw!] and turned away as if undone with us. He seemed to

---

[110] John Milton (1608-1674) describes the angels Ithuriel and Zephon in a contest with Satan in the Garden of Eden. Satan, disguised as a toad, "squat…close at the ear of Eve," to convince her to defy the will of God. However, Ituriel and Zephon find "the Fiend," and Ithuriel touches Satan lightly with his spear [wand], thereby causing Satan to appear in his true form instead of the disguise of the seemingly harmless toad. Idem, *Paradise Lost; an Authoritative Text of the Second Edition*, ed., Scott Elledge (1674. New York: W.W. Norton, 1975), bk. 4, v.v. 788-825. It is interesting that the famed diarist/memoirist South Carolina's Mary Boykin Chesnut (1823-1886), who obviously did not know Apperson, quotes exactly the same image on 29 January 1862 to describe a politician whom she despises, and she longs for Ithuriel to come with his angelic spear and reveal the earthly fiend. Mary Boykin Chesnut, *Mary Chesnut's Civil War*, ed. , C. Vann Woodward (New Haven and London: Yale University Press, 1981) 285.

think we were making fun of him and looked mortified. How he will spend his Quarantine without going mad I can't see. He can't read, no one to talk to, and nothing to draw his mind away to anything except his chance for disease. I know I would have small pox from imagination.

I wrote a letter to Dr. F. to-night informing him of the condition of things and asking him to say to those who seem frightened, not to fear.

The newspapers bring us the news that McClelland [George B. McClellan] is no longer general in the army of the United States. [Ambrose] Burnside has superceded him. The enemy has fallen back from Culpepper towards Washington City. We're [Virginia] not in the crack N. Carolina is now. [111]

CAMP CARTER [CLARKE CO.]

MONDAY, NOV: 17, 1862

Raining some this morning and every appearance of a wet time.

To-day has been a dull one. No papers, no visitors, and no communications any way. Bill the ambulance driver passes to and from the regiment with any business we have to transact. A few of the "Dare Devils" [4th VA Inf. Co. F, Grayson Co.] pass occasionally but as a rule they are an unobtrusive class of men and seem disposed to remain on their own side, little caring about interrupting others or being interrupted themselves.

Our horses are getting better I think. Corrosive sublimate in solution has been applied to Dr. B's horse. I have used caustics to mine until this morning when I made an application of dry calomel. [112] This morning they walk without limping but little.

I have been reading vaccine disease to-day and the theory of contagion. Dr. B. questioned me on Acute Laryngitis and commented. Acute Bronchitis is next lesson.

---

[111] "Little Mac" remained a Maj. Gen., but was unceremoniously relieved of command of the Army of the Potomac without forewarning on 7 November; he said farewell to his emotional men on 10 November. His replacement as commander of the Army of the Potomac, Ambrose Everett Burnside, was not retreating but rather massing for an attack on Fredericksburg. The N.C. coast was largely controlled by Federal navy, with an effective blockade of the important port of Wilmington. Long, 284-90.

[112] *Corrosive sublimate* is a medicine prepared and then suspended in a liquid solution to spread on a wound. The sublimate itself is product of "altering the state of a gas or solid without first changing it into a liquid." *Taber's. Caustics* [from Greek word for burning] are "corrosive and burning; destructive to living tissues." *Taber's. Calomel* [from Greek words meaning, in combination, beautiful and black] is mercurious chloride. *Taber's.* The sublimate and the caustic are strong and harsh medicine, burning and corroding away the diseased flesh.

I do not suppose that Robinson Crusoe was more exiled, or felt worse than Mr. Goins—the man in quarantine. [113] I visited twice to-day. He seems sad, can't read and has no amusement. I would think that such a place would so operate on the mind that some disease would inevitably ensue. I am willing to have sickness but not willing to be exiled.

I am almost insusceptible to any danger from variola. It is not impressed upon my mind that there is any risk from exposure to it here in the open air. [114] If I were to get it or any one of us that stay here I would dislike to destroy my books and clothes—in fact I should hesitate to do so, however imperatively it might be demanded. I have been economical and sparing because of my own necessity, and to loose [sic] what I have selected would not be agreeable to the feelings of any one in my condition.

CAMP CARTER

TUESDAY NOV: 18; 1862

Several of Co "F" [Dare Devils of Grayson Co., 4th VA Inf.] are complaining in a way that might lead to suspicion of the premonitory symptoms of variola. A few days however will decide the question. Vaccinations on some is making appearance [a raised, reddened, bumpy place on the arm, sometimes accompanied by itching, soreness and fever]. In my own arms there is slight impression though I have vaccinated twice before.

I have been reading "Bronchitis" [in Wood's textbook] to-day. It is the hardest matter imaginable for me to concentrate my mind on what I am reading. I go over the work mechanically but without fastening the attention at all. I know that unless there is some change in my course of study, unless I can rivet the attention more firmly on the subject I shall never become proficient in what I would learn. But how is it to be done? How am I to lose sight of the various movings around me and obliterate temporarily impressions that have

---

[113] Daniel DeFoe (1660-1731) described a man abandoned on an island with only his servant for companionship in *Robinson Crusoe* (1660-1731). William H. Goins, age and occupation unknown, was from Smyth Co. and joined Co. F, 4th VA Inf. Dare Devils of Grayson Co. on 20 March 1862. Robertson describes him as "5' 10", dark eyes, dark hair, florid complexion." Released from quarantine, Goins was appointed Cpl. 11 May 1863, shot in left leg, at Payne's Farm (27 November 1863), captured at Spotsylvania (12 May 1864); imprisoned at Elmira NY until 27 June 1865 and then paroled. Postwar story not known. Robertson, *4th VA Inf.*, 52.

[114] "Open air" would not protect him, but lack of exposure to infected men in cramped quarters would; the only real protection was vaccination. Cunningham, passim.

become fixed? or how can I obliviate[115] the sweet morsels of memory, and chain the senses to the work before me without flitting involuntary [sic] from point to point through the immensity of space? This control of the attention, this government of the mind is more important than the gift of memory, and is the greatest victory of our lives. Application must be the first step towards the object to be gained [rather] than the bent of the mind.

Cloudy and rainy to-day as have been for several days.—no papers again to-day—no news—

CAMP CARTER [CLARKE CO.]

WEDNESDAY NOV: 19; 1862

Cloudy this morning. Nothing transpired 'till evening worth noting. Dr. B. read message from H[unter] McGuire [brigade surgeon] asking him if he were willing to take charge of the [general] hospitals at Winchester,[116] if so come and see him. Dr. wrote him a note and went up to see him. I speculated as to what would be the result—Dr. did not seem willing or anxious to take charge of the hospitals without some chance of permanency. When he returned he had accepted the offer and had the order relieving him [sic] duty with the 4th Virginia Regt and assigning him to the post at Winchester. He asked me if I wished to accompany him. I did of course—having wished to get to a hospital for some time. Dr. [A.C.] Smith who has formerly been in charge of those hospitals has been ordered by Surgeon [LaFayette] Guild Med. Dir. of Gen. Lee's army to Culpeper C. H. [117] The post assigned Dr. B. may be permanent and may not. I feel some dread that things will not occur as I would wish. To-morrow we leave the Regt and go to Winchester and I hope all things will work for the best.

---

[115] "obliviate, ob., rare, to forget, to commit to oblivion." *OED.*

[116] A general hospital was a permanent station with a full staff, good facilities, plenty of supplies, and generally was located far from battle lines. Field hospitals were more temporary affairs, usually under a tent, obviously mobile, vulnerable to artillery and other attack, and short of supplies. In the case of Winchester, the inability of either Federals or Confederates to hold the gateway to the Shenandoah Valley made the permanent general hospital there a risky assignment. See Cunningham, *Doctors in Gray*, passim, but esp. 47-69.

[117] See Cunningham's list of medical officers, ibid., 284-90.

Bill, the ambulance driver, came to us after we had retired and seemed very much disappointed that we were going and leave him. It is hard to be left by those with whom we have been associated for some time.

No more cases of variola have occured and I hope no more will. Vaccination is underway pretty effectually, I think. Some dissatisfaction exists, I think in regard to Dr. B's leaving. The men are not so well satisfied with the Asst. Surg: - [La Fayette Hall Jordan[118]]

YORK HOSPITAL, WINCHESTER VA

THURSDAY, NOV: 20; 1862

This morning early we were up and breakfasted. Dr. B. started to Winchester and left me to pack up and come on. After vaccinating several of the "Dare Devils" [Co. F of Grayson Co. in 4th VA Inf.] and extracting a tooth I made preparations to leave. Got Dr. B's books from the Reg't—leaving "Erichsen's Surgery" [119] which Dr. [LaFayette Hall] Jordan did not seem willing to part from.

There is a case of amputating instruments missing and no one knows where it is. It is one that Dr. [Joseph] Crockett captured near Winchester in May [26 May 1862]. The last I remember distinctly about it is when we were at *Aldie* [Loudon Co.; 27 May 1862] and I feel sure that I saw it at Sharpsburg [MD; 17-18 September 1862]—By the way since I commenced writing about it I think that it was put in Dr. [A.C.] Smiths Med. wagon at Sharpsburg.

---

[118] Black's original assistant surgeon Joseph Crockett (1833-1862) was killed at Gaine's Mill (27 June 1862) and buried in Wytheville; see earlier notes. Originally the diarist was critical of Crockett, but had come to respect him by winter of 1862. La Fayette Hall Jordan, age and background unknown, had joined 4th VA Inf. as asst. surg. and became the main asst. when Crockett was killed. On 10 February 1863 Jordan was transfered to the general hospital at Petersburg. Robertson, *4th VA Inf.*, 58.

[119] John Eric Erichsen, *The Science and Art of Surgery; a Treatise on Surgical Inquiries, Diseases, and Operations* (1853. Rev. ed.; Philadelphia: Blanchard and Lea, 1854). Sir John Eric Erichsen (1818-1896) was born in Copenhagen to a Danish banking family, but was educated in London, at University College of London. He studied surgery, and passed the examination for Royal College of Surgeons. He was primarily known for this authoritative textbook, the theme of which was that surgery was a science and not an art. Gaining prominence in Victorian England, he was much studied and quoted in the US when the war began. After the War, Erichsen became surgeon extraordinary to Queen Victoria and was elected president of the Royal College of Surgeons. "Erichsen," *Dictionary of National Biography*, 22 vols. (London: Oxford University Press, 1917), supplement vol. 22. Note that his message—that surgery is an exact science—is taken for granted in the 20th century, but was not really what Hunter McGuire, Harvey Black, or the diarist steward and apprentice surgeon Apperson believed.

I rode up on horseback—my horses feet are improving somewhat—

On arriving at this house I found prospects not flattering—I feel like a poor boy at a quilting—out of place and nothing to say. All the positions that I would have are filled, and it would be a thing unjust to those who are "in" to be compelled to yield to me. I would not do it! Dr. B. said to me to remain that he would want me—I am willing to do anything that is honourable but do not wish to infringe upon the goodness of any one. I would rather be a private in the ranks than a hanger on—a nuisance.

However the whole arrangement is knocked up. Orders have been rec. for the removal, forthwith, of sick to Staunton [General Hospital in Augusta Co]. Everything is mixed and confused—I am a supernumerary [120] and if my trunk was safe for transportation I would not care at all. Dr. B repeated his words again to-night that he not want me to go away. I have nothing to do and am not satisfide [sic].

There are some 400 sick here in Winchester and some two hundred at Middleburg [field hospital in Loudon Co.] and Strasburg [field hospital in Shenandoah Co].

FRIDAY NOV. 21, 1862

YORK HOSPITAL, WINCHESTER, VA [CLARKE CO.]

All day to-day I have been doing nothing. Dr. B. has been disposing of Medical Officers and employees in the hospitals here and preparing to evacuate the place. Most of the employees are being sent to Lynchburg [Campbell Co.] leaving an adequate supply for the requirements of this place. The 1 Div. marched through this morning, A.P. Hill's Div. is on the Berryville Pike [Clarke Co.] and some cavalry force on the Martinsburg Pike [WVA]. I presume that Dr B make [sic] his arrangements to leave in a day or so. Some 200 or 300 sick will be left too unwell to move.

I am boarding at the Hospital, Dr. is Boarding at Mrs. Loring.[121] I have been suffering with headache to-day —

---

[120] "Supernumerary, late L[atin], applied to soldiers added to a legion after it is complete; that is, beyond the number needed, or desired; superfluous; unnecessary. Now rare" Many instances are given for the 19th cent., esp. literary and military. *OED.*

[121] Possibly Mrs. Loving. I could not find any widowed woman named Loring or Loving who held land in Clarke Co. in 1870 VA Census.

I think it to be regreted very much that there is not more rigidness enforced and more correctness and uniformity with regard to keeping regular accounts, records, &c of sick men at hospitals. Several officers have been in the clerk's room to-day inquiring after their men who have died, and in many instances the answers given were not at all satisfactory. The Army regulations is sufficient if properly obeyed.

I have been struck by the ordinary appearance of a majority of the Medical Officers connected with the [General] Hospitals at this place. They are small in stature and don't seem to portray the vivacious[,] energetic character that men ought who are entrusted with the health of an army. The[y] seem too careless[,] almost to look foppish! The whole dread now is that [they] are afraid they will be sent to the field. In times of peace a disabled man was not easy found, but now even the Doctors cry out pittifull [sic] that they are not healthy—too delicate for the field! Aye poor fellows it is a pitty [sic] that fortune should have decreed that you should leave your mama's apron strings! You should have remained home where you could have been nursed and fed and fattened! The trials here are too much for your dainty minds.

YORK HOSPITAL, WINCHESTER VA [CLARKE CO.]

SATURDAY NOV: 22ND, 1862

This morning the town was filled with the shouts of A.P. Hill's and [Richard Stoddert] Ewell's Divisions[122] passing through. I have never seen men in a better humor or higher glee. Every face was bright with a smile and puns and jokes passed from one to the other as they marched rapidly along. Such men can never be conquered. I looked to see some of the evils spoken of lately by some of our Richmond papers and felt gratified to see not a single barefooted man the

---

[122] Jackson's Stonewall Brigade forces were marching toward Fredericksburg to join the rest of Lee's Army of Northern VA at a spot on the Rappahannock River where a great battle was expected with Burnsides's Army of the Potomac. Ambrose Powell Hill (1825-1865) was from Culpeper, VA, a West Point graduate, fought in Mexican War and 3d Seminole War. Resigning US Army comm., Hill took charge of 13th VA Inf., and eventually became Maj. Gen. much trusted by T.J. Jackson. Distinguishing himself with boldness and effectiveness with quick strikes at the enemy, Hill's 13th was noted for successes in Valley Campaign, Peninsula Campaign, and Seven Days Battle. Ewell's men were the 6th Bde, then under the command of Jubal Anderson Early (1816-1894), identified earlier. Richard Stoddert Ewell (1817-1872) the commander of this division lost his leg at Groveton August 1862. He was fitted with a wooden leg and returned to battle 23 May 1863; but he was replaced by Early (1816-1894) in August of 1862 for several months. Edwin C. Bearss, "Hill," and Dale E. Floyd, "Ewell", *Historical Times.*

"Richmond Whig" to the contrary notwithstanding. I saw Eades who told me that the 1 Div. camped near Middletown[123].

Several ambulances loaded with sick were sent of[f] this morning in charge of Dr. J.St.P. Gibson. He will have a tedious time as he got in the rear of all the troops.

I made off duplicate receipts for some medicine gotten from Asst. Surg. W.H. Geddings Med Purv[eyor] some time in August when we were at Camp Crenshaw [probably Orange Co.] for the use of the reg't and forwarded them to the Surgeon General [S.P. Moore in Richmond]. This ought to have been attended sooner but times have been "exciting" which is offered as an excuse.

A member of the Sanitary Committee was here this morning and reports a case of Small Pox among the citizens. [124] Quarantine rules have not been as strictly observed as they ought to have been. Unless much care is observed that loathsome disease will spread throughout our country.

I had a pleasant chat with Dr. Chamberlain Hosp't Steward [illegible; boarding] at this house. I regard him as a nice gentleman.

YORK HOSPITAL, WINCHESTER, VA

SUNDAY NOV. 23RD, 1862

This morning the Church bells were chiming beautifully. How many fond reminiscences it calls up and many pleasing memories it awakens to hear those old bells calling to the peoples to come to the house of God and do Him reverence on this His holy day of rest. But when we scan the condition of the country—how few places are greeted on sabbath morns, how few except the aged and the juvenile and the feminine are called to go [to] the house of God. I ought to have gone this morning but did not. I am sad in heart somehow or other.

---

[123] Middletown, now Middleton, is in Frederick Co. Hummel, *A List.* Eads is probably James M. Eads (born, 1834), a merchant from Rockbridge Co. who joined Co. H, 4th VA infantry and was then detailed as 1st VA brigade postmaster. Robertson, *4th VA Inf.*, 48

[124] Despite official efforts to vaccinate everyone and to quarantine those infected, small pox did spread rapidly among citizens as well as soldiers. For instance, the mayor of Danville (Pittsylvania Co.), Thomas Atkinson, made official complaint of laxness in quarantining, and the press was filled with reports. Cunningham, 198-99.

This morning the enemy's cavalry made a charge on our pickets about 6 mi[les] [from Winchester] and wounded one man. [125] I am really fearful for our things if we stay here any longer.

I have not done much good to-day. Some 25 ambulances came down—this evening—we have some 400 men here at this time.

WINCHESTER VA [CLARKE CO.]

NOV: 24TH, 1862

This morning the clerks[,] stewards and employees in the hospital who had been discharged packed up and decamped. They seem fearful to remain longer. The enemy seems to be threatening this place and the sooner all who [are] not obliged to stay leave, the better. I think Dr. B. proposes to leave day after to-morrow, if not before.

The ambulances brought down yesterday were loaded this morning and started off. I have been doing some writing for the hospital. I went to Mr. Vilwig's shop to-day to get some camp chairs for Capt. A[lbert].G[allatin]. Pendleton[126] aid[e] to Gen. Jackson. Mr. [John] Vilwig[127] charged an enormous price for them—4$ a piece—Capt. [sic.; Maj. Pendleton] sent 20$ and said pay for them. There were six and Vilwig wanted to charge for a table which he said Capt. P. [sic] had gotten before he left, and wished me to pay for them; which I refused to do. I paid 24$ for the chairs and took a receipt.

Vilwig is a cabinet maker from Germany—been in America 10 years. He professes to have been from the outset a firm upholder of the South. But notwithstanding his assertions I should be very particular what sort of information I put into his hands though he may [be] all right. He was very solicitous to find out something from me.

Late to-night news came in that the Batt. guarding the town had orders to move. Our Army is reported to have crossed into Eastern Va at "Thurston's

---

[125] There is report of Federal cavalry skirmish on Saturday near CSA pickets outside Winchester, *Official Records*, 22 November 1862.; and confirmed by Long, 289; but nothing for 23 November.

[126] Pendleton (1836-1901) was an attorney from Smyth Co. and originally Capt. of Co. D, old Smyth Blues; breveted Maj. in 4th VA Inf., Co. D and received confirmation in January 1862; by this period suffering physical disabilities and was given QM post in January 1863 because of disabilities. Robertson, 67. As noted earlier, Pendleton operated a newspaper, *The Visitor*, in Marion. Wilson, *Smyth Co.*

[127] John Vilwig, born 1820 in Germany, lived in Frederick Co. on the outskirts of Winchester. VA Census, 1870.

Gap".[128] Fredericksburg is about to be shelled by Gen. Patrick,[129] yankee, to make Gen. Lee surrender—He refuses emphatically.

[ON ROAD TO MIDDLEBURG; LOUDON CO.]

TUESDAY NOV: 25TH, 1862

This morning everything is quiet [in contrast] to what I expected it to be last night. About 10 o'clock last night news came that the enemy was advancing and the Maryland line was ordered to be ready to move; Dr. B. went to the Provost Marshall's [sic] office and to Gen. [John Robert] Jones' Hd. Qrs. and was told that no danger was approaching.

This morning we sent our baggage off early in the morning. I walked down [the] street. Wagons were being loaded with tobacco that had been pressed to be distroyed [sic; destroyed by burning]. It seems that many speculators have been buying tobacco and bringing it to the place for the purpose of trading with the enemy when he comes in. I hate to see the tobacco distroyed [sic] but glad to see it taken from those who are so careless for the interests of the country. It ought to have been taken and given to our soldiers. I see no plausible reason why they should not have it. The effect of burning it may be better if it had been distributed [sic].

About 2 o'clock we left in company with Dr. [F.H.] Wright.[130] Dr. B. had business at Middleburg [Loudon Co.] and we stopped for the night at Mr. David Miller's house near Middleburg.[131] He is a kind hospitable man—full of interesting humor and chat. I had been at his house and partook of the good things of his table a little more than a year before. There were with me then several who have paid the last debt upon their country's altar.

---

[128] Buckingham Co.; sometimes spelled Thruston, sometimes Thurston. Hummel, *A List.*

[129] Marsena Rudolph Patrick (1811-1888). This Watertown, NY native was a West Point graduate and one time President of New York State Agricultural College at Ovid. He became Provost Marshal General for the Army of the Potomac in October of 1862. John Y. Simon, "Patrick", *Historical Times.*

[130] William G. Bean contributes the name F.H. Wright. Bean, Notes.

[131] There is no David Miller listed in Loudon Co. in 1870 VA Census. He may have moved there after 1860 census and died or moved away before 1870 census.

[ON ROAD THROUGH FREDERICK CO.; SHENANDOAH CO.; APPROACHING WARREN CO.]

WEDNESDAY NOV: 26TH, 1862

This morning we breakfasted, settled our bill, (2$ each)[.] Dr B. paid for himself and me, and were off.

At Middletown [Frederick Co.] Dr. Scarborough was left in charge of the sick that will be left after removing all that are able to go.

At Strasburg [Shenandoah Co.] the hospitals were in an awful condition. Dr. [Black] was not pleased by any means—and Dr. [W.G.] Upshur was ordered to his regiment forthwith and Dr. [S.R.] Swann left in charge. [132] A train [group or line] of ambulances was distributed to the three places and will be sufficient to remove all except 150.

Dr. Wright left us and we moved on up the valley [turned southward]. After leaving the village of Woodstock [Shenandoah Co.] we began to look for lodging. Leaving the Pike, we went on the South side [of the North Mountain] and did not succede [sic] till we got near the mountain to a Mr. Copenhaver—relative of those in Smyth.[133] At one house we stopped and the old woman was not in a very good humor and gave us no encouragement. She seemed very solicitous for us to go to Mr. Copenhaver's where as she said would be almost sure to get entertainment.

Mr. C. was not willing to take us. He is one of those that is always hard up for everything.

The old lady gave a horrible account of the atrocities of the yankees and by her own way of thinking made herself a hero defending the property. She had lost a son in the fight at Kernstown (23 March 1862), and had 5 or 6 children with her then—one a granddaughter. With all their smallness of the natural man we were kindly treated.

---

[132] William G. Bean supplies the initials for Upshur and Swann. Bean, Notes. Neither is listed in regimental lists. Possibly W.G. Upshur is Washington Upshur, born 1830 of Washington Crossing, Richmond Co.; and possibly S.R. Swann is Samuel Swann, born 1812 of Rockingham Co. VA. Census. 1870.

[133] George Copenhaver, born 1849, owned land in Shenandoah Co. in 1870 and was possibly son of the man referenced by the diarist. VA Census. 1870.

[LEAVING SHENANDOAH CO. AND GOING TOWARD FREDERICKSBURG}

THURSDAY NOV. 27TH, 1862

This morning I find my horse had not eaten his feed and seems sick. I was very apprehensive that he would not be a horse much longer. After settling our bill 9$ each (Dr. B paid it) we mounted and rode back to the road passing near the camp of the 6 Va cavalry.[134] Coming in contact with them on the evening before caused us to be somewhat troubled to get lodging. My horse traveled very sluggish. At Mt. Jackson [Shenandoah Co.] we found our baggage and [were] ordered on to New Market[Shenandoah Co.], from where we intend crossing the Massanutten Mountain into Page Co[.] on the track of the army.

Dr. B. stopped awhile and we moved on. My horse came near going down crossing the [Massanutten] Mountain. The scenery from this gap is very fine, but the awful scourge of war has made the picture a sad one. I notice very few straglers [sic] from the army. One poor fellow was about to camp alone in the mountain. That looked like solitude.

We crossed the mountain into "Page Valley" [Page Co.] and began to look for a place to lodge. We called at the 5th or 6th house before we succeded. The army camped in the neighborhood. Mr. Diver said there was a perfect lake of fire around his house, and Mr. Courtz said he would keep us if we could get in no where else.[135] Mrs. [Catherine] Kite[136] agreed to keep us if we could get feed for our horses. We got feed from the miller near Columbian [Foundry] bridge [over North Fork of Shenandoah River]. While we were at supper the ambulance containing our baggage crossed the river and left us. I tried to overtake it to stop it but failed.

---

[134] The 6th VA Cav. was reorganized in late fall 1862. J.E.B. Stuart was in overall command of all CSA cav., but William Edmundson "Grumble" Jones took charge of a new 2d Bde of Cav., which included 6th VA. Jones (1824-1864) was born in Washington Co., VA. He attended Emory & Henry College and then transfered to West Point, graduating 10th in class of 1848. During frontier service in 1852, he married, but his new wife drowned in an accident off the Texas coast, and he was never the same. In 1857, he resigned his commission and began farming in Washington Co., VA. When War came, he joined Washington Mounted Rifles and fought well at 1st Manassas, but feuded with J.E.B. Stuart, his onetime Emory & Henry and West Point classmate. Jackson and Lee admired Jones and appeared to trust him implicitly, but Stuart "could not abide him." Jones drove the 6th Cav. and the entire 2d Cav. Bde. hard, and was described as "the best outpost officer" in the ANV. "Eccentric, cantankerous, with a razor-sharp tongue, Jones cared little for pretense or appearance." Jeffrey D. Wert, "Jones," *Hist. Times.*

[135] There is no Diver or Courtz listed as owning land in Page Co. in 1870 VA Census.

[136] Probably Catherine Kite, born 1797, who owned land in Shenandoah Iron Works section of Page Co. VA. Census 1870.

Mrs. Kite was a genuine old dutch lady, plain in her talk, and frugal in her house arrangements. Two Tennesseeans were stopping there. She and her daughter gave us an extended account of the doings of the yankees and the renegade Dr. Gillispie [137] who lived near.

This old woman had the greatest quantity of bed clothes I ever saw.

[TRAVELING THROUGH PAGE CO. AND MADISON CO. TOWARD FREDERICKSBURG]

FRIDAY, NOV. 28TH, 1862

This morning I went to the miller and gave him 75 cents for 1/2 bu[shel] of corn and an armful of hay. The old lady's charge was 2$ each (I paid it) and gave a boy 25 ct. for attending our horses. My horse was a little better. We started about 9 o'clock and took the road known as Graves' Road across Milam's Gap. The land in the Hawk's Bill" in Page [Co.] is very good. Luray can be seen from the road. Marksdale [Marksville] PO is in this little neck of land. Some 16 good houses can be seen from one point.

The road seems to run into the [Massanutten] Mountain at its highest point. [B]efore getting to the beginning of the ascent one cannot tell where the road crosses. I have never seen a more circuitous route for a road in my life. From the foot on one side to the foot on the other is 14 miles. The road is not steep at any place. The man Grave's, to whose credit the road is placed is certainly an enterprising man to carry a road over the Blue Ridge at that point.

I fell in with the "Orange Rangers"[138] going over and remained with them till I reached the foot on the Eastern side. I found Dr. B. waiting at Mr. Story's a merchant in Madison Co.[139] Here we got put up for the night. The family was mourning the loss of a son and brother who had fallen at Richmond.

Everywhere we go we hear of depradations by the Louisiana Soldiers [Tigers]. I like the men for their bravery, but they are men of little principal [sic].

---

[137] No Gillispie or Gillespie is listed as owning land in Page Co. in 1870. VA Census 1870.

[138] Orange Rangers were Co. I commanded by Capt. G.J. Browning. These horsemen were from Apperson's birthplace, and served in 6th Cav. under Grumble Jones's 2d Cav. Bde. Scott, *Hist. of Oange Co.*, 273-75.

[139] Probably David Story, born 1813, who had a store in Robertson Township in Madison Co.

[TRAVELING THROUGH MADISON AND ORANGE COS. ON WAY TO FREDERICKSBURG]

SATURDAY NOV. 29 [1862]

Dr. paid Mr. Story 2$ each for our Bill and paid a miller $1.75 for food for the ambulance horses. My horse is stiffened up considerably. Madison Co. is rough. Stopped at the C.H. [Orange Court House, Orange Co.] a short time, then went to Liberty Mills [Orange Co.] where we passed the 1 Va Battalion Provost Guard for the Corps.

We overtook two cavalrymen driving two of the 23 NC Infantry before them. One of the N. Carolinians was shedding tears as he moved along, the other looked sad and sick—Dr. B took the responsibility to send them on a permit to Gordonsville [Orange Co.] to the [general] hospital [directed by Dr. B.M. Lebby].

This is what hundreds suffer daily. Every trait of manhood seems to be exhausted and gone and the poor men find solace in nothing but tears.

We found at Liberty Mills that the army was making toward Fredericksburg and we took the left hand road to Orange C.H. Near there we passed A. P. Hill's Division. We intended to camp near the [Orange] C.H. but could not get quarters and we moved onto the south of "Jordan's Lane" and camped in the open air. Lawton's Division[140] was about 3 mi's [miles] below.

I unpacked my trunk and took out such clothes as I shall need and put my books and things that I can spare in it to be sent to my father's [in Locust Grove]. I am afraid I shall lose my books as the roads will be horrid I know. I anticipate going home [that is, the Apperson home place in Locust Grove] to-morrow. Dr. said I could have the opportunity if I chose. I have concluded to leave my horse also if father has feed enough.

The Plank Road is in a bad fix—showing that plank roads are a humbug.

---

[140] Alexander Robert Lawton (1818-1896) was from the Beaufort, SC elite and graduated 13th from West Point in 1839, then earned a degree from Harvard Law School in 1842. Practicing law in Savannah, Lawton became a Georgian and remained politically prominent the remainder of the century; he concentrated on development of and regulation of railroads as a component of economic progress and political programs. When the War came, he was commissioned Brig. Gen. and after capturing Ft. Pulaski "as the first act of war in Georgia," he was ordered to VA, where he served well in Valley campaign, 7 Days Battle, and 2d Manassas. Severely wounded at Antietam, he experienced difficulties in the field and in August of 1863 he became QM of CSA. After War, he lost a contest to Joseph E. Brown for US Senate, "which was viewed as a victory for the 'New South' over the Old." He remained politically prominent, and was chosen president of the American Bar Association, 1882, and was appointed minister to Austria, 1887. Patrick M. McCoy, " Lawton," *Hist. Times.*

[ORANGE COURT HOUSE, ORANGE CO.]

SUNDAY NOV 30TH, '62

Last night I slept cool. This morning our beds were white with frost. I slept badly. We started of[f] early, overtook the Division just as it was going out of camp near Martin's. I pushed on and took the old road at Roache's and went to my father's. I saw F. Johnson at his Tanyard[141] and The Old Grove looks very lonesome to what it used to. I found sister and mother both in bed but better than I expected. Eli has a running sore on his leg which I do not like—he will never be healthy. Father was on the road looking at the army. He is getting along very well and is in good health. Got a letter from Cousin Bettie.

[LOCUST GROVE, ORANGE CO.]

MONDAY DEC. 1ST, 1862

This morning H.D. Roach came over to see me and I spent a very pleasant day. The changes at home are not so great as one would suppose. Mother is up part of the time. Sister will soon be well. Nothing transpired worthy of note. Grandfather came down in the evening—he has changed but little. I leave for the Reg't to-morrow.

Home had but few charms for me. I am sorry to see affliction among my father's folks. Eli is afflicted in a way that I fear will not soon be relieved. Last summer Dr. Q wrote me that he had Erysipelas[142] and now there seems to be some disease of the tibia. The flesh grows up but some internal disease keeps up an issue. Several spicular[143] of bone have been discharged.

Salt is an object with all persons in the country now. 2 oz. to each member of each family at 8 cts per pound distibuted by committees appointed for the purpose. Speculators are selling salt at 1$ per pound. I shall leave my horse, bridle and saddle at my father's. He is careful with horses and by Spring my horse will be worth something.

---

[141] There were many cattle and other domesticated animals raised in Orange Co., and Johnson built a tanyard to cure and tan the skins once animals were slaughtered. Scott, *Hist of Orange Co.*, 132.

[142] From the Greek for *red skin*; "acute febrile disease with localized inflammation and redness of skin and subcutaneous tissue accompanied by systematic disturbance." Now treated successfully with penicillin, it could not be treated in this era and sometimes developed into severe kidney disorders known as nephritis. *Taber's.*

[143] From Latin for *dart*; "needle shaped fragment of bone." *Taber's.*

[ON ROAD TO FREDERICKSBURG FROM ORANGE CO.]

TUESDAY DECR. 2ND, 1862

This morning between 8 & 9 o'clock I started in company with my father to find my Division. He took me on his horse. At Decker's we came upon Gen. A.P. Hill's troops marching towards Fred'g on the Plank Road. About 6 mi's above town he took the right hand road and went in direction of Mr. S. Alsop's. Father went near Mr. Wyatt's with me and I thought it best for him to return. I dismounted and struck for the "Telegraph Road". I gave sister 6$ for a 1/2 bu of dried peaches, and she put them in a worthless sack which was much trouble. I was worried. For a long time I could not get on the track of Jackson's Old Division [that is 4th VA Inf., esp. Co. D]. Some said it was further and some nearer. I walked 'till I was tired. Passed Massaponax Church near sundown and took a left hand road leading to a Mr. Holiday's about a mile and a half below which I found the division.

Dr. B. was at Camp. He has been ordered to take charge of Hospitals for the Corps. Will have to go to Staunton [Augusta Co. to west] to select Hospital supplies.

[GUINEA'S DEPOT, CAROLINE CO. ON ROAD TO FREDERICKSBURG]

WEDNESDAY DECR. 3RD, 1862

This morning Dr. B. started to Staunton to obtain supplies. I have been engaged writing—wrote to Father.

Our camp is in a wood about 3 miles west of Guinea's Depot. This country contrasts unfavorable [sic] with that where we have been for several months past. It is better than the country above this. No news of the enemy. I wrote a letter to Father.

[CAMP NEAR GUINEA'S DEPOT, CAROLINE CO.]

CAMP THURSDAY DEC 4TH, '62

This morning I commenced an inventory of medicines. Dr. [La Fayette Hall] Jordan [Asst. Surgeon to Dr. Black] refuses to take all on hand, and I am separating and giving him such as he wants. I find a better stock on hand than I supposed. Dr. [Samuel Rush]Sayers[144] has two boxes to turn over. Nothing of importance to note to-day. Wrote to Cousin Bettie.

CAMP [NEAR GUINEA'S DEPOT, CAROLINE CO.],

FRIDAY DEC. 5 [1862]

This morning the [1st VA or Stonewall] Brigade moved a few hundred yards from the point first selected for camp; The camp is near Mr. Holiday's. I am not so well—the water in this part [piedmont] of the state is not so good for me as that in the Valley.

I sent, by mail, to Dr. Faris two *vaccine scabs. Variolar*[145] seems to be scattered throughout the country very much, and I think every precaution ought to be used to stop it.

Rain commenced falling which soon turned to snow and hail. A horrible time on us. Dr. [William A.]Holt[146] has been assigned to the 4 Regt. in place of Dr. "B". He was at our tent. He is from North Carolina and is a fine looking man.

CAMP [NEAR GUINEA'S DEPOT, CAROLINE CO.]

DEC. 6; SATURDAY

I am not well this morning. Last night the clouds passed away and the moon shone so brightly that I could have seen a squirrel in any tree.

I have been writing some to-day. Dr. Holt moved up and initiated himself.

---

[144] Samuel Rush Sayers (1833-1914) was surgeon originally with Co. A, Wythe Grays, 4th VA Inf.; transfered to 27th VA Inf., 1 July 1861; promoted to surgeon, then abs. with illness until 31 October 1862. Remained with wounded at Gettysburg (4 July 1863) and captured there. Imprisoned in Baltimore until exchanged, 21 November 1863; transfered back to 4th VA Inf. on 18 January 1864. After War, practiced medicine in Wytheville. Bur., East End Cem., Wytheville (Wythe Co]. Reidenbaugh, *27th VA Inf.*, 173.

[145] "Variolar" is pertaining to small pox, or variola. Specifically, it refers to the pustules. *Taber's*.

[146] William A. Holt, age unknown and hometown in NC unknown; mustered to field and staff, 4th VA Inf. on 1 August 1862 as surgeon. Present for 1st and 2d Manassas, Valley Campaign, and Fredericksburg. Sick and absent during Chancellorsville; transfered to Raleigh general hospital, 23 December 1863. Robertson, *4th VA Inf.*, 57.

I learned to-day that Lt. [John] Bishop of Co. "D" who was wounded at Manassas Aug 30, died at Aldie Va. from his wounds. He was a good man and a model soldier.[147]

The soldiers have been hard at work to-day. Having been ordered to construct huts to afford some protection to the weather. It is truly a sad picture to see those men who have boldly stood the fiery storm of lead and hail in the many battles fought now shivering and shaking around the camp fire: many without shoes and thinly clad. I wonder what the speculating gentlemen at home think when they are sitting around the warm hearthstone with good food well cooked and the wife of some good soldier calls to buy something to keep herself and darling babes from starvation while her husband stands by his post on such a night as this? Does he ask her 20$ per [barrel] for flour and 25$ per hundred for pork? Or does he reflect that were it not for those who are now sacrificing everything that constitutes earthly happiness, all his earnings, gained perhaps by the cost of his very soul's salvation would be swept away by the hand of an unrelenting enemy and instead of wealth, Freedom and luxury[,] subjection, poverty and misery would be their lot? I fear not. The *Almighty Dollar* and their own dear self are all they think of! [148]

---

[147] John J. Bishop (1837-1862) was a cooper who joined Smyth Blues and was ordnance sgt. at muster when it became Co. D, 4th VA Inf. Promoted to 2d Lt. and then 1st Lt. (29 August 1862), wounded and captured at 2d Manassas; exchanged 8 October 1862 and that day wounded again, at Aldie; died from those wounds, 30 October 1862. Robertson, *4th VA Inf.*, 40. Aldie is in Loudon Co.

[148] Cf. the diarist's description here, of men without shoes and adequate coats, with his insistence on 22 November 1862 that none were without shoes or coats. According to regimental histories, Jackson's "foot cavalry" outran its supplies on this hard, wintry march toward Fredericksburg. By late 1863, the CSA would often lack supplies for its troops, but on this campaign, it was more likely problems with logistics than lack of supplies. See esp. Robertson, *4th VA Inf.*, 21-23; Musick, *6th VA Cav.*, 35; and Rankin, *37th VA Inf.*, 55-58. While the diarist blames speculators, it seems more likely that monetary forces, viz., inflation, caused the high prices, since both Federal and CSA treasuries produced paper currency, a supply of money, far in excess of the value of the goods. Both Robert Sharkey and Milton Friedman support the issuance of "greenback" paper money unredeemable for gold (or specie), but both note that far more of the paper money was created than warranted by production of goods and services. See Milton Friedman and Anna Jacobsen Schwartz, *A Monetary History of the United States, 1867-1960*, Studies in Business Cycles, No. 12 (Princeton, NJ: Princeton University Press for the National Bureau of Economic Research, 1963), passim, esp. introd.; Robert P. Sharkey, *Money, Class, and Party; an Economic Study of Civil War and Reconstruction*, Johns Hopkins University Studies in Historical and Political Science Ser. 77, No. 2 (Baltimore: Johns Hopkins University Press, 1959) esp. 50-55.

This is a sad picture, and when we consider that all this suffering is without a murmur—without a dissenting voice we can but praise southern valor and fortitude more than ever before seen. If the North should succeed in subduing us, it will sadden the purest spirits ever given by God to man. While I write though the earth is blacking up with frost and the wind is blowing cruelly and cold, the joyous notes of song float out from many a merry group.

Abe Lincoln's annual message is out in this morning's paper. It is commented upon by our people as being his weakest effort—the most barren, imbecile and worthless composition that his race has ever presumed to send forth to the sovereigns of state—*Haiti* not excepted.[149]

I have been looking for Dr. B but he did not come. I wish he might come in a short time.

CAMP DEC 7; SUNDAY

Last night was a cold miserable night to me—was not well. I have done but very little, if any good to-day. I got a letter from Mrs. Faris. She has returned from her trip to Tennessee—was highly pleased, has bouyant spirits. I am glad she has been [on] the trip. She writes me that there is a case of small pox in the neighborhood. I answered her letter this evening.

Capt. [Joseph M.]Thomas has fallen upon a plan to procure clothing for his men. He went in petition to the court of Smyth for clothes to be sent to him to be distributed and money receipts to pay for them. He wanted me to make off the appeal: I did so in as appropriate language as I could.

---

[149] Haiti, as the world's oldest black republic, was in the racist mind the example of the least intelligently run government imaginable. Comparisons of Lincoln with African Americans were common as insults, despite the fact that Lincoln was himself quite racist. Indeed, in announcing that emancipation would come for slaves of rebel masters commencing on 1 January 1863, the president also called for colonization of the freed slaves so that the US would not be overwhelmed by freed black people. See George Milton Fredrickson, *The Black Image in the White Mind: the Debate on Afro-American Character and Destiny, 1817-1914* (1971. Rev. ed.; Middletown, CT: Wesleyan University Press, 1987) esp. "Prejudice and Reformism," 1- 42; and "Romantic Racialism in the North," 997-129. As for the literary quality of Lincoln's "imbecile" speech, see this excerpt: "As our cause is new, so we must think anew. We must disenthrall ourselves, and then we shall save our country. Fellow-citizens, *we* cannot escape history....In *giving* freedom to the *slave*, we *assure* freedom to the free—honorable alike in what we give and what we preserve. We shall nobly save, or meanly lose, the last best, hope of earth." Quoted in Long, 292.

Gen. [John Buchanan] Floyd has caused our men to suffer. He has only a few soldiers and gets all the clothing made by the people of the Country. His army has never done anything worth doing with good soldiers.[150]

[CAMP NEAR GUINEA'S DEPOT, CAROLINE CO.]

MONDAY DEC. 8TH, 1862

Nothing of interest to-day. Dr. B. arrived from Staunton [general hospital] to-day. He has been successful in obtaining medicine and hospital stores. He was successful. I expect from what he says that the [camp's field] Hospital will be in tents—an arrangement that I do not like very much.

He turned over to Dr. [William A.] Holt such stores as will be needed by the regiment.

I went over to see Dr. Baldwin about the case of instruments that I put into Dr. [A.C.] Smith's med. wagon at Sharpsburg [17 September 1862]. He said that he did not know anything about them and said that he would ask the driver of the wagon. This seems equivocating somewhat. He ought to know all about what is in his wagon. There is one thing I am sure of. I put the case in the wagon and have not seen it since.

The weather is cold. Tents are being constructed by the men. Some are comfortable. The "sick list" of the regiment is very small—most of the diseases are simple. No fevers. Some cases of variola in the Brigade. *Vaccination* has been pretty effectual in all the cases not vaccinated before, and many of those who had been before. The character of the pustule has been severe. Large sores have formed on the arms of a large majority. The healing goes on very slow. It must be owing to the depraved condition of the blood and the want of power[151] in the system.

I drew 12$ of Capt. [James W.] Shields [Bde. Commissary] for commutation of Rations.

---

[150] Although Floyd (1806-1863) did not "cause" the suffering of the Stonewall Brigade, military historians generally concur with the diarist's judgment of Floyd as a commander. Charles M. Spearman, "Floyd," *Hist. Times.*

[151] He has accepted the theory that some of the vaccine is too "weak."

CAMP [NEAR GUINEA'S DEPOT, CAROLINE CO.]

TUESDAY DECR. 9TH [1862]

A cold, frosty morning. I know of no important transactions to-day. Dr. [Black] went to arrange matters for the organization of his [field] hospitals. He has decided that he will go into tents or some dry place.

An accident happened to Dr. [Ezekiel Martin] James of "Smyth Blues" [152] which injured him considerably. All of the shelters made for them to sleep under gave way and fell covering him entirely up in dirt and poles. He is not thought to be seriously injured.

CAMP [NEAR GUINEA'S DEPOT, CAROLINE CO.]

WEDNESDAY DEC. 10, 1862

This morning *Jas Cooley's*[153] time is out—I drew rations for four days—having drawn none since we left Winchester Va.

Our mess is rather a large one. Lt. Col. [Robert Davidson] Gardner, Major [William] Terry, Capt. [John Hall] Fulton, Lt. Fulton, Parson Tibbs, Dr. [La Fayette Hall] Jordan, Dr. [William A.] Holt, and Mr. [William A.] Carrington[154]

---

[152] James recovered from this injury, which apparently cost him no time from service as surgeon. Ezekiel Martin James, age unknown, was physician and surgeon from Jefferson Co., MO; "served as Asst. Surg. of 1st MO St Guard Cav until transfer to 4th VA as hospital steward; performed that duty through 1864." Subsequent career unknown. Robertson, *4th VA Inf.*, 57.

[153] This volunteer James Cooley was one of some 145 "free colored" persons listed in Smyth Co. [838 slaves]. A brick mason, he married Fanny, and they had at least one child; he established a brick laying business, Cooley and Smith, and enjoyed some independent financial success after the War. Cooley was also involved in building a brick church for an independent African American Baptist church in Marion after the War. Another "free person of color" who enlisted voluntarily in the Confederate Army was John Ross. His business was not listed, but he apparently enjoyed some success. Wilson, *Smyth*, 261-65. Notice that Cooley was willing enough to fight for CSA for 20 months, but that he did not re-enlist and returned to Marion to operate his business; notice also that Cooley was respected by the whites of Marion for his years of CSA service and not criticized for leaving when his time was served.

[154] William A. Carrington, based in Richmond, was medical director for field hospitals, Cunningham, *Doctors in Gray*, 285. Robert Davidson Gardner 1830-1906) was carpenter from Montgomery Co. who joined Pulaski Guards of Pulaski Co., which became Co. C, 4th VA Inf.; elected Capt. 25 July 1861; promoted to Lt. Col. 22 April 1862; shot in face at Fredericksburg but continued in field service until 8 April 1864; post commandant, Dublin Depot (Pulaski Co.); after War was carpenter in Pulaski Co. and buried there in Newbern. Robertson, *4th VA Inf.*, 51. William Terry (1824-1888), occupation unknown, was from Amherst Co. and formed Wythe Grays, which became Co. A; Lt. when War started, he was promoted to Capt. 13 May 1861, wounded in left arm and side at Groveton, 28 August 1862 and promoted to Col. Wounded twice more, second time severely. Surviving War, he returned to Wytheville, where he lived until

and myself. We have had potatoes twice in the last week and beans and bacon to-day. "Bull beef" is about all we get. I am anxious to leave. The papers bring us news of a victory by Gen. [John Hunt] Morgan[155] in E. Tennessee.

CAMP [NEAER GUINEA'S DEPOT, CAROLINE CO.]

THURSDAY DEC 11 1862

This morning before day I was awakened by the firing of cannon in direction of Fred'g. It seemed to be from very heavy guns, and continued 'till about 11 o'clock, when it practically ceased, only a shot now and then being heard.

I have been at work on duplicate receipts of store for Dr. [William A.] Holt and invoice for the Surgeon General of Medicine [Dr. S.P. Moore] turned over to Dr. Holt.

Reports from the firing came in about night. The enemy made an effort to cross the [Rappahannock] river in three places on pontoon bridges and were repulsed by our sharp shooters. Gen. Lee is in command in person.

The troops have orders to cook to-day's rations and be ready to move. Afterwards the order was countermanded. It is very much to be regretted that our men will leave their *almost comfortable* huts. There is no doubt a want of blankets in the army but I have no doubt that there are thousands of blankets stored away somewhere that belong to the men. This morning a wagon load of baggage brought from Gordonsville [Orange Co.] was distributed[.] [N]early all the men got blankets, but I see no way that they can be transported. And if

drowning 5 September 1888; buried in Wytheville. Robertson, 76. Capt. John Hall Fulton (1837-1907) was lawyer who joined Wythe Grays, and was appt. 3d Lt. at muster in Co. A. He was promoted to 1st Lt., 13 May 1861, and Capt. 22 April 1862; shot in leg and arm at Groveton, 28 August 1862. At Chancellorsville, he would be shot severely in leg, and his leg amputated, 3 May 1863, and discharged from service. He practiced law in Wytheville, died in 1907 and is buried there. Robertson, 51. I cannot locate a Lt. Fulton in Stonewall Bde. I cannot locate a Parson Tibbs in the brigade. La Fayette Hall Jordan, asst. surg., is identified earlier, as is Dr. William A. Holt, surgeon.

[155] Morgan (1825-1864) was born in Huntsville, Alabama, but was considered a Kentuckian because he grew up in a prominent family in Lexington. A distinguished cavalry officer, he served in the Mexican War, but became most famous for his daring "western" raids, not only in Upper East Tennessee (heavily Federal territory) but also in Kentucky. President Lincoln once wired his Kentucky leadership that Morgan was "having a stampede in Kentucky." William R. Brooksher and David K. Snider, "Morgan," *Historical Times.* Morgan raided forage trains and skirmished along pikes east of Nashville. He was spectacular, but did not fight, much more win, any major engagement in December. Long, 289-94.

Capt. [Joseph M.]Thomas succeeds in getting clothing from the Co. [Smyth, at court session] for his men who can tell how it is to be transported?

I was summoned to appear before an examining committee to testify in regard to the competency character etc. of James Harris. He has lately been chosen a Lieutenant in Co. "D" and some think he is no[t] able to fill the office. I was called upon to tell what I know of him. Capt. [John E.] Roberts, Lt. [Samuel Rush] Sayers [surgeon once with 4th VA Inf. and this day with 27th VA Inf.] and [George Baxter] McCorkle[156]—I know nothing to state. The evidence I heard was not complimentary to his bravery. It is an unpleasant position to be placed in for a person to be compelled to say that which must dampen the prospects of a young man for a long time.

[CAMP NEAR GUINEA STATION, CAROLINE CO.]

FRIDAY DEC. 12; 1862

Orders were last night for reveille at 5 this morning and move at 6. The troops marched in direction of Fred'g. Dr. B. determined to move to the house he had selected as a hospital. He rode off and directed me to come on. I went but got lost, or rather I took the wrong road. When I got to Guiney [Guinea] Station I found Dr. Sydnor who informed me that Dr. had rec'd orders to follow the army. I went on and put an ambulance in the train of ambulances belonging to the hosp't dept. in charge of Surg. Black. I found several of the employees—Chamberlain[,] [Harvey Allen] Jameson and [James Henry]

---

[156]James F. Harris (born1835, death date unknown) was a farmer from Smyth Co. who joined Smyth Blues, which became Co. D, 4th VA Inf. Although voted Lt., he was not confirmed after this hearing. Subsequently, at Chancellorsville, he suffered severe wound in leg, 3 May 1863. From 15 November 1863 to 1 March 1864, he was listed as AWOL. Returning and pardoned, he was captured at Spotsylvania, 12 May 1864 and imprisoned at Elmira, NY until after War. Paroled on 11 July 1865, with no records of peacetime life in Smyth or elsewhere. "5'9", gray eyes, dark hair, florid complexion." Robertson, *4th VA Inf.*, 55. Capt. John E. Roberts (born 1838, death date unknown) was a farmer who joined Grayson Co. Dare Devils, and was elected Lt. when it became Co. F, 4th VA Inf. Promoted to Capt. 17 September 1862; later captured, at Wilderness, 5 May 1864; imprisoned at Ft. Delaware, Del. until 16 June 1865, peacetime record in Grayson Co. or elsewhere not found. "5'8", hazel eyes, light hair, florid complexion." Ibid., 70. George Baxter McCorkle(1842-1895) was a student who left school to join Rockbridge Grays, who became Co. H of 4th VA Inf. Enlisted as pvt., but breveted 3d Sgt. at once and then elected 2d Lt., 20 April 1862, 1st Lt., 25 August 1862, and Capt., 20 April 1863. Captured at Gettysburg, 4 July 1863, he was imprisoned at Ft. Delaware Prison, Del., but exchanged 14 March 1865 and returned to unit for surrender. After the war, he lived in Rockbridge Co., and is buried there at Falling Spring Presbyterian Church. Robertson., 62.

Noland—also Dr. Wilkerson.[157] We moved towards Fredericksburg. At several places, [there were] cemetaries in the woods. I saw ladies and children making their way from their homes in the ill-fated city of Fredericksburg. What a sad spectacle! What a distressing thing to see our people this oppressed by so unholy a war.[158]

We got to "Hamilton's Crossing" about 2 o'clock and camped for the night. Some occasional shots were heard principally on the left where [James] Longstreet was. He was along the hills from the Spottsylvania Road to the river above and [T.J.] Jackson's Corps from Longstreet's right to the river below—perhaps Gen. [J.E.B.] Stuart had his cavalry division next to the river on Jackson's right.[159] The position arrangement and disposition of our troops have not been superior for fighting since the war began. A semicircle of hills is strewn around Fredericksburg and the crest of the hills is lined with our batteries. The enemy may break through our lines on the right near the river and turn our right; but it would be accomplished at a terrible loss. Our men are sanguine of success—very few are falling back.

We went into camp just below Mr. Yerby's[160] house about 4 miles from Fredericksburg. Dr. Hagy came up with some stores—such as blankets, bed

---

[157] Harvey Allen Jameson (born 1841, death date unknown) was a farmer who joined Pulaski Guards, which became Co. C, 4th VA Inf. He served as hospital steward for undetermined time, but "through at least Apr. 1864." Robertson,58. James Henry Noland (1841-1906) was a machinist from Charles Town [now WVA] who joined Botts Grays of Charles Town, which became Co. G of 2d VA Inf. Pvt. assigned to Col. James Walkinson Allen (1829-1862) headquarters of 2d Inf., he was sick in field hospital November and December 1861; subsequently with medical department. After War, returned to Charles Town and worked as machinist and died and is buried there, Edge Hill Cem. Denis E. Frye, *2d VA Inf.*, Virginia Regimental Histories Series (Lynchburg, VA: H.E. Howard, 1984) 122. I cannot find Dr. Wilkerson or a soldier named Chamberlain in the Stonewall Brigade.

[158] Ambrose E. Burnside had built up a large force on the Rappahannock and on 21 November 1862 called for the surrender of Fredericksburg. He was persuaded by town officials to let women and children evacuate, and he was also persuaded to allow officials time to consider conditional surrender. Officials were probably stalling, waiting on Jackson's forces to march in from the west to form a right flank for Lee's sizable force. James Longstreet was already present, dug in with a force on Marye's Heights overlooking the Rappahannock. Long, 288.

[159] J.E.B. Stuart [described earlier] directed artillery on the Confederate right. He did so very ably, and after this battle, he and his cavalry guarded passes on the Rappahannock River during winter of 1862-1863 and kept R.E. Lee and ANV fully informed of Federal movements. Long known for bold rides and unorthodox maneuvers, Stuart here demonstrated tactical competence of a high order. John D. Kallman, "Stuart," *Hist. Times.*

[160] Probably John P. Yerby (born in 1827) who had house at Cortland Township in Spotsylvania Co. outside Fredericksburg. VA Census. 1870.

sacks, pillow ticks,& c. also 20 hospital tents. One of these we pitched and had quite a comfortable [sic].

Dr. [Hunter Holmes] McGuire [chief surgeon of Bde.] was around—after supper all of us laid down upon our blankets, all expecting to-morrow to be a day of bloodshed.

[CAMP NEAR YERBY'S, OUTSIDE FREDERICKSBURG]

SATURDAY DEC. 13TH 1862

This morning the whole earth was shrouded in a canopy of smoke and fog.

Nothing could be seen more than a few hundred yds. We ate breakfast and put things in order to move as soon as it may be necessary. The two armies lay last night within 400 yds of each other face to face.

Precisely at 20 min to 10 o'clock the first gun fired—and the fight soon became general. Dr. moved us in above Mr. [John P.] Yerby's and pitched his Hospital tents and by noon the wounded commenced coming in. Dr. Chamberlain was placed in charge of the ambulance train. The heavy guns of [James] Longstreets and our lines were thundering heavily till late at night. The sufferers were chiefly artillerists it being the greatest artillery fight we have yet had. The Rockbridge Artillery[161] was hotly engaged and suffered deeply. Robert Frazer[162] from Orange was wounded and brought to the hospital. Being a citizen of my native county I felt under some obligation to give him some special attention. He seemed heartily thankful for any little favor done him.

A.P. Hill's division became hotly engaged with small armes during the day. The soldiers from North Carolina have sometimes not fought as well as they might but to-day has fully placed their reputation above question. They have

[161] Rockbridge Artillery was formed in Lexington [Rockbridge Co.] with the Rev. William N. Pendleton, rector of Lexington Episcopal Church serving as Capt. Many of the artillerists were students from Virginia Military Institute, but many farmers and tradesmen of Rockbridge and Augusta Cos. also joined. They were immediately assigned to Gen. T.J. Jackson and fought in his Bde. Robert J. Driver, Jr. *The First and Second Rockbridge Artillery*, Virginia Regimental Histories Series (Lynchburg, VA: H.E. Howard, 1987), 1-7.

[162] Robert Frazer (1839-1917) was from Orange Co. and knew Apperson before War. Student at University of Virginia, he left school to enlist in Co. B, Rockbridge 1st Artillery. Wounded at Kernstown, 23 March 1862, he recovered but was sick and missed action in late spring of 1862. At Fredericksburg, he suffered compound fracture of the forearm and a wound in the leg, 13 December 1862. He was sent to general hospital in Gordonsville and then Charlottesville, and discharged for disability 31 August 1863. He returned to University of Virginia and became physician and teacher in Culpeper Co. until 1900, then moved to Farmville in 1900. Driver, ibid., 65.

fought like veterans to-day, and won for themselves everlasting laurels. The troops from Georgia fought well and suffered very heavily, especially the 60th & 61st Regts.[163]

The infantry was not generally engaged, Gen. [T.J.] Jackson's division was in the R Road and did not fight except in skirmishes.[164]

There are a large percent of the wounded by cannon shot. Many operations were performed—I notice that the prostration from wounds is very severe and [the wounded men are] hard to rally. Anesthetics have been administered in all the important cases. We have a good supply of stimulants[,] sedatives and antiseptics.

All the wounds were attended that could be and we lay down at 1 o'clock to rest—one of the stewards staying up to see that the nurses gave every attention necessary. The night is cool—every one expect[s] the battle to commence again as soon as daylight is seen.

[FIELD HOSPITAL NEAR YERBY'S, SPOTSYLVANIA CO.]

SUNDAY DECR. 14TH 1862

This morning a few more wounded were brought in who had been picked up.

The fight was not resumed—occasionally a shot was fired. [Ambrose E.] Burnside is panicked—he is evidently brought to a check—he dare not come farther.[165] Nature seems to have thrown these hills around Fredericksburg for the very purpose to which they have been applied.

---

[163] Casualties for these two units under command of Alexander Rober Lawton (described earlier) were very heavy; 60th suffered 78 casualties and 61st 100 casualties. La Fayette Guild, "List of Killed and Wounded....," 13 December 1862, *Official Reports*, Ser. I, Vol. 21, 557-62.

[164] "The fog of war" noted by Douglas Southall Freeman has again confounded the diarist. In fact, Jackson's VA Bde suffered a major assault from William Buell Franklin (1823-1903) and briefly fell back; however, a vigorous counterattack by the Bde restored the lines. Patricia L. Faust, "Fredericksburg Campaign," *Hist. Times.*

[165] Burnside wanted to attack the following day but was dissuaded. The Federals had taken a portion of the city, and their artillery barrage had destroyed much of the town's businesses, churches, and homes. Finally persuaded to leave, Burnside's huge Army of Potomac was able to escape during a tremendous rain storm. T.J. Jackson pressed R.E. Lee for a vigorous pursuit, but Lee declined because of the positioning of the Federal artillery. While McClellan was faulted for being overly cautious, Burnside's recklessness in assaulting virtually impregnable fortifications on hills and across the Rappahannock River proved even more disastrous for the troops. Burnside resigned in disgrace, and took full blame for the debacle. Lee's star rose even higher, as did Longstreet's and Jackson's, and Stuart had shown himself capable of working effectively within a broader plan; yet the CSA was damaged in this fight, for Fredericksburg lay waste and the Army of

Lt. Col [Robert Davidson] *Gardner* of the 47 Regt was seriously wounded yesterday by the bursting of a shell. A fragment struck him in the face and fractured the inferior *Maxillary* and lacerated his face very much.[166] A few others of the regiment were slightly wounded. None of the "Blues" were injured I think.[167]

The day has been spent in operating. I have not been present to assist in many owing to the fact that no one rests where one of our medical officers is. Some of the operations were very interesting. Amputations[,] excisions[,] *Syme's[,] Choparts* and a *Pirogoff* operation.[168] We rec'd more stores to-day.

[FIELD HOSPITAL NEAR YERBY'S, SPOTSYLVANIA CO.]

MONDAY DEC 15TH 1862

A flag of truce has been pending to-day for the enemy to bury his dead. The wounded at this [field] Hosp't are being sent away—taken to the R Road and sent to Richmond and then distributed to the [general] Hospitals.

We have here some 8 or 9 yankees who are claiming the attention of our surgeons. I admit that my feelings towards them are not such as should belong to anyone towards an enemy. But who can forbear to feel hatred towards such a

---

the Potomac remained a huge and well-drilled fighting force still intact and capable of doing terrible damage to Virginia. Faust, "Fredericksburg Campaign," op. cit. Official casualties were 12,653 for Federals and 5,309 for Confederates, a very bloody day's work, Thomas Jonathan Jackson, "Report No. 303," 31 January 1863, *Official Records,* Ser. I, 21:635; Ambrose Everett Burnside, "Report No. 4: Returns of Casualties in the Union Forces," 3 April 1863, *Official Records,* Ser. I, 21:129-45.

[166] See earlier description; Gardner was with Pulaski Guards of 4th VA Inf., not 47th VA Inf. "Inferior maxillary" is "a structure below the structure" of the upper jaw, and indicates a profound wound. "Inferior," "Maxillary," *Taber's.* Gardner never fought in the field again, but continued with staff service.

[167] The 4th VA Inf. in which Blues served suffered twelve casualties, low compared to the artillerists and to GA's 60th and 61st, and of course very low compared to Federal casualties. L. Guild, ibid., 557-62.

[168] "Syme's operation. [James Syme, Scottish surgeon, 1799-1870] 1. Amputation of the foot at the ankle joint with removal of the malleoli[protruberance on both sides of the ankle joint]. 2. Excision of the tongue. 3. External urethrotomy." *Taber's.* Probably amputation of the foot, given the nature of field hospital operations. Cunningham, *Doctors in Gray,* 221-22; 227-30; 268. "Chopart's amputation. [Francois Chopart, Fr. surgeon, 1743-1795]. Disarticulation [amputation through a joint] at the midtarsal joint[in middle of bones connecting ankle to lower leg]." Ibid. "Pirogoff's amputation. [Nicolai I. Pirogoff, Russ. surgeon 1810-1881] Foot amputation at the ankle, removing a portion of the os calcis [opening, or mouth of, the heel bone]." Ibid.

race[169] [?] It requires more than humanity to bear the sight of those who burn our homes [and] turn our mothers and sisters out in the woods for shelter in dreary winter all for the purpose of making us slaves to an infernal theory that "all men are equal". Here now they share the attention of our surgeons and nurses while our own wounded suffer, the few medicines that we catch and grab at different points and now must be used for the purpose of saving the life of the very men who would starve us for the want of it. The northern journals set up a most heart rending howl throughout this land because we amputate the limbs of their men without an anesthetic and give them no opiates (in which they lie) but suppose they did not—How are we to get it while every spring branch inlet is guarded.[170] Well may they fear us: well may their tyranical administration and *cabbalistic* congress[171] fear for the welfare of their keeping. Every act I extend towards the abolitionist is prompted by my feelings of humanity, and while I wait on and administer to the wants of the wounded invader, I feel that how much I would that he were dead.

[FIELD HOSPITAL NEAR YERBY'S, SPOTSYLVANIA CO.]

TUESDAY DECR. 16TH 1862

More sick were sent off this morning. The general impression is that Old Burnside has decamped [evacuated] the other side. I wonder if he is frightened!

---

[169] The diarist in typical nineteenth century language is not speaking of racial identity but of national identity, and regards the American race as a different nationality or "race" contrasted with the southern nationality or "race."

[170] Lincoln's blockade based on Winfield Scott's "anaconda strategy " for using the navy to control the coast and the river highways.

[171] "Cabbalistic. Pertaining to, or of the nature of, or like the Cabbala or cabbalist; having a private or mysterious sense; mysterious." *OED.* The US Congress, with only a few southerners representing border states, was reorganized on wartime footing with a few powerful committe chairpersons, mostly from the Republican Party, and they produced high tariffs, a transcontinental railroad, the Morrill Land Grant college fund, and a number of things that southern Democrats had long blocked; and of course Lincoln took extraordinary actions by executive fiat as commander in chief during a wartime emergency when Congress was not in session. By contrast, the CSA granted very little power to its president, and its congress was inefficient, perhaps owing to the regnant theory of state rights that kept most power effectively at the state level with individual governors and general assemblys instead of at Richmond. Allan Nevins, *The Statesmanship of the Civil War*, The Page-Barbour Lectures of the University of Virginia Series (New York: Macmillan, 1953); Frank Lawrence Owsley, *State Rights in the Confederacy* (1925. Reprint ed.; Gloucester, MA: Peter Smith, 1961); and most thoroughly, Emory M. Thomas, *The Confederacy as a Revolutionary Experience*, New Insights of History Series (1971. Reprint ed.; Englewood Cliffs, NJ: Prentice-Hall Spectrum, 1978).

Poor fellow! We will deal far more gently with him than his people will unless he pushes in to Richmond without stopping at all the Hills and Rivers.

This evening the army is in motion. The enemy have all left. The army [T.J. Jackson's VA Bde.] moves down toward Port Royal [on the Rappahannock in Carolina Co]. Dr. [Hunter Holmes] McGuire [chief surgeon of Bde.] sent an order to Dr. B. We move with our Hosp't arrangement after the army. We have about 31 wounded and sick men to be sent off—All the boxes are packed.
Wrote to Dr. F: Father and cousin Bettie.

[ON ROAD TOWARD PORT ROYAL, CAROLINE CO.]

WEDNESDAY DECR. 17, 1862

This morning before sunrise we were driving on after the army. All our stores packed in ambulances and wagons. Crossing the RR, and marching S.E. we struck the Port Royal [road] leading from *Guiney* [Guinea] Station [Caroline Co.] to Port Roy[al]. About 2 o'clock we camped about six [miles] to *Guiney.* We pitched our tent in the pines and had good fires made. Rails of course if there were many lying over near were burnt. This look[ed] hard [as in harsh or cruel] to a poor Old gentlleman [who] came to us praying for the last bit of fence he had. He said he was low on fuel. His farm was out in the *community[,]* his four sons in the army and no one to look after his property but him. I never look at this picture but I feel a deep sympathy for the suffering of those in Virginia. But what does this sympathy do? Is it in keeping with the spirit of the times? Sympathy does well when peace reigns in our land—when poets roam at eventide and listen to the voice of rocks[,] trees[,] hills and vales; but now when humanity [humane behavior] is obsolete, kind feelings are dead and honesty *gone[,]* sympathy does but little—is alone and silent.

Our camp—a piece of pine forrest where the winds cannot strike.

[CAMP ON ROAD TO PORT ROYAL, CAROLINE CO.]

THURSDAY DEC. 18: 1862

Last evening Dr. "B" received orders from Med: Dir: [Hunter Holmes] McGuire to turn back to *Guinea* Station and erect or organise a "receiving Hospital." Bright and early we were up and on the road towards the station. I walked with S[amuel]. Mohler[172] . The road was very rough and frozen. We took

[172] Samuel Mohler (1840?-1864) was carpenter probably from territory that became WVA who enlisted at Romney [Hampshire Co.] in Co. I Frontier Rifles of 13th VA Inf. as Pvt., was

a wrong road and had to walk a few miles out of our way. At the station there [were] large quantities of stores, some disable[d] guns and sick men. There are several stores with prices like a piece of ~~stretched~~ india rubber—stretched to suit the purse. Apples worth 1 copper doz. Cakes 4 for a dollar—sausage 1$ per lb. and other things according.

We moved accross the [Rappahannock] river to a house belonging to Col. White.[173] Here we occupy one room as our office and one as a dispensary: all others are use[d] for patients. A family of refugees[174] lives here in the house. Dr. B. does not expect to remain at the house long but will stay if the Med: Dir: [Hunter Holmes McGuire] agrees, if not he will move to the station and pitch tents near the R. Roads.

The Richmond Papers are jubilant over the success at Fred'g. There is *no* doubt but our success is far greater than we are aware. Burnside seems to have retired somewhere perhaps to pine over his misfortune. The loss of the enemy is reported to be 20,000—our loss is reported 2000—I think there are more.[175]

[Field Hospital in Col. White's Home, Caroline Co.]

Friday, Dec. 19th, 1862

This morning we opened a set of books and commenced to organise the hospital force.—The attendants are 27 in number. I have to take charge of the books, a thing not very agreeable. [Dr.] Chamberlain [physician steward] has charge of the ambulance train—[Dr.] *Sydnor* [surgeon] to receive and distribute the sick—[Samuel] *Mohler* [enlisted man] Gen: Ward Master—Collins druggist[176] and [Harvey Allen] Jameson a supernumerary [superfluous detail worker].

---

promoted to Cpl. and then demoted to Pvt. Wounded at Cedar Mountain (9 August 1862), he was hospitalized and then returned to duty for Fredericksburg march and battle; killed at Lynchburg, 18 June 1864. Riggs, *13th VA Inf.*, 129.

[173] Probably Col. Hugh R. White, born 1806, who had a home in Madison Township, Caroline Co., VA Census. 1870.

[174] Families were permitted by Burnside to evacuate Fredericksburg before he began his attack.

[175] Official casualties for Federals were 12,653 and for Confederates 5,309. See earlier note.

[176] Probably Van Buren Collins, (age unknown, born 1837?), farmer who enlisted at Culpeper C.H. in Co. C [no nickname], 7th VA Inf. as pvt.; "served in commissary dept. considerable time," [and thus likely to become druggist]; captured at Sayler's Creek, 6 April 1865; oath of allegiance to US 19 April 1865; postwar record unknown, Riggs, *7th VA Inf.* Possibly Daniel M. Collins, age and hometown unknown, enlisted with Co. L Blacksburg [no nickname], 4th VA Inf.; wounded, 5 Septemer 1862; Robertson, *4th VA Inf.*, 45; transfered to Co. F Winchester Riflemen

Some 25 men reported to-day. Some poor fellows were scarcely able to move — their faces flushed, voice weak and stammering, eyes dull in expression[,] watery and red. These poor fellows have done their duty and many of them are leaving to return never more.

James Cooley went home to-day and promised to return in 10 days. Dr. "B" paid him $31.50*c* for his services. I am still messing with Dr. B, [Dr.] Hagy and [Dr.] *Purifoy*—I do not like the arrangement much—think I shall board with the stewards and ward masters.

I sent to Luther B. Faris a book—"Sanford and Martin"[.] I think it a good book for boys of his age. The weather is very cold. I think as soon as Dr. B. make[s] all the arrangements we will be more nicely situated.

I have not looked around but think I will at some not distant [time]. If we can get stoves for the tents we will then be perfectly satisfied.

HOSPITAL 2 CORPS A.N.V. [WHITE'S HOUSE, CAROLINE CO.]

SATURDAY DEC 20TH, 1862

Yester-day we receiv'd some 25 men. Many efforts will be made out for the men on the day after they are received. We will be able to make a large difference if let alone. Some of those rec'd are horrid looking cases.

I am somewhat doubtful whether I shall be much pleased with hospital duty.

I have nothing [to] note that will be worth the troubles.

[HOSPITAL, WHITE'S HOUSE, CAROLINA CO.]

SUNDAY DEC. 21ST '62

To-day has been spent much as yester-day. A case of variola was brought in to-day—D[rury] W. Venable [identified earlier] paid me $35.50 to-day being the full amt. of all he owes.

From the accounts in circulation I am led to believe that the battle of Fred'g resulted in a most successful affair for us. Burnside had as well to give in.

---

of 2d VA Inf. on 8 April 1863. Captured at Spotsylvania, 12 May1864 and joined US service, 8 June 1864. Frye, *2d VA Inf.*, 90.

HOSPITAL 2 CORPS A.N.V. [CAROLINE CO.]

MONDAY DEC: 22ND, 1862

To-day differs none from days passed. We are having several cases of varioloid[177] & variola to-gether, every day. There is but very little difference in the movements, of the nurses of the Small Pox wards and the other wards. This is a thing that perhaps does not make a great deal of difference. The disease has spread all through the country, and if a patient fails to take it here he will contract it elsewhere. The disease is going lightly so far with those infected.

I wrote to Mrs.Tomlin to-night. I have my hands full—am busy during the whole day nearly. There are a few hours about noon that I am not as much engaged. In the morning I make out morning reports, and [illegible verb] returns if any are required and mark the departure of all patients sent off, and make off a list for the medical offices on board ambulance train. All deserters and men returned to duty are so marked, and notices furnished to company commanders. *Other work comes then*—copying orders, letters, & c. At night the distributor of patients [Dr. Sydnor] brings in his list and I register the names and examine the certificates. This usually occupies my time 'till about 8 o'clock. I read awhile, write in my diary and retire.

HOSPITAL 2ND CORPS A.N.V. [CAROLINE CO.]

TUESDAY DEC 23RD 1862

Dr. [Hunter Holmes] McGuire Med: Dir: was here to-day. Seemed satisfied with the arrangement of the Hosp't. He requests that a report be made of the news sent from the different regiments. This is going to be a tedious job. I shall be obliged to have the number of the reg'ts and the divisions to which they belong.

There was a R.R. accident somewhere near here yesterday or last night—we have one of the wounded here—~~right~~ left arm and leg fractures.

Dr. Wilkerson put on straight splints. He is from Georgia—the accident killed three and wounded several others.

---

[177] Varoloid, "of or related to variola." Fevers possibly related to smallpox. *Taber's.*

WEDNESDAY DEC 24TH 62

HOSP'T 2ND CORPS A.N.V. [CAROLINE CO.]

I witnessed an operation on one S.W. Adams of the 26th Ala. for fistula in ano[178] . The patient was placed upon a stretcher and chloroform given. Dr. B. performed the operation. I think it one of the dirtiest I have seen; but perhaps unnecessarily so. The openings were one on either side and all above oposite the coccyx—all [illegible word]—they were opened deeply and fearlessly with very little hemorraging [sic].

This is Christmas Eve. To-morrow is a day that has been regarded longer than any festival known. How it will be spent by our brave boys who sleep on the banks of the Rappahannock I cannot say—and how it will be spent by the good folks at home is not for any of us to say. I doubt not but many nice things will be prepared at home but will be of but little interest to the mothers and sisters of the soldiers. How I do wish to be at home! How I would like to meet some social, favorite ones and enjoy the purest pleasures of the mundane sphere! How I long to see a gathering of ladies and listen to the sweet call of feminine voices chanting the melody of some of our spirited national anthems.

I did not send my letter to Mrs. Tomlin and will do so to-night.

The news this morning is of a most exhilerating kind. The whole North seems to droop beneath the awful blow that has been given [Ambrose E.] Burnside at Fredericksburg. The Federal cabinet is about to split—[William Henry] Seward and [Salmon Portland] Chase[179] about to quit—Can we look for peace at no distant day?

---

[178] "Fistula. [L., pipe]. An abnormal tubelike passage from a normal cavity or tube to a free surface or to another cavitiy....[that] may result from abscesses, inujuries, or inflammatory processes. Ano. is probably short for anus, and this fistula may be an abnormal tubelike passage from the anus to a free surface resulting from a wound. *Taber's.*

[179] Secretary of State William Henry Seward (1801-1872), a self-made man from New York and a great power in the new Republican Party, was more conservative than most Republicans by this phase of the War; although opposed to extension of slavery, he was no abolitionist. Deft in diplomacy, he receives much of the credit for keeping the British and the French out of the War, and for restoring American and British relations to good order after several disastrous confrontations. Absorbing much criticism for the string of northern military defeats, Seward did proffer his resignation, but Lincoln was able to "balance" that moderate's offer to resign with the offer of Salmon Portland Chase (1808-1873) to resign as Secretary of Treasury. Edward G. Longacre, "Seward," *Hist. Times.* Chase, once governor of Ohio, was a rising star in the more radical, aboltionist wing of the new party, and in 1855 wrote an article in the *New York Times* that "at once laid out the bedrock gospel of the fledgling Republican Party." Twice a rival of Lincoln's for presidential nomination and often intriguing against him, Chase despised Seward, but his military strategies and wartime policies threw him into allegiance with Lincoln and Seward in the

HOSPITAL 2ND CORPS A.N.V. [COL. WHITE'S, CAROLINE CO.]

THURSDAY DEC 25 '62

To-day memorable for the nativity of Christ finds [us] as did the last covered with the "crimson tide of war." The star of Bethlehem shines through a dark, misty veil. Last 25 [December 1861] Jackson was at Camp Stephenson below Winchester [Clarke Co]. We looked ahead then as we look ahead now—with hopc.

The boys have been preparing for a dinner to-day—were up early and were beating and working eggs for nog—I did not partake. The day has been far too merry with us for the times we have. Boys in full glee while the lifeless body is being carried along to the "dead house"—Death no longer brings these feelings of the condition of the living—No lifeless frame can touch upon the feelings of a hardened soldier.—Several of the boy[s] have been a little "in the wind." [drunk]

We lost 2 patients yester-day and two more to-day, and there are others very sick. Not one single thought is expended about the awful condition of the fickleness of man's life.

Dr. B. was invited to dine out to-day but declined. We had a good dinner—turkey—chicken pie & pudding.—At night we had a good oyster supper.

We sent to Lt. Jno. John's[180] the money for some articles for the use of the hosp't.—1 Bl. molasses, 30 lb coffee and 30 lb rice. Dr. B. requested the receipts with the requisition. Lt. Johns is in the Comissary Dep't. at Richmond. We also forwarded duplicates of invoices of Med's turned over to surg. [William A.] Holt.

Cabinet debates. Chase is credited with creating a modern financial system, based on issuance of "greenback" currency not held to the gold standard, heavy borrowing by sale of government bonds to investors, and bold expenditures both on the military and on such projects as the transcontinental railroad and the Morrill Land Grant for agricultural colleges. John E. Stanchak, "Chase," *Hist. Times*. See also Sharkey, op. cit. Lincoln's skill in keeping such disparate and even untrustworthy characters on his team during the difficult days after the Battle of Fredericksburg is detailed fully by David Herbert Donald, *Lincoln* (New York: Simon & Schuster, 1995).

[180]Probably John Johns, born 1832 in MD. and living in Madison Ward of Richmond in 1870. Johns was Lt. in commissary of Richmond. VA Census. 1870. Apparently not related to John Johns (1796-1876), Episcopal Bishop of VA (1862-1876) and former president of College of William & Mary (1849-1862).

HOSP'T 2ND CORPS A.N.V. [COL. WHITE'S, CAROLINE CO.]

FRIDAY DEC. 26, 1862

Those who seemed to enjoy the holiday festival yesterday are not so gleeful this morning. I have not yet had any time to engage in any spirit.

I saw a *post mortum* to-day of one soldier who died yeterday of pneumonia He seemed to be suffering with some affliction of the brain—being delerious for the whole time. The caput[181] was removed and the brain taken out. Some adhesions were visible—perhaps incipient in their nature. When the sternum with the covering was removed the lungs were shown to be in horribly congested condition—the texture in some places broken down[,] the extremities of the *liver hepatized,*[182] and the entire lung black and gangrenous. I was busy and did not pay as much attention as I would like to have done, or read the case either. There are a great many men dying here—about 2 a day—some die as soon as they are brought in. The cases seem to be of a very severe form, especially those *inflamatory diseases* of the lungs. The patients die rapidly. This is partly owing perhaps to the depraved condition of the blood and as sure as the lungs become disease[d] pure blood becomes less and less every breath and hence the patient with a previously shattered, emaciated condition soon gives up. The variola cases are doing well. None have died—some 10 on hand now. We receive and send off some 60 or 75 each day—.

I rec'd two letters from home to-day—one from Mrs. F. & one from Mrs. [Mary] Tomlin[183] —. Mrs. F is in fine spirits, Mrs. [Mary]Tomlin not so much so—I do long to get out there this winter—

No news from the enemy at this time I think.

HOSPITAL 2ND CORPS A.N.V. [COL. WHITE'S, CAROLINE CO.]

SATURDAY DEC: 27, '62

The weather is very warm for December. Some clouds passing—rain expected.

I have been very busy to-day. Commander of 37 N.C. Reg't sent for some of our ambulance drivers to-day who had left their regiments without leave.

---

[181] "Caput. L....the head." *Taber's.*

[182] "Hepatitis." "Inflaming" of the liver, whether by bacterial or other infection probably unknown to these physicians. *Taber's. McGrew's.*; Cunningham, 164.

[183] Apparently Mary Tomlin, born 1810. See p. 117n.

I made out weekly statements of sick and wound[ed] rec'd in hosp't for the week ending Dec. 25th. Whole number for 4 Div: 463—(Jackson's 53 - D.H. Hill's 107 - "Early's" 107 A.P. Hill's 110 —). This shows a large ratio of mortality among southern regiments compared with Jackson's Old Div., which is comprised almost entirely of Virginians. D.H. Hill's are mostly North Carolinians.

HOSPITAL 2ND CORPS A.N.V. [COL. WHITE'S, CAROLINE CO.]

SUNDAY DEC 28TH, 1862

This morning is fine, warm and nice. The same influx of patients to-day as yesterday and the same disposal made of them. I have spent the day in such duties as are incumbent daily—I rec'd a letter from Father's folks—Mother & sister are[illegible, possibly traveling] to-day.

MONDAY DEC. 29TH 1862

This morning a case of pilfering came up in the hospital. One Thomas of 26 Geo Infty came in last evening and while here purchased a pr shoes from one Hart[184] of 11th Va Infty for 10$. When he paid for them he exhibited a tolerably large ammount[sic] of money—about 100.00/100. After lying down he was awakened by some one attempting to get their hands in his pocket. This morning his purse was gone, and Dr. B. instituted a search. In the boot of Hart was found a sum of money corresponding with the amt. lost. Hart made a very poor defense—gave several conflicting statements about it. He told the examiner however before he was searched that he had his money in his boot.

Thomas and Hart are both retained and Dr. has written Col: [David Funsten] of Va Regiment [11th Inf.] giving him a plain statement of the case. It remains yet to be seen what will be done.

[George] Pickett's Div, in which my brother is, is in the camp near the station. I would like to see Nat—I wrote him to come up.

News from the West is good—we are gaining on the yankees.[185]

---

[184] Patrick S. Hart, born 1838, was a farmer who enlisted in Lynchburg Rifles, which became Co. E, 11th VA Inf. However, regimental histories show Patrick S. Hart discharged because of sickness before this incident. Robert T. Bell, *11th VA Inf.*, Virginia Regimental Histories Series (Lynchburg, VA: H.E. Howard, 1985) 77.

[185] William Tecumseh Sherman (1820-1891) with more than 31,000 effectives was marching toward Vicksburg and was stopped in a fight at Chickasaw Bayou, MS. by John Clifford

[HOSPITAL AT COL. WHITE'S, CAROLINE CO.]

TUESDAY DEC 30TH 1862

Nothing to change the former routine—Hart came in the office this morning and made a confession of his guilt. He is a hard working man. I told him that the only way for him to do was to confess his fault and try to do better in the future. Thomas is an ignorant man and perhaps is very poor. I would think so from his appearance. Dr. Hagy went away to-day to see Dr. [A.C.] Smith. I wrote to [sic; left uncompleted]

I have been suffering with pain in the head to-day.

HOSPITAL 2ND CORPS A.N.V. [COL. WHITE'S, CAROLINE CO.]

WEDNESDAY DEC 31ST, 1862

To-day closes the old year and places it in the chronological table. I might make a long comment upon what has taken place during the last year but I cannot now —

We are losing a good many of our cases now—no cases of variola died to-day. I have been busy in reports—will have several to make out to-day—got invoices from surg H[unter] McGuire for Battlefield supplies—he is unjust in his requirements. The supplies were distributed to the field hosp'ts and expect[s] Black to receipts for him. I wrote to Mrs. F. to-night. I am unwell.[186]

HOSPITAL 2ND CORPS A.N.V. [COL. WHITE'S, CAROLINE CO.]

THURSDAY JAN'Y 1, 1863

The New Year was ushered in by a charming morning. The air is cool and bracing, and the sky clear and beautiful. We have entered upon another year. Our national affairs are far more promising now than at the same period a year

---

Pemberton (1814-1881) and about 14,000 effectives on 29 December 1862. Pemberton's position on the cliffs of the bayou gave him a great advantage, and cost Sherman 1776 casualties, while Pemberton lost around 200. John Hunt Morgan (already identified) "was still skirmishing near Johnson's Ferry or Hamilton's Ford on Rolling Fork, and he captured a stockade at Boston, KY." Generally, however, the western fighting was dominated by Federal forces thorughout December, and these CSA successes on 29 December were exceptions to the pattern. Long, 301-02.

[186] On this day, Lincoln signed into law a bill creating WVA as 35th state; also, he signed an agreement with a promoter offering a place in Haiti for American slaves of seceding southerners; such slaves were scheduled to be freed on 1 January 1863. Long, 303.

ago. May the national horizon continue to brighten 'till this fratricidal war has closed, and may the world never see another year of so much bloodshed.

To-day has passed like all the days since we have been here. I have been busier than usual making out weekley [sic] statements of sick and wounde[d]. The[y] report a considerable dimminish[ment] in the sick reports. I wrote some more for Mrs. Faris.

HOSPITAL 2ND CORPS [COL. WHITE'S, CAROLINE CO.]

FRIDAY JAN'Y 2ND '63

The papers this morning bring tidings of glorious work in Tenn: Bragg has attacked the enemy[187] and drove him from every position except his extreme left. Though we rejoice we fear that the news from "the left" will not be so good tomorrow. The northern mind seems to have been deeply aroused. Every paper brings tidings of the work of our Privateer [Raphael]Semmes[188] . Ship insurance goes up rapidly. There are good times ahead of us.

HOSPITAL 2ND CORPS A.N.V [COL. WHITE'S, CAROLINE CO.]

SATURDAY JAN'Y 3RD, 1863

This morning Dr. B. concluded to remove the Small Pox ward farther from the hospital. I have been sleeping with Dr. Purifoy who attends the small pox cases and if there is any susceptibility to the disease in me I stand a good chance to contract it. I have been too much crowded in the room [where] I staid and concluded to pitch a tent and stay in that. Dr. Purifoy had one put up for him and myself. I can get pure *fresh air.*

This evening a young lady made her appearance in our midst. Many young love lusted chaps are prancing around like game chickens [fighting gamecocks]. She gives us apparently a great sweep and acts in a manner not becoming [a proper lady of the Old South].

---

[187] "Bragg's Confederate Army of Tennessee, despite apparent victory in the first stages of the battle, withdrew from Murfreesboro toward Tullahoma, Tenn." Long, 308.

[188] Raphael Semmes (1809-1877) was born in MD but considered himself an Alabamian. An officer in US Navy and decorated for bravery in Mexican War, Semmes also earned a law degree and he practiced law in Mobile after Mexican War. A commander in CSN, he had support of CSA Secretary of Navy Stephen Russell Mallory (1813-1873) to "weaken the North's overseas trade" with "commerce destroyers." "For nearly 2 years he succeeded in evading his pursuers, even sinking a US warship, the *Hatteras*." He was defeated 19 June 1864 in battle off port of Cherbourg, France, by *USS Kearsarge*. Notice that Apperson uses the term "privateer," a kind of pirate, which was the designation ruefully given Semmes by US Secretary of Navy Gideon Welles (1802-1878).

HOSPITAL 2ND CORPS A.N.V. [COL. WHITE'S, CAROLINE CO.]

SUNDAY JAN'Y 4TH 1863

I have been busy all day making reports for the remnants of the past month. The day is very fine—Dr. Purifoy moved over into the pines and has his department reporting from there. Sent to Dr. [E.] Giddings Med. Purveyor's Office for some articles but failed to get them because the requisition lacked formality. Dr. J.B. Gilkeson left here this morning for Staunton [Augusta Co.]—Mr. Harry Earhart[189] was sent to Montgomery Co. yesterday to buy provisions for Hosp't. The number admitted was smaller yesterday and to-day than at any day previous. Dr. Graham is here on a visit to his Brother, who is very sick in Hosp't.[190]

I have finished a letter to Mrs. Faris and wrote one to home, also wrote Capt. R[obert] H Dungan 48 Regt asking him to save $10.00/100 for me from [John G.] Thomas from his company.[191]

HOSPITAL 2ND CORPS A.N.V. [COL. WHITE'S, CAROLINE CO.]

MONDAY JAN'Y 5TH 1863

To-day has passed as usual—about 40 were admitted at Hosp't. & about the same number was sent away. The weather threatens to be bad.

---

[189] Henry Earheart (1836-1892) was from Blacksburg section of Montgomery Co., occupation unknown. He joined Co. L [no nickname], 4th VA Inf. as foot soldier, but was detailed 31 December 1862 as "agent to buy hospital supplies and continued in that job to end of war. Buried in Blacksburg." Robertson, *4th VA Inf.*, 49.

[190] Possibly Joseph Draper Graham (1835-1898), physician from Pulaski and attached to Co. C, 4th VA Inf. Dr. Graham was wounded at 1st Manassas (21 July 1861), captured at Kernstown (23 March 1862); exchanged, 5 August 1862; and transfered to 37th VA Cav, 28 February 1863; after War practiced medicine in Draper (Wythe Co.], buried in Oglesby Cemetary, Wythe Co. His brother may have been David Calvin Graham (1841-1865), occupation unknown but also from Pulaski who joined Pulaski Guards, Co. C of 4th VA Inf., was wounded at Groveton (28 August 1862) and unable to return to active duty until 31 August 1863. Once he recuperated, he was wounded again, at Winchester (19 September 1864), captured and imprisoned at Point Lookout Prison, MD, and never regained his health; exchanged 10 February 1865, he died 28 February 1865. Robertson, *4th VA Inf.*, 52.

[191] Robert H. Dungan, captain of Co. D, 48th VA Inf. is his old correspondent who had attended Emory & Henry College; John G. Thomas, age unknwon, was farmer from Seven Mile Ford and pvt. in Co. D under Dungan; Thomas had been in general hospital in Charlottesville in May 1862 before returning to duty for these campaigns. John D. Chapia, *48th VA Inf.*, Virginia Regimental Histories Series (Lynchburg, VA: H.E. Howard, 1989) 119, 157.

Dr. [Hunter Holmes] McGuire sent for the names of medical officers who send their men to hospital that are in 24 hours after admission. I made out a list and sent him but did not make it as full as I perhaps ought to have done. Dr. McGuire had sent some papers—invoices for Dr. B. to sign but they called for so much above what he rec'd that he informed McGuire of the fact and Dr. McGuire send for them to-day saying that he will sign the whole thing himself.

HOSPITAL 2ND CORPS ANV [COL. WHITES, CAROLINE CO.]

TUESDAY JAN'Y 6TH, 1863

News from Tenn. this morning is not so flattering. Gen. [Braxton] Bragg has fallen back from Murfreesboro to the neighborhood of Shelbyville bring[ing] 4000 prisoners and 24 pieces of artillary. The enemy admits a loss of 30,600 - many Gen'l officers killed.

James Cooley came down to-day. He continues with us—Henry Johnson a brother in law of his came with him and was given employment in the Hosp't as a washer at 20$ per mo.[192]

The young lady here on a visit is a *menace*—I do not understand her—she presents several counterfeits of character. The boys still flock around her. I have been invited in to-morrow—I must acknowledge that I have not a very good opinion of any of [the] lot. I should not be at all surprised if the boys bring down a strong reproof from Dr. "B." for the noise they make every night.

The usual number of patients were rec'd to-day I think. I have been reading "The Light of the Harem" in [book title illegible] and am writing now at 11 o'clock. Dr. Sydnor heard the death of his father last evening and that together with dys[entery] keeps him down somewhat.

---

[192] Note that Cooley had joined as a volunteer, and now returns to work, for money, but evidently without status as a soldier. Henry Johnson is a different story. Also a "free man of color," Johnson faced the strict new laws in VA by which the Commonwealth responded to Lincoln's Emancipation Proclamation, in effect 1 January 1863. Slaves had to be accurately registered, and could be "drafted" away from masters to serve on work details for the army. Free persons of color had to be watched closely, and a free man such as Johnson, or Cooley for that matter, was safer working for pay with a CSA hospital than back home where he might be picked up and beaten by patrols. For Smyth Co. story of patrols after January 1863, see Armstrong, *Smyth Co. Hist.*, vol. 2, *Antebellum Years*, 129-30. These two cases show that the story of African American soldiers in the Confederacy is a quite complex one, not by any means fully told.

HOSPITAL 2ND CORPS A.N. VA [COL. WHITES, CAROLINE CO.]

WEDNESDAY JANUARY 7TH, 1863

No new scene has passed to-day. The work of one day is much like that of another. To-day the ~~monthly~~ weekly statement of men received in Hospital is due. I have been engaged at it.

HOSPITAL 2ND CORPS ANV GUINEY'S STATION [CAROLINE CO. VA

THURSDAY JAN'Y 8TH, 1863

To-day as yesterday—Dr. B sent [Henry] Johnson ["free man of color" employed at field hospital]down to Richmond to procure some supplies.—such as Stoves, Blankets, etc.

Miss Mollie [Mollie Graves, alias Miss Walker, the mysterious visitor of "counterfeits"] still has a large share of the home appropriated to her. She is quite a myth—I am at a loss to know how to decide for I would be very unhappy to decide against her character and very much to blame to decide for it under the present modus operandi.

I finished weekly statement to-day. It shows the number of 311 rec'd during the week–13 of that number died. The fatality is large. The weather continues fine.

HOSPITAL 2ND CORPS A.N. VA. [GUINEY'S STATION, CAROLINE CO.]

FRIDAY JANUARY 9TH, 1863

This morning the sky was overcast with clouds and some appearance for snow. [Harvey Allen] Jameson did not return to-day. Dr. [Joseph Draper] Graham came from the camp of the first Brigade and says that orders have been issued for so many to have furloughs. I am wanting one and think I cannot let the opportunity pass. I hate to say so to Dr. B. for I cannot well see how I am to leave. I am not prepared to go it is true.

Andy [Andrew Tate] Sanders left for home to-day. He procured a substitute and left the service. I wrote a note to him yesterday for him to come by and see me but he did not do it.[193]

---

[193] Sanders (identified earlier) was still listed on rolls of Co. D, 4th VA Inf. through December 1864, possibly because his paid substitute was not properly enrolled. Robertson, *4th VA Inf.*, 71.

I got a letter from cousin B. to-day—I had a few hours with Miss Mollie—am more perplexed than ever about her —Mollie, oh what a pity that every woman will not place herself above suspicion.

HOSPITAL 2ND CORPS A.N.V. [CAROLINE CO.]

SATURDAY JAN'Y 10TH, 1863

This morning rains commenced falling and fell until late in the night. The number of patients rec'd are not very large now.

This morning Miss Hester White came in search of her brother J[ulian]. I[vanhoe]. White who is sick here. [194] I was called upon to wait on the young lady which I did with a great deal of confusion I know. She is a very good looking lady—I suppose about 20 years old and has a very decided manner as if when she had made up her mind to do a thing she went about [it] with whole soul and body. When I first met her she was in tears. I first took her in the office and then in Miss [Kezia] Shepherd's room and went to my tent and got my register and found her dear brother's name among the living. O What a relief! What a load was thrown from her poor groaning heart! She cried more eranestly than she did before. I went into the ward and found him and then took her in and left without staying to witness the meeting. She had come from Buckingham County alone.

I was highly pleased with her[,] I admit[,] for such a woman cannot fail to reap the purest blessing that a country can afford. After she had taken some refreshments and rested awhile I went into the room where she was and had a dear old-fashioned conversation on sensible matters. What a contrast between her & Miss Mollie who was constantly bursting out in the most masculine laughs!

---

[194] Julian Ivanhoe White (1835-1910?) was one of three brothers from the White family of New Canton [Buckingham Co.] who served in Co. C Travis Rifles of 44th VA Inf. A day laborer, J.I. White was only 17 when he joined Travis Rifles. His brothers were Samuel Easton White (1841-1932), an infantryman who was wounded and then imprisoned at Elmira Prison, NY after capture at Spotsylvania (12May 1864) and Fountain Edlow White (1848-1910?), who was barely 15 when he joined Co. C, 44th.

All three brothers are listed on Confederate Roll of Honor. J.I. White was removed from this field hospital to the Scottsville general hospital near Charlottesville and then the larger Chimbarazzo general hospital in Richmond. On his recovery, J.I. White was transfered to Co. I in 44th. Kevin C. Ruffner, *44th VA Inf,* Virignia Regimental Histories Series (Lynchburg, VA: H.E. Howard, 1987), 112.

I spent nearly the whole evening with Miss Mollie and must say my opinion of her is not much improved.

HOSPITAL 2ND CORPS ANVA [CAROLINE CO.]

SUNDAY JANUARY 11TH, 1863

This morning Miss [Hester] White and Miss Mollie left for Richmond. Miss White got her brother [Julian Ivanhoe White] off [to Scottsville general hospital]. I had a pleasant shake hands [sic; his phrasing] with her before they started. I almost wished she could have been forced to have remained longer. She lives near New Canton in Buckingham County. Her brother belongs to the 44th Va. I received the kindest thanks for what little I did for her.

[Harvey Allan] Jameson [steward] arrived from Richmond this morning but did not succeed very well with the object of his errand [to pick up medical supplies]. The requisition we sent down some time back has now arrived.

I got a letter from D.F. Hagy to-day bringing me the sad news of the death of Mrs. Beaty, sister of my friend Cap't [Joseph M.]Thomas [identified earlier].

I am getting somewhat homesick and will ask for a furlough to-morrow I think.

HOSPITAL 2ND CORPS A.N. VA. [CAROLINE CO.]

MONDAY JAN'Y 12TH, 1863

Nothing worth noting passed to-day. The character of the diseases of the men is very malignant—many die a short time after being brought in.

I wrote to cousin Bettie this morning. Had a settlement of my accounts with Dr. Black—owe him $5.69c.

[FIELD HOSPITAL, CAROLINE CO.]

TUESDAY JAN'Y 13TH, 1863

I am somewhat lazy in rising most mornings—retired late at night though.

Maj. [Wells Joseph] Hawks commissary[195] sent up his account current for the month of January but it does not compare with mine exactly. Some 500 lbs more of flour is charged than we rec'd.

---

[195] Wells Joseph Hawks (1814-1873). Born in MA, Hawks "[m]oved to Winchester circa 1843 and then to Charles Town. Bought an old church in Charles Town and converted it into a carriage

We got from Asst. Surg [E.] Giddings a small lot of medicines. When we made the requisition we called for some 6 or 10 quires [sets] of paper[196] . Stationery is a thing that we are hard up for.

[Harvey Allen] Jameson has been sent over to the Small Pox ward by Dr. Black.

I have determined to make an effort to get a furlough.

I wrote to [Dr.] Snidow to-night.

Witnessed a Post Mortem examination of a case of pneumonia. The patient died last night with all the symptoms of *congestion*, the substance of the lung was dark and on being opened bloody serum exuded. In the 2nd stage of Pneumonia.

[FIELD HOSPITAL, CAROLINE CO.]

WEDNESDAY JAN'Y 14 '63

To-day is the last day of the third week—or the day on which the weekly statement is due. I have been posting the books so as to be able to make up a report promptly.

[FIELD HOSPITAL, CAROLINE CO.]

THURSDAY JAN'Y 15TH, 1863

This morning the wind is blowing furiously and tents are tossed about and several are down. Hospital tents do not [do] much good in windy weather.

Orders from Gen. Lee this morning require [Arthur E.] Collins druggist , [William N.] Foreman [of hospital] ward[,] Master Sgt [Francis]Benson [197] commissary to report to the 9th Va forthwith.

---

manufacturing establishment. Served as commissioner and superintendent of the public schools of Jefferson Co., as mayor of Charles Town, and was elected to the VA House of Delegates in 1855 and 1857. M. (1) Mary Smith, (2) Sarah Smith, (3) Sarah B. Worthington. Commissary Capt. of 2d VA Inf. Commissioned Maj. and served as Gen. [T.J.] Jackson's Chief of Commissary, 10/22/61-5/10/63; also on staffs of Generals Ewell, Early, and Lee. Postwar, returned to Charles Town. d. 5/28/73. bur. Edge Hill Cem., Charlestdon, WVA. Frye, *2d VA Inf*, 104

[196] "Quire....A set of four sheets of parchment or paper doubled so as to form eight leaves. . . hence any collection or gathering of leaves, one within the other, in a manuscript or printed book. Also twenty-four (formerly twenty-five) sheets of writing paper." *OED.*

[197] Arthur E. Collins, age unknown, was druggist who enlisted in 4th VA. Inf. but was transfered to Co. K, 9th VA Inf.; also posted to general hospitals as druggist; captured 1 April 1865 at Five Forks, imprisoned at Point Lookout, MD, and released 2 June 1865. Benjamin H. Trask, *9th VA Inf.*, Virginia Regimental Histories Series (Lynchburg, VA: H.E. Howard, 1984) 59.

I finished and handed in report for the week—229 received—22 died. A long report of deficiency disease was made out which was a very horrible and worthless job.

Pres[ident Jefferson] Davis message is in papers to-day it is among the ablest papers of our brighter days. It is lofty in sentiment, sanguine of purpose, consolatory in effect, pregnant with independence, warlike and fearless in spirit and full of encouragement and hope. [198] He thinks one year more will chronicle the end of the war. Great God grant that it may be so—that the cannon that now frown upon our battlefields will no more belch forth the thunder of fanatacism, that all of us may return to our homes and from beneath our own vines and fig trees look out upon the world as it is.

HOSPITAL 2ND CORPS ANVA [CAROLINE CO.]

FRIDAY, JAN'Y 16, 1863

The wind blew furiously last night and the rain beat upon my tent very heavily. I suffered a great deal of uneasiness about it blowing away and subjecting us to the mercy of the storm. I was very much aggravated this morning with our boy Jim [James Cooley]. [199] I got no fire or water 'till after breakfast.

Nothing of any importance has transpired.

William N. Foreman, age unknown, was ship joiner who enlisted in unknown Co. before transfered to Co. K; before transfer, wounded at Seven Pines (1 June 1862); hospitalized; released and transfered to 9th, to work with patients in field hosptials, then wounded again, 13 April 1865, and hospitalized/imprisoned at Petersburg until paroled, 17 May 1865. Ibid., 65 Francis L. Benson, age unknonw, was plasterer who joined 4th VA Inf., became Sgt., but was detailed to field hospitals; and on this day, Benson was assigned to hospitals serving 9th Inf, until February 1864; nurse and guard in Winchester and then Petersburg general hospitals before discharge, 28 February 1864. Died 27 October 1901. Ibid., 52.

[198] Davis had returned from a tour of troubled west, during which time he reorganized western army and gave commander of west Joseph Eggleston Johnston (1807-1891) the command: "To *hold* the *Mississippi* is *vital.*" Speaking in Richmond before a "serenading crowd," Davis declared that CSA was the "last hope" for "the perpetuation of that system of government which our forefathers founded—the asylum of the oppressed and the home of true representative liberty." Of the Federals, Davis was not quite as "consolatory" as the diarist says: "Every crime which could characterize the course of demons has marked the course of the invader." Quoted in Long, 308-10.

[199] Note the fall in Cooley's status, military career over and no longer a soldier, now day laborer for wages from Dr. Black; he is virtually a servant, and is here called *boy*.

News from the army is to the effect that the enemy is making some move. Things begin to assume an active appearance. Ah! How I will dislike to break up and leave here now.

[FIELD HOSPITAL, CAROLINE CO.]

SATURDAY JANY 17TH, 1863.

There is some rumor that the army is about to move, & that the enemy is making demonstrations at Fred'g again. This is as I expect and is very plain. He will make a threat here while his forces will be moved in another direction. The next battle may well be for the coast of N. Carolina.

The number rec'd in Hospital to-day is much larger than usual.

Sgt. [Francis L.] Benson the commissary here has broken out with variola. [William N.] Foreman one of the ward masters is very much complaining. I expect every one at this place will take the disease. The work of Dr. [Exekiel Martin] James [surgeon] seems about to end in humbug. [200] Vaccination seems to exert but little protective influence.

I wrote to Dr. F to-night—have been reading some to-day.

[FIELD HOSPITAL, CAROLINE CO.]

SUNDAY JAN'Y 18TH, 1863

This morning I imitated home as much as I could by changing my clothes. The day has been tollerably [sic] busy for me. I did not copy the names of those received and have it to do this morning. The result of my neglect is that I made a mistake in making out provision returns of 19 men.

Dr. Purifoy sends off five of his cases to-day—back to duty.

I received a message from Dr. [La Fayette Hall] Jordan [staff officer, asst. surgeon] to-day to the effect that Dr. [A.C.]Smith of the 33rd Va says that I am mistaken about leaving a case of instruments in his wagon. I am willing to swear that they were put into his wagon and that I have not seen it since.

I spent a part of this evening in the ward room. Two of our tents caught fire from the stove and are almost ruined.

Ward master [William N.] Foreman was sent over to the Small Pox ward.

---

[200] Ezekiel Martin James, age unknown, was originally in Jefferson City, MO cavalry unit as surgeon; transfered as hospital steward and assistant surgeon in 4th VA Inf. on 15 May 1863 by official records, but apparently serving as surgeon before May on this mission after Fredericksburg battle. Remained with Dr. Black's team through 1864. Robertson, 57.

HOSPITAL 2ND CORPS A.N. VA. [CAROLINE CO.]

MONDAY JANUARY 19 1863

This morning the wind blows cold. Dr. Black & [Samuel] Mohler are at work in the semi-annual return for property.

Rec'd a letter from cousin Bettie—no news —.

HOSPITAL 2ND CORPS A.N. VA. [CAROLINE CO.]

TUESDAY JANY 20TH 1863

Early this morning a venerable old man came in the search of B. T. Turner who poor fellow died some time ago. The old gentleman was a plain or rather rough though a professed Methodist minister from Carrol Co[,] Ga. In the evening Mr. Darden 13 Ga. Infty came here to look after some relatives. He lives in Terrell county[,] Georgia and has a son-in-law in the small pox ward. He proposed to mail a letter for me to Uncle Bill so I wrote one and [gave] it to him to be mailed near Albany. I have heard nothing from Uncle since I have been in service and why I am not able to say. I write him now for the last time *I think*—I do not wish to be importunate.

Orders were rec'd from Corp's Hd. Gen's forbidding officers and men leaving *Guiney* Station without Surgeon's Certificates and the approval of Division Commanders. This is a *stunner*. Here we have some 132 men to be disposed of and which it will be impossible almost to obtain the approval of Division Commander, and to-morrow others will come in when every place we have is full. Dr. Black dispatched a courier to the Med: Dir: asking for instructions. The cause of this order has arisen out of the reports we made relative to the lists sent with sick men for admission here.

The wind and rain to-night are disagreeable. Our tents flap and flutter in the air like so many sails in a storm and the rain batters against the tent in a manner not pleasing to the ear.

HOSPITAL 2ND CORPS ANVA [CAROLINE CO.]

WEDNESDAY, JNY 21ST, 1863

Today "Judge" Noland[201] came and reported to Dr. "B" for duty in Hospital. He has been acting as clerk for Dr. Smith for some length of time & I suppose feels as if the Hospital Department is under some obligation to him for employment. I suppose that Dr. will give him some employment however.

Mr. Thomas from Montgomery Co. was here to-day looking for Lt. Howe. He learned a lesson I think while here although he is old enough to be familiar with the walks of the world —. He requested that I should peruse the register to find what day the Lieutenant was sent here & what direction & time sent off. I did as he desired but did not find the Lt's name on the book & remarked to him that perhaps he had not been sent here; but he insisted that he had as a brother written so to him and that brother never made a mistake in his life, and spoke it in a tone a little noisy. I remarked that he was one out of the small number that never made a mistake. Before he left he found out that the Lt had never been here at all and was probably in camp, & while at dinner I hinted that the "*correct brother*" had made a slight mistake this time to begin upon.

James Cooley was taken this morning and seems to be ailing considerably. I hope he will not be ill long.

Rain has been falling all day and the wind blows very strong. Mr. [Henry] Earhart [procurement agent] returned from the upper counties to-day with a pretty good supply of provision I believe.

Very few new [patients] were sent in ~~this morning~~ to-day.

HOSPITAL 2ND CORPS ANVA [CAROLINE CO.]

THURSDAY JANUARY 22ND 1863

To-day has been a damp rainy day. I made out weekly statement of sick and wounded for the week which shows 280 received—a few less than last week. Part of the day I was engaged at semi-annual return of property. Have

[201] The title *Judge* is ironical. James Henry Noland (1834-1898) was machinist from Charles Town who served in Co. G in field officer's headquarters and then was hospitalized. Only unofficial records place him in medical department, until he is recorded officially as postwar member of Turner Ashby Camp, Winchester. Diarist entry confirms the unofficial record and explains the experiences that Nolan would offer in postwar service. Buried in Edge Hill Cem., Charleston, WVA. Frye, *2d VA Inf.*, 122.

commenced reading the life of [Horatio] Nelson by [Robert] Southey[202]—have little time to read—my tent is frequently overflowing with a boisterous crowd and though I like company it is not agreeable to be crowded regardless of whatever I have to perform.

HOSPITAL 2ND CORPS A.N. VA. [CAROLINE CO.]

FRIDAY JAN'Y 23RD 1863

This morning the air is warm—some fog, and everything is damp.

Not withstanding orders that have been issued from General [T.J.] Jackson's Hd Quarters regarding the necessary papers for sick & wounded to carry with them, I see but very little, if any change for the better, and until those orders are obeyed by surgeons of regiments it is impossible to obey it here. The Medical Department has a way of doing matters up loosely, more so than any class of men I know of.

Part of to-day was spent on the "Returns." [official reports from his field hospital] I have read several pages of the life of Nelson—bought a "Webster's unabridged Dictionary" of [General John Robert] Jones for 5$. He has [Charles] Dickens Works that I would like to possess but I fear to buy now under the excitement of the times.[203]

I understand that the army is under marching orders. Dr. B rec'd some important orders from the medical director [LaFayette Guild]—I look for a move soon.

Rec'd two letters —one from Sister Mary & one from S.K. Sanders.

---

[202] Horatio Nelson (1758-1805), British hero of the Napoleonic Wars, was memorialized by the romantic biographer Robert Southey (1774-1843) in *Life of Nelson* (New York: Harper & Bros., 1836). Southey closes this way, quoting the pre-Homeric Greek poet Hesiod [as translated by Allan F. Westcott]:

> Thus it is that the spirits of the great and the wise continue to live and to act after them; verifying in this sense, the language of the old mythologist [Hesiod]:
> These god-like spirits, through the will of almighty Zeus, are beneficent,
> and remain on earth as the protectors of mortal men.

Note that the extant editions of *Southey's Nelson* available to Apperson concluded with Hesiod's Greek, and not with a translation. The diarist seems to have known some Greek.

[203] Charles Dickens (1812-1870), the English novelist and reformist of the Victorian Era, was by far the most popular novelist in the US at the time of the Civil War. The diarist probably read Dickens's works serialized in magazines, and now he wishes to buy the bound novels; he, like most Dickens fans of the era, liked to read and re-read favorite novels.

HOSPITAL 2ND CORPS A.N. VA.

SATURDAY JAN 24TH, 1863

No new thing to-day. Prospect for moving is not so good plain [sic].

Dr. Hagy is unwell yet and it seems indeed that he will not get out again soon. He is an odd one I might say and with all deference to his virtues and amiable qualities, there are few men who present so many charcteristics of a dotage man [sic; a man in his dotage, or senility]. Simple as a child is his wishes and whimsical as some old spinster in the most famishing times of our country. His skill as a physician is good and gained as fit [or propitious] by the dint of much study & application will be better appreciated in a country practice than here in the army.

Dr. Wilkerson is a different man in more respects. Diffidence is his most prominent characteristic—he has a large capacious brain and it is well stored with medical fact, which is useful at all times, not only to himself but to all around him. I have been tempted to call him lazy but perhaps without justification. Passionately fond of gunning [hunting] he is out nearly every day. But I forbear to say more—If other eyes should fall on this I should regret it.

HOSPITAL 2ND CORPS A.N. VA. [CAROLINE CO.]

SUNDAY JAN. 25TH 1863

Another Sunday has come and gone. No marked notice is appreciable between Sunday and week days. Last night I went with some boys "around town" and returned tired & muddy and no successful enterprise to boast of. All young men should remember that impertinent dogs and divers[204] mud puddles await them in their nocturnal peregrinations.[205] Such at least is my experience.

I have been reading the language of flowers[206] to-day from a book kindly borrowed by Miss Keziah [Shepherd]. The poetry is truly sentimental but some of the expressions are full.

---

204 *Divers* is the correct nineteenth century spelling for *diverse*, and still accepted, though rare, today. *OED.*

205 Journeys, with a sense of almost piratical derring-do. The tone is ironical, since neither mud nor dogs slow pirates on a peregrination.

206 *The Language of Flowers: With Illustrative Poetry; to which is Now Added The Catalogue of the Flowers and the Dial of the Flowers* (7th ed.; London: Sanders & Otley, ca. 1840). This volume, available in many editions, featured pictures of flowers, folk-sayings about flowers, and a section "Poetry of Flowers," all in high-Romantic style appropriate to a Victorian audience.

HOSPITAL 2ND CORPS A.N. VA. [CAROLINE CO.]

MONDAY JAN. 26 1863

More men than usual were rec'd yesterday & I was busy this morning to ensure the proper execution of my duty. Part of the day I was engaged on property returns and at night at divers disputes and debates on various subjects. My opponent in every instance was Lt. [Norman DeV.] Howard[207] of 2nd Va Infty, who by the way is a sensible chap of more than ordinary comprehension; who has no doubt had fine opportunities for natural culture.

The principal matter in dispute and in which I stood alone, was the proper course to pursue in cases of seduction. The policy opposed to me was that the law of the land is not sufficient ~~enough~~ in its penalties to protect helpless females from being injured by degraded men; and that in such cases the friends & relatives of the injured one should take summary modes of punishment.

This I object to at first reflection without being able to set forth much argument in favour of the ground which I selected. To give freedom on a full scope to the revenge that seems to cry out from the blasted virtue of a relative would be giving license to a passion ten times more disastrous and alarming in effect than the crime it is intended to destroy. If the restraint of virtue and esteem for pure women and all the laws society has dictated with the moral teachings are not sufficient to break up the lust for defilement no fury and useless revenge will avail anything.

In the first place what woman allows her confidence to be handled by one whom she does not know to have the proper appreciation of her worth[?] Let her watch him in his advances and when the bounds of reason are overreached turn from him as she would from the serpent that will sting to death. Let her relatives not be lured by false appearances which in these cases often prove the bitter cup and with the penalty of our laws and disatisfaction of society & womans own value of her chastity & I assert there will be but little use for the dagger of revenge in the hands of an infuriated brother or injured father.

---

[207] Norman DeV. Howard (1842?-1900?) was a schoolteacher from Washington, D.C. who had moved to the lower [northern] Shenandoah Valley. He apparently had more training in medicine than Apperson, although it may have been informal training. When War came, he enlisted in Clarke Rifles, which became Co. I, 2d VA Inf. After several sicknesses, he was transfered to work as clerk in general hospital at Staunton and sometimes at field hospitals. In May of 1863, he was transfered to work as hospital steward with 33d VA Inf, and was soon promoted to asst. surg. After War, he practiced medicine in St. Louis, MO, and in parts of FL. He was apparently still living in FL in 1900. Frye, *2d VA Inf.*, 107.

That it will in any way change the occurrence is at once false, for he who disregards truth and honour so far as to defy knighthood's faith will not be scared by threats of summary treatment, unless he be a weak imbecile creature. You make a desperado of yourself, and a prominent individual of him you would punish, and publish to the world the stain on the character of the injured one.

[FIELD HOSPITAL, CAROLINE CO.]

TUESDAY JAN. 27TH, 1863

To-day is a damp day—nothing of importance passed. The number of men rec'd to-day is much larger than ever before in consequence of the probability of moving, perhaps to-ward the enemy. There is much talk about the enemy crossing the Rappahannock in front of our army. The correspondence of the northern journals meditate a move, and indeed say that their army is moving with Pontoons.

I am not able to say but in my own reflection I cannot believe but that the yankee Generals are endeavoring to shroud a move elsewhere which in their opinion is more useful to them. To cross here in front of General [R.E.] Lee at this season of the year would be the second attempt at suicide. No army in the world can brave the storm and tramp the land of this country and successfully operate on our works and on our army in its present sanguine condition. Let the enemy come in to his own destruction, and ere he reaches 15 miles of Fred'g toward Richmond he will turn [aside] with a shattered beaten army.

HOSP'T 2ND CORPS A.N.VA. [CAROLINE CO.]

WEDNESDAY JANY 28TH 1863

This morning snow was falling rapidly and continued to fall during the whole day. Our usual number of sick were rec'd.

D[rury] W. Venable [ambulance driver of 4th VA Inf.] was over. He is doing well.

A gentleman named W.W. Pegram from near Clinton N.C. was here with Mrs. Strickland, whose husband had died a few days previous. He tendered me an invitation to come to his house, which I shall most assuredly accept when it [illegible; sense is, when peacetime allows such travel and visits].

Miss Mollie returned to-day—the boys seem to have quite a jubilee. I received a letter from Mrs. [Mary] Tomlin. Dear old lady she wishes me to come out and how dearly I would go if I could!—how I would enjoy about a month! It might not be that she would be so great a friend as she would make me believe she is, but I have no reason to doubt her sincerity. Her letters are always full of expressions that make me believe that she is just such a friend as I dearly love—helpful in time of need, cheering when despondency would destroy hope, and sympathetic when sorrow would assail the breast.

There are some ties that bind me to that country [Smyth Co.] which I am not capable to account for. *Sporadic* as are [sic] I have never had any cause to doubt the permanency of their nature. The ties binding a person to his native place are and have allways [sic] been represented as stronger than all other ties. I have often exclaimed "whence cometh this love of country", the love that glowed in the breast of a Tuscan, [208] glows in the breast of every fine man of our country; but my case may be an exception—the home of my adoption I love. Its high mountains & shady valleys, its babbling brooks & crystal streams, meandering through the gorgeous depths of the mountain passes and gushing out in the valley beyond: its beautiful landscape as far as the eye can reach presenting a panoramic view where vision can feast untiringly throughout the short space of life, and then with open-heartedness & *unostentatious* habits of of [sic] the people are enough to warm the heart of the coldest . Such is the house I adopted[,] such is the house I left, and such is the house for which my soul yearns.

HOSP'T 2ND CORPS A.N.VA. [CAROLINE CO.]

THURSDAY JANY 29TH, 1863

To-day has passed as others have done before it, leaving only here and there a mark on *memory's* tablet. This evening I spent a couple hours in Miss K's [Keziah Shepherd] room with Miss M[ollie]—I am sorry my *good* opinion of her is unshaken—she is still a myth. Things passed that will do only for memory—do only to be locked up in the recesses of the heart. Oh! for that

[208] Tuscany is a province in northwestern Italy, whose most famous city, Florence, has since the twelvth century been the center of artistic, scientific, and political expression for much of the continent. The Risorgimento (1815-1861), an effort to unify Italy under republican institutions had just come to an end, and Italy was unified, albeit without much reform or republicanism. Many Confederates spoke of Italy's efforts to free itself from the Habsburg Empire, drawing parallel lines between southern nationalism and Italian nationalism, and the diarist may be confounding romantic expressions of intellectual and artistic inspiration from Tuscany with the effort to establish an autonomous Italian republic. The diarist in other places refers to rebellions scattered throughout Europe in 1848, not only Italian, but also Polish.

"gift" so ardently longed for by the poet that our own actions might be scanned by ourselves before they are unfolded to the criticising gaze of the world.

HOSP'T 2ND CORPS A.N. VA. [CAROLINE CO.]

JANY 30TH, 1863

This morning Capt Beck 44 Geo came in my tent & he is [sic; he has] a private house in the neighborhood—and some remark brought Miss M[ollie]. on the floor as a topic. He declared himself at once as being in for an introduction and a trial of her speed, setting to-night after tea as the hour that she would come over. A Mrs. Allen whose husband is in Genl. [Jubal Anderson] Early's division stopped here to communicate with him. She is apparently a nice and good lady—and I am by no means to[o] bold in making a bold wish for those whom I think worthy.

The day passed[,] night came and with it Capt Beck ready to launch out upon a new sea with smiles for oars in flattery's boat. He was by some means thrown in close proximity with Mrs. Allen and for three mortal hours a continuous conversation was kept up. Like Dr. Coleman the language just pours out, sensible, logical, and interesting--The many hair breadth escapes, the desperate fights and gallantry of himself and troops, then the prospect before us, the lights ahead and the desolation of our land, especially Virginia were topics mingled together in a manner that was to some extent pleasing. Touching the last resting place of the gallant dead he paid some nice and appropriate remarks. Mrs A[allen]. appreciated all, I listened to all and Mollie for one time was muted.

We left. Capt B[eck]. found on arriving at his house that he was too late for admission[209] and he returned to my tent. Very little sleep did we get—speculating [about rumors of advances and retreats to come in Jackson's strategy]

Capt B[eck]. knows my uncle's family in Georgia. Spoke of them in terms of warmest friendship.

HOSPITAL 2ND CORPS A.N. VA. [CAROLINE CO.]

SATURDAY JANY 31ST 1863

Following the bent of inclination last night, of course my work was left undone for this morning. Such is too often the case I know with all in my fix.

[209] The homeowner would not let him in at such a late hour.

Cap't B[eck] left and returned in the course of the hour—Miss Walker [actually Mollie Graves] with him. I went out shooting [hunting] with Mrs. Allen. She is as fearless with a gun as any gentleman. A very good shot too.

The boys had a droll comic tableau this evening in one of Miss K's [Keziah Shepherd] rooms. I went some time after they had commenced but am forced to say that beyond the social company of Mrs A[llen] I did not enjoy it. I took a seat near her, one too that had just been vacated and soon we were wrapped in each other's thoughts. It seemed that my reflections, which are melancholy in their nature found a responsive manner from her breast. The mountains, the country, and pure, unsophisticated sentiment she seemed to love. The nature that all must love had an ardent admirer in her breast, and her intelligent eye seemed to pierce my soul & her open and candid expression seemed to invite [me] to lay my thoughts at her disposal and bid me go on never fearing but that in her I would find one whose appreciations were holy.

While the others were jesting and passing away every moment with many frivolous words, I sat in a dreamy mood listening to her voice. I remarked to her that I had no taste for that manner of living—too light for me, too gay[210] to last. She seemed to seize upon the expression in a moment and for some length of time we conversed easily in what a young lady should be to be useful & admired. "Oh!" said she "that my sex would so conduct themselves that no eye of suspicion should ever rest upon them."

She has a cough and she asked me to prescribe for her. I left her at about 11 P.M. with an engagement to visit the graveyard on to-morrow.

HOSPITAL 2ND CORPS A.N.VA. [CAROLINE CO.]

GUINEY DEPOT VA FEB'Y 1 1863

This morning as soon as i could leave I walked over to see the last resting place of many a poor soldier. Mrs Allen & myself & Cap't Beck & Miss Mollie [Graves].

I read over the names upon the various headboards; Oh what a sad walk—we returned—I gave her my card, she having asked it of me.

The day wore away. I had a short walk in the evening and after supper went into Miss K's [Kezia Shepherd's] room and was soon t^ete `a t^ete with Mrs Allen. At first she was laughing at reminiscences of the rustic habits of the

[210] In nineteenth century, the word means happy and frivolous, with no connotations about sexuality.

mountain people, and finally coming into that same sad reflecting mood of last evening. The many sincere regrets of her life and her manner of living[,] the confessions of her heart, the conceptions of her mind and the tyranny of her will. She has servants [slaves] that are not as servants [slaves] ought to be, and which she acknowledged to fear [in potential revolt]. She seems to crave a heart to beat in unison with hers, and one that was pure and holy in its intentions and declaring before the heavenly father that every word she spoke was from the depths of her heart. She was drawn up by a question on the moral effect of conscience—She had no hesitation at first in saying that it was correct; but after a while she guessed it ought to be studied.

I left the room precisiely at 10. and just here I ought to say a few words that I may read in after days and know what I thought now. Mrs A[llen] is, I [have] no doubt a virtuous woman[.] Her husband cannot be good and kind to her—She is in trouble—her affections to me are prompted momentarily because of the sympathy I feel for her: If this should turn otherwise I will know afterwards. It is now midnight. I lay down revolving in my mind the impropriety of the evening. I must acknowledge that my feelings are more touched with the words of that lady though she is a married lady (?) than they have ever been before. [211] My feelings are pure, uncontaminated by the devilish workings of thoughts which are at enmity with virtue and courtesy.

HOSPITAL 2ND CORPS A.N.VA. [CAROLINE CO.]

MONDAY FEBY 2ND, 1863

Another day has passed and I take my seat by the rude table to place a few vagrant thoughts on these sanguine leaves.

The report of sick and wounded for the past month is done—I have been working on the register nearly all day.

Dr. B rec'd communication from H[unter Holmes] McGuire [chief surgeon of Bde.] to move the hospital because the bridge across the river is in such a condition that crossing is considered difficult and dangerous. I do not think that another place can be found in the neighborhood with as much convenience as is here, and here it is scarce. Dr. B & Dr. H[agy] rode out to select a place.

Miss Mollie [Graves] and Mrs. A. (?) came to my tent and spent 1/2 hour—Mrs. A gave me some cakes. I asked her to take a walk which she

[211] The diarist inserts the parenthetical question mark. He often punctuates her name thus, because he begins to doubt that he knows her true identity.

consented to do. We went a short way down the road but the wind compelled us to return.

Here now I may drop a few words almost in secret to myself—I am not inclined to give credence to "romance founded on fact," and believe that the basis of romance as was written by the many, who have written works[,] is nothing more than imaginary! Yet there is something connected with Mrs. A (I do not believe this is truly her name) that causes me to pay her strict attention. But this attention is with as pure motives as ever prompted the will to plan or the hands to do. She has doubtless met with misfortune. Her appearance is that of one who has seen some of the better society, but her hands look as if they have lately been toiling. Her expression is careworn and confiding and she has so casually a bright, and I must say sweet smile always about her face—shows plainly that she has a heart untainted by some of the follies of her sex. I fear she is too confiding though she professes not to be and seems to try to act her part as a lady should.

When we were nearing the house on our return she told me that she was now witnessing the setting sun for the last time from this house. She could not tell—her plans here had not been accomplished and it might be that she would be compelled to return and if she did she would tell me some secret that will astonish me! And after night she came into the room and soon arranged things so that I was thrown near her. She reverted to what she told and I asked[,] why not tell me now[?] She replied that she had concluded to do so and trust to my honour, which she was bound to say that her judgment of human nature had caused her to rely upon, to be a friend to her. And asked me too not to think any less of her afterwards though I might be astonished at many revelations she would make—stating that her life was one of mystery and adventure. To this, of course I would have been guilty of inhumanity and unfeeling heart for women if I had not encouraged an open confession of her troubles, with the promise to give my assistance wherever it would be of service, and a pledge of friendship so far as consistency would allow. She spoke of circumstances and persons as connected with her troubles. To-morrow a walk is agreed upon as the time that she will reveal her secret. Now to all this what am I to say by way of comment?

There is some foreboding in my mind I must admit, and who would not? Does she not speak of things that have not transpired? Does she wish to throw any trouble around me or does she wish to open her heart to me that the load will be lighter? Why is it that she has singled me out of the whole number of men for her purposes? Am I, in her opinion more easily duped or does she rely on me as more capable to bear part of her load? What can I do for her but listen to her tale of sorrow? Will I get into a difficulty and lose my reputation? Is she poor and needy, or are her circumstances as adequate to her wants! These are questions recorded as they present themselves, and which can not be answered only by time. I am enlisted in her sympathy and as far as rectitude will allow I am her friend.

HOSPITAL 2ND CORPS A.N. VA. [CAROLINE CO.]

TUESDAY FEBY 3RD, 1863

This morning the wind was blowing furiously and the snow flying in all directions, and the air continued to grow colder as the day wore along, though the snow stopped falling. Of course the subject of yesterday's notes was uppermost in my mind and my thoughts were as turbulent as the wind. In addition to what had transpired last night I learned early this morning that Dr. Black addressed a note to Miss Keziah [Shepherd] last night relative to some things that had been going on and afterwards had an interview with her, which as I learned amounted to a decision that "Mrs. A." should leave forthwith.—Miss M[ollie Graves] is also going to-day. An[d] yesterday while I was walking I met Dr. B & thought something shone in his countenance not very agreeable. He was pacing the porch also for some time - I would like to know his feelings towards me. All this taken into consideration I did not wonder much at his proceedings.

I feel badly about the matter and more interested than ever. I went into Miss. K's [Keziah Shepherd's] room and had been there but a short time when in came Dr. B. This was too bad! I almost exclaimed—caught again! I left the room and went to my tent and took up a piece of paper and commenced writing a note to "Mrs. A," but before I had written half dozen sentences I rec'd a message from her to meet her in her room. I went forthwith. She says "I am going this morning. I have a box here which I shall leave in your care to be sent to Lt. [Tinsley Linsley] Allen Co. "A" 58 Va. Infty[212] and a letter, which by your doing

[212]Tinsley Linsley Allen (1830-1909) was then 1st Lt., Co. F, 58th Va Inf. A farmer from Buffalo Springs [Amherst Co.] he joined what was then Long Mountain Boys at War's coming, originally as a corporal. Elected 2d Lt. 1 May 1862 and 1st Lt. 18 July 1862. Later, he was hospitalized in Richmond general hospital, 17 April 1863–28 February 1865. Elected Capt. on release, he was "retired to Invalid Corps the same day." After War, he was merchant, Amherst Court House, and became Vice President, Amherst National Bank in 1884. Died in Roanoke, 1909, and buried at Lynchburg Presbyterian Cemetary. Some of Allen's corr. survives, and it includes this enticing fragment in a letter to his mother, dated 14 October 1861: "I also saw a young lady that I love very much." Otherwise, Allen describes daring actions by the 58th, another unit in T.J. Jackson's "Foot

for me I shall be ever grateful." She then gave me a letter directed to Lt. [Tinsley Linsley] Allen. Tears would have welled up I know but she restrained them. I told her that it was with the deepest regret that I could not hear what she had to reveal—She promised to write me—I asked her for her address—She took a piece of paper and wrote unhesitatingly "Mary J. Camden Richmond Va. Box 187" and remarked as she handed it to me that that was what she wished to tell me that she had assumed a false name for only a short time but it was with pure motives. Lt [Tinsley Linsley] Allen was not her husband as she had represented but her cousin, and matters of vast importance required her to see him.

I was willing to do anything I could to benefit her, and help her in what she was trying to do.

She and Miss Mollie [Graves] started off together. When the ambulance train started—I went to the ambulance and bade her good by [sic]—I gave her 10 bits [$1.25, CSA dollars] and she accepted it.

As the ambulance rolled away I felt relieved—But who would not have been astonished to see her back again in less than an hour with a stalwart officer by her side? This indeed proved to be, in reality, Lt. [Tinsley Linsley] Allen. Now comes mystery again. How are they to do___ ? [Apperson's punctuation] Will they play out the part of man and wife? In a few moments she came to my tent and asked me to please send her box which I did. Near night she came to my tent twice and I was absent each time, but she left a message that I should come in her room. I went in and she asked if Lt. [Tinsley Linsley] Allen could get lodging with me—of course I did not object. She also asked me in to become acquainted with the Lt. I went in after a while. He is a stout built man with nothing very intellectual about his countenance and I think has some hesitation in his speech. He conversed with some diffidence and awkwardness. I remained but a short time, and told the Lt. that he could come to my tent and I would furnish him a place to lie down. I left them and I suppose they are still talking. It is I am sure midnight and he has not made his appearance yet. Let things be as they may, there is mystery sure. There is some extreme circumstances or she is as _______________ [Apperson's punctuation]. I am determined to find out. She plays the part she has undertaken rather badly.

Cavalry" active at Manassas, the Valley Campaign, Seven Pines, and Fredericksburg before he was sent to hospital. Robert J. Driver, Jr., *58th VA Inf.*, Virginia Regimental Histories Series (Lynchburg: H.E. Howard, 1990) 89; 15, 19; quoted, 4.

I have done no work scarcely to-day, and I wish this affair was over. I hope she will leave to-morrow. I am really become fearful of the true history of her life—.

HOSPITAL 2ND CORPS A.N. VA. [CAROLINE CO.]

WEDNESDAY FEBY 4TH, 1863

Last night the Lt. came in my tent, I am sure after midnight. He seems meditative this morning and left soon after breakfast. She sent for me and I have never seen so apparently as grateful person in my life. I could not find [several illegible words, sense of which is that he could not find words to say], for hope and fear were at a full pitch. She told me that she would write me and inform me where she lived and that her house should be my home.

She left for Richmond. I went to my work—Reports are made off for month of January—1295 rec'd. during the month & 90 deaths. After night I commenced a letter to her —

HOSPITAL 2ND CORPS A.N. VA. [CAROLINE CO.]

THURSDAY FEBY 5TH, 1863

This morning I wrote a letter to "Mrs. Allen" [Mary Camden][213] of which I kept a copy—my mind is not at all satisfied in regards to the occurrences of the past week. To distrust what I have been told would be unjust but to believe what my eyes tell me is wrong would be equally so. Time will prove the true nature of the affair, perhaps to my sorrow, but at all events I am determined to push my investigation as far as possible, or until my mind is satisfied. I asked her in my letter to let truth, *candor* and cincerity [sic; sincerity] have full sway in whatever passed between us. I shall make it my business to visit her if nothing transpires and [then] compare appearances to representations.

I wrote a letter home—to father —.

Snow commenced falling this morning and afterwards rain.

I made off weekly statement to-day—141 received —

---

[213] Mary Camden also liked to be called Mollie, and sometimes The Other Mollie. Since Mollie Graves remains in communication with the diarist, and he feels it necessary to refer to Mary [Mollie, the other Mollie] Camden as Mrs Allen or Mrs A to protect her, these things grow no simpler.

HOSPITAL 2ND CORPS A.N. VA. [CAROLINE CO.]

FRIDAY FEBRUARY 6TH 1863

To-day is wet and bad—S[amuel] Mohler [214] went home this morning on sort of a leave of absence.

I have been straightening up books—it is very difficult to keep books correct at a hospital of this kind.

Dr. Hagy and myself have determined to spend at least two hours each day on anatomy & surgery —. We are now working in conjunction on ["]Practice of Medicine in Neille & Smith".

HOSPITAL 2ND CORPS A.N. VA. [CAROLINE CO.]

SATURDAY FEBY 7TH, 1863

To-day Dr. Sydnor & myself rode over to Capt [John] Glaize[215] to obtain some clothing—I purchased a jacket at 10$.

The roads are almost impassable. I do not comprehend how it is possible for transportation of the army to be conducted in the present condition of the country—for an army to attempt to move now would be folly. Rec'd a letter from Mrs. F and two pr socks & mufflers from Howard [Faris].

HOSPITAL 2ND CORPS A.N. VA. [CAROLINE CO.]

SUNDAY FEBY 8TH, 1863

To-day Dr. Sydnor started to Richmond—I loan[ed] him 50$ - the new theatre opens to-morrow night and I presume he will have a good time. I would like to visit Richmond myself but perhaps my motives are selfish.

Today has seemed like Sunday—Dr. B. & Dr. H[agy] went to church. I spent a short while in Miss Keziah's [Keziah Shepherd] room. I fear the old lady

---

[214] Samuel Mohler, identified earlier, would return to duty 18 November 1863. Riggs, *13th VA Inf.*, 129.

[215] John Glaize (1822-1901) was farmer apparently from Winchester (Clarke Co.) who may have joined Winchester Riflemen militia serving as militia's QM; this unit became Co. F, 2d VA Inf., and Glaize may have been unofficial QM for Co. F. On 28 April 1862, Glaize officially became QM for Valley District with rank of Capt.; he was also Asst. QM to Forage QM of ANV. He was paroled by Federals on 9 April 1865 when Winchester passed into Fed. hands permanently. "Postwar, in lumber business in Winchester, sheriff, treasurer, jailor, and magistrate in Winchester; on City Council of Winchester, 1887-90....bur. Mt. Hebron Cem., Winchester." Frye, *2d VA Inf.*, 100.

regards me rather a hard lot. I saw an article in the "Illustrated News"[216] that I have half a mind to answer and were it not for the repulsive idea I have of "love sick sentiment" I would not hesitate.

HOSPITAL 2ND CORPS A.N.VA. [CAROLINE CO.]

MONDAY FEBY 9TH 1863

I have no news to record to-day—one day passes much as another. I rise and write the names of patients rec'd the previous day if not done the night before. After making off morning reports and taking the books over *to suit the manners of the surgeons dinner comes on and sometimes* I am dainty and sometimes voracious. After dinner Dr. Hagy with "Neille & Smith" occupys [sic] two hours which I divide as near as I can between him and old Morpheus [sleeping][217]—especially when I have a full stomach. Another hour is spent in gossip and supper is announced after which "Neille & Smith" is again in demand. Afterwards a little *otium cum dignitate*[218]—I wrote to Mrs [Mary] Tomlin—and to father.

[FIELD HOSPITAL IN CAROLINE CO.]

TUESDAY FEBY 10TH 1863

To-day I fully expected a letter from "Mrs. Allen" [Mary Camden] but failed to get one—time enough has elapsed since I wrote for a reply—perhaps I may never hear more from her and I am not sure but it would be better for me not to hear more of her.

There seems to be some probability of movements with the army. Some skirmishing above Fred'g, occasioned by an attempt on the part of the enemy to prevent entrenchments being thrown up.[219]

---

[216] A popular magazine often featuring articles about young lovers in various dilemmas, some of them no more far-fetched than the diarist's own relationship with Mary [Mollie, Mrs. A] Camden.

[217] Morpheus was the god of dreams, and was the son of Somnos, the god of sleep. However, in poetical allusions of the 19th cent., esp. those of romantic vein, Morpheus became the god of sleep itself, as Apperson uses the image here. "Morpheus," *Bulfinch's*.

[218] Literally, respite with full dignity; connotation is well-earned leisure in between difficult tasks. "otium," *Oxford Latin Dictionary*.

[219] On 6 February 1863, there was skirmishing at Wiggenton's Mills, Aquia Creek [Stafford Co.] feeding Rappahannock above Fredericksburg, *Offiical Records* 1, vol. 25:1:10-11.

[FIELD HOSPITAL, CAROLINE CO.]

WEDNESDAY FEBRUARY 11TH, 1863

To-day has been cloudy—I sent an article to the "Illustrated News" this morning—I was very well pleased with some parts of it but others I expect will secure its fate—the scrapbasket.

To-night we had a bit of fun in the shape of a court martial for G. W. Boteler[220]—one of the Wardmasters—he came out not guilty of the charge preferred.

No letter [from "Mrs Allen" Mary Camden] again to-day—To-morrow I look for "Cid"[221] [Dr. Sydnor] , and perhaps he will bring some intelligence of things in general.

[FIELD HOSPITAL IN CAROLINE CO.]

THURSDAY FEB 12 1863

I have done a good day's work to-day, though I did not rise very early. After making out the usual paper for transfer of sick and wounded, I made off weekly statements for the medical director [La Fayette Guild].

The report shows 124 rec'd [,] 14 returned to duty[,] 1 absent without leave, 15 died and 126 remaining—last month 125 remained.

I looked for Dr. Sydnor to-day, but he did not come for some cause or other. I presume that some ties held him. I looked also for a letter [from Mary Camden] but looked in vain.

Mrs. Catlett sent a garment over this evening on which she had been sewing for me—I am very well satisfied with the job—both work and price.

---

[220] Records are unclear. I can find no G.W. Boteler in Jackson's Bde. In Hokee's Bde, Early's Div., 2d Corps, there was an Alexander R. Boteler, Jr. (1843?-death date unknown) who served as Ward in Ordnance from April 1863; this same soldier, a "cadet" from Virginia Military Institute was unofficially ward master in ordnance with Rockbridge Artillery, 2d VA Inf. at this time in early 1863, and could be the wardmaster "tried by courts martial" in mock trial. Frye, *2d VA Inf.*, 85.

[221]He has begun to call Dr. Sydnor "El Cid," after the popular Romantic Era novel of the crusader El Cid (1808) by Robert Southey, whose work on Admiral Nelson he had already read. El Cid was the 11th cent. Spanish nobleman Rodrigo Diaz de Via, whose military exploits in The Crusades were immortalized in an anonymous poem, or song of 12th cent. Spanish literature [ca. 1140]. A French play (1637) by Corneille and some anonymous oral traditions added a love interest to the songs, and Southey incorporated this story in his popular novel. The idea of crusading on behalf of Christianity and on behalf of a fair damsel were both popular among young literati of the Civil War such as Apperson. Richard Garnett, "Robert Southey," DNB.

I am too *decrepit* in my journal to do anything properly or to make it interesting and useful to me hereafter—I commenced saying what I had done to-day and before I had scarcely completed the sentence I was on something foreign to it. After making out reports, I perused surgery & anatomy a while for the benefit of Dr. Hagy who intends appearing before the board of examiners for a commission. I commenced reading "Waverly" the first book of the works entitled "Waverly Magazines"[222]—I do not expect to [be] much interested in it or much benefitted.

[FIELD HOSPITAL IN CAROLINE CO.]

FRIDAY FEB'Y 13TH, 1863

This morning I rec'd a letter from Mrs. Faris dated the 8th inst —. She says she has dispaired [sic] seeing me until the war ends. I rec'd another from B[enjamin F[ranklin] *Leonard*[223] [called Frank Leonard] of Co. "D" 4 Va Infty—for a long time he has been unwell - unable to do anything because of Rheumatism. Some time ago I sent him word to come to the *r'giment*, he being then at [field] Hosp't, and some effort would be made to give him a discharge, this was before the System of Medical Boards was innaugurated, and while we were at the regiment. He informs me that he has gone before the Board[224] and was ordered on duty, and appeals to me for assistance to ameliorate his condition. I am sorry for Frank for while there seems to be but little evidence of disease from external appearance, yet he is a man of too much character to feign

---

[222] Sir Walter Scott (1771-1832) wrote the sequence of Romantic era novels called Waverly Novels, of which the first is *Waverly.* Set in Scotland, the novels chronicle Scottish characters in nationalistic vein that was warmly received among rebellious southerners, esp. in the era of the Civil War, when readers sympathized with all characters fighting for self-rule and independence, and particularly so if the characters were noble fighters who told a good tale. Leslie Stephen, "Walter Scott," DNB.

[223] Benjamin Franklin Leonard (1841-death date unknown?) was Smyth Co. farmer who joined Smyth Blues and then served in Co. D, 4th VA Inf. Wounded at 1st Manassas, he subsequently developed chronic rheumatism, and was discharged from further duty on 2 April 1863. Robertson, 61.

[224] CSA Army Medical Boards were set up to examine candidates to serve as physicians or surgeons, and Cunningham shows evidence that the boards were generally exacting and painstaking in their examinations. Connected to those boards were local field medical boards who examined patients to see if applicants who wanted to be discharged were sufficiently disabled to be pardoned from further duty. Cunningham, *Doctors in Gray*, 32-35; 286. Some of the local field examining boards were thought to be unfairly tough in allowing deferments and pardons for dismissal.

a thing of the kind. If it is possible I will get him a place in [field] Hosp't [of Caroline Co.] & I will talk to Dr. Black for him.

I rec'd a copy of the "Southern Literary Messenger"[225] from some unkown hand. I can trace it to no one but "Mrs. Allen" [Mary Camden] which may be a freak of vanity, for she has not written me.

The journal promises to be one excellent this year—[Robert Reid] Howison the author of the History of Va. has commenced a history of the war[226] which from the pains the author seems to take will be valuable. Another article entitled "Jackson's Part of the Maryland Campaign" does honor to the old hero and his troops. I have not had [sic] read all yet—I hope the generous person who sent it will continue, if not I will subscribe.

I wrote to Mrs. Faris.

[Field hospital, Caroline Co.]

Saturday Feby 14th, 1863

This morning Dr. B. rec'd notice that he had leave of absence for 20 days. Dr. Walls takes his place until he returns. This is a damper to me. I have been feasting my fancy with the prospects of a furlough but I feel doubtful now that there is any chance for me.

I have been reading "Waverly" nearly all day—can't say that I am much pleased—the awkward words tire me.

[Field Hospital, Caroline Co.]

Sunday Feb'y 15, 1863

This morning Dr B left. I spoke to him about going home, he at first thought that I might go, but then said he wished me to stay till he returned. I shall do so, but I greatly fear that before he returns furloughs will run out with General [T.J.] Jackson.

---

225 *Southern Literary Messenger; a Magazine Devoted to Literature, Science and Art* was edited by G.W. Bagby and published in Richmond by MacFarlane & Ferguson. It was virtually the only general-interest magazine for intellectuals that survived any length of time in the South and it featured essays, articles concerning scientific discoveries, and literature. Hereinafter SLM. Archives, Emory & Henry College.

226 Robert Reid Howison (1820-1906) wrote the series on the war for SLM, 1863-1864. He wrote *A History of Virginia: From Its Discovery & Settlement by Europeans to the Present Time*, 2 vols. (Philadelphia: Carey & Hart, 1846-1848).

To-day while at dinner a letter was brought from the Post Office for me. On opening it I found it was from "Mrs. Allen." [Mary Camden] To give an analysis of its contents would perhaps be unjust as the contents of this book may someday meet other eyes. The writing was in pencil and to preserve the letter I shall be under the necessity of transcribing it.

The story she tells I am constrained to believe is sad as it is. The composition of her letter does well enough but the writing and spelling show a want in that respect; however if the story is true, the reason has been given. I must say that I have thought that something similar was her history. She indulges in some affectionate remarks which seem to have a good motive. I am not satisfied yet; and I am not sure but that it were best for me to remain so and drop the matter where it is, though I have firmly resolved to find out everything.

I learned to day that she represented me as being her nephew to Mrs. [Harriet] Catlett.[227] What that *motive* could have been for I know not. I shall write her in a day or so. She did send me the "Messenger" and some papers—the latter I have not gotten.

Pickett's Division is moving to-day. I wrote by [Van Buren] Collins to Nat [Cincinnatus Apperson, his brother]: [Van Buren] Collins [228] staid with me last night —

I was in Mis' K's [Keziah Shepherd] room sometime this evening.

James Cooley went as far as Lynchburg with Dr. "B" and will be back in 3 days. I loan[ed] him 5 dollars—making 13 he is due me.

[FIELD HOSPITAL, CAROLINE CO.]

MONDAY FEB'Y 16TH 1863

To-day I have felt very unwell—late in the evening I felt better and visited Mrs. [Harriet] Catlett in company with Miss Keziah [Shepherd]. On the way she told me of something that Mrs. Allen [Mary Camden] said that of course I am not very well satisfied with. I am truly afraid that Mrs. A. [Mary Camden] is

---

[227] Probably Harriet Catlett, born 1810, who still had a home in Port Royal Township, Caroline Co. according to 1870 records. VA Census. 1870.

[228] The 7th VA Inf. was mostly Orange Co. boys known well to the diarist; during reorganization, it was placed under a new division commanded by George Pickett, and maneuvered alongside Jackson's Bde. at Fredericksburg and in these campaigns. Cincinnatus Apperson was a farmer who rose to Sgt. before being penalized by courts martial; he later commanded a post-war trainor camp. Van Buren Collins, already identified, was serving with commissary and could visit with hospital stewards easily between campaigns. Riggs, *7th VA Inf.*, 17-19, 61, 69. Scott, *Orange Co. Hist.*, appendix.

deceptive in practice. I shall watch very closely every passing event in my connection with her. I have determin[ed] to keep an exact copy of what passes between us. Dr. Sydnor arrived from Richmond to-day—He states as a reason for his stay that no requisition has reached the Quartermaster with whom he was to transact business.

He gives a favorable account of Miss Mollie [Graves].

The papers brings[sic] us news of great disaffection in the North West states of the U.S. government[229]—rumors are also ripe that the enemy are fading back—Frank Watson[230] of 7 Va. was at my [field] Hospital—I had a long chat with him.

[FIELD HOSPITAL, CAROLINE CO.]

TUESDAY FEBY 17TH 1863

This morning when I arose I found the ground white with snow, and it continued to fall all day with rain and hail.

Dr. Hagy went up to the examining board to-day but it did not convene [CSA surgeons had to be re-examined periodically by board, under guidelines provided by by Dr. A.N.Talley, president of the board). I have been reading "Waverly" [1st in *Waverly* series by Sir Walter Scott] Have a very severe cold.

I commenced a letter to "Mrs. Allen" or rather "Mollie" [Mary Camden] as she is known to me now. It may be that I am doing wrong in writing her but I hope not—I wish to continue correspondence with her until I find out whether she has deceived me and shape my action accordingly. Only 1 man rec'd to-day.

---

229 There was general dissatisfaction everywhere in the North because of the "Fredericksburg debacle," and the US Senate passing (16 February 1863) of The Conscription Act, a draft of soldiers for the Federal forces, was not popular in some places. Finally, there was contention over the Emancipation Proclamation, with abolitionists, primarily in the Northeast, saying that it did not go far enough, and pro-Union people, with no particular geographical location, saying that it went too far. There was, however, significant support for the Republican Party in the Midwest, and Lincoln's position was reasonably secure given the bad news from Fredericksburg and the widely publicized bickering between Federal officers. Above all, there was growing anger throughout the northern states from east to west about the CSA and its armies. This anger was unifying in its own way for the US. For a summary, see Long, 283-317

230 Benjamin Franklin (Frank) Watson, perhaps born in 1840, death date unknown, was a friend from Orange Co. who joined Hazelwood Volunteers, which became Co. E of 7th VA Inf. when organized at Culpeper CH. Watson was a farmer known to the Appersons in the Wilderness area of Orange Co. He was wounded at Williamsburg (5 May 1862), but recovered and served out the war with 7th Inf, being paroled on 16 April 1865 after the ANV surrendered at Appomattox Court House. Riggs, *7th VA Inf.*, 98.

[FIELD HOSPITAL, CAROLINE CO.]

WEDNESDAY FEBY 18TH, 1863

This morning I find myself rather unwell with a severe cold. Snowed some last night and soon commenced raining and continued to rain all day.

I finished "Waverly"—think very well of it. In the evening I went through *Materia Medica* with Dr. Hagy—he returned from the Crossing [Hamilton's Crossing on the Rappahannock] again to-day without seeing the [examining] board.

James Cooley ought to have returned to-day but did not. He is almost worthless—I have trusted him too much. Should not be surprised if I loose[sic] 13$ by him.

[FIELD HOSPITAL, CAROLINE CO.]

THURSDAY FEBUARY[SIC] 19TH, 1863

Dr. Hagy passed the Examining Board to-day for "Surgeon"—He merits it I think. The sun came out this evening and I felt some hope that we may have some fair weather.

I was called upon to visit a black girl over at Mrs. [Harriet] Catlett's this evening to stop *bleeding*—it had ceased before I arrived.[231]

The water is rising very fast in the river and I expect will be very high—it will cause a removal of the [field] hospital I expect.[232]

I commenced reading anatomy to-day. I wish to follow it during my spare hours until I finish it. I know I am not half studious enough for I have more spare time now than I have had since I have been in service and ought to make good use of my time. It is so hard though for me to concentrate my mind while so many are passing to & fro.

---

[231] Though clearly a racist who supports slavery of black people, the diarist generally deals with the illnesses of black patients in a Christian and compassionate, if not by any means a professional way—the era's practitioners deal with very few patients in a professional or scientific way, but rather in an "artistic" and "sympathetic" and "holistic" approach of another time when physicians held little professional standing and no more prestige than the personal affection that they earned from neighbors. See Steven Stowe, op. cit.

[232] February in Virginia, especially along the Rappahannock, was wet, with very heavy snow and much rain. Burnside and his successor Joseph Hooker (1814-1879) spoke of the "mud march," for the Army of the Potomac, and even Jackson's Bde., the famous "foot cavalry," was slowed by soggy ground, high rivers, and a preponderance of mud and snow and ice, all in amounts far greater than normal for the Commonwealth. Long, 321.

[FIELD HOSPITAL, CAROLINE CO.]

FRIDAY FEBRUARY 20TH, 1863

This morning is a pretty morning though cool. Dr. Walls and Dr. "Syd" [Sydnor] went to Richmond. Dr. W[alls] asked for me to go with him, but I declined.

Last night I told Dr. "Syd" about "Mrs. Allen" [Mary Camden] and I felt to-day that I ought not to have done so while to have kept the whole from him I could not well have done. She made me pledge her secrecy before she told me what she did but afterwards she put a responsibility on my hand that I could not keep secret from him. If she is as I would like her to be I will make all straight with her, and if she is not then I need not regret. "Syd" will look for her but I hope he will not succeed in finding her 'till I have heard from her.

I rec'd a letter from Dr. F: to-day—more of a good friendly letter than have received for some time. It sounded so much like him—like the manner in which he used to talk —. He is very anxious for me to come home—which I will do the first opportunity.

James Cooley came back to-day. I walked over to Mrs. [Harriet] Catlett's with Judge Noland and spent an hour or so —. Mrs. Catlett is a relative of Rev. Thos. Catlett[233] of Washington Co.

[FIELD HOSPITAL, CAROLINE CO.]

SATURDAY FEBY 21 1863

This morning I was up pretty early and read anatomy awhile—Dr. H. questioned me on it awhile.

The papers bring very good news to-day. The disaffection of the Northern army and the states of Indiana, Illinois, Kentucky & New Jersey seem to be doing good work. A gunboat has been captured from the enemy at the mouth of Red River. Foreign intervention is running high—[234]

---

[233] . I could not find the Rev. Thomas Catlett in the 1870 census for Washington Co., VA, and I could not find him in Lewis Preston Summers's list of antebellum ministers of all faiths in Washington Co., 1777-1870, in idem, *History of Southwest Virginia, 1746-1786; Washington County, 1777-1870* (Richmond, VA: J.L. HIll, 1903) 844-46.

[234] Confusion over naval events: On 17 February 1863, "*Indianola* posted itself at the mouth of the Red River on the Mississippi below Vicksburg in its operations against Confederate riverboats. Confederate guerillas attacked the Federal boat *Hercules*, and Federals burned Hopefield, Arkansas, near Memphis, in retaliation." As for foreign intervention, Queen Victoria on 5

I got a letter from "Mrs A" [Mary Camden] to-day. She has surely gotten impatient—Her conclusion is that I have decided unfavorable [sic] to her and wish to drop her acquaintance, which I have done by not replying to her letter—. I wrote her on the 17th and I presume she has not gotten it. I wrote her this evening informing her that I had still the same opinion that I had when she was here and when I changed that and concluded to drop the correspondence I would give her my reasons, for so doing and asked her to do the same. I told her that I had told "Syd" [Dr. Sydnor] something about her—

I do not know what to conclude as regards her. I shall continue writing to her until I find out something. Her letter seems somewhat disappointed with me.

To-night the boys had a mock trial—in which J[ames] H[enry] Noland [medical department with Bde.] was Plaintiff. [illegible; Thomas R.?] Howard in the part of the commonwealth attorney [prosecuting attorney], H[arvey] A[llen] Jameson [steward in Co. C, 4th VA Inf.] & myself in the part of the accused[235]—witnesses were examined before the jury and the case opened—after some rough sport the jury was called in for a verdict—not guilty.

Since dark snow has commenced falling and has fell [sic] rapidly and continuous [sic].

Orders were rec'd for us to remove the hospital—the river is impassible—most of the sick was stopped at the [Guinea's] Depot to-day and placed on the cars.

Dr. Walls did not return to-day as we expected.

"Aunt Kesey" [Keziah Shepherd; "aunt" is an affectionate term here] is unwell —

February 1863 addressed the British Parliament to state that Great Britain was *not* going to intervene in the fighting, "because it has not yet seemed to Her Majesty that any such overtures could be attended with a probability of success." There were mass demonstrations in British cities by labour groups and others celebrating Lincoln's Emancipation Proclamation. Long, 318-19.

[235] Thomas R. Howard, age unknown, was asst. surgeon with staff, 9th VA Inf., Trask, *9th VA Inf.*, 73; Noland of med. dept. already identified; and Jameson, steward in Co. C, 4th, already identified.

[ON THE MOVE IN CAROLINE CO.]

SUNDAY FEBY 22ND 1863

To-day has been the most disagreeable day I have seen for a long time. The wind blew rapidly from the north and wind and hail fell all day. The snow drifts about very much —

The cars did not come up from Richmond to-day until about night. I have spent the day in reading and sleeping when I was not *bored* by some of the boys who were too lazy to keep fires in their own apartments. During the evening I was sleeping.

This has truly been a day for sad reflection. How many poor soldiers are to-day shelterless. Longstreet's corps being on the march. To-night when they stop, if they started at all to-day, where will they repose their weather-beaten & wearied limbs...[diarist's elipsis marks] But is there not a sadder picture yet? Does not the poor widow and orphan suffer from this chilling wind[?] Does not the poor wife whose husband is far away in camp look at her darling babes with the strong affection of a mother's love and feel that this storm is an awful visitation of God's power[?] To whom does the widow, who[se] only son has laid his life on his country's altar, or now stands on the banks of the Rappahanock watching the moving bodies of the motley race for the opposite shore and warn them that he still watches at his post[?]—I say what does his poor helpless mother rely on for wood and water and provision while this storm rages[?] Oh 'tis sad.

Aunt Kesey is something better to-day—I was in her room twice.

[ON THE ROAD IN CAROLINE CO.]

MONDAY FEBY 23RD 1863

This morning Dr. W[alls]. and Dr. Syd came from Richmond—Dr. S. was "booming" as the boys say.

The morning is quite clear and cold. The snow is about 8 inches deep —. Orders were received for the Hospital to be removed as soon as the condition of the weather will admit. Also orders from Dr. [La Fayette] Guild [ANV medical director in the field] for all the ambulance wagons to be repaired.

Dr. Walls has concluded to send Dr. Syd down to the [Guinea's] Depot with a few tents and receive and send off such men as come there for transportation—Now this arrangement is sure to work badly. It is with a great deal of difficulty that any system is observed here where all work to-gether and for one part to be there—and the other here: I feel very doubtful of the result.

I rec'd of Cousin Bettie 2 pr nice socks with a letter—she is a kind, good girl. Have been reading Dr. Dick's work on *Benevolence and Education.*[236]

[TEMPORARY FIELD HOSPITAL, TENTS, CAROLINE CO.]

TUESDAY FEB'Y 24, 1863

This morning Dr. Syd moved down—I think from the array of nurses that they intend to enjoy themselves. [Probably male nurses, and the enjoyment is most likely drinking and gambling; the context of other remarks is that the culprit here is the male nurses and not Dr. Sydnor]

I have been reading a work on "Marriage as it is and as it should be."[237] I am not well conversant with the standard that such works should come to; but I feel sure that the work is one of merit. It is dedicated to "My affectionate wife Lizzie Lee."

I received a letter from *Mollie* [Mary Camden, Mrs A]. Indeed I do not know what course to pursue. For me to throw out any inducements that would lead her to presume upon my affection, except as a friend would be unpardonable in

---

236 Thomas Dick (1774-1857) was a Scottish astronomer responsible for publicizing and popularizing astronomy in a number of books and essays accessible to the "lower and middling classes" of the British population. Son of a linen manufacturer in Scotland, Dick was raised in strict Calvinist religious traditions and was always as much interested in religion as in science. Defying his father's wishes, he studied science rather than working in the family linen manufacturery, and he became a school teacher determined to do two things: 1) show the "connexion of science and philosophy with religion" and 2) to make astronomy something that the average British citizen could understand and enjoy— and within a context of believing Christianity. To accomplish these goals, he left the Scottish schools and moved to London, where he studied the "sidereal and celestial universe" with powerful telescopes and wrote extensively. Author of highly regarded scientific papers, he was elected to the Royal Astronomical Society by practicing astrophysicists who admired his research, but he was granted honorary doctoral degrees because of his activites in popularizing science and in promoting the "connexion" between science, philosophy, and religion; his first honorary degree came from Union College in NY, and he from the late 1830s was refered to as Dr. Dick. He helped start a magazine, *Educational Magazine and Journal of Christian Philanthropy,* personally editing the first three volumes (1835-36) and contributing speeches and editorials thereafter until his death in 1857, one of which may be this pamphlet concerning benevolence and education that the diarist is reading. Agnes Mary Clerke, "Dick," DNB.

237 John Bayley, *Marriage as It Is and as It Should Be* (New York: M.W. Dodd, 1857). John Bayley (born 1814) wrote this widely disseminated book of some 117 pp on the morality of marriage in the Victorian Era. He apparently was not related to the great British jurist Sir John Bayley (1763-1841) who wrote on legal matters but also wrote on moral matters for the Anglican church; and he apparently was not an ancestor of the 20th century essayist and novelist John Bayley.

me; if she has deceived me in regard to the position she occupies in life that that [sic] friendship would not find accordance in my heart. I shall continue some further, and visit her when I have an opportunity to do so and then I can decide what course to pursue.

I was introduced to Mrs. Hagy to-night—she came here day before yesterday—she seems to be a good cheerful lady—very good looking.

[TEMPORARY FIELD HOSPITAL IN TENTS, CAROLINE CO.]

WEDNESDAY FEB'Y 25, 1863

This is a beautiful morning. Almost warm enough without fire.

Sgt. Nelson[238] of Capt. [John] Glaize forage train came in my tent this morning and we got into conversation. He asked me to write him after the war. He gave me his address—"J.P. Nelson, Prof. of Math & Nat. Science, Martinsburg, Va." He is looking to a situation as professor in some college after the war. I know nothing of the gentleman except to recognize him when I see him. I expect however that he is a very nice gentleman. He is a married man.

I was called over to Mrs. [Harriet] Catlett's this evening to open a large abscess[239] in the side of a child's neck. I went over and had a chat with Mr. C[atlett].—the first time I have ever [met] him—was introduced to a Mr. Johnson. Had a game of backgammon with Miss Annie [possibly the daughter of the Catletts] opened the abscess and returned. Wrote a letter to Cousin Bettie[,] settled with my washer woman and retired—suffering very much with head-ache, from a cold.

[FIELD HOSPITAL IN TENTS, CAROLINE CO.]

FEBY 26TH 1863 THURSDAY

This morning I rose with a very disagreeable head-ache and felt very unwell for some time after noon. I took a large dose of Morphia [a form of morphine used for painkilling] which helped me somewhat.

---

[238]There is no J.P. Nelson recorded in 2d VA Inf., from which Capt. John Glaize (identified earlier) formed the forage train for the Bde on this march. The Nelsons listed in 2d VA Inf. are not sergeants and are assigned to other duties at this time. However, the forage train apparently kept inexact records, and there may be no full list of the personnel working on Capt. Glaize's forage train on this campaign. See Frye, 2d VA *Inf*, passim.

[239] "Abscess,....L., abscessus, a going away, a localized collection of pus in any part of the body which is the result of disintegration or displacement of tissue." *Taber's.*

Miss Mollie Graves came to-day —. Somewhat surprised I was to see her—I got a letter from Mrs. [Mary]Tomlin—Dear old lady she never writes a letter but she touches upon the preparation that all of us should make for the grave. She informs me that Dr. Beatie[240] died in Richmond on the 15th with Small Pox. This is a very sad death. He had been married only a few months to a lovely young lady. Now he is in eternity before the throne of justice. Oh! how I wish I could live a holier and better life.

Mrs. T [Mary Tomlin] wishes me to come out [to Smyth Co]. She says she will speak a good word to Miss *Amelia* for me if I will determine not to marry any of her kith[241]—This gets me. I did not know that she would have thought such a thing. I wonder who she would select for me of her numerous connections.

I wrote to Miss Mollie [the "other Mollie," Mary Camden, Mrs. A] to-night. I am getting somewhat distrustful about the propriety of my course. I do not see [any]thing to where I am to blame—It is a private correspondence and with pure motives on my part—I am more and more of the opinion every day that she is leading a romantic life—and perhaps in circumstances that are somewhat embarrassing.

I was in "Aunt Kesey's" [Keziah Shepherd] room and she showed me a letter that she had gotten from Mollie [possibly Mollie Graves, but more probably Mary Camden, Mrs. A]—I of course read it with interest. I made off weekly report to-day—115 rec'd[,] 4 returned to duty[,] 102 sent to *Gen* Hosp't and 8 died during the week.

I am much better to-night.

---

240 Possibly Claiborne Watkins Beattie of Chilhowie, a descendant of Col . Robert Beattie who had helped found the town of Chilhowie. Local-historian Goodridge Wilson, who was always very careful in such matters, appeared to think that Dr. Beattie was a different person than Claiborne Watkins Beattie, and Wilson was uanble to find full identification of this other Beattie who was a physician. Wilson, Smyth Co..

241 *Kith* originally refered to *fellow countrymen*, that is, neighbors of the countryside. During the late-nineteenth cent. the word came to mean friends and acquaintances, and by the turn of the century, the phrase *kith and kin* refered so broadly to relatives that *kith* was sometimes used by itself to refer to relatives. *OED*. Apperson is obviously quoting a lady's use of the term as the term is changing its meaning. Given the context of Mary Tomlin's remarks recorded elsewhere in Apperson's memoirs, she seems most likely to be using the term to mean those of the same class or "quality," viz., with some landed property and slaves as well as some education, membership in a Protestant church, and "prospects." She seems to say , thus, that "Amelia" is not the "right kind" of person for Apperson to marry, being too poor.

HOSP'T 2ND CORPS A.N. VA. [TEMPORARY TENTS, CAROLINE CO.]

FRIDAY FEBRUARY 27TH, 1863

This is a damp morning—The business of to-day has been small—The river has been too high to allow the sick to cross to the [Guinea's Depot].

I have been doing nothing of any importance to-day. The boys had a bogus court's martial and had some fun. Dr. Wilkerson[242] made an inefectual[sic] attempt to send up a paper ballon—it took fire soon after it started up.

I spent a short while in Mrs Keziah's [Shepherd] room—Miss Mollie [Mary Camden] does not seem well disposed to-wards me.

I loan[ed] "Judge" Noland[243] 10$ to-night not altogether in accordance with my feelings—he promised to return it in two days. Here lies one of my weak points. If a person asks me to loan money I almost involuntarily do so. I have tried to save my wages and have been successful to a satisfactory degree but the way of letting Tom, Dick, and Hary[sic] have money is doing myself great injustice. There is due me at this time over 100$ loan money and most of it in small ammounts. How I am to collect this I do not exactly see. A hundred dollars to me is a good deal, and the loss of it would be keenly felt.[244]

HOSPITAL 2ND CORPS ANVA [CAROLINE CO.]

FEBUARY[SIC] 28TH 1863

To-day I have been working on monthly report. None of the sick could be sent away because of the water being too high.

---

[242] Possibly William H. Wilkerson (1838-1895) a salesman in Farmville (Prince Edward Co.) who enlisted in Randolph Guard of Prince Edward Co., which became Co. G, 44th VA Inf. He later served as nurse and in medical dept. throughout War, although there is no record of him being trained as a physician. He did attain officer's rank on staff, possibly as Capt., definitely as 1st Lt. After serious wound at Spotsylvania (10 May 1864), his leg was amputated, and he worked as clerk in Richmond medical offices after hospitalization. He was granted a CSA pension by VA and lived out his life after War in Farmville, but there is no record of practicing medicine in postbellum years. Ruffner, *44th VA Inf.*, 112.

[243] So-called because he served as judge in some of the mock courts-martial trials the boys held. Probably James Thomas Noland (1832?-death date unknown), a laborer from Gordonsville (Orange Co.) who strung telegraph wire for 13th VA Inf. and then drove ambulance wagons for Jackson's Bde on this campaign. Spelling of surname unconfirmable. Riggs, *13th VA Inf.*, 131.

[244] Even in this time of rising inflation for CSA currency, one hundred dollars could still buy almost a full month's room and board;or it could buy a month's worth of servant's labor (as from James Coolley); or it could buy several pair of pants and shirts—or the tuition charges for a semester's "readings" at the Medical College of Virginia—the most likely object of Apperson's efforts to save money.

I rec'd another letter from Mollie [Mary Camden]. She seems to rely upon me as a gentleman and gives her reliance as a reason for the confidence she placed in me. Her letters are very much wanting in correctness—both in spelling and composition. However it will not do to judge by this of her character and standing for I have known several estimable ladies that were deficient in that. That she is pure in principal [sic] she seems to declare and wishes me to visit her in Richmond.

There are two things that prompt me to pursue the course that I do. Curiosity and high regard for female worth.—Curious to know what her true standing is. [T]hat I may not do injustice to human nature and my regard for female character and feelings prompt me to continue that every suspicion may be laid aside, or if unfavorable to give proper attention to my steps hereafter. I wrote to Dr. Faris to-day. [Moot trial official] Judge [James Thomas] Noland paid me the 10$ he borrowed last night.

Mr. [J.P.] Nelson [would-be professor] of Q.M. Dept is a guest of mine to-night.

HOSPITAL 2ND CORPS A.N. VA. [CAROLINE CO.]

SUNDAY MARCH 1ST 1863

This is another sabbath. With us it has not been spent as profitably as it should have been. I do feel that I ought to consider more about my prospects to leave this mundane sphere. I was reading Dr. [Thomas] Dick's "Proofs of a Future State" this morning, and was struck with the force of the argument that only three states can exist—only three dispositions can be made of man [:] Heaven or Hell or Annihilation.

A book entitled "Grace Truman" [245] was handed me to-day and, I soon became interested in it. It is a *religious* publication—or a sort of theological fiction—or religion and romance combined and very sectarian.

[245] Sallie Rochester Ford, *Grace Truman, or Love and Principle* (New York: Sheldon & Co., 1857). This 499 page novel was widely distributed for more than 50 years, the later editions including an essay "How I Came to Write Grace Truman," by the author Ford (1828-1910), a believing Baptist. In later years the novel was distributed by the American Baptist Publishing Society. The novel deals with questions of sin, redemption, and a radical conception of salvation by grace alone accomplished by adult baptism. When the diarist refers to the sectarian focus and to the group interested, he is talking about the Baptists.

Aunt Kesey [Keziah Shepherd] and Miss. M[ollie Graves] came in my tent and spent several hours—Dr. Walls was in also. I went in the house and joined in singing a couple of hymns:

No mail to-day—I learn that a RRoad Bridge has been carried away by the late freshet, and the cars will not be up for several days—perhaps.

[FIELD HOSPITAL IN TENTS, CAROLINE CO.]

MONDAY MCH: 2ND 1863

This morning I commenced the monthly report and by evening I was ready to put it to-gether, but on reflection I find there was no blanks on hand and I defered it to obtain one from the Medical Director [La Fayette Guild].

I have read nearly half through "Grace Truman" [by Sallie Rochester Ford]. As to the merits of the work I cannot say much. I cannot exactly reconcile novel reading [and] religion—although most of our light reading on sacred subjects is imaginary.

Baptism seems to be clearly proven, and as a matter of course close communion follows in its wake. I have no doubt the work will do much good for the church [American Baptist] it is intended to favor. I bough[t] a lot of books for Aunt Kesey to-day—Paid 20$. I am satisfied with the purchase. The works of Dr. [Thomas] Dick, Dryden, Josephus (several)[,] Franklin, and Clarke's *Commentaries* are among the most important[246] .

---

[246] Thomas Dick was already identified; these are religious tracts concerning charity and benevolence, scientific reason and Christian belief. John Dryden (1631-1720) was poet, dramatist, essayist, and critic of the English Restoration period for the Stuart kings; he fell out of favor after Glorious Revolution of 1688-89, but continued to write poetry of highest quality. Of his *Collected Poetry* [which is probably what the diarist is reading], James Kingsley says, "He set the tone of English poetry for nearly a century." Quoted, Kingsley, "Dryden," *Collier's Encyclopedia.* Flavius Josephus (37-100) was a Jewish soldier and historian born to a noble family who reluctantly joined a Jewish rebellion against the Roman Empire. A poor general, he and his fellow rebels lost, as he feared that they would; and he entered into service to Roman noblemen, sometimes in the Emperor's court, esp. after 70 CE, when Jerusalem was destroyed by the Empire. He wrote history of Jews, *The Jewish Wars* (ca. 90; English trans. and reprint, ca. 1860) and *Antiquities of the Jews* (ca. 90; Eng. trans. and reprint, ca. 1860) and wrote defenses against anti-Jewish prejudice, *Against Apion* (ca. 90; Eng. trans. and reprint, ca. 1860) and his autobiography, *Apologia Pro Sua Vita* (ca. 90; Eng. trans. and reprint, 1860); widely read and quoted, his works make fine reading and have an inspiring, even bracing teleological dimension, but are not reliable as to chronology or facts. Benjamin Franklin (1706-1791) was the Renaissance person of the Revolutionary and Early National periods of US history. Author of many scientific papers and political essays, his most widely distributed *Poor Richard's Almanack* (1732; constantly reiussed) established a cultural norm for American ideals of hard work, thrift, industry, study, dedication, and common sense

I was invited over by Mrs. [Harriet] Cattlett to meet some young ladies. I was introduce[d] to Miss Mary *Tattaille* , a very handsome nice lady—returned about 11 o'clock and retired.

HOSPITAL 2ND CORSP A.N. VA. [CAROLINE CO.]

TUESDAY, MARCH 3RD, 1863

To-day the hospital is being moved. I do not like to leave the present place. I took the Books I purchased and put my name on the first leaves and packed them away to be transported.

Miss Mollie [Graves] came in my tent to-night and for once she talked quietly for a short time. She promised to look after the other Mollie [Mary Camden]. I did not give her any clue that will implicate me in any way. I will not prove traitor to any confidant[e] [person who confides] [,] though of [sic; if] M[ollie]. G[raves]. can find out anything it will be thankfully received and properly appreciated. She formed a better opinion of "Mrs. A" [Mary Camden] than did anyone else.

I wrote Mollie C [Mary Camden]. a letter to-night. I looked for one from her to-day but none came.

James Cooley went to Richmond to-day without saying anything to me.

HOSPITAL 2ND CORPS, A.N. VA. [CAROLINE CO.]

WEDNESDAY; MARCH 4TH, 1863

This morning the weather is cool—I finished "Grace Truman" [by Sallie Rochester Ford]—I did not read it as carefully as I ought to have done and hence was but little benefitted by the arguments on baptism between [fictional characters] Mr. Lewis and Mr. Jordan. There are some fine characters in the book and things are so intricately interwoven with romance that any reader may become interested in the disputes. I am unable to give any opinion that would be of any value in discussing the merits of the work. There is perhaps a little too much coloring in the story.

---

within a context of republican virtue and natural philosophy. Adam Clarke (1727-1832) was a British theologian educated by sponsorship from Charles Wesley. Clarke was an astute scholar of the Bible, and he provided a scholarly foundation for Methodist interpretations of Christian belief. His commentaries on the texts, esp. of the New Testaments, were very influential for all Protestants of the Civil War era. Idem, *The Holy Bible...with a Commentary and Critical Notes...*(2d rev. ed.; New York: G. Lane & C.B. Tippett for the Methodist Episcopal Church, 1847). Hereinafter *Clarke's Commentaries.*

I made preparations for moving over this morning but did not go. To-morrow I guess I shall move off.

Quite a gay party assembled in Mrs K's [Keziah Shepherd's] room. Some very good songs were sung—"Do they miss me at home"? "Gentle Annie", "Twenty years ago"—"Good by [sic]" —

I wrote a letter to Mrs. Wainscott of Little River, Alexander Co. N.Ca. in answer to inquiries about the death of her husband who died a few weeks ago. It is with deep regret that I could not give her such information concerning the last moments of the life of her husband. It is impossible for us to know what [was] the last messages of the dead —The nurses may at times know the last words but soon it will be forgotten. —

HOSPITAL 2ND CORPS, ANV [CAROLINE CO.]

THURSDAY, MARCH 5, 1863

This morning early, I struck my tent and moved over to the new site for the hospital. I have never seen roads in such a condition as they are now. None can form any idea of their true condition unless used to them.

The spot chosen for the hosp. is a bleak, barren ridge. When the wind blows from the west nothing interrupts its course 'till it strikes our tents, and I expect they will soon be torn into shreds —

James Cooley has not returned yet. I am resolved to hire him no longer —.

To-day the weekly report is due but I could not make it —

I received letter from Mollie [Mary Camden] to-day—. She seems very solicitous for me to pass through Richmond. I am growing colder in my feelings to-wards her. I fear she cannot keep up what she professes to be—some of that dignity that makes woman beautiful in the eye of man is wanting.

I received $11.25c. of Maj. [Wells Joseph] Hawks [commissary] for commutation of Rations not drawn while traveling from Winchester to the army near Fredericksburg.

[FIELD HOSPITAL, CAROLINE CO.]

FRIDAY, MARCH 6, 1863

This morning I arose with a severe cold. The wind threatens to upset the whole concern and cuts very keenly—. Very few sick are sent in now. I made out weekly statements to-day—158 recd [,] 5 Re[turned to] Duty [,] 137 sent to Gen'l Hospt. and 13 died.

Nearly all the Hospt. property is moved over —

HOSPITAL 2ND CORPS, ANV [CAROLINE CO.]

SATURDAY, MCH. 7, 1863

Dr. Hagy came from Richmond to-day. Jas. Cooley went home. This is as I expected. He cannot be depended upon. I have favored him in every instance that I could and now he has shown himself ungrateful. However, I am glad he has gone as it saves me the trouble of refusing to hire him ever and I will save my money. He was owing me 13$ but Dr. Hagy did not settle with him so I am safe [Hagy can deduct the debt from what he pays Cooley]. He has allowed Dr. Black's saddle to be misplaced and his horse to be used scandalously. This though is not Cooley's fault entirely. The horse was left in charge of Dr. Walls. I know Dr. B will be angry when he returns.

Henry Earheart [Co. L, 4th VA Inf.] , agent to purchase supplies[,] returned to-day from the lower end of Wythe County.

Dr. Hagy brings us the news that Chamberlain of this corps who has been attending medical lectures [at Medical College of Virginia, Richmond] passed for an M.D. at the course examinations at the close of the sessions.

I am glad to hear it. While I am envious and self accusing, I must do something for myself. I ought to have made some effort to have attended lectures this past winter myself. I am unpleasantly situated. I fear that one on whom I look as a friend [Dr. Harvey Black] is careless of my interest while he is very anxious that I should remain with him that my services may be available. I am determined to busy myself to some purpose next fall. I have saved money enough to take me through one course and I am going to get it if there is any possible chance. Another thing [is that]I ought to apply myself more diligently while here.

I finished monthly [reports] to-day—The number received during the month is 493—57 deaths occurred—31 of which were from variola. This disease has been very fatal. The percentage is about 33—Whether this is owing to a want of attention or to the exposed condition of the hospital I am unable to say.

Dr. Syd[nor] went up to Hamilton's Crossing [on the Rappahannock River] to-day—sent a requisition by him for 1 bbl of whiskey—got 20 gallons.

I have been feasting myself on the anticipation of a trip home as soon as Dr. B returns—I cannot say whether I shall be successful or not.

I received a letter from Cousin Bettie to-day —

[FIELD HOSPITAL TENTS, CAROLINE CO.]

SUNDAY, MARCH 8, 1863

Another sabbath has come and gone, another week of our life is measured of[f], and the shore of that boundless sea, eternity, is drawing nearer and nearer as the weeks come and go. How many since the last sabbath has [sic] left this mundane shore and launched out on that limitless ocean? How many too are there that have made preparation for the voyage? Have for their pilot Him whom the wind and sea obey? How many are now struggling with the waves of despair and longing for help when no arm can save them, and crying out, "lost, lost!"

To-day I read in the papers that three citizens of my county [Smyth] came to a most shocking death by falling on a mill wheel while in motion, they being in an inebriated condition. Deplorable indeed are their vessels for this ocean wave that tossed them into the presence of their maker. Oh! How sad! I see around me each day promising young men degrading their character, dissipating their money, wasting the precious times of youth, and drowning their intellect by the intoxicating bowl. God grant that I may ever have the spirit to refuse a participation in so abominable and sinful a habit. How I wish I were a Christian and could leave off the sins that I know I commit every day.

I received a letter from Mollie [Mary Camden] to-day. The last letter I wrote her seems to have disturbed her mind very much. She writes me a long letter giving her reasons for coming up here and her business with Lt A [Tinsley Linsley Allen]—she also assures me of the honorable position she holds in society [and] refers me to Dr. Brown[247]. I am somewhat convinced that at least a part of what she says is correct. I can never give up [the fear] that she is not a pure woman until I see for myself. She writes like a woman that has been bowed down by sorrow and whose spirit is brave. I feel deeply for her and oh! that I *knew* that all I have heard is true. I answered her letter as best I could—I do not wish to commit myself in any way for if I find out that after her repeated pledges of sincerity and truth she has intended to deceive me I shall give her some wholesome advice and retire. My feelings towards her are those of sympathy.

---

[247] Possibly Dr. Bedford Brown, a surgeon based in Richmond during the War who sometimes served in the field. Bedford Brown, a North Carolinian born in 1825, eventually made his home in Alexandria. VA Census 1870. Cunningham, 185, 187n.

I looked for Dr. [Bedford?] Brown to-day but he did not come.

The day has been very good—a bit windy—. I have been reading the description of the Texans from Texas to Fred'g. I am prejudiced against the work as everyone will be who is not a Texan. I will not criticize any point of it.[248]

HOSPITAL, 2ND CORPS ANV [CAROLINE CO.]

GUINEY'S DEPOT, [SUNDAY] MRCH 9, 1863

This is a lovely spring morning—so much like the weather I allways [sic] loved at home [Smyth Co.].

Dr. Chamberlain came up to-day. Although he took the degree of M.D. he pronounces the course there [at Medical College of Virginia, Richmond] emphatically a humbug. He says the standard is low and very little is learned. This I am sorry for I do hope the standard of medical education will be raised. I have the fierce ordeal to pass through and I wish to have a fair trial at some good school, I hope.

Dr. B did not come to-day —. I finished the Texas Campaign to-day. Sent Surg. Gen. [S.P. Moore] duplicate receipts of articles received of Med. Dir. [La Fayette Guild] and forwarded acknowledgments to him of the receipts.

The boys have all gone to the old hospital [the private home in Caroline Co.] to give the parting trick to Miss Mollie [Graves]. I am below par there, I know, and therefore I did not trouble anyone with my presence.

---

[248] Texans at home were overwhelmed with frontier fights against Native Americans, but they were generally successful at holding off Federal forces, retaking any positions lost until 1864. More famous, or infamous, were the two large Texas units who went east, one under the transplanted Kentuckian John Bell Hood (1831-1879) and another under Texas sugar planter Benjamin Franklin Terry . Effective in combat, the troops were notorious for reckless maneuvers in the field and untrammeled behavior in camp and countryside between campaigns. Terry's Texas Rangers were a feared cavalry unit, widely credited for popularizing the "Rebel Yell," and his Rangers "ride like Arabs, shoot like archers at a mark, and fight like devils," according to a Federal officer. The Rangers generally fought in the western campaigns east of the Mississippi River, distinguishing themselves at Shiloh, Perryville, Stone River, Chickamauga, Knoxville, and Atlanta. Hood's Texas Brigade was much more active in VA, "and because it repeatedly saw frontline action, its total losses were staggering," esp. at 2d Manassas and Antietam. Indeed, at Appomattox Court House, only 617 veterans survived of Hood's 5,300 enlistees, a record of sacrifice even greater than the Stonewall Bde of VA. Patricia L. Faust, "Hood," "Hood's Texas Bde," *Hist. Times.* Jeffrey D. Wert, "Terry's Texas Rangers."

[FIELD HOSPITAL, GUINEA'S STATION, CAROLINE CO.]

TUESDAY, MCH 10, 1863

To-day Dr. B returned.—3 days over time. I was glad to see him—perhaps because I hope to get off myself.

Snowing this morning. I have been suffering with a cold again.

I shall put in an application for furlough to-morrow. I am not well[.] [I would be] pleased to get 20 days . . . [diarist's ellipsis mark]

"Judge" [James Henry] Noland will take my place [as steward serving Harvey Black.] It is a question with me whether I ought to stop in Richmond. I have resolved to find out more and I do not know how I could do so better than by going to see her [Mary Camden]—. She may be in better circles than I imagaine. If so, it will not be easy to say what I plan, and if she is in low society, which I do not think can be, I will be mortified. I will best decide when I start [on furlough, if granted].

[FIELD HOSPITAL, GUINEA'S STATION, CAROLINE CO.]

WEDNESDAY, MCH 11TH, '63

This morning I made preparations to go over to Hdqrs of the 2d Corps with my application for leave of absence.

I saw Dr. [Hunter Holmes] McGuire [medical director of 2d Corps] and got his approval. The application must go up to Gen'l [R.E.] Lee's quarters. Maj. [Alexander Swift "Sandie"] Pendleton promised to return it in three days. [249] Dr.

---

[249] William Nelson Pendleton (1809-1883) was a rector at Grace Episcopal Churchin Lexington, VA and also an instructor of artillery at Virginia Military Institute. Trained at West Point, he graduated 5th in class of 1830, but spent much more time in the pulpit than in the field prior to the war. Fifty-one when secession came, he served as "nominal chief of artillery,"performing well in terms of staff administration, organization, and coordination, but was "only average" in the field itself. He often preached to large gatherings of soldiers. After the war, Willian Nelson Pendleton returned to Grace Episcopal Church, and his vestry included R.E. Lee, who became president of Washington College. Pendleton's son Sandie [Alexander Swift] Pendleton (1840-1863) was raised in Lexington and educated at Washington College in that town, where he joined a literary society that included Thomas Jonathan Jackson. Teaching at Washington College for several years, he entered graduate studies at The University of Virginia to improve his teaching credentials, but had to leave in order to join the CSA effort. He became Maj., and was appointed T.J. Jackson's main officer for ordnance, being trusted by Stonewall Jackson "to convey his orders clearly and concisely, in routine paperwork and under battlefield conditions." After Jackson's death following Chancellorsville, Sandie Pendleton became Lt. Col. and chief of staff for Jackson's successor, Lt. Gen. Richard Stoddert Ewell. Subsequently, he became chief of staff for Lt. Gen.

McGuire wishes a return of medical officers. Moses Gibson is a clerk for him. [250] Leonard Mohler went over. [251] He was to accompany me but went over before I was ready—He found me at Hdqrs —

I visited the 4th [VA Inf.] Regiment [Smyth Co.]—it was on picket duty. I know several of the boys. Went over to the 48th [VA Cav.] Reg't and saw Capt. [Robert H.] Dungan. I was very proud to learn that he received a promotion to Lt. Col. of the Regiment. I have always esteemed him, and prophesy for him a brilliant & useful life. He is a model of a man and deserves the esteem of his friends and countrymen.

The rations to a soldier have been reduced to 1/4 lb. bacon and 3/4 lb. flour per day, yet all seem fat and healthy. All are anxious for Joe Hooker to come forward and give a showing. [252] The monotony of winter quarters has been dispelled by court martial of the officers of the army. Those who so dastardly left their comrades to fight the foe while they lurked in the rear during the fights of last summer have been brought to the realization of the fierce demands of justice.

The penalties inflicted have in some cases been severe. The whipping post and hard labor under confinement, and confiscation of wages in others. I do not feel any sympathy for them.

Jubal Anderson Early for detached duty in the Valley after December 1863 and again the following June, 1864. Sandie Pendleton was killed Fisher's Hill (22 September 1864), and was eventually buried near T.J. Jackson in Lexington. In 1883, the surviving rector and military veteran Willian Nelson Pendleton was buried alongside his son. Patricia L. Faust, "Pendleton," *Hist. Times.*

[250] Moses Gibson (age unknown) originally joined 2d VA Inf. and transfered to 4th VA Inf. 31 October 1862; he became clerk to Hunter Holmes McGuire, director of Bde surgery. On 30 April 1863, Moses Gibson was promoted to steward, Apperson's rank. Robertson, *4th VA Inf.*, 52.

[251] Probably Samuel L. Mohler, already identified.

[252] Joseph Hooker (1814-1879) of Hadley, MA was a grandson of a Revolutionary War hero of same name. This 19th cent. Hooker was a West Point graduate and veteran of Second Seminole War and Mexican War, where he was breveted Capt. for gallantry at Monterey, Maj. at Natural Bridge, and Lt. Col. at Chapultepec. His courage under fire at Williamsburg (5 May 1862) during Peninsula Campaign earned him nickname "Fighting Joe." He suffered defeat at Fredericksburg, and criticized Ambrose E. Burnside, his superior. Lincoln replaced Burnside with Hooker, but did so reluctantly, because he worried about Hooker's ambitions and intent to make himself "dictator" over the Army of the Potomac. At this point in the diary, Hooker is maneuvering his troops for a major engagement at Chancellorsville, where he will be outgeneraled in strategy by R.E. Lee and overmatched by T.J. Jackson in the field. John D. Kallman, "Hooker," *Hist. Times.*

I saw B.F. [Frank] Leonard [already identified] to-day. Poor fellow[.] I do wish I could do something for him. He can scarcely move about at all [because of rheumatism].[253]

I enjoyed the ride very much—the roads are almost impassable[.] A road has been made for many miles by laying pine poles and brush on "sleepers" [that is, a bed of brush at the base of the poles and brush] which forms a very good passage for wagons.

Several cannons were headed towards the enemy's lines. The misery of tooth-ache is mine.

[FIELD HOSPITAL, GUINEA'S STATION, CAROLINE CO.]

THURSDAY, MARCH 12, 1863

To-day I received a letter from sister Mary containing one mother had received from Uncle Charles [Jones of Mississippi]. His address is Parischall Camp, Lt. Gant's Squadron, 1st Miss. Cavalry. He says he has been in several fights and had some narrow risks.

I am spending my days not very profitable [sic] now. Have been reading the Apocryphal New Testament some to-day—a very strange work.[254]

To-day is very cold.

---

[253] Benjamin Franklin Leonard was discharged on 2 April 1863 because of rheumatism. Robertson, 59.

[254] The diarist uses *profit* and its forms in a nonmonetary, almost Biblical sense (at least as the Jacobeans translated the Bible]. The adjective *profitable* to him means being brought in closer, and more proper, relationship with God, usually thorugh some processes of prayerful study and sanctified learning. Although not a member of any particular sect, Apperson is close enough to predominant Methodist and Baptist and "New Light" Presbyterians to declare a profound suspicion of, if not hostility to, the Jewish Apocrypha and the New Testament Apocrypha. He says thus that reading the "very strange work" of the New Testament Apocrypha brings him no closer to a right relationship with God, and is thus not a particularly sanctified activity, that is, "not very profitable now" in spiritual sense.

[FIELD HOSPITAL IN CAROLINE CO.]

FRIDAY, MARCH 13, 1863

Nothing new to-day. I got a letter from Mollie [Mary Camden]. Some of it [seems to be] significant.

Think! I wonder if she will deceive herself. I looked for my furlough to come to-day —

I wrote [illegible remainder of sentence]

HOSPT. 2ND CORPS ANV [CAROLINE CO.]

GUINEY'S DEPOT, SATURDAY, MCH 14 [1863]

I looked for my furlough to-day, but it came not. Nothing of unusual interest occurred —

[Illegible name of a washerwoman] brought my washing.

[FIELD HOSPITAL, CAROLINE CO.]

SUNDAY, MCH 15, 1863

Another sabbath. It has been spent partly in reading Dr. Ralston on "Free Agency."[255] In the evening, we were apprised of the fact that a sermon would be preached at the Widow Thornton's near our hospital. Several of the boys went over. As a general thing, the people of this section live in old houses, though they are comfortable and convenient. Mrs. Thornton seems to have a great many servants around her and mostly young negroes [sic].[256]

---

[255] Samuel Ralston (1756-1854) was a theologian active in early 19th cent. in the many debates concerning free will, predestination, "free agency," infant baptism, and adult baptism. Born in Ireland, he was educated in Scotland and earned theological degrees at the University of Glasgow as a Presbyterian divine. Coming to the US, he entered freely in many debates, and published many tracts. In 1822 he was granted an honorary doctorate by Washington College of Pennsylvania (today Washington & Jefferson University), and was generally refered to as Dr. Ralston thereafter. See his letter on Free Agency, the possible source of this pamphlet in *Debate on Christian Baptism; Between Mr. John Walker...and Alexander Campbell...*(2d ed., enlarged, with strictures in 3 letters respecting said debate published by Samuel Ralston; Pittsburgh, PA: Eichbaum & Johnston, 1820), Emory & Henry College Archives.

[256] Probably Frances Thornton, born 1820, a widow who had property in Reedy Creek Township of Caroline Co. in 1870 Census. In that same township are a number of black freed people with surname Thornton, as suggested by the diarist's notation. VA Census 1870.

At the house when we arrived, some ten or fifteen soldiers were gathered together. The porch was fixed for our accommodation until the service commenced.

[Illegible section in which Apperson seems to be describing the house interior.]

I looked too into the room when it was open to catch a glimpse of some of the fair ones of earth—only three were there besides the old lady, who, by the way, was by no means inferior [Frances Thornton was then 43 years old]. One, a little girl ten years old, I presume, another a daughter about 14, good looking, and a lady from appearance about 22. She had a good face and wavy hair. I looked at her for some time and would pronounce her "good looking" too had I not learned that she was the minister's wife, and he, I would suppose, 65 years old.

"Come unto me all ye that are weary and heavy laden and I will give you rest." was the text selected.[257] The sermon was very brief, though perhaps an earnest one. The chief plan was that we were weary and heavy laden and that Christ had promised us security [and] peace by application [by believers asking for grace]. Thus, He said that nothing made us gloomy and dissatisfied as the assertion that there was no peace for him hereafter—that Death gave the judgment and [illegible] were before everyone. [Real peace can come only through accepting the grace freely given by Jesus Christ in his passion, resurrection, and ascension; death of the body cannot end a soul's existence, provided that the person who owns the soul has asked for forgiveness in corporate worship involving confession and baptism before other believers]. He called on all to come now [to be baptized] while he was there.

We returned to Hospital [field hospital near depot station]. Snow and hail are falling —

NO FURLOUGH TO-DAY.

I wrote a letter to send to Uncle Charles [Jones of Mississippi]

[257] Matthew 11:28. "Come unto me all ye that labour and are heavy laden, and I will give you rest." (KJV). Generally used by Apperson.

HOSPITAL 2ND CORPS ANV [CAROLINE CO.]

GUINEY'S DEPOT, [MONDAY] MCH 16, 1863

To-day nothing passed of any importance. Very heavy cannonading was heard in the direction of Fredericksburg. It is said that the Yankees are engaged in target practice. Whether or not this is so we are unable to say.[258]

[FIELD HOSPITAL, CAROLINE CO.]

TUESDAY, MCH 17TH 1863

This evening again the cannonading was heard more clearly than yesterday. Many rumors afloat—Troops are under marching orders. I may bid adieu to furlough now since for me all authorized leave is over. This is truly hard.

[FIELD HOSPITAL IN CAROLINE CO.]

WEDNESDAY, MCH 18, 1863

We learned this morning that Fitzhugh Lee had an engagement with the enemy at Kelly's Ford in Culpeper [Co.][259] Lee lost very heavily [that is, not the battle, but in numbers of troops]. The enemy is certainly making demonstrations. Genl. [R.E.] Lee passed up the railroad this morning. No passenger trains—the cars have been impressed to bring up Genl. [John Bell] Hood's division [Hood's Texas Bde].

We may look for work here [as surgeons after battle] ere long.

---

258 Target practice was likely. Gen. Joseph Hooker was massing his forces of the Army of the Potomac for another major engagement along the Rappahannock; Gen. R.E. Lee was massing his own Army of Northern Virginia forces for such an engagement, and T.J. Jackson's Brigade of "foot cavalry" in the ANV was marching to support Lee's troops, but also on maneuvers. Both sides were reluctant to begin a major engagement during winter, and some late snow and cold weather had slowed the coming of the next big eastern battle. Meanwhile in the rivers campaigns, Gen. US Grant and Gen. W.T. Sherman were laying siege to the City of Vicksburg, the last major Confederate stronghold on a major "western" river and the key to opening up the "Mississippi Highway" to Federal control.

259 Kelly's Ford was a crossing point on Rappahannock River. Federal cavalry under William Woods Averell (1832-1900) crossed the river at the ford in an assault on Confederate forces near Culpeper Court House. Fitzhugh Lee (1835-1905) met Averell's cavalry with his own cavalry near the Wheatley Farm. The Federal cavalry were driven back across the Rappahannock, but casualties were heavy for such a brief fight: 78 Federals, 133 Confederates. Although the CSA celebrated the victory, it was costly for another reason: John Pelham (1838-1863), known as "Gallant Pelham" and already marked as a great prospect for the Confederate army was killed in the battle. Long, 329.

B.R. Jones received a letter from Mollie [Mary Camden] to-day [260] I am almost determined to let her slide for reasons known to myself.

Dr. Black has been giving the Hospital attendants a short lecture. As he says, things are becoming too loose. Not only are they becoming too negligent in the lower departments, but some of the higher officials are wanting in interest, I think.

Capt. [Robert Henry] Dungan sent his brother John here to-day. [261] He [Capt. RHD] wrote me a note asking that he [JRD] be sent to Charlottesville [general hospital]. I did what he requested. He states that Laura Faris, he learns, was to start to the Asheville Female Institute to-day. [Drury] D.W. Venable [of 4th VA Inf.] came to the hospital. He paid me 20$ that he collected for me—10$ each from S.M. Sexton [262] & W.A. Griffith. [263] He [Venable] gives me some points about the Camdens in Amherst [the family of Mary Camden, Mrs. A or Mollie] [264]

I have commenced reding [sic] the "Partisan Leader"[265] —

---

[260] Beverly Randolph ["Bev"] Jones (1832-1912) was apparently from Darkesville [Frederick Co.], a farmer, and originally served with Co. B, 1st Artillery of Rockbridge. From 26 October 1861 to 7 May 1862 he served with QM dept. of Stonewall Brigade.; then he served as hospital steward with Apperson under Harvey Black. "Light complexion, blue eyes, dark hair." In 1864 he was promoted to Capt. and transfered to local defense troops for Nitre Bur., Rockingham. After War he farmed in Winchester until 1912, and is buried at Mt. Hebron Presbyterian Church Cemetary. Driver, *1st and 2d Rockbridge Art.*, 69.

[261] John R. Dungan (1834-1863) also from Seven Mile Ford was 5th Sgt. with Co. D Lee Co. Guards. Fell ill with typhoid fever and on 22 March was reduced to Pvt. during lengthy illness. Transfered to Charlottesville general hospital, he died of typhoid fever on 1 April 1863. Chapla, *48th VA Inf.*, 119.

[262] Solomon McDonald Sexton (1842-1863), an original Smyth Blue, was in Co. D, 4th, listed as student at War's start and held rank of Cpl. Promoted to Sgt. in June 1863, he perished at Gettsyburg, 3 July 1863. Robertson, 72.

[263] Probably William A. Griffith (1845-1922), likely from Floyd Co., occupation unknown. Pvt. with Co. F, 2d. Co. of 14th VA Cav., Montgomery and Roanoke Cos. [no nickname]. Later captured at Cedarville (12 November 1864), he was exchanged and released, but had to enter one of Richmond's general hospitals, 27 February 1865. Discharged and pardoned in Roanoke, he lived there until 1922 and was buried at Roanoke City Cem. Driver, *14th VA Cav.*, 129.

[264] Mary Camden was listed in 1870 census as living in Amherst Co. after the War. Census VA. 1870.

[265] Nathaniel Beverly Tucker, *The Partisan Leader: A Key to the Disunion Conspiracy* , ed., Thomas A. Ware (Secretly Printed in Washington [1836] by Duff Green, for circulation in the Southern States, but afterwards suppressed; reprint ed.; Richmond: West & Johnston Press, 1862), Special Collections, Emory & Henry College, also available on computer files, Academic Affairs Computer for Documenting Southern History, University of North Carolina, Chapel Hill. Duff Green (1791-1875) was a Democrat active in Andrew Jackson's "Kitchen Cabinet," and Tucker (1784-1851) was from a famous VA family of jurists and academics. Tucker was disturbed by the

[FIELD HOSPITAL IN CAROLINE CO.]

[THURSDAY] MARCH 19, 1863

I made out the weekly reports to-day. It shows 113 received—57 sent to General Hospital[266] 19 Returned to duty, and 5 died.

The army has become quiet again, I think.

I wrote a letter to Dr. Faris to-night. Dr. B says he has written to Dr. [Hunter Holmes] McGuire regarding my application for furlough.

Snow is falling very rapidly—This could put an end to military operation for a time.

I finished "The Partisan Leader" to-day—of its merits I cannot speak satisfactory [sic]—I hardly know what to think of the work myself—it closes very unsatisfactory [sic]—leaves the reader on the pitch of excitement to draw any conclusions he chooses.[267]

---

crisis created over the Tariff of Abominations and John Caldwell Calhoun's (1782-1850) nullification proclamation (1832) and the resulting threat to the union and wrote this novel as a warning about the folly of such sectional controversies. Green and Tucker were supporting Calhoun as next president after Jackson, and they attacked Martin Van Buren of NY, the eventually chosen successor because of his personal rivalries with Calhoun and his strong NY identity. Green originally edited and published the *US Telegraph* as an organ for Jackson, but he had to relinquish the newspaper because of ill health, and the *Washington Globe* became the Jacksonian Democratic organ. In the novel, a thinly disguised Martin Van Buren has become president and wages bloody war against the southern states; Tucker here made a stand for slavery, where his forebears had been eloquent against the peculiar institution.

[266] Probably in Richmond, where there were ten permanent structures. Cunningham, 284-87.

[267] Only a committed poststructuralist would agree with the diarist that the reader could "draw any conclusions he chooses." Author Tucker, sponsor Green, and reprint editor Ware were all celebrating victory by the partisan southerners who are on their way to achieving independence. Although the novel ends with the outcome of the Civil War untold, the Union general, who consistently misrepresents his failures in the field as successes, has been killed in battle, and the southern partisans are otherwise victorious in recent battles and quite optimistic. There is a striking exchange between the cruel president and the female partisan Delia who is confirmed "in all her detestation of the cold, selfish, and crafty politician, whom she now beheld for the first time [218]." To drive home his point further, Tucker concludes with an author's statement that he has set this book "forth as the first *Bulletin* of that gallant contest in which Virginia achieved her independence; lifted the soiled banner of her sovereignty from the dust, and once more vindicated her proud motto, which graces my title page,—SIC SEMPER TYRANNIS! AMEN. SO MOTE IT BE." [220] Ware in his introduction to the 1862 edition that Apperson reads makes it clear that he sees the novel as a prediction of eventual southern partisan victory: "I commit the great work, in its original form, to its own vindication, trusting to the intelligence of the reader to apply the coincidences which mark its fulfillment as a political prophecy." [VIII] Tucker, ed., Ware.

[FIELD HOSPITAL, CAROLINE CO.]

FRIDAY, MARCH 20TH [1863]

To-day has been one of the most disagreeable. Snow, rain, and hail. Indeed a storm quite characteristic of the month. I have been reading some little of one thing on a condition of another—My mind is restless and unstable—Truly has it been said that the hardest battle man fights is with his own rebellious mind, and the greatest victory ever won is when the mind is fully disciplined. My mind has never been under proper control and now it is worse than ever before.

I wrote to cousin Bettie to-night. I find it easier to write letters than to do anything else. Here a little of the [illegible; sense is, *the pleasures of reading gossip and light observations in correspondence*] keep me employed.

No men were sent to the General Hospital to-day.

HOSPITAL 2ND ARMY CORPS [CAROLINE CO.]

SATURDAY, MARCH 21, 1863

The weather continues to be bad, though somewhat warmer.

Dr. B rec'd communication from HdQrts. to-day but no furlough for me. I gave it up, though when I yield, I am forced to think hard. I am a little inclined to feel cold towards Dr. B. He does not seem to care anything about my going [home on furlough] or anything about my desires. He is to me cold and indifferent. Why is it? I have never labored harder to please anyone than I have him, and up to now I have tried to show him constant respect. He does not seem to appreciate my efforts at all, and rather appears to me as if he takes it for granted that because it is my duty, I must do it. This I will admit, but my duty was not to wait last winter until he could spare me better to go home, or this winter for him to return before I went, and then seem unconcerned or rather glad that I cannot go. One thing, I have done everything I could to please him and have never asked any special favors of him, and do not think I shall ever be obliged to do so. My nature is odd in this respect. When I do my duty towards a person, I expect to be treated dutifully, and in the same faith that I extended my services.

Dr. Walls returned from Richmond to-day.

To-day's papers contain a very fine address from ex-Governor Seymour of Connecticut.[268] It is down on the [Lincoln] administration, justifies the South,

---

[268] Thomas Hart Seymour (1808-1868) was three-times governor of Connecticut and founder and leader of the Connecticut Peace Democrats. Growing up in Hartford, CT, he attended a

and advocates [illegible] and cessation of hostilities. [William Henry] Seward [U.S. Secretary of State] & Count [Edouard Henri] Mercier[269] seem to be yawling[270] at each other.

I wrote a letter to father to-night and one to Mollie [Mary Camden]—the latter was very spare—I cannot write her with the same feeling that I once did.

I commenced [Sir William James Erasmus] Wilson on "Diseases of the Skin"—[271]

---

military college and had a military career as well as a legal and political career. A decorated veteran of the Mexican War, he also published a Democratic "organ" newspaper, *The Jeffersonian*, and he served in US Congress in the 1840s, always as an ally to the southern wing of the Democratic Party. Three times he was elected governor of CT in the 1850s. He was out of office when War came, but founded the Peace Democrats and tried to persuade northerners to let southern states secede. His popularity rose with Confederate victories, such as Fredericksburg, but it fell with Federal victories, particularly Gettysburg. He failed to win the governorship in a close race in 1863 and ended his political career in some disfavor as northern excitement over the great victories overwhelmed memories of earlier unhappiness and protest. "Seymour." *Cyclopaedia of American Biography.*

[269] Edouard Henri Mercier (1816-1886) was French minister to the US during Napoleon III's rule. Son of a diplomat, he was born in Baltimore while his father served in the US; a clever and fortunate diplomat, Henri Mercier survived the upheavals of French politics and international relations before and during Napoleon III's reign but did not survive the debacle of the Franco-Prussian War (1870). In the Civil War, Mercier was generally thought to be pro-southern, advocating recognition of the Confederacy as a belligerant, visiting Richmond in 1862, and once proposing a kind of common market for CSA and France for trade and credit during the War. However, he was a realist and after the Battle of Sharpsburg (17 September 1862) and the popular European response to Lincoln's Emancipation Proclamation, he understood that French and British public opinion had swung to the side of the Federals, and he also understood that the CSA would not succeed in an invasion of the North. He brought an offer from Napoleon III to mediate an end of the war in 1863, but Seward angrily rejected the offer, which is the episode to which the diarist refers. Frustrated with his diplomatic efforts, Mercier persuaded Napoleon III to reassign him, to Spanish relations at the end of 1863. Despite the public "yawling," Mercier enjoyed warm relations with Seward and could deal with him successfully on major issues throughout the time period. Daniel B. Carroll, *Henri Mercier and the American Civil War* (Princeton: Princeton University Press, 1971).

[270] "Yawling, intrans. v....to cry out loudly from pain, grief, or distress." The usage is most likely picked up from Daniel De Foe, *Robinson Cruesoe* [which diarist had been reading]. "They all ran skreaming and yawlling away." *OED*..

[271] Sir William James Erasmus, *On Diseases of the Skin* (5th American ed. of 5th English edition; Philadelphia: Blanchard & Lea, 1863). Erasmus Wilson (1809-1882) was a Scottish surgeon who was son of a surgeon; he became a world authority on skin diseases and wrote the textbook for his era. A Fellow of the Royal Society of Surgeons, Erasmus Wilson joined the Royal College of Surgeons in London and served as benefactor and publicist as well as main researcher and master practitioner of skin surgery and the study of dermatology. With his own money he established an endowed professorship of dermatology at the Royal College, and with his skills he established the field as one respected in medical science. D'Arcy Power, "Wilson," DNB.

[FIELD HOSPITAL, CAROLINE CO.]

SUNDAY, MARCH 22ND [1863]

To-day has been a beautiful day. The snow melted rapidly under the rays of the sun and by noon had nearly all disappeared.

I have been reading something of different books, pamphlets too. I took a walk in the evening and was at the "Small Pox" ward. Dr. Purifoy is quietly, snugly fixed up. Mrs. Crump from Natchez, Mississippi was there—She came to wait on young [George] Perry from Charlottesville who is very low with variola.[272] I had a short conversation wtih her. She is well acquainted with Jas. Dungan[273] and his wife. Mrs. Crump has had variola very badly and is much disfigured. I spent an hour—I do believe it is becoming a very weak point with me to idolize woman's company. However comely they may be, there seems to be a soothing [element] in their voice and a sweetness in their expression that wins my devotion at once.

Capt. [Robert La Fayette] Francisco [QM] came on his way from home [Smyth Co.] He gives a doleful account of the money worshippers in the country. Dr. Sydnor came also—He has been home on furlough. He slept in my tent.

[FIELD HOSPITAL, CAROLINE CO.]

MONDAY, MCH 23, 1863

I rose this morning with the determination to make the proposition to Dr. B to send up another application for furlough, but after reflecting upon it, I determined not to do so. I do not feel that I have the right to ask it again. This is one of my weak points. Anything that I feel is due me justly is the thing that I am most dilatory in pressing. I have an inner sentiment that whatever is due from one man to another will be given without repeated demands. I am now satisfied that I shall get no furlough and have not many regrets to make about the failure. I have had some very sweet anticipation of home and friends and felt

---

[272] George H. [or P.] Perry, possibly born in 1839, was a farmer from Albemarle Co. who enlisted in 7th VA Inf. at Culpeper Court House as Pvt. in Hazlewood Volunteers, who became Co. C. "Listed as absent sick, autumn 1861 to 8/64." Riggs, 88.

[273] James W. Dungan (1833-?) was a carpenter from Smyth Co. who joined Lee County Guards, who became Co. D, 48th VA Inf. as Pvt. He was hospitalized in Charlottesville in February 1863 and then detailed as nurse and wardmaster in general hospital in Charlottesville until end of War. Chapla, *48th VA Inf.*, 119.

that I would see them all. But now I will be content to remain 'till the war is over. The campaigning of another summer is before us, and I expect doing my share of it.

This evening I visited Mrs. [Frances] Thornton in company with G.W. Botelere and Dr. Thomas. The evening was pleasantly spent about as follows —.

We arrived at 8 o'clock—Mr. [James Henry] Noland and S[amuel] Mohler were already there—having gone over ahead of us. At first we felt some delicacy at entering a parlour where we had been preceded by those whom we did not expect to see.

After going through the formalities of an introduction to two little girls, mere children, one of them drummed a while on the piano forte. Aunt Kesey [Keziah Shepherd] was there (she has moved across the [Rappahannock] river to Mrs. [Frances] Thornton's and is cooking for the small pox patients) and expressed herself as being very glad to see me. Well I suppose it was so. Supper was announced. We, of course, had supped. Mr. Hoyt of the Ordnance train is boarding there. He was pleasant and acted gentlemany. Mr. [James Henry] Noland's voice powers were enduring beyond anything I have seen.

After supper Mrs. [Harriet] Catlett was introduced. She is a tall pale lady with a pale complexion belonging to the ladies of these lowlands and very gray hair. I was not in her company much and could judge but little of her disposition. Next came Mr. Catlett, a merchant at Port Royal, a brother to Mrs. [Frances] Thornton. He is quite a dignified looking gentleman, well dressed and mannered. His hair is about gray enough to influence one to deep regard. Mrs. [Frances] Thornton came in next and took a seat in a distant corner. She is sedate and I presume reserved. She has quite a charge to keep, in the way of running servants and such things as running a farm. I believe she has a son in the army.

There were others, Mr. Newman and Mr. Carson. This latter gentleman seems to be disposed to give special attention to the daughters of Mrs. [Frances] Thornton. He, [Mr. Carson] I understand, does not meet the full measure of Mrs. [Frances Thornton] T's desires. Last, not least, came the minister's young wife, Mrs. Friend. I have before spoken of the difference in their ages. She was the center of attention. She sat before the piano and requested to know what the company wished for their entertainment—What sort of songs. "Judge" [James Henry] Noland decided love and sentiment—love and sentiment we had. I must own, I neither admired the oral or instrumental performance though the lady is proficient in both. I called for one piece, "Fisher's Hornpipe" which was played.

After the music was over "Judge" [James Henry Noland] and [Samuel] Mohler withdrew. I took a seat by Mr. Catlett and had an interesting chat on the prospects of coming prosperity of the nation and the gloomy condition of Virginia. He has a good tact at conversation. Mr. [G.W.] Boteler cornered the minister's wife [Mrs. Friend]. She is a great belle, I understand.

At a late hour we left. All were pleased. Will go back soon.

[FIELD HOSPITAL, CAROLINE CO.]

TUESDAY, MCH 24, 1863

Nothing unusual transpired to-day. I received a letter from Nat [brother Cincinnatus Apperson]. He is near Petersburg VA.

I wrote a long letter to Mrs. T [Mary Tomlin] to-night —The weather is quite wet and rainy.

[FIELD HOSPITAL, CAROLINE CO.]

WEDNESDAY, MARCH 25, 1863

This is the most changeable weather I have ever seen. Raining last night and this morning clear and sunny one hour, the next hour hail & snow.

I was asked to see one of the "Dare Devils" [Grayson County, 4th VA Inf.] in Team Master [QM Robert La Fayette] Francisco's train. I went after dark with Mr. [G.W.] Boteler—found him slightly sick. From there went to Mrs. [Frances] Thornton's. Captain Montgomery of the 4th La. Infantry was in the parlour, t^ete `a t^ete with Mrs. Friend [young wife of elderly minister]. I did not enjoy myself a great deal. Not because Capt. [Montgomery] or anyone else was present, but did not feel easy there or rather feel welcome. The piano was open and Mrs. F[riend] performed. She asked me for a selection of pieces. She does not know that my knowledge of music is limited to none at all.

The [Thornton] family is very much averse to persons from S[mall] Pox hospital coming near their house. Capt. M[ontgomery] is an officer of the guard and put some very impertinent questions to me. One was soon after I went into the room [:] If I had anything to do with the small pox patients[.] I did not mind the question. It is but the manner of asking, as if to take me unawares and in case I should [fail] to reply to request [the Thorntons] to send me away. This was my inference however erroneous it may be. I answered him as I was bound to do

[FIELD HOSPITAL, CAROLINE CO.]

THURSDAY, MCH 26, 1863

To-day is raining—I went over to see my patient [Daredevil from Grayson Co., 4th Inf]. Found him better. Spent an hour or so with Capt. [Robert La Fayette] Francisco [QM] and Mr [Henderson] Snodgrass[274] and returned to camp.

News in to-day's paper is good. The enemy's gunboats have been repulsed at Vicksburg[275] , and one sunk. The expedition of the enemy in Yazoo Pass [276] is also in critical condition.

[FIELD HOSPITAL, CAROLINE CO.]

FRIDAY, MARCH 27, 1863

To-day has been set apart by our president [Jefferson Davis] for thanksgiving and prayer.[277] However it may be observed at home [Smyth Co.] where churches are plenty and meetings in vogue, I know no attention is paid to it

---

[274] Henderson Snodgrass (1838-1865) apparently from Wythe Co. was a teacher who joined Wythe Grays, who became Co. A, 4th VA Inf. On 10 September 1862 he joined staff as QM Sgt. working with Capt. Francisco. Killed at City Point in Prince George Co. across county line from Petersburg (20 April 1865) of gunshot wound to head. Robertson, 74. Snodgrass did not die in official combat with 4th Inf., but he may have died from hostile fire since some fighting continued.

[275] Federal gunboats north of Vicksburg at Steele's Bayou had been attempting to assault the city from the waterways. On 25 March, the *Lancaster* was sunk, and the *Switzerland* was disabled, and the remaining gunboats withdrew. "It was the last of a number of unsuccessful efforts to find entrance to Vicksburg, the last before the slowly mounting major effort under [US] Grant." Long, 331. *Civil War Naval Chronology*, ed. Eller, pt. 3, 53.

[276] Yazoo Pass was another water entry to Vicksburg; it too was blocked off by the actions at Steele's Bayou. President Lincoln, in some exasperation, asked Maj. Gen. Stephen Augustus Hurlbut (1815-1882): "What news have you? What from Vicksburg? What from Yazoo Pass? What from Lake Providence" What generally?" Hurlbut, in overall charge of the base camp at Memphis presided unsuccessfully over the "widely dispersed 16th Corps" in this phase of the siege. It would take a land assault by Grant to take Vicksburg, and the city would hold out until the fateful day of 4 July 1863. Long, 330. See also Stewart Sifakis, "Hurlbut," *Who Was Who in the Civil War* (New York: Facts on File, 1998).

[277] Both the US and the CSA tried out different days of thanksgiving. Davis had earlier proclaimed 28 July 1861 as such a day, and Lincoln had set 28 November 1861 as a day of thanksgiving and prayer. In July of 1864, Lincoln set 6 August as a new day for thanksgiving and prayer. In Octobe r of 1864, Lincoln established the final Thursday of November as the Thanksgiving Day, although that day was not widely observed in the postbellum South until the 20th cent. Long, 1102-03.

here. I have been closely engaged reading Bulwer's novel, "Strange Story". It is very interesting and if read by one who could appreciate a novel for anything else except the excitement of the imagination caused by sympathy for or hatred of the characters, it is, I expect, a good thing.[278]

Weekly statement due to-day. 129 Rec'd, 138 to G.H. [General Hospital]; 10 RD [returned to duty]; & 7 died. Firing has been heard in the direction of Fredericksburg, yester-day and to-day. A few more days, and I look for movements of some importance. One party or the other must strike, and if the blow is given by our side, we may look for a terrible one.

I received a letter from C.E. Collins containing the account with the hospital department enclosed for my rearrangement. He says all the troops except his Brigade have been sent toward N. Car.—that Bde. is near Petersburg, Virginia.

I rec'd a letter from Mollie [Mary Camden]. Its tone and sentiment seem on a par with its predecessors. I sometimes wish I had never undertaken a correspondence with her. I see I cannot get out of it now without some pain to her, i.e., if she is truthful in her assertions. Her letters cannot be any pleasure to me when I know she writes the same to one other person [Beverly Randolph "Bev" Jones, already identified]. Because what a correspondent says to me of attachment more lasting than for any other person and then breathes the same words to as weak a creature as the one [Bev Jones] to whom I alluded there—I, of course, lose the interest I first experienced. I almost abhor the flattery that is lavished on all alike. I have been reading "The Strange Story" and it is *strange* indeed!

[FIELD HOSPITAL, CAROLINE CO.]

SATURDAY, MCH 28, 1863

Raining very rapidly nearly all day. Lt. [Robert C.] Vaugh, Smyth Blues, was sent up here to-day with continuous fever. [279] He says preparations were being

---

[278] Edward Bulwer, Baron Lytton, *Strange Story* (London: S. Low & Son & Co., 1862). First published in *All the Year Round* magazine, 1841, available, General Microfilm Company, Cambridge, MA. Usually called Edward Bulwer Lytton or Edward Lytton, the novelist was born in 1803 and died in 1873. His novels were very popular in the period, and this one was reprinted and issued in New York by A.L. Burt in 1842 and kept in circulation for decades thereafter by that house and by others; Apperson may have read the version issued for southern distribution by S.H. Goetzel Publishers in Mobile, AL, issued in 1863.

[279] Robert C. Vaugh (born 1837), spelled in Regimental records as both *Vaugh* and *Vaughan*, and listed in local histories as *Vaugh*. He was a tinner from rural Smyth Co. who joined Smyth Blues, who became Co. D, 4th Inf. Appointed 2d Lt. 29 August 1862, he was promoted to 1st Lt.

made in camp for a removal of baggage to the rear. He and I had a long talk of the company and its officers. I regret very much on account of the company that Capt. [Joseph M.]Thomas is forced to resign. I know though that his health is such that he is incapable of doing duty in the field. [280] The question is on whom does the care and interest of the company fall? This is a question of much importance to anyone that feels any ties to a company that has been so long in the service and stood with others at the post of danger. Many noble spirits have left it for the land where "the wicked cease troubling and the weary are at rest."[281]

One of the original members of the company, I am pained to hear, is now flaunting the streets of Marion regardless of the fact that he was once a "Smyth Blue". With a high head and proud heart, he claims the patronage of the citizens of Smyth and while he passes the patriotic sons stand by in silence. The day of retribution will come nevertheless.

I finished Bulwer's "Strange Story" to-day. I did not read it as carefully as I ought to have done. It is a good thing! More of the theatrical than is usually found in works of fiction. The chief purpose of the work is in opposition to materialism. And also aims a hard strike at skepticism and superstition. [illegible sentence] It leaves the reader to decide without any evidence [illegible]. [Four illegible sentences]

I rec'd three Magnolias [blossoms] from Richmond to-day [probably a gift from Mary "Mollie" Camden, then in Richmond]. I have a better opinion of the magnolias than I have of the "News". [*News* refers to contents of the letter]

[illegible sentence]

[FIELD HOSPITAL, CAROLINE CO.]

SUNDAY, MARCH 29 [1863]

This morning the wind blows cold. I dressed in clean clothes before breakfast. After duties of the day were over, I took [Flavius] Josephus' History

---

on 8 April 1863 during this march toward Chancellorsville. He was captured at Gettysburg (4 July 1863) and imprisoned in Ohio until after War, released on 10 June 1865. "5' 7 1/2", hazel eyes, auburn hair, fair complexion." Postwar career and death date unknown. Robertson, *4th VA Inf.*, 78. On spelling, Armstrong, *Hist.*, vol. 2:232-33.

[280] Joseph M. Thomas, already identified, officially resigned on 8 April 1863 during this campaign "because of 'insipient Pthisis'". He lived out his postbellum life in St. Albins, WVA. Robertson, 76. Probably incipient ptosis, a persisting dropping of the eyelids, esp. troublesome in mornings on awakening because the eyelids appeared to be stuck shut. "Ptosis," *Taber's*.

[281] Job 3:17 : "There the wicked cease from troubling; and there the weary be at rest." (KJV)

[identified earlier] to read some. We do not dine on the Sabbath until 3 P.M. and have no supper.

I went over to Mrs. [Frances] Thornton's on an errand for Dr. Black. I had an hour's conversation with Aunt Kesey [Keziah Shepherd]. She told me some things that I will not suffer myself to believe—for fear of flattery to myself.

Presumption is said by some to arise from ignorance and to lead to the ridiculous. I heard a good joke on one of our "would be" doctors this evening. Many of the hospital attendants have been introduced as Doctor. Mr. M [sic—I cannot identify] went to a house in the neighborhood with a caterer and was introduced as Dr. M. The lady in the kindness of her heart asked him to take some lily leaves over to the [field] hospital to dress blisters, stating that they were better than cabbage leaves. He says, "Yes, I believe they are better than mustard."[282]

I will never assume that which I am not prepared to act out. I am getting in the habit of running with the other boys, and I think it will stop.

[FIELD HOSPITAL, CAROLINE CO.]

MONDAY, MCH 30, 1863

To-day has been mild and sunny—G[ideon] Hale of the "Dare Devils" called in to-day[283]—Newton Umbarger of Co. D, 4th Va was sent to this hospital for lacerations of the toe.[284] Charles M. Bordan of Co. "E" has been here several days. He is very low. I visited him this evening. He knows me, but from his looks, dissolution was not distant.[285] To-day the Provost General made a descent

---

[282] Mustard, sometimes in paste, sometimes in powder, was used as "counter-irritant, emetic, stimulant, and condiment." "Mustard," *Taber's*. It was applied in a variety of forms, but was never used as a dressing [bandage or wrap].

[283] Gideon Hale (born 1832) was a farmer from Grayson Co. who joined the Grayson Dare Devils, which became Co. F. He was detailed as regimental wagonmaster in this period of the march to Chancellorsville and Fredericksburg. On 25 September 1863, he was AWOL, "but returned to duty after producing an 'order of detail' covering the time he was absent"; wounded in left arm at Payne's Farm (or Locust Grove, Apperson's birthplace) in Wilderness Campaign, 27 November 1863; to Chimborazo General Hospital, Richmond. No information on postwar activites or death date. Robertson, *4th VA. Inf.*, 53.

[284] Possibly Abram Newton Umbarger, age unknown. Infantryman with Co. D who was detailed as nurse in April 1863 [possibly after severe wound]; captured at Greenwood Depot (2 March 1865); imprisoned at Fort Delaware Prison, paroled and released on 21 June 1865. "6' 0" , gray eyes, dark hair, sallow complexion. No postwar information. Robertson, ibid., 77; and Armstrong, *Hist.*, vol. 2, 223.

[285] Charles E. Bordan (1840-1863) was stone-mason from Montgomery Co. who joined Highlanders, who became Co. E, 4th VA Inf. Wounded at Groveton (28 August 1862), he died of

upon a cutler's establishment[286] and confiscated his entire stock [of cutlery, tobacco, whisky, foodstuffs, and other goods] and put him in the ranks. The offence was smuggling whisky. Some 20 gallons was found among his goods, packed in rice and corn. About $1800.00 worth was sent to the [field] Hospital. Among other things, a box of tobacco. this pleased the lovers of the weed.

Some would-be musicians with a crippled accordian and half a strung guitar were making a wretched display of musical talent around our quarters. Though Uterpe [sic; Euterpe] was not very lavish with her gifts upon me nor was Juno on a spree when my endowments were issued, and therefore I ought not to criticize.[287]

I wrote a short, cold note to Mollie [Mary Camden] to-night.

[FIELD HOSPITAL, CAROLINE CO.]

TUESDAY, MARCH 31, 1863

This morning Dr. Wilkerson informed me that he was going to Richmond and said he would call on "Mrs Allen" [Mary Camden; Mollie] if I would tell him where she lived. I gave him a letter of introduction to "Mrs Allen". How far this will agree with her feelings, I am very anxious to know. It may place her and him in somewhat an awkward position, not knowing aught [288] of each other. I wrote her a letter explaining the course for her to follow towards him, but I fear she will not get it before he goes. She may blame me if she is disposed to do so. It will subject me to the necessity of making an explanation. I wish to know the

---

this fever. "5' 9", blue eyes, fair complexion." Robertson, 40. Official records incorrectly show him dying on 23 March, when he clearly is still alive on 30 March.

[286] Cutler is derived from French and Latin words for knife; "one who makes, deals in, or repairs knives and similar cutting utensils." *OED.*

[287] Euterpe was one of 9 daughters of Zeus, king of all gods in Olympos, and Mnemosyne (goddess of Memory). Originally the 9 daughters, or Muses, were indistinguishable from each other; but over time each took on a particular quality or attribute, Euterpe's being the gift of lyric poetry. Juno is the Latin name for Hera, Zeus' wife. In Roman mythology, Juno provided gifts of attractiveness, or "radiant grace" to shine on the visage of a mortal, usually a male, as she did for Jason. Edith Hamilton, *Mythologies* (Boston: Little, Brown, 1942) 40-43; 173; 322. The diarist is saying that he cannot sing or play an instrument and that he is not even particularly attractive to women, and thus should not criticize musicians.

[288] "Aught...anything whatever; anything. In interrogative, negative, and conditional sentences....In Shakesp[eare], Milton, Poe, [the verb] ought or [noun or adjective] aught occur indiscriminately." Phonetically and etymologically aught and ought are related but different. *OED.*

state of her social circle, and her appearance at home. I cannot continue a correspondence with her on an uncertainty.

Sgt. [Henderson] Snodgrass [QM Sgt. with QM Capt. Robert La Fayette Francisco] came to see me this evening. James Eads[289] Co H 4th Regt. took dinner with me.

Charles Borden [already identified] of whom I spoke died last night. "Judge" [James Henry] Noland invited me down to Mr. Dabney's—agent at the [Guinea Station] Depot. I went and had an hour or so with a Miss Ball—not pretty though. She caused me to break a rule of mine—that of playing cards. I have never made a pledge to quit anything of the sort, but simply left [sic] the habit die. She invited me to play and I did so. I may deserve censure.

"Judge" Noland was not satisfied until we went seranading. At Major [Wells Joseph] Hawks' [Commissary, already identified] tent, we found Mr [Charles H.] Gallaher [290] with a violin—He and "Judge" play very well a guitar—[Illegible words in sentence; sense is, Noland played guitar and Gallaher played violin and all sang.] "Lone Starry Hour", " Music in the Air" and "Home Sweet Home" were all tortured on the violin strings and we wound up by singing "Good By". Back to the [Guinea Station] Depot and the same under the young ladies['] windows—the curtain drawn aside once or twice is ample recompense.

Snow was an inch or two deep on the ground this morning. I wonder how it will be to-morrow morning.

I have a large lot of work [sic] on hand now in the way of reports. It is near midnight I guess—I go to bed—I will sleep all [next] day, I fear.

---

[289] James M. Eads, born 1834, was a merchant, probably from Rockbridge Co., who joined Rockbridge Grays, who became Co. H., 4th VA Inf. "[D]etailed as brigade postmaster some time after Apr., 1862; on duty through at least Feb. 1864." End of War and postbellum career unknown. Robertson, *4th VA Inf.*, 48.

[290] Probably Wells Hawks' fellow West Virginian from Charles Town and clerk in Commissary Charles Horace Gallaher (1839-1911), a clerk in Charles Town (Jefferson Co., later WVA), who joined Botts Grays, which became Co. G in 2 VA Inf. Promoted to Sgt. and serving with Commissary. "[F]lorid complexion, blue eyes, amber hair....Wded. in head at Payne' Farm" (27 November 1863). General hosps., Richmond Chimborazo and Staunton. Returned to duty 2 November 1864, captured at Spotsylvania (12 May 1864), imprisoned at Elimira, NY; exchanged 20 February 1865; paroled at Winchester, 30 April 1865 at Staunton. Moved back to Charlestown, now in WVA, and worked as clerk until death, 29 January 1911. Buried at Edge Hill Cemetary, Charleston,WVA. Frye, *2d VA Inf.*, 99.

[FIELD HOSPITAL, CAROLINE CO.]

WEDNESDAY, APRIL 1, 1863

This is all fools day. When I rose the cooks and workers were trying their skill at deception on each other as Dr. Black made his appearance. He had many calls unsolicited by them from the duped

I finished monthly reports to-day. Also monthly returns of medical offices. The number rec'd into the [field] Hospital this month was 543. Of this number, there were 31 deaths—variola. I had but very little trouble with the report of this month.

[QM] Capt. [Robert La Fayette] Francisco took dinner with me. The greater part of the boys have gone to Mrs. [Frances] Thornton's to-night. I had an invitation to go along but excused myself. Dr. Sydnor and I walked out some distance and had some fun. Perhaps I may regret it.

[FIELD HOSPITAL, CAROLINE CO.]

THURSDAY, APRIL 2, 1863

Old Ulyses (?)[291] has allowed all the winds to escape him to-day—a perfect hurricane is raging—tents are capsized and torn—Dr. Black's was first down—He moved into mine—The weather is warmer.

Mr. [G.W.] Boteler and myself took a long walk up by the mill pond and up the creek. It is so pleasant to stray around and view the grounds so far from our house. It brings to memory the days of yore.

I have quarterly returns to make out, but can do nothing towards it to-day—too windy. Dr. B has been reading Cross on baptism[292] and having lately read "Grace Truman" [identified earlier] he is somewhat interested in the subject. He does not exactly believe that baptism can be emblematical of the death, burial, and resurrection of the Saviour, and the Eucharist typical of the same. I hold that the Eucharist is only in commemoration of the death of Christ, while, if Baptism may be emblematical of the death(?), burial, and

---

[291] Apperson wrote the question mark. He knew he was misspelling Ulysses (or Odysseus). He also probably realized it was not the demi-god hero who unleashes wind but Aeolus , god of wind. It is possible that he was thinking of Agamemnon, who prayed for wind to launch his ships in the Trojan War, but promised a sacrifice of his daughter, for which crime he was duly punished ten years later on his return. "Ulysses," "Aeolus," "Agamemnon," Hamilton, *Mythologies* and *Bulfinch's*.

[292] William G. Cross, *Christian Baptism* (Richmond: C.H. Wynne, 1859).

resurrection of Christ, the Lord's Supper is only in memory and strengthens faith and enhances grace. [Apperson supplied the parenthetical question mark about death.][293]

[FIELD HOSPITAL, CAROLINE CO.]

FRIDAY, APL 3D 1863

Nothing new to-day—The wind continues to blow. Mrs. Faris wrote me to-day, or rather I received a letter from her. [illegible sentence]

News is scarce—[illegible sentence] Dr Wilkerson returned from Richmond to-day & a gang of [illegible adjective] prostitutes, hag Irish, and dutch [sic] Irish had a considerable [sic; noun missing] in Richmond on yester-day—called it a "Bread Riot". Dr W[ilkerson] says it was no small affair. The papers are entirely reticent about it. Dr. [Wilkerson] thinks it is no bread riot as jewellers and dry goods stores were broken into more frequently than any others. Thousands of dollars of commissary stores were issued to them, but they seemed to pay no attention to it. This is a disgrace. Genl. [John Henry] Winder, Gov. John Letcher and President [Jefferson] Davis harangued the people. Force was a necessity.[294]

---

[293] Cross was a Methodist minister, and he here takes a mainstream nineteenth century Methodist approach to baptism, as Apperson quotes for his own creed. Cross is enrolled in the Virginia Annual Conference of Methodist Ministers and described in an introductory remark by Leroy M. Lee. Harvey Black's position, at least as quoted by diarist, is congruent with Old Light, or more traditionally Calvinist, Presbyterians, as is most of Black's recorded creed. The diarist is generally skeptical of ritualism and attracted to pietism, while Black is much more sympathetic to ritualistic expressions of creed. See Cross, "introduction by Leroy M. Lee." Membership rolls, Virginia Annual Conference, 1860, EHC Archives.

[294] John Letcher (1813-1884) was already identified as a states rightist and pro-slavery intellectual who tried to avoid War; he was also identified by Patricia L.Faust as one enmeshed in details who administered the Commonwealth poorly during War and who resigned as governor in 1864 and failed of election to the CSA House. See Faust, "Letcher," *Hist. Times.* John Henry Winder (1800-1865) was a MD native who graduated from West Point with expertise and indeed considerable competence in artillery. He resigned US commission as Maj. of artillery in order to join CSA and became a Brig. Gen. assigned as provost marshal and prison commandant in Richmond. As provost marshal, he was also responsible for security in Richmond; accused of high-handed tactics, Winder was particularly criticized for his civilian detectives who spied on Richmonders and enforced the system of internal passports. In this case of the Bread Riots, Winder had to enforce the civilian government's decision and the military officers' desire to keep

[FIELD HOSPITAL, CAROLINE CO.]

SATURDAY, APRIL 4, 1862

To-day the wind blows harder and harder and more of it. There is so much dust in my tent that I do hate to take hold of anything that dirt will soil. Dr. Chamberlain [the young man and fellow steward recently passing examinations at the Medical Collcgc of Virginina] went before the Medical Board [of Virginia] and passed for assistant surgeon. He went to Richmond to-day in sort of a jollification.

At night, snow commenced falling and when I retired it was accumulating very rapidly. The "Richmond Examiner" reports the riot sarcastically. [295]

[FIELD HOSPITAL, CAROLINE CO.]

SUNDAY, APL 5, 1863

This morning the snow is about 8 inches deep. The wind still blowing. This is Easter and I hope the old notion that a storm at Easter closes the winter will hold good. I am very tired of this place. Henry [Thomas]—our washer man—went home to-day and I gave him $2.50 to take the books I wanted to send home and my map. I directed him to leave the books in care of Mr. Bates

---

news of the Bread Riot out of daily press coverage so that northerners would not learn of the incidents. Emory M. Thomas, "Winder," *Hist. Times.* Of the incident itself, Faust describes the events of 2 April 1863: "[A] crowd of several hundred women, boys, and a few men began an orderly march from Richmond's Capitol Square to the city's business district. They were going, one woman told an on-looker, to the bakeries to get bread. The crowd, quickly swelling to more than 1,000, engaged in widespread, indiscriminate looting. When Pres. Jefferson Davis learned of the unrest, he went to the scene and urged the crowd to stop its lawlessness. Reason failing, the president ordered the rioters to disperse within 5 minutes, after which time a military company [under command of Gen. John Henry Winder] would be prepared to fire on them. Realizing the men might be forced to shoot, the crowd scattered. By 13 Apr. several participants had been arrested and either released or held for trial; eventually the principals were convicted and given sentences of varying severity.

"Wishing the North to have no further knowledge of conditions in Richmond, the government requested that newspapers refrain from reporting the event at all; instead, they printed exaggerated accounts. The *Richmond Examiner* blamed the trouble on Yankee agents. Davis, along with other observers, believed the rioters merely wanted an excuse to pillage. The needy, meanwhile, were no better off than before their protest." Idem.

[295] Note that Faust and other careful researchers think that the *Examiner* was engaging in something closer to "yellow journalism" or tabloid sensationalism rather than sarcasm. See Faust.

in Marion.[296] I am very much gratified to know that I have gotten this off my hands here.

Mrs Keziah [Shepherd] and Mrs. [Frances] Thornton were at the [field] Hospital to-day—Mrs T[hornton] insisted I pay her a visit. Sgt. [William H.] Thomas[297] came to-day. I wonder if I could not get off.

[FIELD HOSPITAL, CAROLINE CO.]

MONDAY, APRIL 6, 1863

This morning the weather seems to promise something better in a few days. Dr. Sydnor went to Hdqers to-day. Capt. [Robert La Fayette] Francisco [QM] paid me a visit. Parson Tibbs came here sick.[298] Rev. Mr. [Beverly T.] Lacy[299] came to the [field] Hospital for the purpose of appointing a Chaplain—took dinner. Sgt. [Henderson] Snodgrass [QM Sgt] was at my tent. He is a good fellow, high toned, honorable and generous. I have often thought he would make one of the warmest friends. He says though that he has a powerful dislike to anyone that may once have caused him to be cross. It is my own position too. I can never feel again towards anyone after a difficulty as I did before. The disagreement may be settled and matters adjusted and seemingly move on smoothly as they did before, but nothing but a formal intimacy can exist between us again. The thorn may be extracted and the wound healed, but the

---

[296] I cannot find a man named Bates in Marion in 1863. The local historians Wison and Armstrong list no family named Bates in Smyth Co. There is no Bates in the census for this decade; either he was missed or he moved out of Smyth Co. before census was taken; the only Bates listed in Sturgill and Sturgill, *Smyth Co. Cemetaries* is Solomon Bates, who was born in 1882.

[297] William H. Thomas, born in 1836, was merchant from Montgomery Co. and joined Montgomery Highlanders, who became Co. E, 4th VA Inf. Promoted but then reduced in rank, he was Sgt. for a period; transfered to 14th VA Cav. Robertson, *4th VA Inf.*, 76 . Co. G of 14th Cav. was called Border Rangers and comprised many re-enlistees from 4th Inf. who transfered. He was detailed to shoe horses during part of this period; his own horse was killed at Port Republic, 26 September 1864 , and he paid $2,500 for cav. substitute and left 14th Cav. No further records of military service. Postbellum, he became a sales person in Blacksburg, retiring there and still listed in directory in 1917. Death date unknown. Driver, *14th VA Cav.*, 192. Not to be confused with another William H. Thomas, same age, who served in 4th VA Inf. but was discharged in 1862 because of illness. Robertson, 76.

[298] A civilian minister apparently not on regular chaplain assignment; possibly Richard Tibbs, born 1804, and still resident in Goochland Co. in 1870. VA Census 1870.

[299] Beverly T. Lacy, age unknown, was chaplain-at-large for the Second Corps of the ANV. He had a supervisory role over chaplains in the 4th and 7th and other regiments in 1st VA Brigade. There is a charming story of an interaction with Gen. R.E. Lee in which Lee demonstrated his simple faith—and his dependence on the chaplains to minister to him. Pitts, 62, 147.

scar will remain to renew the recollection. I am sorry this is my disposition. It would seem that I have no forgiveness. I do forgive but not forget. The impression once made upon the mind that the person with whom you deal is not true, you watch him involuntarily.

I have been working on quarterly reports to-day. Read W.S. Oke on Erythemia[300]—I liked it tolerably well—am a little interested.

News in the papers this morning brings in a telegram from Genl. [Richard] Taylor. He has captured the Yankee gun boat "Dianna".[301] Capt. [John

---

[300] Erythemia is the disease caused by overproduction of red blood cells, though that cause was not well understood in 1863. The condition of erythema marks the disease erythemia. It was not until 1891 that "true erythemia" was isolated and identified as a set of discrete diseases. In the diarist's Civil War era, the terms are used interchangeably, and no real differentiation is attempted since cause was unknown, and no real cure found. Both condition and disease are marked by macules, or spots, on the skin; and the macules show "diffused redness over the skin." See "erythema," Taber's. and "true erythemia," *McGrew's*, 34, 133. W[illiam] S[amways] Oke, *Practical Examination of the Immediate Treatment of the Problems of Eczema that Occur...[in] Surgery & Midwifery* , 2 vols. (London: Longmans, 1831-35), chapter "On Erythema." See also idem, "Notes on the Treatment of Erythemia...," *Association Medical Journal* (1853). Oke (1785-1886) of Southampton Medical Society in England was prominent in treatment of skin diseases, with monographs on erythemia and a textbook on skin diseases. The diarist is apparently reading a chapter in Okes's textbook. Other prominent authorities of the era still in print on the subject of erythemia and erythma were the British practitioners and scholars George Hume Weatherhead (1790-1853), James Begbie (1798-1869), Henry Samuel Purdon (cannot find dates), and the German Albert Wyttenbach (born 1833). Only Okes seems to have an extant textbook with chapter treatments in 1863.

[301] Richard Taylor (1826-1879) was a fine combat leader from "Springfields" near Louisville, KY. He had almost no prior military experience in 1861, but this relative of former president Zachary Taylor and Union general Joseph P. Taylor and onetime relative by marriage of Jefferson Davis, was educated at Harvard and Yale and on the European continent, and took full advantage of his connections, his training, and his native intelligence. Rapidly promoted, he was Lt. Gen. during this engagement on the Miss. River, and his excellent memoirs, *Destruction and Reconstruction* (1879) indicate a confidence that the CSA forces could have won the river campaign if not for the "stupid, pig-headed, and obstinate" character of his superior Gen. E. Kirby Smith (already identified) who detached troops from Taylor at a crucial moment in defense of the river. He later was given command of a district in LA. Fred L. Schultz, "Taylor," *Hist. Times.* On 28 March 1863, CSA Naval and forces under Taylor defeated Union gunboats at Pattersonville LA and in process captured *USS Diana.* Long, 332. *Diana* was under temporary command of Acting Master Thomas L. Peterson who was "reconnoitering the Atchafalaya River...and reported that ship's 'tiller ropes were shot away, the engines disabled, and she finally drifted ashore when it was impossible to fight or defend her longer, and she ultimately surrendered to the enemy.'" *Civil War Naval Chronology*, ed. Eller, 54

Singleton] Mosby has done it up for the Yankees again [at Fairfax Court House].[302]

[FIELD HOSPITAL, CAROLINE CO.]

TUESDAY, APL 7TH 1863

Parson Tibbs left this morning. I gave him some directions to the houses of R. Richards and V. Quisenberry [civilian physicians in Orange Co. and family friends] as he went towards Charlottesville [general hospital]. Dr. Chamberlin [the young associate recently receiving credentials as a physician] has been ordered to a cavalry regiment in the Valley. [303] Dr. Magruder has been assigned to duty at this [field] Hospital. Several of the boys are on a [drinking] spree.

Dr. B paid off Hospital attendants. I received $42 for 2 months. [304] There is bill pending in the Confederate Congress and has passed one house to raise the pay of soldiers and non-commissioned officers to four dollars more per month [viz., $25 per month instead of $21]. This with the clothing commutation raises our wages to quite a respectable amount.

---

[302] John Singleton Mosby (1833-1916) was born near Richmond and attended University of Virginia until imprisoned for shooting a fellow student. The incident and the subsequent trial interested him in law, and he studied and passed the bar and began practicing law in Bristol, VA. Joining a cavalry unit, he soon fell in with Brg. Gen. J.E.B. Stuart and gave that Cav. leader the idea for the "ride around" Geroge Brinton McClellan's entire army. Late in 1862 he became more autonomous and led Partisan Rangers in independent raids. "He and 29 men stole into Fairfax Court House, VA, and captured Union Brig. Gen. Edwin H[enry]. Stoughton [1838-1868]. Quickly Mosby became the bane of the Union, his activities in northern VA so successful that Lt. Gen. US Grant ordered him, and his followers, when captured, hanged without trial." They were never captured and this officer, "mentioned in Gen. R.E. Lee's orders and reports more than any other Southern officer" survived the War to become a successful attorney in Warrenton, VA—and postbellum friend of US Grant. Virgil Carrington [Pat] Jones. "Mosby," *Hist. Times.*

[303] I cannot find him listed in the regimental histories for CSA cavalries.

[304] $21 per month remained Apperson's base salary from enlistment. He did receive a $50 dollar bonus for re-enlisting on 12 November 1862, and he was on occasion reimbursed for extraordinary expenses involved in travel while on steward's duty. The clothing commutation was a credit for clothing needed in line of work, and was sometimes handled as a reimbursement, sometimes as a credit and sometimes as an "advance" on payment. Prior to this year, there were "stoppages," that is deductions from his base salary of $21 for clothing bought in line of work. As noted on 12 November, such "stoppages" often amounted to $7.00 per month; giving him back this money from 1863 had the effect of raising his monthly salary 50%—or more, if he received commutation but did not spend all of it on clothing.

I got a letter from Mollie [Mary Camden] to-day. [Bev] Jones got one too. She gives me some very broad hints that my last letter does not chime so well. I am sorrowful that I ever commenced a correspondence with her. I am inclined to "cut" it and it would be a blessing to me if she would "cut" mine. She evidently makes one assertion that I do not think coincides with her desires. She calls [Bev] Jones an "affected boy". Why does she encourage that affectation? She says she has closed all her correspondence but myself [sic]—does she think I believe this? She says she has lost another relative. In [Bev] Jones' letter nothing is said about it.

Dr. Hagy and I visited Mr. Motley's [305] this evening. Spent a few hours very pleasantly with Mr. and Mrs. Motley in the parlour. I did not have the pleasure of the company of his daughter. He has a very nice parlour—2 settees, one common table, one sun table, books in shelves. The windows nicely arranged with beautiful muslin curtains and brass fenders before the fire, etc.

He invited us to return again and promises to visit in the [field] Hospital to-morrow. He has evidently been a gentleman in times past, and I have no right to say he is not now. Quite an old Virginia aristocrat, I think. I have been reading "Neligan on the Skin". [306]

[FIELD HOSPITAL, CAROLINE CO.]

WEDNESDAY, APL. 8, 1863

This morning looks much like a good spell of weather will come now. The papers bring the news that the fight in Charleston [SC] has commenced [sic].[307]

---

[305] Possibly John L. Motley, born 1817, who had land and a home in Bowling Green Township of Caroline Co. in 1870. VA Census 1870.

[306] John Moore Neligan, *A Practical Treatise on Diseases of the Skin* (3d American ed.; Philadelphia: Blanchard & Lea, 1863). Neligan (1815-1863) was a British authority on skin diseases whose textbook was widely used in Civil War era.

[307] The fight was actually over on 7 April, but the *Richmond Whig* reported that the fight began on this day. Charleston Harbor was site of major naval assault by 9 Federal ironclads commanded by Flag Officer Samuel Francis du Pont (1803-1865) on 7 April 1863. Du Pont's ships attacked Ft. Sumter, but batteries on both Ft. Sumter and Ft. Moultrie returned fire; Ft. Sumter was heavily damaged, but the batteries on the harbor forts inflicted greater damage, throwing some 2209 shells as compared with 154 from the ironclads. Five vessels were disabled, and the *USS. Keokuk* sank on 8 April. Human casualties were light in this fighting, but damage to vessels was so heavy that du Pont withdrew that evening, having "decided that Charleston could not be taken by naval force." Long, 335-36. *Civil War Naval Chronology*, ed. Eller, pt. III, 59-62 [includes picture of *Keokuk* and Adm. du Pont].

A desperate conflict is expected. I visited Mrs. [Frances] Thornton's in company with Dr. Thomas and Mr. [G.W.] Boteler. I was introduced to a Miss [Eve] Thornton—had a chat.

I ought not to have left this evening. The quarterly report demands my time, and I had to write hours after my return. I find a mistake in the report for March. I do hate to see these mistakes.

[FIELD HOSPITAL, CAROLINE CO.]

THURSDAY, APL 8, 1863

This morning I finished and handed in quarterly reports.

In the afternoon Dr. Wilkerson, Henry Mohler,[308] Chaplain [Jaquelin Marshall] Meredith,[309] and [G.W.] Boteler and myself went fishing. Mr. Meredith is Chaplain of 4th Regt [sic] and is temporarily placed here. I was informed by Mr. [G.W.] Boteler that there were some ladies at Mrs. [Frances] Thornton's and I was expected over there at night. The ladies I expected were not there, but I had a very pleasant evening with Mrs. Friend [young wife of an elderly Caroline Co. minister]. She says it is as common for the married ladies to have attention paid them as it is for the single ones. This reflection is to some extent particular to her as she is so fond of company. Our friend, "Judge," [James Henry Noland] was not treated with very much respect and he left

---

[308] Probably William Henry Mohler (1833-1912) of Kerr's Creek Confederates, Rockbridge Co., which became Co. G of 58th VA Inf. A farmer from Kerr's Creek area of Rockbridge Co., Mohler was brother of James H. Mohler (1839-1862), of same G Co., 58th Inf. who was killed in action at Fredericksburg (3 December 1862). William Henry Mohler was promoted to Sgt., but was reported AWOL from 7 June 1862 to 1 August 1862 when he returned and was reduced to Pvt. He would be captured in Fredericksburg in May in aftermath of Chancellorsville, sometimes called 2d Fredericksburg and imprisoned in Ft. Delaware, Del. Exchanged on 23 May 1863, he was returned to combat action until captured yet again, Spotsylvania Court House (12 May 1864) and kept until June 1865 after CSA surrender in April 1865. After War, again a farmer in Kerr's Creek area of Rockbridge Co. until death in 1912. Buried at New Monmouth Presbyterian Church Cemetary, Rockbridge Co. Driver, *58th VA Inf.*, 123.

[309] Jaquelin Marshall Meredith (1833-1920), apparently from Stafford Co. along Potomac River, was an Episcopalian clergyman appointed chaplain of 47th VA Inf. on 1 May 1862 and serving until 1 May 1864. After War he married Ellen Bankhead and served Episcopal churches in Norfolk area, dying in VA Beach 6 November 1920 and being buried in Aquia Episcopal Church Cemetary. Homer D. Musselman, *47th VA Inf.*, Virginia Regimental Histories Series (Lynchburg, VA: H.E. Howard, 1991) 142. Also, Pitts, *Chaplains*, 149. Meredith was never listed as chaplain of 4th Inf., but perhaps diarist means to say that the chaplain's assignment with 4th regt ["here"] is the temporary one.

unceremoniously. Mrs. Friend excused herself from playing [the piano] because she had been traveling. She played one piece of which I think the words are very touching. The chorus is this:

I will love you as long as I live
But when that brief season is o'er
Ah! do not disparagingly grieve
For I can love evermore —

After she left the parlour, I passed a few commonplace remarks with Mrs. [Frances] Thornton and proposed to leave. Mrs. Friend is a lady that has been a great deal into company and understands the fashionable [things to do]. I like her conversation very much, if it will last.

[FIELD HOSPITAL, CAROLINE CO.]

FRIDAY, APL 10TH, '63

To-day we had an exhibition of the fair but ugly. Mrs. Schultz and daughters Mrs. ___ , and Miss ______ [Apperson's blanks]—I can't begin to name them all—came over to the [field] Hospital. Mr. [G.W.] Boteler and myself saw them home. I walked with Miss Mollie Thornton—a very modest, unassuming young lady. At Mrs. [Frances] Thornton's we found Mrs. Friend [young wife of local minister], Capt. Montgomery [already identified] , and a Capt. [Charles Jones] Green.[310]

---

[310] Charles Jones Green (1839-1909) was born in Falmouth (Stafford Co.) and graduated from Virginia Military Institute in 1859 (as had his older brother William James Green). He joined Stafford Rangers during the John Brown insurrection at Harpers Ferry and helped to capture Brown. After Brown's trial and execution, Green moved to New Orleans, apparently working as a merchant. When War came, he returned to Stafford Co. and helped form Co. A of 47th Inf., becoming its Capt. by election. Records indicate that he was wounded seven times during War., including wounds at Gaines Mill (27 June 1862), Chancellorsville (3 May 1863), and Spotsylvania Court House (19 December 1864). Eventually promoted to Maj., he was wounded yet again at Ashland (29 April 1865) as War ended and was paroled by Federal Govt. on that date. After War, he returned to Stafford Co., became a farmer and a merchant and married Virginia Whittmore in 1872; in 1873 he and his wife moved to Dallas, TX, where he farmed and sold merchandise. Died 1909 and buried in Greenwood Cemetary, Dallas, TX. Musselman, *47th VA Inf.*, 126.

[FIELD HOSPITAL, CAROLINE CO.]

SATURDAY, APL. 11TH [1863]

There are times in the history of all men when they seem to have forgotten the true position they occupy—I find myself to-day in an engagement to go to Mrs. Motley's. Of course went—was introduced—had a very pleasant time. Miss Sue [Motley] plays "Whist" and "Sledge". We returned about dark.

The boys [of the Medical class taught at field hospital] had "taken up a subject" [a corpse] and were dissecting it. I went and looked on for some time. Dr. Black rec'd a communication from [Medical Director] Surg[eon] [La Fayette] Guild to-day with a copy of a letter from a Surgeon [possibly J.L. Cabell] of Richmond[311] relating to the manner in which sick have been sent to a hospital. Often, he says, in "Articulo Mortis"[312]—and having no descriptive list—their graves are often left unmarked. This is a thing much to be regretted and should be remedied as soon as possible. The hardest blow is on regimental surgeons. I have been culling the registry for evidence [so that regimental surgeons in his field hospital do not send corpses unidentified by properly kept list or manifest to general hospital].

I rec'd a letter from Cousin B[ettie] to-day—

[FIELD HOSPITAL, CAROLINE CO.]

SUNDAY, APRIL 12, 1863

Spent the day in camp until near night. Most of the time I was in the "dead tent" watching the dissection of some important anatomical parts, also some amputations and resections and ligatures. [313]

Near night S[amuel Leonard] Mohler and myself walked over to Mrs. [Frances] Thornton's and sat an hour. I like the modesty of Miss Mollie Thornton, and when I see a young lady, free from affectation and whose whole manner seems one of kindness and warm heartedness I cannot fail to admire her. Our friend [G.W.] Boteler seems taken.

---

[311] Possibly Dr. J.L. Cabell, surgeon stationed in general hospital at Charlottesville. Cunningham, 287; also possibly Dr. Gabrell, whom I cannot find in records.

[312] Latin, "at the time of death," *Taber's.*

[313] *Resection* is Latin for "cutting off," and is "partial excision of a bone or other structure"; *ligature* is Latin for "a binding," and "is process of binding or tying...sometimes strips of fascia [fibrous membrane covering, supporting, and separating muscles] obtained from a patient are used as ligature." Ibid.

D[rury] W. Venable was to see me to-day—Capt. [QM Robert La Fayette] Francisco was here also.

[FIELD HOSPITAL, CAROLINE CO.]

MONDAY, APL 13TH, 1863

To-day is beautiful. The sun shines cheerful. The fields seem to smile again. Miss Keziah Shepherd and Miss Mollie [Graves] came up from Richmond. Took dinner with us.

Miss Mollie [Graves] will count on a high time with her beaux, Dr. Wall and Dr. Wilkerson, two amorous swains bowing before the altar of love. In the evening we walked over. All had a very interesting time; had some chat with Miss Mollie Thornton—made an engagement to go fishing. I will write her when she leaves. She and Miss Susan Catlett tried to have a bit of fun with myself and Mr. [G.W.] Boteler by sending some bogus pills over. Small puffs, they were filled with cotton seed. I was not deceived. The appearance outwardly was enough.

Dr. "Wilk" [Wilkerson] of course was discovered with Miss Mollie [Graves] all evening and Aunt Kesey seemed delighted as much as Mrs. [illegible] ever was.

I loan [sic] Capt. [Robert La Fayette] Francisco $140.00 to-day. He gave his due bill for the unit.

I rec'd a letter from home [probably Mrs. Faris] to-day —

[FIELD HOSPITAL, CAROLINE CO.]

TUESDAY, APL 14TH [1863]

This morning the sun shone brightly and I expected a beautiful day. Towards noon, the air grew perceptibly cooler and some indications of clouds.

Our fishing party for this evening is broken up—Mr. Friend [the minister and husband of the socialite Mrs. Friend] preaches at Mrs. [Frances] Thornton's at 1/2 past 4 [PM] Miss Susan [Catlett] and Miss Mollie [Thornton] made attonement [sic] for the cotton seed puffs to-day by sending some very nice sweetmeats.

I am loosing [sic] time that should be spent reading and studying. The ladies are kind to me and insist that I should come often.

We walked over before [the Rev. Friend's] service—had a chat with Mrs. Friend—Dr. B was over.

The sermon was preached from the 22d Rev. & 17 verse "And the Spirit and the bride say, Come."[314] I did not get the meaning of the sermon—remained after services and diverted myself in teasing the girls [Mollie Graves; Susan Catlett; possibly Mrs. Friend].

[FIELD HOSPITAL, CAROLINE CO.]

WEDNESDAY, APL 15 [1863]

Soon after morning rain commenced falling and with the wind made one of the most disagreeable days. I had the pleasure of receiving a letter from Mrs. Faris and Laura Faris. Dr. [William Faris] has rec'd one package of my books—perhaps all of them. I did not understand it so, though. Mrs. Faris informs me that Dr. [Caliborne Watkins] Beattie's Books will be sold in a few days and wanted to know if I wanted them. I wrote to her to tell Dr. [William Faris] to buy them. If I get out of the army, I will want them. If I do not, money will be of no use to me.

Laura [Faris] says she expected to start to Ashville, Ala[bama] to the female institute the Tuesday [21 April 1863] after the date of her letter. She asked me to write her. I will do so, I think. I am not sure I ought to without the consent of her ma [Mrs. William Faris]! Though my feelings towards her will be those of a brother to a sister.

The uninvited "Mrs. A" [Mary Camden] is on hand again. Dr. B rec'd a notice that a lady was at the [Guinea Station] depot and wished to see him. He sent Sgt. Horn [315] over who failed to give any satisfaction. He mumbled a curse and went down, but came back in a great rage—Dr. B gave an order to Horn to report to his regiment [possibly 29th Inf.] at once. Horn wanted an explanation but Dr. B told him that he [Horn] did not—[Harvey Black did not] wish to be trifled with. Horn was ignorant of who the woman was that traveled in and Dr. Black and I stated it to him, disarming any intention to deceive or jest. Dr. Black withdrew the order [for Sgt. Horn to leave the hospital area at once] and

---

[314] Revelation 22:17: "And the Spirit and the bride say, Come. And let him that heareth say, Come. And let him that is athirst come. And whosoever will, let him take the water of life freely." (KJV).

[315] Possibly J.D. Horn (birth date unknown, killed in action, 20 May 1863) of Smyth Co. who served with Co. B, 29th VA Inf. Alexander Smyth, *Smyth Co.*, ed. Presgraves, 18.

seemed satisfied. In the meantime Dick [Richard M.] Jones[316] came up with a card addressed to me and [Jones also escorted in] a gentleman whom he intimated was Mr. Dabney.[317] The lady was none other than "Mrs. Allen" and she was asking us for an interview. Mr. D[abney] wanted a statement. They are stopping at Mr. Dabney's. I sent a note that I would be over at 8 o'clock. I had ten thousand thoughts. What can the message mean? Why does she let that ignoramus [sic] [Richard M.] Jones into anything? He published it [talked about her message to the diarist] as soon as he got to the [field] Hosp't. This vexed me. I was expecting every minute for Dr. B to call upon me for some explanation. I determined to go over and not say anything about it to him. I had an engagement to go [to] Mrs. [Frances] Thornton's with Dr. Wilkerson and so I started with him and went down the road to Mr. Dabney's [in Port Royal Township of Caroline Co]. I found the road in a horrid conditiion and rain fell in torrents. They were sitting in a small room. The meeting was rather cool. I soon found there was no chance for a private interview [with Mary Camden]. I moved my seat near her and we had some conversation but upon nothing that was to give me any satisfaction.

Her explanation for her trip up here is that Lt. [Tinsley Linsley] Allen has some papers that she needs and she is after them. This does not seem very plausible, as the division that Lt. Allen belongs to is at Hamilton's Crossing [an upper ford on the Rappahannock River in the area where Gen. Joseph Hooker's Army of Potomac cavalry was maneuvering preparatory to a major engagement at Chancellorsville and a planned second assault on Fredericksburg] and she ought not to have gotten off the [railroad] cars at Guinea's [Station depot]. She says she is compelled to be in Richmond by 8 o'clock to-morrow night and she still intends going up to Hamilton's [Crossing] to-day and return on the evening train. She cannot visit the Regiment [Lt. Tinsley Linsley Allen's 58th Inf.] during the stay of the train at Hamilton's.

---

[316] Richard M. Jones (1833–?) was a student who joined Montgomery Fencibles, which became Co. G of 4th Inf. After wound at Groveton (28 August 1862) he left Inf. and entered "detached service" with QM. Later captured, 5 May 1864 at Wilderness and imprisoned, Elmira NY. Paroled after War, 19 June 1865. "5'11", blue eyes, light hair, florid complexion." Postwar record unknown. Robertson, *4th VA Inf.*, 58.

[317] Two possibilities are Charles Dabney, born 1834, and Joseph Dabney, born 1829; each man owned a home and land in Port Royal Township in Caroline Co. and was civilian in status in 1863. However, given Mary Camden's sense for intrigue and misidentification, Dabney may not be the real name for the gentleman escort and host. See "Dabney," VA Census. 1870.

If she intends to go up to Hamilton's why did she wish to come to the [Guinea Station] Depot?—She says that she will be in a tent [at Hamilton's Crossing] although her escort is Mr. Dabney [who is said to have a home in this house in Port Royal Township section of Caroline Co.]

But after all I cannot think but that she is better than my friends think she is. She betrays too much sorrow, too much agitation to be a base woman—She may have those fears too—She gave me a hug when I started and I saw the tears in her eyes.

She seemed to be much affected of [sic] the gentleman ["Dabney"] that was with her. He watched her closely too. I would have given anything for an hour's interview.

She gave me a letter stating that she would probably never have another chance to see me. The writing was on the back of an old letter written by a Mr. Dorman of Co. "J" 2 La. Infty [apparently one of the Tiger units of Louisiana said to be reckless both in battle and off-duty]. I went back to my tent and wrote a letter to send to her. I stated the suspicion that was out on her and asked her to say nothing before [Richard M.] Jones [the "ignoramus"]. I have no ill feelings towards him, but he is not the person to be privy to any grave matter. Mr. Dabney is among us in the morning —.

I have some dreads and regrets in this matter. Some of my friends may think I am playing a bold hand [gambling]. The ladies [Mollie Graves, Mrs. Friend, the Catlett matriarch and the Catlett daughters, the Thornton matriarch and the Thornton daughters and cousins] may get wind of it and *that* I don't want.

[FIELD HOSPITAL, CAROLINE CO.]

THURSDAY, APRIL 16TH 1863

This morning Mr. [Feldburg?] came over.[318] I had made preparations for him as I expected him. I heard that they ["Dabney" and Mary Camden] went up to Hamilton's Crossing and returned on the evening train to Richmond. This is some relief to me I am sure.

To-day is the birthday of Miss Eve Thornton. The boys had an invitation to go over. When evening came several walked over. Mr. Catlett from Port Royal was there and with the ladies we had quite an agreeable party. I enjoyed the

---

[318] Apparently a relative or friend of "Dabney." I cannot find anyone named Feldburg listed in 1870 Census for Caroline Co. or any neighboring county.

company of Miss Mollie [Thornton] much to the discomfort of my friend [G.W.] Boteler.

I have been surprised at Dr. "Wilks" [Wilkerson]. He promised me he would say nothing of "Mrs. A" [Mary Camden], but he did to Miss Mollie [Thornton]. She asked me about it. I do not care so much. I know my intentions are good.

Miss Mollie Thornton is a very quiet girl and is deserving of high regard. Her modesty makes up fully for what she lacks in beauty. Miss Susan Catlett is loquacious indeed. Miss Keziah [Shepherd] seemed to rule with becoming dignity. Mrs. Schultz was a mute spectator. Dr. Purifoy and his wife entertained each other with amiability. Mrs. [Frances] Thornton stood by the piano and enjoyed the music when anyone was performing. Mrs. Thomas and the young ladies—Miss Anne Catlett & Miss Eve Thornton—were arranged in a triangular form. Dr. Jamison was on hand too for a while. Miss Mollie Graves was a supernumerary[319] for once.

Egg nog and cakes were served. I regret most sincerely that I was prevailed upon to take a glass. I felt that to refuse to taste any would be slighting the hospitality of the lady of the house [Frances Thornton].

The company broke up about 10 o'clock. Friend [G.W.] Boteler was a little luny—so was "Judge" [James Henry] Noland.

[FIELD HOSPITAL, CAROLINE CO.]

FRIDAY, APL 17, 1863

This morning is cool—To-day already, I have had to take a short nap—rec'd a note from Miss Mollie Thornton that she had an invitation to visit Mr. Motley's and requested us to come over and go with them. I obtained permission from Surgeon Black for [G.W.] Boteler and myself to go—went.

At Mrs. Motley's we enjoyed ourselves very much—A Band from a Georgia Regiment came after supper and gave us some good music. Soon after the members of the band were introduced and things became quiet indoors the sounds of violins were heard outside.

Mr. Motley might have been frightened—enough to wake him [viz., raise him from the dead]. The company was a gay[320] one and deported themselves

---

[319] He uses the military term for redundancy in ironical fashion; usually the charming Mollie Graves dominates parties, especially where young soldiers are attending.

[320] Happy and joyous; no sexual connotations. See earlier note.

very well. A Capt. Lockett[321] was the only name I learned. Miss Motleys are indeed very interesting girls—Miss Gwynn [Motley] is quite deserving respect: Miss Sue [Motley] is more vain. The violin crowd was brought in—"Judge" [James Henry Noland] found the most important individual in the lot. Miss Galleher [possibly Gollehon] was along. They were much surprised to find a regular band present when they stepped in—Cake and Wine were served—I took no wine.

We returned to camp about 10 o'clock. Dr. B spent his time yesterday evening composing a schedule of rules for the government of the Hospt; the only clause affecting me is "No employee will leave the Hosp't without permission of the Surg: in charge:" This is right. I have been going enough now to stop awhile.

[FIELD HOSPITAL, CAROLINE CO.]

SATURDAY, APL. 18, 1863

This morning promised a pretty day.

We went fishing in the afternoon. Dr. Jamison and some others went into the water and hauled the seine. We caught a very pretty string [of fish] [.] The crowd that went into the water got "tight" [drunk] and of course was very witty—

There was a general invitation extended to the Hospital boys to visit Mrs. [Frances] Thornton's to-night at a tableau.[322] I felt ashamed to go but on learning that there were some strange ladies there I could not decline. Dr. Hagy, Dr. McGuire [possibly Hunter Holmes McGuire], Dr. Wilkerson, Dr. Magruder and indeed all except Dr. Black went. I had to introduce the gentlemen and one lady said I surely had a shower of doctors on hand.

---

[321] Among VA officers, at least in Stonewall Brigade, the only officer named Lockett I can find is Samuel D. Lockett (1833-1864), a former merchant of Grayson Co. who joined Smyth Blues as Cpl., then served 4th VA Inf. in Co. D as Sgt.; in 1863 he resigned 4th Inf., went to Wythe Co. and joined 22d VA Cav., being elected 1st Lt. This Lockett was killed in action at Lynchburg on 18 June 1864. Jeffrey D. Weaver, *22d VA Cav*, VA Regimental Histories Series (Lynchburg, VA: H.E. Howard, 1991) 96. Robertson, *4th VA Inf.*, 61.

[322] A costume party, generally built around a theme, in this case a wedding scene in which St. Paul's descriptions of the kinds of love are personified. "tableau vivant (French lit. living picture)—a representation of a personage, character, scene, incident etc. of a well known painting or statue by one person or a group of persons in suitable costumes." Plural, tableaux vivants, tablee. *OED*.

I can't say that I care much for tableaux or tablee. It may be pleasant to the participants, but not to the occupants of the room. The marriage was conducted very well—indeed looked natural. A representation of Faith, Hope and Charity was the best, Miss Mollie Graves representing Faith. Her countenance was composed and looked forward on the beholders with a confident air—(may that air never have cause to be otherwise) Miss Eve Thornton represented Hope, the best performer present. She stood between Faith & Charity, her hands clasped and eyes upturned towards Heaven. She seemed to gaze on scenes beyond this vale of tears. Miss Anne Catlett represented Charity. She seemed busy scattering crumbs around and dispersing gifts to the poor, unconscious of who was looking at her.

I enjoyed myself with the ladies promiscuously. I was a little ruffled in temper at "Judge" [James Henry] Noland. I do not like monopoly and wished to take a young lady in the room as a friend of hers expressed a desire that I should entertain her for a while. I got the young lady—Miss Buckner—to change her seat and sit on the sofa. She did so and I took a chair in front of her. Judge took a seat by her side and seemed to me to be somewhat presumptuous. Proposed eating a philopena which she did.[323] I spoke to her several times but my voice was soon drowned by his. I left in disgust, for I thought she felt herself in a disagreeable place.

Miss Bucker is a very nice lady—very delicate and dignified. Miss Jessee is large, and not so finely featured nor has so nice an expression of countenance as Miss Buckner. Drs. Wilkerson and Miss Mollie [Graves] of course were entertainment for each other. The old ladies hung around till midnight and disappeared. Aunt Kesey [Keziah Shepherd] was exuberant. The party broke about 10 o'clock. I got a letter from Mrs. [Mary] Tomlin to-day—also a paper from Mrs. Faris.

---

[323] This was a game for two only, and the diarist was right to recognize monopoly, albeit with the young woman's clear consent to be with Noland alone; Apperson thinks Miss Buckner finds herself in a "disagreeable place," but the nature of the game suggests she wanted Apperson to leave so that she could be with Noland. Philopena is a "corruption of Greek [words not joined together in the Greek] for *much loved* and *penalty*, from an idea that the gift was a penalty of friendship or love." The game involves two people sharing food, usually twin kernels of the same nut. After eating the philopena, the two contest with words, for instance the loser being the first one to answer "yes" or "no" to questions in a series, the first one so answering forfeits the last kernel. *Webster's 2d Intl.*

[FIELD HOSPITAL, CAROLINE CO.]

SUNDAY, AP. 19 1863

This is Sabbath. I slept late this morning. We had just finished sweeping out when the ladies appeared. Miss Keziah [Shepherd}, two Mrs. Thorntons [one probably Frances Thornton], Miss Eve Thornton and Miss Mollie Thornton, Miss Sue [Catlett] and Miss Anne Catlett. [G.W.] Boteler had rece'd a permit from Dr. B to go to Hamilton's Crossing, and the ladies concluded to go. They went to the [Guinea's Station] depot, but soon returned. The conductor said he could not put them off where they wished to be put off. I finished my morning's work and walked over with the ladies. Miss Mollie Thornton, I am vain enough to think, has considerable affection for myself, but I cannot encourage it. I parted with her probably never to see her again. She requested me to write frequently.

I took a nap in the evening. Before I awoke the Miss Motleys [Gwynn and Sue] were announced. I rose and went to them—took a stroll with them, and I accompanied Miss Gwynn [Motley] home, Capt. [John] Glaize,[324] Miss Sue [Catlett] and Motley the youngest [Sue Motley]Lt. Col. [Alexander] Peck came and I thought we had better leave. This gentleman I have met before and I distrust him perhaps.[325]

"Judge" [James Henry Noland] & myself had a considerable flare-up. He was reproaching me for something I had said in the presence of Mrs. Galleher [possibly Gollehon] last night. I told him that I was ruffled last night, and that I did not think he acted the part of a dignified gentleman and told him when the occurrence took place again, I would insult him since he spoke somewhat disrespectfully to me. I asked him to walk out of the tent. I am a good friend of "Judge's" and will do as much as anyone for him, but I like for a man to know

[324] John Glaize (1822-1901, occupation before war unknown) apparently born and/or raised in Winchester. Joined Winchester Riflemen, which became Co. F, 2d VA Inf. Appointed Capt. and Asst. QM to VA Militia guarding Winchester after 1862 Valley Campaign. QM Dept. as Capt. of Valley District 28 April 1862. On 15 September 1864 joined ANV Forage QM corps and served with ANV until surrender. Paroled at surrender. Married Selma Baker and after War established lumber business in Winchester. Elected to Shenandoah Co. offices: Sheriff, Treasurer, Jailor, and Magistrate; City Council of Winchester, 1887-1890. Buried Mt. Hebron Cemetary, Winchester. Frye, *2d VA Inf*, 100.

[325] Possibly Alexander H. Peck of 14th VA Cav. Peck (1835-?), was laborer from Montgomery Co. who joined Ft. Lewis Volunteers, who became Co. B of 4th VA Inf. 1st Sgt. at muster, he was elected 1st Lt. but resigned Inf. 21 April 1862. Joined 14th Cav. sometime in spring or summer 1862 and rose in rank. Robertson, *4th VA Inf.*, 67.

what he is doing. Noland is one of the queer genii.[326] I know I talked to him too plain but unless talk is plain, he will misunderstand it. I wrote two letters to-night, one to Miss Laura Faris, and the other to Miss Kate Dunn of Richmond, Va. in D[rury] W. Venable's name and for the purpose of finding out something of "Mrs. Allen" [Mary Camden]. Miss Dunn is Venable's cousin.

[FIELD HOSPITAL, CAROLINE CO.]

MONDAY, APRIL 20, 1863

This morning rain commenced falling very rapidly, and continued during the day. Nothing of interest occurred.

Dr. Hagy took some of the boys and went fishing. They were not very successful. I was in the water Saturday evening. The water is too cold to stay any great while, and the pond is too rough for the seine.

I wrote to Cousin Bettie and to father. I asked father to turn my horse on grass as soon as it came, and I would pay the pasturage. Dr. Syd[nor] & [William H.]Thomas[327] went over to see Miss Mollie [Graves]. I do not care much about her.

Not many sick are brought in now. There are a great many cases of dropsy of some form or another. Dr. B. rec'd an order from Surg. Gen. [La Fayette] Guild directing him to exercise more care in selecting patients for transportation. This will give us a much larger number of patients here for treatment, and will require much more room for accommodation of the sick.

---

[326] Arch phrase meaning *strange type*, but more in the nature of sui generis or eccentricly individualistic than anything judgmental or even evaluative. "Queer," like "gay," had no particular sexual connotation in the Civil War Era.

[327] William H. Thomas (1836-?) was merchant from Blacksburg who enlisted in Montgomery Highlanders, who became Co. E of 4th VA Inf. He rose and fell in noncommissioned ranks in 4th Inf. and then on 26 September 1862 he transfered to Co. G, 14th VA Cav. He served in Cav. until his horse was killed at Port Republic on 26 September 1864, although part of that service was on "shoeing detail" rather than combat. After his horse was killed, he paid bounty of $2,500 and left service. In Blacksburg, he worked as a salesman and was still living in 1917 according to city records. There is a William H. Thomas who died in 1918 who is buried in Blacksburg, but Robertson suggests that he is a different man [in ordnance, and born in 1837]. Driver, *14th VA Cav.*, 182; Robertson, *4th VA Inf.*, 76.

[FIELD HOSPITAL, CAROLINE CO.]

TUESDAY, APRIL 21, 1863

This has been a chilly day. The spring is very backward, very few trees show any inclination to bud, and fields are almost as bare as they are in winter. I have been reading [John Julian] Chisholm's "Manual of Military Surgery" to-day.[328] I had a chat with some of the boys in regard to forming a class of students for the study of some branch of medicine. There are now about 10 medical students on duty here, and with that number, a very respectable class could be formed. In joining it I think it necessary to go into some sort of organization that will insure order and dignity and compell each member to study to maintain a fair standing in the class. To do this we must have a set of rules. When these are adhered to, we might hope for something interesting and instructive. I proposed that we have a meeting to-morrow night and come to some conclusion. I know that some encouragement is necessary for judicious study for myself and it is much the same with others. Dr. Hagy and Dr. Wilkerson both promised aid.

I wrote to Miss Mollie Thornton to-night. I don't know that I was doing right though. I can only promise her the hand of friendship, more, she cannot expect. Although she is a nice, good girl and would make anyone a worthy helpmeet,[329] it is wrong for me to give her any grounds for claim for more than a friend. [G.W.] Boteler got a letter from [Mollie Thornton]. I believe she likes Boteler, but I would not care. She said enough to me to satisfy any doubts.

Several of the boys are over at Mrs. [Frances] Thornton's to-night. If she has not an extra amount of endurance, she must surely wish for this Hospital to move away.

---

[328] John Julian Chisolm (1830-1903) was a surgeon from SC, originally with Medical College of SC in Charleston and later medical purveyor for CSA in Columbia, SC. He wrote one of four scientific treatises authorized by the Surgeon General La Fayette Guild to instruct surgeons of the CSA. His treatise, *A Manual of Military Surgery for the Use of Surgeons in the Confederate Army* (Richmond, VA: Medical Services of Surgeon General, 1861, 1862, 1864) was issued in at least three editions and was more widely used than the other manuals. After War, he returned to Medical College and enjoyed a distinguished career with national recognition. Of Chisolm's manual, Cunningham notes that "[Chisolm's] books were 'in the pockets' of medical officers, and early in 1864 the Army of Tennessee's medical directors acknowledged receipt of 433 copies of the manual written pursuant to the Surgeon General's orders." Cunningham, quotation, 219; 248; 147; 270-71.

[329] In the KJV the phrase is "an help meet for him," meaning that Eve was help appropriate or fit or apt for Adam. Southerners of Civil War Era and later ran the two words together and generally spoke of all wives as being *helpmeets* for their husbands, and sometimes also transliterated things a step farther and described all wives as *helpmates.* Gen. 2:18 (KJV). See "meet," *OED.*

[FIELD HOSPITAL, CAROLINE CO.]

WEDNESDAY, APRIL 22, 1863

This morning Miss Mollie [Graves] & Aunt Keziah [Shepherd] came over. They took dinner with us. Miss M[ollie Graves] is as gay as ever and quite fascinating or so she thinks. She has a very great influence over Dr. "Wilk" [Wilkerson]. He is with her at all times. What his intentions are I cannot say. I do not think they are pure. A fishing party is on hand for the evening.

I got a letter from Mollie [Mary Camden]. The representations of her condition are deeply affecting indeed. She seems to have felt a painful force in what I told her while she was up here, and when she wrote, she was in bed. I do not know how to take her. Sometimes I think her a woman that attempts to make some impression and become a heroine. She has a mania for something. I wrote her a letter stating that my opinion of her was not such as that of others and I would not change till I had cause.

We [the would-be medical college students] had a meeting to-night and came to a sort of conclusion about the class. Astrology [sic][330] forms the subject of a lesson to-morrow night. I fear that there will be a want of unity and order under our present arrangement.

[FIELD HOSPITAL, CAROLINE CO.]

APRIL 23D, THURSDAY [1863]

Raining very hard this morning. No sick sent off. I was engaged most of the day in studying anatomy. I read Gray and Richardson [texts identified earlier].

I rec'd the nicest bo[u]quet from Miss Mary Battaille & Miss Susan Catlett this evening. It is indeed the most lovely thing of the kind I think I have ever seen.

The class met to-night at the hour appointed. Dr. Black was present and was invited to make some sort of address which he did in plain candid style. He said he was heartily glad that we had formed ourselves into a class for the purpose of doing something for our advancement. He stated upon consultation with the Medical Director [field director Hunter Holmes McGuire, overall director La

[330] The diarist writes *astrology*. However, his next entry discusses surgical anatomy as the topic of study, and William G. Bean suggests that the diarist simply wrote down the wrong word, since there is no other mention of studying astrology. Bean, notes.

Fayette Guild][331] it had been decided to have detached a number of young men who had been Students of Medicine and have them attached to the [field] Hospital. This had been done and by careful attention a vast amount of useful information might be gathered by us, and of that character that could be found nowhere else. He asked the hearty cooperation of everyone in making the sick and wounded comfortable, and pointed out the advantages that must inevitably accrue from a firm determination to study. He suggests a study of surgical anatomy, as looking to the probability that we soon may be called upon to act at some post in the field of conflict. His remarks were very apropos. He and the other medical officers then left us and we proceeded to quiz. Dr. Ellsberg quizzes [asks worthwhile questions in examination] very well. Most of the boys answered well to[o] except Judge [James Henry] Noland—makes an ass of himself wherever he goes, and in whatever he does.

I am quiz master for Saturday night and the subject reaches from the cocyx to the frontal bone.

[FIELD HOSPITAL, CAROLINE CO.]

FRIDAY, APL 24, 1863

This has been one of the changeable spring days. Rain falling in torrents one minute and the sun shining brightly the next, now a gust of wind sweeping over our tents and making ropes and "flies" [tent coverings without sides] tear and flap and presently a still quiet comes.

The mail brought me another letter from "Mollie" [Mary Camden]. She says nothing of her health this time. This chimes badly with [six illegible words] in her last [letter] I rec'd. The same expressions of grief are again re-iterated and the repitition of good wishes for me. She hopes I will not be troubled about her sorrows and wishes to know if I wish to discontinue writing her. She still persists that if I could see her in Richmond, I would be convinced of her innocence. This is premature. I have never intimated that I believed anything derogatory about her character.

The report from our lines in the neighborhood of Port Royal [also in Caroline Co.] is that several boat loads of Yankees crossed the Rappahannock and captured several wagons belong to Maj. [John M.] Preston Q.M. News from other parts of the country is very quiet. [James] Longstreet and [Daniel Harvey]

[331] The context does not make it clear which directing officer he is talking about.

Hill have both failed to do anything on the southern and eastern coasts. A[mbrose] P[owell] Hill's division is moving. [332]

I have been reading some 'till to-day. Dr. Wilkerson, I think, will lecture to-morrow night.

[FIELD HOSPSITAL, CAROLINE CO.]

[SATURDAY] APRIL 25, 1863

The weather is better to-day. Among the arrivals on the train of indisposed [soldiers] was Lt. [Tinsley Linsley] Allen [supposed cousin and probable lover of Mary Camden in her "Mrs. Allen" role, and very briefly, tentmate with the diarist]. I at first thought I would go down and see him but afterwards thought differently. I went down to a tent, and he was there, but he did not seem to recognize me and I passed by in silence. I may have acted properly and I may have not

Our meeting came off to-night. Had a very interesting meeting. Dr. Wilkerson lectured on "Surgery". He first gave definitions of the word and then the practice and duties of a surgeon in times gone by. He placed the surgeon as the "tool of the physician" and spoke very exhaustively of the progress and perfection made of it as a branch. Gunshot wounds then formed the subject of his remarks. He conflicts with the teaching of [John Julian] Chisolm [author of the most widely used surgeon's text in CSA medical corps] in the extraction of [minie] balls. Dr. Wilkerson says, if a ball is submerged in bone, leave it. Dr. Chisolm says it is not the question, Can balls remain enclosed in the tissues, but *do they*? and advises extraction wherever there is the least chance to do so.

After the lecture the quiz was conducted and answered. I acted as quiz master. Our next is Dr. Hagy to lecture and the frontal and temporal bones for the quiz.

---

[332] A federal expedition concluded a successful raid ending in Port Royal between 22 and 24 April 1863; the incident with John Preston's wagons is not recorded in *Official Records*. Federal forces skirmished in Suffolk Co. in southeastern Tidewater, and were essentially unchecked by CSA forces. A. P. Hill's march along the Rappahannock preparatory to the fighting at Chancellorsville is among the most justly storied of his career, and it contributed greatly to T.J. Jackson's fame as a fast-marching "foot cavalry." See E.B. Long, 340-42; Edwin C. Bearss, "Hill," *Hist. Times*.

[FIELD HOSPITAL, CAROLINE CO.]

SUNDAY, APRIL 26, 1863

It was understood last evening that we have preaching to-day at 11 o'clock but owing to the indisposition of Mr. Patterson [sic], the minister, it was postponed. Mr. [W. Gaines] Miller, who arrived to-day, agreed to preach this evening at 4 o'clock.[333]

Mrs. Keziah [Shepherd] and Mrs. [Frances] Thornton came over. Miss Mollie [Thornton] and Eve [Thornton] also. They returned home to dinner, to return again to evening service. After dinner Mr. [G.W.] Boteler and myself walked up to Mr. Motley's to come with the ladies. Had a walk with Miss Gwynn [Motley].

Unpleasant things will happen to all of us at times. Miss Mollie Graves did not come in the tent where the young ladies were until after preaching and when she did it was in such a manner that I was unable to find an opportunity to introduce her. She left the tent and threw out some very curt insinuations. I have written an apology but do not blame myself as much now as I did at first, and don't feel much inclined to apologize. We went home with the young ladies. Miss Sue [Motley] is quite lively. Miss Gwynn [Motley] is more reserved. Dr. B thinks we were guilty of a very grave injustice to the young ladies in not introducing them this evening. I hope not. the day has not been spent as pleasantly as I would wish.

The sermon was plain, preaching from a well-known text[,] "Come unto me all ye that are weary and heavy laden and I will give you rest." He first spoke of the burden we bear naturally and spiritually, then of the comparison with [illegible adjective] allusions in the old Mosaic law—in calling upon them he said[,] ["]Take my yoke, for it is easy["]—that is easier than the Mosaic law—the laws of the gospel could be borne more easily. Thus those whom he called had the glory of that rest.[334]

---

[333] I cannot find a minister named Patterson serving ANV at this time; more probably, it was Peter Archibald Peterson, who was assigned on regular basis as chaplain in ANV. W. Gaines Miller was chaplain regularly assigned to 46th VA Inf. Pitts, 150-51.

[334] Words ascribed to Jesus Christ quoted in Matthew 11:28-30: "Come unto me, all ye that labour and are heavy laden, and I will give you rest. Take my yoke upon you, and learn of me; for I am meek and lowly in heart: and ye shall find rest unto your souls. For my yoke is easy, and my burden is light." (KJV). It is the doctrine of Christ's grace offered because people are unable to follow the laws given by Moses [Mosaic Law]. Pitts (in *Chaplains in Gray*) notes such verses concerning grace and forgiveness were the most common themes among CSA chaplains in the sermons he examined: "The main burden of the chaplain's message, however, dealt with sin and

Preaching has been appointed for 4 o'clock to-morrow.

[FIELD HOSPITAL, CAROLINE CO.]

MONDAY, APRIL 27, 1863

More men came to-day than usual. I was very busy 'till afternon. I excused myself of my engagement to go to Mrs. Motley's after the girls. They came down for the preaching. Mr. Patterson [sic; possibly chaplain Peterson], the Baptist, preached from the text, "This is my beloved son in whom I am well pleased."[335] I have not heard a better sermon for a long while. He spoke then of God and his attributes, first claimed as [illegible], then the divinity acknowledged. Arguments from the historical, natural, and spiritual world were given [illegible adjective] force [illegible noun]. The belief of the [illegible] voice, i.e., that is the belief of the [approximately fifty words concerning sermon are completely illegible].

He has been unwell and did not talk as long as he would have.

I walked home with Miss Gwynn Motley. She is a good girl, very modest and dignified. I returned about sundown. Spent the evening in packing [because of reports that a major battle was coming soon, and the field hospital would be moved].

[FIELD HOSPITAL, CAROLINE CO.]

TUESDAY, APL 28, '63

To-day passed quietly. No news of importance. I wrote a letter to Mrs. [Mary] Tomlin this evening.

[FIELD HOSPITAL, CAROLINE CO.]

WEDNESDAY, APL 29, '63

This morning early the sound of cannon was reverberating along the shores of the Rappahannock. A courier soon came with some orders for Dr. Black—It stated that Dr. B should be ready to move his hospital near the field. Dr. went to make preparations to obey orders. Another came, ordering the ambulance train

---

retribution, pardon and salvation. This was the message that he, by personal conviction, by the situation of battle, or the desires of the soldiers, felt compelled to bring." Idem, 111.

335 Matthew 3-16-17. God's words, spoken when the Heavens parted after John the Baptist baptized Jesus Christ; the "Spirit of God descending like a dove, and lighting upon him. And lo a voice from heaven, saying, 'This is my beloved Son, in whom I am well pleased'." (KJV).

up. By 2 P.M. the wagons were ready to move. [G.W.] Boteler and myself called at Mr. Motley's. The old gentleman seemed very much grieved. Rain commenced falling. We remained 'till nearly night. I am sure even that late I did not wish to leave Miss Gwynn [Motley]. But duty called and I could not refuse to go. Taking the wrong road we missed the wagons at Hamilton's Crossing and had a severe trip. Weary and footsore we found the camp about midnight and lay down to sleep on the wet ground with nothing under except a tent "fly." Before morning rain fell and drenched us. The camp was at the house of a Mr. Alsop.

In wandering around we passed the old Brigade [1st VA or Stonewall Bde]—I saw the 4th [VA Inf. comprising Smyth and neighboring counties] and had a cordial meeting with many of the boys.

There was considerable fighting to-day near Fredericksburg which resulted in some thirty killed, wounded and captured from our side. The loss is principally from 6th LA & 13th GA.[336]

[CAMP AT ALSOP'S, CAROLINE CO.]

THURSDAY, APRIL 30TH '[18]63

To-day spent in camp speculating what would be done. The morning was very foggy and rainy. As soon as the fog cleared up firing commenced and was kept up through the day, though not briskly. The enemy keeps close to the river under his guns out of danger. Our line and theirs are not far apart. The artillery firing was at too great a distance for much harm to either side.

---

[336] On 28 April, Joseph Hooker's Army of the Potomac "crossed the Rappahannock in the Wilderness [Apperson's birthplace], upstream from Fredericksburg. Meanwhile, a large force still confronted the Confederates across from the city. A flank attack by the Federals was obviously planned. At Fredericksburg early in the morning the bell in the Episcopal church rang out the alarm." The particular fighting that Apperson heard was likely at Franklin's Crossing or Deep Run just below Fredericksburg; it could also have been from White Oak Run or Fitzhugh's Crossing. George Stoneman's cavalry "operated against" R.E. Lee's communications while skirmishing broke out at several crossing points on the Rappahannock upstream and downstream from Fredericksburg. Stoneman (1822-1894), a native of Busti, NY and a distinguished West Point graduate with rank of Maj. Gen., would become quite infamous in Apperson's adoptive home for "Stoneman's Raid" in 1864. On this occasion, his "lackluster" cavalry leadership on this particular maneuver against Lee was heavily criticized. Meanwhile, R.E. Lee "probed and planned" in Fredericksburg. On 30 April, Hooker addressed his Federal forces and congratulated them on the three days of maneuvering, telling them that the enemy forces of the ANV "must ingloriously fly, or come out from behind their defences and give us battle on our ground, where certain destruction awaits him." Hooker closed with the prediction of "splendid success." Long, 340-45.

The chief opinion is that we will fall back. The enemy is only making a feint here while the main body is crossing at Kelly's [Ford of Rappahannock] and at Germanna [Ford of river].

Dr. Hagy was sent back to Guinea['s] [Station Depot] this morning to send all baggage to Hanover Junction [in Hanover Co. south of camp on a main railroad line and near North Anna River].

The signal lights are busy all along the line. There are two or three [military] bands of music performing near our camp. The feelings aroused by hearing the "Marseilles" [sic; song *Marseillaise*] and seeing ten thousand campfires burning at the same time is very striking.[337]

Dr. Gilkerson came up on to-days train and reported to Dr. [Hunter Holmes] McGuire [medical director in field for ANV] who ordered him to report to Dr. Black [chief surgeon in ANV]. He has passed the board of examiners [test] at Richmond for an assistant surgeon.

I rec'd a letter from Miss Mollie Thornton to-day and answered it. I also got one from Mrs. Faris and Mollie [Mary Camden] yesterday.

[CAMP AT ALSOP'S, CAROLINE CO.]

FRIDAY, MAY 1ST, 1863

Orders were received early this morning from Dr. [Hunter Holmes] McGuire to move. Following close in rear of [Isaac Ridgeway] Trimble's Division.[338] We passed up by Yerby's house and out to the plank road near Mr. Wyatt's. "Mose" Gibson[339] fell in with us. Near the Telegraph Road we obtained

---

337 The French Revolutionary fight song was popular with CSA troops who looked on the War as a fight for independence; it was also a symbol of the lingering hope that Napoleon III was going to help the CSA in the War.

338 Isaac Ridgeway Trimble (1802-1888) was a West Point graduate and distinguished engineer from Maryland with 10 years of army engineering and 29 years of civilian engineering. When War came, he "burned bridges north of Baltimore to disrupt the passage of Union volunteers to Washington, D.C." In CSA, he served first as Col. of engineers, helping with defenses at Norfolk and then commissioned Brig. Gen. under Gen. Richard S. Ewell. He fought well in Valley Campaign, Seven Days, and Cedar Mountain, but was severely wounded at 2d Manassas (29 August 1862). He was not available to lead his Division on this campaign, but did return for the Gettysburg Campaign. Jeffrey D. Wert, "Trimble," *Hist. Times.*

339 Moses Gibson (birth and death dates unknown, but alive in 1906), nicknamed Mose, joined 2d VA Inf. at Darkesville and then transfered Oct. 1862 to Co. D, 4th VA; on 31 October1862 he was detailed as clerk to Surg. Hunter Holmes McGuire, and probably came to know Apperson then. On 30 April 1863 he was promoted to hospital steward. Frye, *2d VA Inf.*, 100; Robertson, *4th VA Inf.*, 52.

forage for our team. The artillery of Col. Brown detained the ambulance train for some time. I was surprised to see the fine condition of the artillery horses and the new guns. The troops seemed in full spirits and were marching rapidly.[340]

At the Telegraph Road we turned to the left at Mr. Wyatt's and out to the plank road [from Chancellorsville to Fredericksburg] at Tabernacle Church. At a little house near the [Tabernacle] Church some wounded were brought belonging to [R.H.] Anderson's Division [of James Longstreet's corps][341] , and a little lower down was the [field] hospital of [William] Mahone's Brigade.[342] Several Squads of prisoners were brought back—it looked natural to see "blue Jackets" going to the rear. Dr. Sydnor amputated several fingers for a Yankee.

We moved across the plank road and a little up to the right of the road going west and camped. Dr. [Hunter Holmes] McGuire, Dr. Coleman, Col. Abner Smead[343] and several others were to supper. Dr. B expressed some dissatisfaction at his mess being so large and his feelings as regard Commissioned & Non-Commissed officers messing to-gether—I quit the mess. [Apperson would have been the only Non-Commissioned person in that list.]

News from the front is that the enemy is falling back before our skirmishers.[344]

---

[340] W.G. Bean notes that R.E. Lee sent T.J. Jackson with the divisions of A.P. Hill, R.E. Rode, and R.E. Colston from Fredericksburg to Chancellorsville "to engage Hooker's advance guard which was marching eastward from Chancellorsville toward Fredericksburg. Jubal A. Early's division of Jackson's corps and other troops remained on the heights overlooking Fredericksburg." Bean, notes.

[341] Anderson's forces had been guarding the fords upstream from Fredericksburg. Bean, notes.

[342] William Mahone (1826-1895) was from Southampton City [Southampton Co.], a graduate of Virginia Military Institute, and a respected civil engineer and president of Norfolk & Petersburg Railroad when War broke out. He was appointed Col. of 6th VA Inf. and rose in rank throughout the fighting. He "was one of the officers of the ANV who emerged as leaders of high rank and reputation in the campaigns after Chancellorsville (1-4 May 1863). From the Wilderness to Appomattox, Mahone's troops were considered some of the best fighters in the army, making their commander one of Gen. Robert E. Lee's most trusted generals." After the War, he reestablished his RR and entered VA politics. Elected to US Senate in 1880, he was a Readjustor, VA's "version of the Republican Party." "The control of state politics was virtually in Mahone's hands for a time...." J. Tracy Power, "Mahone," *Hist. Times.*

[343] W.G. Bean identifies Abner Smead as a native of GA, a West Point graduate of 1854, and inspector general of T.J. Jackson's corps. Bean, notes.

[344] When Joseph Hooker's troops marching on the Plank Road and Turnpike encountered T.J. Jackson's forces, the Federal General withdrew the Army of Potomac to Chancellorsville and entrenched there. It was not a retreat, but the maneuver probably cost the Army of Potomac the opportunity for the bold initiative that Lincoln wanted for his army in this long-planned

[FIELD HOSPITAL ON THE PLANK ROAD, CAROLINE CO.]

SATURDAY & SUNDAY, MAY 2 & 3, [18]63

This morning we moved about sun rise.[345] Some cannon and small arms were heard on the old pike. On the hill near Mr. Perry's our army seemed to have staid last night. Over towards McGhee's[,] pickets were firing and some heavy artillery. Two of our caissons were blown up by the enemy—The troops marched up the plank road to "new store". Here were a great many wounded. The house bore unmistakable marks of a conflict near-by. Heavy cannonading towards the Old [Catharine] Furnace. I have feared the enemy would get those hills and give us trouble to dislodge them. The ambulance train took the old Catharpin road [Catharpin was in Prince William Co.] and went up to Todd's Tavern [Spotsvylania Co.][346] I was on horseback. There we took the road known as Brock's and travelled it about a mile. The troops came out from the [Catharine] Furnace, crossed Brock's Road and left it [turning] to the right. We came near having a panic here. The enemy, I suppose, perceives our forces crossing beyond the [Catharine] Furnace and decide [sic] to cut of[f] our wagon trains—several horses were wounded and some wagons turned back. Dr. B directed us on a left-hand track up by Wm Stephens [sic][347] and by Mr. Trigg. I began to expect that the fight would occur at Wilderness [his birthplace and site of his family's church in Orange Co.] being the best position I know of in the section of [Orange] county.

Passing the old Hawkins place [two miles west of eventual battlesite], I could but notice a great change. The fields had grown smaller and the road seemed shorter. Trees had sprung up and grown up since last I saw the place; the old [Hawkins] house was gone. The little mounds still stood in the yard, though,

---

engagement. See Long, 347-50. Chancellorsville was a community built around Melze Chancellor's [born 1815] home in Spotsylvania Co. It was listed in census as Chancellors Township of Spotsylvania Co. VA Census 1870.

[345] W.G. Bean writes, "This was the beginning of Jackson's daring flank movement on May 2, 1863. Lee, after ascertaining that Hooker's right flank was unprotected, directed Jackson to attack it. The next morning, May 2, Jackson, marching by way of the Catherine Furnace through the Wilderness to Hooker's rear and right flank, surprised the Eleventh Federal Corps and routed it. Meantime, Lee, with his other troops, remained on Hooker's front, simulating attacks, to cover Jackson's flanking maneuver." Bean, notes.

[346] W.G. Bean reports that Todd's Tavern [Spotsylvania Co.] was on the Brock Road connecting Chancellorsville to Spotsylvania Court House.

[347] More likely, William A. Stevens, born 1821, who owned a home in Chancellors Township in Spotsylaniva Co. VA Census 1870.

marking the resting place of the old people who lived so long ago. The old free Negroes' house looked familiar. When we reached the Plank Road cannonading had commenced in direction of Mrs. Jones' old place. I supposed it was there [at that house] but I afterwards learned better. We passed the old schoolhouse where I studied the rudiments of spelling and arithmetic in 1845—almost 18 years ago. My feelings were such that I seem not able [to] discuss them. The firing grew desperate—Dr. B was ordered forward to establish a [field] Hospital [at Wilderness Township of Orange Co.] and send the ambulances on the field. When we reached the old turnpike [where Apperson's father had once driven wagons for hire] the ambulances were sent down and the loaded wagons went to Wilderness. Out tents were pitched along a Guly where I have enjoyed many, many plays at "Gully Keeper". [a game something like "King of the Hill," but with the "king" standing above the gully and "keeping subjects" down in the gully instead of at the base of the hill]—The wounded commenced coming in—and we went to work.

It seems that Jackson commenced upon them as soon as he came up, and the enemy made tracks [ran away]. Our troops fought almost recklessly. The enemy left his works [entrenchments and tents].

The saddest event of the day is a wound rec'd by Gen. Jackson—Several of us were sitting around the fire and one of the boys remarked jestingly that a tent had been put up for Gen'l Jackson, that he had fought so well that we could afford to Give him one. Another said he was wounded—Had his leg shot off. He did not mean it—several of us laughed at the idea of Jackson being wounded —knowing that he had escaped in so many hard fought battles.

But the truth is too painful to write—he was wounded in the left arm and amputation was necessary—Dr [Hunter Holmes] McGuire operated. [348] I got

---

[348] The operation was performed at once. Dr. McGuire was assisted by Dr. Black, Dr. Walls, and by Dr. Coleman. As far as medical records can show, and in Apperson's "Reminiscences," the operation was successful, and T.J. Jackson could have returned to duty after recuperation, as had other field officers who had suffered severe wounds such as William Mahone and Jubal A. Early; indeed, as noted earlier, "Old Bald Head" Richard S. Ewell lost a leg and returned to field leadership riding horses and leading in place of the slain T.J. Jackson. What killed Jackson was not the operation, but the disease of pneumonia that he contracted in hospital during recuperation. As often happened to Civil War surgeons, it was not their operating-tent surgery that failed, but their recovery-tent or recovery-house field hospital after the surgery. The authority on Jackson, James I. Robertson Jr. affirms everything that the operating surgeons claimed in their reports and that the steward-diarist records in diary and in "Reminiscences." Robertson, *Thomas J. "Stonewall" Jackson; the Man, the Soldier, the Legend* (New York: Macmillan, 1997); and idem, *Stonewall Brigade.*

about a[sic] hours sleep and it was day and the cannon booming very heavy. The wounded commenced coming. The Enemy's strong works had been stormed and taken principally by [Isaac Ridgeway] Trimble's Division under command of Brigadier Gen'l [Raleigh Edward] Colston.[349] The "Stonewall Brigade" covered itself in glory while its chief officer lay suffering in hearing of the guns. The enemy had entrenched himself from Jenny's Old House in Chancellorsville. Rev: Melzi [sic; Melze] Chancellor lived at Bullard's old place and earth works were all around.

The loss in the 4th VA Regt is almost appalling—went in with 365 and lost 162. The [Smyth] "Blues & Grays" [most of whom were in Co. D of 4th; Wythe "Grays" were mostly in Co. A, but Apperson knew little of them and probably confounded his adoptive home Grays with the Wythe Grays] lost over 50.[350] The Brigade charged the enemy works 3 times before it was successful. Genl [Elilsha Franklin "Frank"] Paxton was killed. He was a brave man.[351] Capt. [Milton Hall] Harmon[352] of the 4th Reg't was killed. Capt. [John Hall] Fulton lost a leg.[353]

---

[349] Raleigh Edward Colston (1825-1896) was born in Paris and adopted by a VA physician in 1842. A graduate of Virginia Military Institute, he taught French at the Lexington school until the War came. He rose through ranks in major battles, and Gen. T.J. Jackson chose his former VMI faculty colleague to command a brigade and then, on Trimble's wounding, a Div. In the fighting at Chancellorsville, Colston was involved in controversy because his troops did not advance as quickly as Jackson originally thought necessary, although of course there is no way of knowing Jackson's actual judgment of Colston's performance. On 20 May 1863, Colston was relieved of divisional command. He later served, without criticism, at Petersburg in 1864; and he was commanding CSA troops at Lynchburg when War ended. After War, his career became the stuff of legend: He joined Egyptian army and suffered a bad fall from a camel in 1879 and returned to US an invalid. He died penniless in the Confederate Soldiers' Home in Richmond. Jeffrey D. Wert, "Colston," *Hist. Times*, s.v

[350] Robertson does not count casualties by unit per engagement, but confirms that deaths in 4th were the most severe among CSA troops at Chancellorsville, and estimates that casualties and morbidities were highest. Ibid.

[351] Elisha Franklin Paxton (1828-1863), nicknamed "Frank" or "Bull" was from Rockbridge Co. and a graduate of Washington College in Lexington who had practiced law in Ohio prior to joining 27th VA, the old Rockbridge Rifles. See earlier notes. Paxton's appointment by Jackson was controversial, even leading to the resignation of Andrew Jackson Grigsby. Jackson was convinced that Paxton would do well, and he did fight bravely, but his death in this engagement and Jackson's own subsequent death makes it impossible to render meaningful judgments on Jackson's decision in this case of an unpopular promotion. See Wert, "Paxton," Hist. *Times*.; Reidenbaugh, *27th VA Inf.*, 72, 80, 168

[352]Milton Hall Harmon (1838-1863) was a farmer, apparently from Montgomery Co. who joined "Montgomery Fencibles," which became Co. G of 4th VA Inf. He was elected2d Lt. on

At the [field] hospital we were soon cramped. Something to eat was the main consideration.

These were trying scenes on ground once so familiar. I looked in vain for some familiar face of some citizen. I came to the conclusion that they too had been taken by the enemy or were afraid to come out.

Many sad scenes were brought up during the day and at night we were wearied and took some rest. The time passed rapidly—days hardly noticed [in their passing].

[WILDERNESS FIELD HOSPITAL, PLANK ROAD, ORANGE CO.]

MONDAY [MAY] 4, 1863

Nothing outside of the usual course of such stirring events passed to-day.[354]

---

joining and promoted, becoming Capt. on 22 April 1862. Killed 3 May 1863, Chancellorsville. Robertson, *4th VA Inf.*, 55.

[353] John Hall Fulton (1840-1907) was an attorney from Wytheville who joined Wytheville Grays, who became Co. A, 4th VA Inf. Appointed 3d Lt. on joining, he was promoted rapidly, becoming Capt. on 22 April 1862. He was wounded before, at Groveton (28 August 1862) in leg and arm; on 3 May 1863 at Chancellorsville, he was wounded so severely that doctors amputated his leg. He was discharged as disabled on 1 August 1863 and returned to Wytheville, where he practiced law until death in 1907. Buried in Wytheville. Robertson, 51.

[354] *Official Records*, May 4, 1863 show 1,665 CSA troops killed, 9081 wounded, and 5919 missing, from "effectives" of some 60,000; Federal casualty lists show 1,606 killed; 9762 wounded; 5919 missing from a huge "effectives" of some 133,868. The percentage for CSA are thus more than twice as bad. Some authorities consider the fighting at Fredericksburg to be a separate engagement, called 2d Battle of Fredericksburg, but it is very hard to disentangle the casualty lists for those two episodes that can properly be considered one long engagement, lasting from 27 April to 11 May and one farflung engagement up and down the Rappahannock River. In the Fredericksburg city fighting, Jubal A. Early's troops were driven from Marye's Heights, but Hooker's subsequent withdrawal back across the Rappahananock allowed CSA troops back into the Heights and the whole city. Jefferson Davis sent a wire to R.E. Lee: He said the southern people are "reverently united with you in giving praise to God for the success with which He has crowned your arms." Lincoln, for his part, tried to encourage Hooker, but was clearly dismayed. He met with Hooker on several occasions, trying to arrange another major attack across the Rappahannock. In summer when Lee began marching toward MD and PA on a desperate northern offensive, Hooker asked for an additional 10,000 troops from Harpers Ferry to help him, and when refused, he angrily resigned his position with Army of Potomac, so that the great Battle of Gettysburg was led at the North by George Meade instead of Hooker. Hooker took reassignment in western campaigns. Military historians praise Lee for the bold gamble of dividing his forces by sending Jackson on a flanking maneuver that left Lee's main body of 14,000 facing most of Hooker's 133,000 effectives; they praise Jackson for his most masterful "foot cavalry march"; they praise J.E.B. Stuart for his effective replacement of Jackson; but they roundly condemn Hooker for retreating to entrenchment when he first encountered a major force of CSA troops, thereby losing the offensive initiative; and they are scathing in denunciation of him for

I saw some of the Misses Hawkins and thought I knew them. A servant came along and informed me that I was right. I sent them my card & compliments. I went to Lt. Col. [Robert H.] Dungan to-day[355] He was wounded by fragment of a shell striking him in the breast. No outside damage—spilling some blood. This evening Dr. B & myself walked over to 1st Brigade [1st VA, or Stonewall Bde] Hospital, at Woodville Mines [Rappahannock Co.] farm. There I found many of my old associates and friends mutilated and torn—Horrible War.

There have been some preparations for receiving a visit from the Yankees here. [George] Stoneman with a division of Yankee cavalry made a raid through Louisa and Hanover Counties—tearing up the Central [Rail-] Road near Trevillian's Depot [Louisa Co.] and the R.P. & F.R.R. [Richmond, Petersburg & Fredericksburg Railroad] near Ashland [Hanover Co.] and then went towards James River to Columbia [Cumberland Co.][356]

This is something more bold than usual for the enemy though there is nothing daring. Our whole army was engaged here with [Joseph] Hooker and [George] Stoneman could go over our country unmolested. He met with no opposition—meeting but women & children & defenceless citizens. Noble work! Daring deed! Valorous Stoneman! His name will be sung far and wide among his northern brethren. The damage done was to capture a train of sick, burn the cars, and tear up the R. Roads. I hardly think he will visit us.

The fighting has nearly ceased. Our army is about 1/2 mile in advance of Chancellorsville and the enemy between that & the [Rappahannock] river. It is also reported that our force at Fredericksburg has been dislodged and the heights around Marye's have been captured.[357]

---

failing to attack Lee's exposed force of 14,000. See Long, 333-50; and John D. Kallman, "Hooker," *Hist. Times.*

[355] Robert Henry Dungan, a correspondent of antebellum days when he studied at Emory & Henry College, has already been identified. He was promoted to Lt. Col. on 2 January 1863 by unanimous vote of board of officers responding to Gen. Turner Ashby's enthusiastic recommendation. This wound, evening of 2 May 1863, involved a minie ball shot from some distance that "struck in the breast by a solid shot, but fortunately, so far spent that it broke no bones." He returned to action in June, commanding Brigade and sometimes Regt and achieving promotion to Col. Postwar teacher in Chilhowie (Smyth Co.) and then founder of Jonesboro (TN) Male Institute. "A staunch Democrat" and member Missionary Baptist Church of Bristol. Died 6 November 1903 in Bristol and buried there. Robertson, *4th VA Inf.*, 119.

[356] Dr. W.G. Bean notes that Columbia is in Goochland Co., but in Hummel's *List of Places* for antebellum years it was listed in Cumberland Co. [and another Columbia in Fluvanna, but that could not be the site]. Hummel, *A List*, 41; cf Bean, notes.

[357] As noted, this report was accurate, but the Federals abandoned Marye's Heights when Hooker moved the entire Army of the Potomac back across the Rappahannock.

It has been freely asserted that [James] Longstreet has come up.[358]

[FIELD HOSPITAL, WOODVILLE MINES FARM, RAPPAHANNOCK CO.]

TUESDAY, MAY 5, 1863

To-day we were busy. Dr. B sent Dr. Hacket and myself over to the [Woodville Mines] Farm to assist Dr. [John Alexander] Straith. On our way over, we met father, Mr. Henry Roach, his wife and wife's sister, Mrs. Sanders. Of course, all were glad to see me, or seemed so. They had been to the barn [serving as field hospital] and seen the wounded. I went in and met John F. Payne, Wm. Reynolds, & [illegible, possibly Abner; possibly Benj.] Sisson.[359] Dr. [John Alexander] Straith put me to work on some mutilated hands. I took off a number of fingers, and one was taken out in the middle of the metacarpal bone.[360]—This was Martin Roan, Co "A" 4th VA Infty[361]—I extracted a ball from among the tarsus[362] in the foot of Sam Byars.[363]

---

[358] James Longstreet was called to abandon siege of Suffolk in order to come to Fredericksburg area along Rappahannock and rejoin the ANV. He left Suffolk on 3 May 1863. Long, 348.

[359] Bean identifies Payne, Reynolds, and Sisson as boyhood friends from Orange Co. Scott lists John Payne as Pvt. with Co. A, 13th VA Inf, the original "Montpelier Guard'; William H. Reynolds as Pvt. in Peyton's Battery, later Fry's, in Cutshaw's Bn; and Abner Sisson as Pvt. in Co. I, 6th VA Cav., originally "Orange Rangers." Scott, *Hist. of Orange*, 264-77. John Foster Payne (no birth and death data) is listed as member of 13th VA Inf. and noted as hospitalized, Riggs, *13th VA Inf.*, 133; Abner Sisson is listed as Lt. in 6th Cav. who "resigned 12/4/62 for 'failing health & a wish to gratify my company and a total disqualification to do justice to myself or those under my charge" and could not be the Sisson listed here; but Elhannon Benjamin Sisson (1845-1914) seems likely, listed as Pvt. in 6th Cav. from Orange Co. who later was hospitalized, November 1863 with gonorrhea and April 1864 with rubeola; postwar, Elhannon Benjamin Sisson lived in Louisa Court House until 1914 and is buried in Fairfax City Cem., Musick, *6th VA Cav.*, 155; William H. Reynolds (no birth and death data, but noted as still living in 1902 in Orange Co.) is listed in the Orange Artillery, originally Peyton's Artillery by Gregory J. Macaluso, *Morris, Orange, and King William Artillery*, Virginia Regimental Histories Series (Lynchburg, VA: H.E. Howard, 1990), 102. If this is Apperson's friend William Reynolds, he is also listed as one who had suffered from gangrene, was captured and imprisoned and released early in 1863 and then sent to hospital where he remained until early 1864 (which would fit the diarist's notes here).

[360] "Metacarpal bones" are in the hand "after the wrist." *Taber's.*

[361] Martin Roan, born in 1847 in Smyth Co., was a brick-mason who joined Smyth Blues, which became Co. D. He is listed as wounded at Chancellorsville (3 May 1863); "detailed by surgeon for conscript duty in Smyth Co. [until 1864; no further records]. Robertson, *4th VA Inf.*, 70. Possibly returned to Smyth Co. postwar, but not listed as buried in Smyth Co. Sturgill and Sturgill.

[362] "Tarsus," one of "seven bones in the ankle." *Taber's.*

[363] Samuel A. Byars, born 1849 [but no death date], was a "brickman" from Smyth Co. who had been captured at Kernstown (23 March 1862) and held until exchanged, 5 August 1862. He is

These old acquaintances of mine were standing by. I do not wish to boast or show any egoistic proud spirit; but this was one of the most pleasing moments of my life. The men who stood around me were those who once looked upon me as an infant, and one had treated me disrespectful [sic]. Now I was regardless of him [ignored him]. I looked to men in higher positions and was familiar with men in standing beyond any he could expect to reach. I could also show that what I had undertaken was not on my part a trifle—empty [illegible, sense is task or mission]—but that I had made progress and looked to higher position and brighter days.

I suppose there is in the breast of everyone a secret pride when placed in a similar position. I have not gone as far as I ought to have gone but with my limited means I have gone as far as I could.

We got through about dark and went back to our [field] Hospt [on Plank Road in The Wilderness, Orange Co.]

Our army is in front of Chancellorsville—all quiet!

[FIELD HOSPITAL, PLANK ROAD, WILDERNESS, ORANGE CO.]

WEDNESDAY, 6 [MAY] [18]63

This morning rain began to fall and soon the whole place was one mudpuddle. I saw Lt. Col. [Robert Henry] Dungan and proposed that he go to my father's [in Locust Grove in Orange Co.] for a few days. He agreed to do so; but before he got off new orders came for the wounded to be sent to Guineys Depot [Caroline Co., site of field hospital where diarist served long weeks earlier]. He went in an ambulance to Guineys. Dr. Hackett & myself went over to the barn [field hospital building for Woodville Mines Farm in Rappahannock Co.] again. Nothing much to do and I went up home [Locust Grove in Wilderness, Orange Co]. My father had been down and brought me some things and had gone to the battlefield. He was not at home when I arrived. An officer from one of the Louisiana Regiments was there sick. Two young Ladies under the signature of "F:H" & "A.C." sent me a plate of rice, chicken—I returned my thanks to the unknown persons and sent the dish to some wounded of my Regt [4th VA Inf]. At home I found nothing new—The yard around the house was beautiful—as green as as [sic] could be.

I sat up late and went to rest with a cheeful good will.

---

listed as wounded in left foot, Chancellorsville (3 May 1863). Upon recovery, apparently AWOL according to records, from 15 November 1863 until at least 30 April 1864. No further records. Robertson, 42. Not listed as buried in Smyth Co., Sturgill and Sturgill.

To-day I meet an old servant that had served under my father[364]—He was glad to see me.

[FIELD HOSPITAL, PLANK ROAD, WILDERNESS, ORANGE CO.]

THURSDAY, MAY 7, 1863

This morning by light I was up and off to my post [at field hospital]. Arrived there before some had left their beds. I passed James Dempseys[365] and Mrs. Jacobs hailed me.[366]

I met Mr [James Garland] McCleary,[367] husband of one of Proctor Becker's Daughters at our Hospt [on Plank Road in Wilderness, Orange Co]. I procured a pass for him from Dr. Black to stay at James Dempseys for two days —

A. Jones called to see me to-day.[368] I was too busy [to] pay much attention to him. Henry D. Roach was down in the evening—N. Jones[369] invited me over to see him [Henry Roach]—I got permission of Dr. B to meet. The old fields as I went along were familiar to me.

To-day I performed my first important operation—took off a Yankee's leg below the knee. Dr. Wilkerson[very much the veteran surgeon and one who helped teach the aspiring medicla college students] stood by—I felt no embarrassment whatever.

---

[364] I do not think that the Appersons owned slaves in Orange Co. When Apperson means *slaves*, he says *slaves* and not servants. The diarist probably means to say that someone else's slave had been hired out by his father, possibly when his father worked with the turnpike-stage company or possibly for seasonal work on the family farmlands at harvest time.

[365] James A. Dempsey, born 1825, had a home in Orange Court House dist. of Orange Co. VA Census, 1870.

[366] James Jacobs, born 1811, had a home and land in Orange Court House dist. of Orange Co. at this time, near Dempsey's, and this could be his wife. I cannot find her name. VA Census 1870.

[367] James Garland McCleary (1844-1924?) was farmer from Orange Co. enlisted in Co. A, 7th VA Inf. as Pvt. Survived major battles, including Chancellorsville and Gettysburg, but captured at Milford Station or Point Lookout (21 May 1864) and not exchanged until 14 March 1865. Postwar career unclear; possibly farming in Orange Co. and buried there in August 1924, or possibly the James Garland McCleary farming in Fredericksburg and buried in that city in August 1924. Riggs, *7th VA Inf.*, 84.

[368] Possibly A.J. Jones (no birth or death data), an orderly from Orange Co., antebellum occupation unknown, who worked directly under Col. James Lawson Kemper in 7th VA Inf. Riggs, ibid., 82.

[369] Probably Alphonso Napoleon Jones, perhaps born in 1842 (no death data and no postwar data), a farmer who enlisted as an officer in Co. K of 7th VA Inf. and was promoted to Capt. In June1862 he had been captured and was held POW until exchanged in August 1862. He commanded 7th briefly after Gettysburg (4 July 1863) and "wrote rgt.'s official report of Pickett's charge." "Florid complexion, blue eyes, sandy hair." Riggs, 82.

Mrs. Jones gave me a full history of Yankee vandalism. It is truly distressing. No people can prosper whose propensity for wanton destruction of our property and oppressing defenceless women is so great. How the blood is made to boil at such atrocities—such acts of inhumanity.

[FIELD HOSPITAL, PLANK ROAD, WILDERNESS, ORANGE CO.]

FRIDAY, MAY 8, 1863

I returned early this morning. Dr. B rec'd orders to send off all those wounded that could bear transportation and then move his hospital back to Guinea [Station, Caroline Co.] Dr. went away and asked me to stay in the rear. Nearly a hundred wagons reported to carry the wounded to Hamilton's [Crossing]. I distributed the wagons to the different Hospitals. I am somewhat pleased at going back to Guineas—there are such pleasant associations there. I have been very busy all day—Saw John F. Payne [identified earlier] Harrison Payne[370] and several others.

I went up home again [to Locust Grove] this evening. Was very tired when I got there: I had thought to have brought my horse with me [back to field hospital in Caroline Co.] but he is in low condition and father wishes to use him so I concluded to leave him. I was offered 250$ for him and I do not know but that I ought to sell him but if he gets the grass of summer he will be worth more next winter or be worth nothing [the horse may recover with summer feed in warmer weather and become much more valuable; or he may become listless and fail to recover at all]. Father wishes to work him too. There is some risk in leaving him when the enemy is apt to make raids.

To-morrow we leave this field of late conflict and go back to a quiet retreat [at field hospital in Guinea's Station, Caroline Co]. Many are the scenes we have witnessed here, many are the sad reflections that must follow us after this. Here the distinction between the wealthy and poor, the learned and ignorant, the distinguished and the unknown are merged into one lot. The friend and foe lay side by side suffering similar agonies at each other's hands.

My heart has grown callous to the suffering of the enemy. I am sorry for it too—We have in our hospital a Surgeon Hartman from the 11th Corps of [Joseph] Hooker's army [Army of the Potomac]—he is shot through the body, intestines—injured, feces passing from the wound. I have see him several times.

---

[370] I cannot find Harrison Payne in Orange Co. Artillery or 7th VA Inf. or 4th VA Inf. No Harrison Payne is listed by Scott among Orange Co. citizens serving in other VA units.

He asked me for the sake of humanity not to let a brother in the profession suffer for attention [not to be ignored or slighted by CSA physicians], but I am too incredulous to look upon him with much pity. He is in my hands and he pleads for mercy [.] [A] few days ago he was in yonder army, and had fate been otherwise some poor rebel would have seen him pass haughtily by. He is doing well and perhaps his condition in diet & c[etera] may save him. He is very abstemious [abstaining from unhealthy food and drink and other bad habits of diet].

[FIELD HOSPITAL, GUINEA'S STATION, CAROLINE CO.]

SATURDAY, MAY 9TH, 1863

This morning I rode down to camp[,] my brother accompanying me to take the horse back. We started with our wagons abouat 9 o'clock. I was lame from a tight shoe and could not walk very well. In company with others we walked down to Chancellorsville. The battlefield, like others, were [sic] well-strewn. The works taken by [Isaac Ridgeway] Trimble's division [commanded at Chancellorsville by Elisha Franklin Paxton, who was killed in the engagement] were very strong—Made of large logs and brush in front of them. After passing through this, the batteries on the hill at [illegible; a hill across the Plank Road and behind the Federal entrenchments] threw a sheet of bomb, [illegible, sense is some sort of ammunition such as cannon balls], and grape that riddled the roads. I regretted very much to see the fine mansion here burned. Mrs. [Melze] Chancellor was living there at the time and lost all her furniture—she is a widow. Our wagons came up and I took a ride. Just below New's Store Capt. Horn[371] took a right hand road and traveling was tollerably [sic] good—in the Plank Road it was horrible.

We passed Spotsylvania Court House and down by Mr. Anderson's to near Massaponax Church [Spotsylvania Co. east of the Court House] where we camped for the night. Camping out in the forest in the clean grass is very pleasant.

I had been suffering with Head ache but with the help of a dose of Morphia I was better at bedtime—We slept near our fire in the open air.

Dr. Gilkerson & [Samuel] Mohler, John Wilkerson & myself composed our immediate party. All the nurses and cooks of the Hospt. were along.

---

[371] I cannot find a Capt. Horn, Horne, or Hern in this Div., but he could be in another Div. since he is only by coincidence offering the diarist a ride.

The weather has become fine and looks like spring. We should be thankful to our Dear Master for the blessings he gives us.

[CAMP, MASSAPONAX CHURCH, SPOTSYLVANIA CO.]

SUNDAY, MAY 10TH 1863

This morning we left camp and came in across the Telegraph Road towards Guinea Station. Yester-day my feet were so sore that it was with much difficulty that I could walk. This morning I feel much better. S[amuel] Mohler and myself concluded that we would call at Mr. Motley's as we passed but did not.

Very little was done when we reach[ed] the [field] Hospital. Here tents were pitched for our comfort.

We heard that Genl [T.J.] Jackson was very low at the house of a Mr [Thomas Coleman] Chandler with Pneumonia.[372] [Samuel] Mohler & myself walked over to Mrs. [Frances] Thornton's and when we returned word had come that General T.J. Jackson was no more. Oh! What a blow this was! What a loss! How disheartening.

But God gave him to us and He has taken him from us and we should trust to Him to raise another in his stead. His death will cause a nation to mourn for no man of the war has so completely won the affection of the people as Jackson.

I got a letter from Miss Mollie Thornton to-day—She seems to be a good girl. [A]lso one from Mrs. Faris.

[FIELD HOSPITAL NEAR GUINEY STATION, CAROLINE CO.]

MONDAY [MAY] 11TH [18]63

This morning I commenced a tedious job—putting the books to rights. No record has been kept since we went away and things are confused, and it falls to me to bring order out of this confusion. Great many men have died and no note kept. I sent to [Harvey Allen] Jameson [hospital steward in field] for his report—

---

[372] Thomas Jonathan Jackson was removed from the field hospital to the house of Thomas Coleman Chandler at Guiney Station (Caroline Co.—the depot that the diarist often spells Guinea or Guiny). As noted, he had contracted pneumonia, and on this Sunday in the middle of the afternoon he passed on. As also noted, Robertson agrees with the contemporaneous medical authorities—including Apperson's diary and "Reminiscences" that he made use of—that it was the pneumonia the general contracted and not his wound and not his operation that killed him. Thomas Coleman Chandler was born in 1798 and maintained a home in Port Royal Township of Caroline Co. according to 1870 Census. VA Census.

Nothing of any importance transpired. I went to the [Guiney Station] Depot to see the body of Gen'l [T.J.] Jackson leave. A detail had been made from his Old Brigade [The 1st VA Bde, which included 4th Inf comprising Smyth Co. troops] to escort the body down, but it was late arriving. The body went early on special train. I regretted very much that the escort did not get to go. The Old Brigade has stood by the old hero since the beginning of the War, and fought boldly.

Severe have been the criticisms pressed upon its merits but the last fight closes the mouth of slander in many. I learned that Gen'l [J.E.B.] Stuart expressed himself as having nothing more to say against that Brig. At a very momentous hour in the day, when several Brig's were drawn up ready to grapple with the enemy Gen. [J.E.B.] Stuart rode in front of the line and ordered the Column forward two or three times. The shot and shell were tearing and striking through the air and sweeping everything before them. The colmns stood motionless—The Gen. [J.E.B. Stuart] drew his sword and called to the "Stonewall Brigade" to forward, and it did forward, though almost in the jaws of death. Three times did they rush forward leaving the ground strewn with the flower of their ranks but finally the enemy gave way and the victory was ours.

[FIELD HOSPITAL NEAR GUINEY STATION DEPOT, CAROLINE CO.]

TUESDAY, MAY 12, [18]63

To-day I have been writing all day. Miss Keziah [Shepherd] & Mollie [Graves] came over in the evening. I wrote a letter to Mollie [Mary Camden]—one to Dr. Faris[.] [A]lso one to cousin Bettie. Good many sick are arriving. Dr. Hagy has a hospital at the [Guiney Station] Depot in which he has some 200 or 300—that will be broken up and moved here soon.

[FIELD HOSPITAL NEAR GUINEY STATION DEPOT, CAROLINE CO.]

WEDNESDAY, MAY 13 [18]63

To-day I had some difficulty with reports from the small pox hospital. I am vexed sometimes. Rained this evening.

[FIELD HOSPITAL NEAR GUINEY STATION DEPOT, CAROLINE CO.]

THURSDAY, MAY 14TH, 1863

To-day I have ben busy—have nearly got my work done.

The air is very cool —

[FIELD HOSPITAL NEAR GUINEY STATION DEPOT, CAROLINE CO.]

FRIDAY, MAY 15, 1863

To-day I finished monthly reports and handed them in. Miss Molie Thornton sent me a message that she was in the neighborhood. I concluded to walk over—Dr. Black had borrowed a book from Mr. Motley and asked me to take it home.

I ought to have gone over before but could not muster the courage. I went and found the young ladies very interesting—took a stroll with Miss Sue [Motley].—Mr. Wilson came and took Miss Gwynn [Motley].

Mr. Motley came a short while before I left and seemed very solicitous that I remain longer.

Mr. [Samuel] Mohler & myself walked over to Mrs [Frances] Thornton and spent a very pleasant evening

[FIELD HOSPITAL NEAR GUINEY STATION DEPOT, CAROLINE CO.]

SATURDAY, MAY 16, 1863

We got our Hospital to work again and transfered some men to-day.

The weather is very warm. Dr. Sydnor's Brother came up from Richmond. Mr. [Samuel] Mohler & myself went to Mrs. [Frances] Thornton's again. Went fishing—no fish caught.

I wrote a letter home to father.

[FIELD HOSPITAL NEAR GUINEY STATION DEPOT, CAROLINE CO.]

SUNDAY, MAY 17, 1863

This has been a very pleasant day. I was in camp 'till evening. [Samuel] Mohler & myself walked down to the widow's [Frances Thornton]. Dr. B did not want us to go and soon sent for us after we went. A train of ambulances were[sic] expected from Wilderness [Orange Co.] with wounded. They did not come however—William Stuart[373] and several others were here.

---

373 William Stuart (1839-1888) was apparently a clerk from Wytheville. He joined Wytheville Grays, who became Co. A, 4th VA Inf. 2d Cpl at muster, he was elected 3d Sgt and then 2d Sgt but reduced in rank, 17 April 1862. Probably working with supply at time of this visit. Became acting Ordnance Sgt. 24 November 1863; promotion permanent 8 March 1864 and attached to Field & Staff. Buried in Wytheville. Robertson, *4th VA Inf.*, 75.

This morning Dr. B sent [for] a large number of the helpless that Dr. Hagy had at the [Guiney Station] Depot. Gus [Augustus Oury] Saunders [sic; Sanders][374] was among the number.

Mrs. [Frances] Thornton[,] Mrs. [Mary] Schooler [,][375] Miss Keziah [Shepherd] were over this evening. Mrs. [Mary] Schooler is a very nice old lady. Just such a one as we can love with enthusiasm.

[FIELD HOSPITAL NEAR GUINEY STATION DEPOT, CAROLINE CO.]

MONDAY, MAY 18TH, 1863

This morning about 10 o'clock the ambulance train arrived with the wounded expected last night. They were of the 1st Brigade [Stonewall Bde], in charge of Surgeons Walls & [Samuel Rush] Sayers [376] of Wytheville. Capt. [John Hall] Fulton was one of the number and Col. [James Kerr] Edmondson of the 27th VA. another.[377]

They seem to be doing well. They were immediately sent on. I was very busy 'till evening. There is a pic-nic on foot [being planned] here among the fellows.

---

[374] Augustus Oury Saunders[sic] (1836-1909) was from Smyth Co. and joined Smyth Blues, who became Co. A, 4th VA Inf. No official record of this wound, but a record of "accidentally wounded" at Malvern Hill ((1 July 1862) almost ten months earlier. Later became commissary Sgt. Robertson, 71. Sturgill & Sturgill find him buried in Elizabeth Cemetary, Marion, Smyth Co., and tombstone spells name *Sanders*. Smyth, Armstrong, and Wilson also spell name *Sanders*.

[375] Mary Schooler, born in 1800, was listed as owning a home and land in Bowling Green Township of Caroline Co. in 1870 Census. VA Census 1870.

[376] Samuel Rush Sayers (1833-1914), a physician and trained surgeon, apparently from Smyth Co., was surgeon at muster in 4th VA Inf. He transfered to 27th VA Inf. in July 1861, but transfered back to 4th on 18 January 1864. He went to Wytheville to practice medicine after War and lived there until 1914; buried in Wytheville. Robertson, 71. Records of 27th Inf. indicate that Sayers was captured while tending wounded at Gettysburg (4 July 1863); imprisoned in Baltimore, MD until 21 November 1863; released and served until transfer to 4th Inf. Buried East End Cemetary, Wytheville. Reidenbaugh, *27th VA Inf.*, 173.

[377] John Hall Fulton, already identified, had his leg amputated after severe wounds at Chancellorsville (3 May 1863); he returned to practice law in Wytheville, and lived until 1907 in Wythe Co. James Kerr Edmondson (1832-1898) was Col. with 27th VA Inf. Born in Buena Vista (Rockbridge Co.), he attended Washington Col. and held Lexington City offices upon graduation in 1853. He joined 2d H Co. as officer, was soon elected Capt. and soon after that appointed Adjutant for 27th Inf. Elected full Col. to rank from November 1862. At Chancellorsville (3 May 1863) he was shot in breast and left arm, and left arm was amputated. He was absent wounded until resigning commission on 12 December 1863. Postwar held many Lexington City offices and returned to Washington Col. to attain LLB and later practiced law in Rockbridge Co. Member VA Leg., 1870-80; trustee, Washington Col.; Mayor of Lexington and County Judge. Buried Stonewall Jackson Cem., Lexington. Reidenbaugh, 142.

Miss Keziah [Shepherd] went to Richmond this morning to procure some things. I was engaged in writing the invitations but did it without regard to form. No one seemed to be principal in the arrangements and they were sent out without a signature of any kind. What the ladies will think of it—Will they come?—

[Samuel] Mohler & myself went over to Mrs. [Frances] Thornton's again. I was entertained by Miss Mollie [Thornton] 'till near mid-night—The parlour was left to us entirely—I ought to stop going over there so much. Miss Mollie [Thornton] is too nice a girl for me to bear the idea of making any impressions unless I was situated [to] reward them.

She is my *beau ideal* of an *unalloyed* woman—I do not think she has ever been taught household duties very much, or at any rate has never labored very much.

I wrote a letter to Mrs. [Mary] Tomlin—Rec'd one from Laura Faris at Ashville [Alabama school] and one from Cousin Bettie.

[G.W.] Boteler came over to-day and of course went to Mr. Motley's.

I learned to-day that Stephen E. James and E[phraim]. Hogston of "Smyth Blues" had died of their wounds. James was one of the best soldiers I have ever seen. Poor fellow, he was wounded through the center of the back at Malvern Hill (probably 3 July 1862, when Federal forces took it and held it until 7 August 1862).[378]

[FIELD HOSPITAL NEAR GUINEY STATION, CAROLINE CO.]

TUESDAY, MAY 19, [18]63

This morning the sun found me in bed. So much for my late hours last night.

I got permission of Dr. B. to go to the pond and clean out a place for the pic-nic. The spot selected was not a very nice one, it is true but does very well. If our crowd is as respectable and our fare as good as the ground I shall be satisfide [sic].

---

[378] Stephen E. James (1838-1863) was a farmer from Smyth Co. who joined Smyth Blues, became provost guard with Co. D, 4th VA Inf., appointed Cpl. 18 April 1862. Wounded in hip at Malvern Hill (1 July 1862). Diarist is apparently wrong; James recovered from wound in hip at Malvern Hill and was appointed Sgt. He fought in Chancellorsville and died of unspecified wound, perhaps it was the wound in the back. Robertson, 58. Ephraim M. Hogston (birth date unknown-1863), probably Smyth Co., occupation unknown, Pvt. in Co. D, died from unspecified wounds at Chancellorsville. Robertson, 56.

We went in fishing—the water is very cold—caught a very nice mess [of fish].

Our medical class was again organized to-night. The same plans were adopted for our study.

[FIELD HOSPITAL NEAR GUINEY STATION DEPOT, CAROLINE CO.]

WEDNESDAY, MAY 20TH [1863]

This morning Aunt K. [Keziah Shepherd] came back from Richmond, and brought Miss Mollie [Graves] & Miss Emma [Graves], Miss Mollie's sister.—The pic-nic fever is getting up somewaht —. I fear it will be a failure at a heavy cost.

Dr. Wilkerson & myself went over to the widows [Mrs. Frances Thornton] to-night. Dr. Ellsburg was over also. I enjoy Miss Mollie T's [Thornton] company as usual.

We get news of a defeat to our army at Jackson Mississippi which hurts.[379]

[FIELD HOSPITAL NEAR GUINEY STATION DEPOT, CAROLINE CO.]

THURSDAY MAY 21, [18]63

This morning everything was astir—The pic-nic was first on docket. Some of the boys went over early. I could not go until after the sick were moved off. Drs. Walls & [John Alexander] Straith came down—I was so delighted to see them. They ate a snack and we went over. I was agreeably surprised to find as nice a crowd. More ladies than I really expected.

Gentlemen were escorts of the ladies—There was Miss Mollie Thornton first—as modest and tender-hearted as a lilly—Then Miss Anne Catlett with her profusion of curls—Miss Evie Thornton too had curls—and moved about with the lofty Mr. [Samuel] Mohler. Then Miss Mollie Graves flitting from place to place dallying with one here and one yonder, asking a word with one and

---

[379] US Grant was advancing steadily and unremittingly in Mississippi as part of the eventually successful land siege of Vicksburg [after Federal naval assaults had failed]. Grant sent James Birdseye McPherson (1828-1864), commander of 17th US Corps and William Tecumseh Sherman (1820-1891), commander of 15th US corps of his army to Jackson, state capital of MS. On 14 May 1863 CSA Gen. Joseph Eggleston Johnston, "knowing it was futile to oppose Grant with twelve thousand men, began to evacuate vital supplies and withdrew to the north. He left two brigades to delay the Federals," but these were quickly overwhelmed. Grant was now free to advance into a major engagement at Vicksburg, while Sherman remained in Jackson to destroy CSA supplies and installations. Long, 353-55.

making a wry face at another—then her sister [Emma Graves] with the homeliest beauty I ever saw—looking dejected[,] disappointed and over-rated. These were all the ladies with whom I was acquainted—No, I forget. There were the Misses Motley [Gwynn and Sue Motley]—the first of all in accomplishments. Miss Gwynn [Motley] wore a Yellow dress, which with her expression compared very well. She is calm and dignified—Miss Sue [Motley] looked less mischievous than I have seen her before. I found them sitting with with [sic] Miss Mollie Thornton in a shallop [boat] [380]—I looked at Miss Gwynn's [Motley's] independence, Miss Sue's [Motley's] mischief, and Miss Mollie's [Thornton's] modesty—Now the ladies that I was not acquainted with—Miss Jessee had been introduced before—I do not think her handsome—and have not seen enough to think her amiable. She [Miss Jessee] had two or three sisters along—or they were Misses Jessee anyway [possibly cousins]. A Miss Anne Thornton was entertained by Dr. Ellsburg when I arrived. I afterwards became acquainted. She is a trump—as gay as a lark—Talked incessantly, and is good looking.

Two Miss Williams were charming ladies. Not too reserved or too gay—animated enough to be pleasant. Several Misses Farish—I made an accidental acquaintance with one—She stammered. Several others were there—The old Ladies were too—Mrs. Catlett and Mrs. Shutre & Aunt K[eziah Shepherd]. I enjoyed the old Ladies society as much as any. The party had a dance. Two violins—very little spirit [alcohol] was used.

Dr. [John Alexander] Straith talked to Miss Sue Motley & Dr. Walls to Miss Gwynn [Motley]. [G.W.] Boteler came and took Miss Sue [Motley] away.

The evening passed very pleasantly—. I walked over to the [field] Hospt with Drs. [John Alexander] S[traith] & W[alls].

The ladies—a portion of them—went up to Mrs. [Frances] Thornton's and the Hosp't crowd [male nurses, other stewards, and orderlies] went over[.] We had a very nice time—Perhaps a little too gay. Too much spirit and wordly amusement.

---

[380] The image is odd; a shallop is a small boat, possibly set in the pond. It may be that he intended to write *shallow*, in noun form a shallow place in a pond, but that too would be an odd image since they are dressed up nicely for a pic-nic instead of for fishing [where the women too sometimes went knee-deep into the water with a seine]. It could be a *shale*, in noun form a rock made of shale and big enough to sit on, but the letters do not look like *shale*. See *OED* for synonyms used here.

[FIELD HOSPITAL NEAR GUINEY STATION DEPOT, CAROLINE CO.]

FRIDAY, MAY 22D, [18]63

To-day was busier than usual. Yesterday was my regular day to make out weekly statements but as we generally do I let the pleasures of the moment divert my time to enjoyment.

News from our western army is not flattering—I have long feared some disaster there. When Vicksburg is gone we are then cut off from Louisiana & Texas. I wrote a letter to Laura Faris [in shool in Ashville, Alabama].

[FIELD HOSPITAL NEAR GUINEY STATION DEPOT, CAROLINE CO.]

SATURDAY, MAY 28TH, [18]63

This day has been a warm one. I walked down to see Capt. [John] Glaize [QM] in regard to pay of clothing not drawn upon 8th Octr 1862—He says that he will pay anything that is due. I went by the widow's [Mrs. Frances Thornton] and had several hours with the ladies. I do believe I am fond of their company—Why should I not be?—I returned to the Hospt at dark and Miss Keziah [Shepherd] insisted that I should go over with her—I did so—the Misses Graves [Mollie and Emma Graves] have been at the Hosp't all day—

The young gentlemen came over with the violins and went into a regular dance[.] I was somewhat doubtful of the propriety—I did not dance or sing—Miss Mollie [Thornton] was my companion for the evening, and her quiet manner suited me for I felt somewhat meditative or rather pensive.

[FIELD HOSPITAL NEAR GUINEY STATION DEPOT, CAROLINE CO.]

MONDAY, MAY 25TH, 1863

To-day has been one of the warmest days. I remained in camp all day. Dr. [William D.] Christian[381] of Appomattox came to our [field] Hospt. in quest of a Mr. Driver and his son—Driver had died of S. Pox and his son had not been to the [field] Hospt.[382] He then wished to go to Gen'l [Ambrose Powell]Hill's HdQers and failing to procure a conveyance he remained with me.

---

[381] William D. Christian, born in 1810, was a physician who practiced and lived in Clove Hill Township of Appamattox Co. VA Census 1870.

[382] Possibly William H. Driver, birth and death data unavailable; from Isle of Wight. If the diarist means to say that William H. Driver's father died in the Small Pox Hospital, and the soldier had been unable to visit his civilian father prior to his death, then the diarist is talking

The old gentleman was a great talker and seemed to be well informed on most topics.

The Misses Graves [Mollie and Emma Graves] went home to-day. I commenced a letter to Mrs F[aris]—did not finish it.

[FIELD HOSPITAL NEAR GUINEY STATION DEPOT, CAROLINA CO.]

MONDAY, MAY 25TH, 1863

Last night the air turned very cool and the wind blew hard. The morning was so cool that I put a stove in my tent. The air was cool during the day—the sun shined dim—a little mist at morning—cleared up towards noon.

Dr. [William D.] Christian left for Hamilton's Crossing —

I understand that Miss Mollie Thornton is unwell to-day—Dr. B Had [sic] an invitation to a dining party about 8 miles distant [.] I was invited also but could not go—Capt. [Robert La Fayette] Francisco [QM] came by for Dr. He went—I have been reading [John Julian] Chisolm [authorized military text on surgery] to-day. News from the west is very cheering: Joe [Joseph Eggleston] Johnston had repulsed [Ulysses S.] Grant's army and all are sanguine of a brilliant victory.[383]

Dr. Wright reported at our [field] Hospt. for duty, I think—I have not seen his orders though.[384]

I finished my letter to Mrs. F[aris] and wrote one to "Mollie" of Richmond [Mary Camden].

---

about this man. Driver was a non-com. with 9th VA Inf. who in June of 1863 would transfer to the CSA Navy. Trask, 9th *VA Inf.*, 62. If the diarist means to say that a soldier named Driver has died of Small Pox, then I cannot confirm that any soldier named Driver in the 1st brigade did so, and cannot identify these people.

[383] On19 May 1863 Grant sent three divisions in a sudden land assault on Vicksburg's defenses, commanded by John Clifford Pemberton. Strong attacks were repulsed, with about 1,000 Federal casualties. On 22 May 1863, Grant attempted a second assault, this one almost suicidal, costing the Federals 3,199. Having failed by water assault and by land assault, Grant "began the siege in earnest, digging approach trenches and building artillery positions." Joseph Eggleston Johnston, in overall command, had little to do with the repulse of these two assaults; in fact, President Davis anxiously wrote to Johnston and to other CSA field offices to get Pemberton some help by attacking Grant. After Grant saw the futility of this sort of attack, he doggedly prepared a siege that was bound for success. Long, 353-58.

[384] Possibly Dr. James H. Wright of Smyth Co. who had been on general hospital duty in Richmond; he was not officially sent to Regt until 3 July, but often the diarist reports cases in which someone has changed duty long before official records note the changes. This Wright was wounded and captured, at Morton's Ford (6 February 1864) and died from wounds, 22 April 1864 at Kalorama Hospital, Washington, D.CRobertson, *4th VA Inf.*, 82.

To-night several of us went serenading—I got a bouquet with the compliments of the Ladies—chance that I got it. [He presumes that some kind of random drawing led the "Ladies" to send him the bouquet].

[FIELD HOSPITAL NEAR GUINEY STATION DEPOT, CAROLINE CO.]

TUESDAY, MAY 26, 186[3]

The air is more moderate this morning.

No news from Vicksburg. This evening I went over to see Miss Mollie [Thornton]—She is better than she was Yester-day, but has not entirely recovered from the effects of the medicine she took yester-day. Took a walk with her.

Drs. Black & Hagy went up to Dr. [Thomas Coleman] Chandler's [house in Port Royal Township of Caroline Co., where T.J. Jackson died of pneumonia while recuperating from the amputation of his arm].

The girls are expecting a crowd over at the widows [Mrs. Frances Thornton] to-night.

Our class met again to-night or rather about half of it and recited the lesson.

Most of the boys went over [to the party at Mrs. Frances Thornton's house].

[FIELD HOSPITAL NEAR GUINEY STATION DEPOT, CAROLINE CO.]

WEDNESDAY, MAY 27, 1863

This morning the news from Vicksburg is still encouraging—The day has been warm—Miss K[eziah Shepherd] sent for us to come over[,] that some nice company were up at the widows [Mrs. Frances Thornton]. [Samuel] Mohler and myself went over—Mrs. [Frances] Thorntons son and niece Mollie Thornton's brother were there—Also Mr [Thomas?] Catlett from Port Royal and daughter [Sue Catlett]—I enjoyed myself as much as I could reasonably. —

The boys have on foot another pic-nic—I am opposed to it for various reasons.

[FIELD HOSPITAL NEAR GUINEY STATION DEPOT, CAROLINE CO.]

THURSDAY, MAY 28, 1863

This morning I was loath to leave my bed—Late hours last night make a late riser next morning. To-day is the day for the elective franchise to be cast throughout the State—our people have not lost all that party feeling that in days gone by moved them to great exertions at the polls. The last sparks of party have been kindled to burn for a short time—soon they will fade again and we hope never again to be fanned into life—I cast my vote for Extra Billy Smith [William Smith] for Gov;[385] Jno Echols for Lt. Gov; W[alter]. Preston for Congress and Ran. Tucker [John Randolph Tucker] for Att'y Gen'l[.] [Thomas] Flournoy is Smith's opponent and [John Daniel] Imboden is [John] Echol's.[386]

---

[385] The Whig Party was no more, and CSA Virginians thought of themselves as old style *republicans*, that is, citizens without partisan affiliation. Actually, however, the remnants of the Whigs were still around, emphasizing a message of assisting business and developing transportation, commerce, banking, and industry while still supporting slavery. The Democrats, more vocal in support of secession, were now apt to talk most forcefully about agrarian values and defending the rights of farmers even at the expense of developing business interests. In these races of 1863, Washington Co.'s Walter Preston was an old Whig, as was Thomas Flourney of Halifax Co.; and it is interesting that Apperson, given his lifelong interest in economic diversification and business development, supported Preston, the old Whig dedicated to such pursuits. Otherwise, the remaining candidates were Democrats, all solidly pro-secessionist, and Apperson probably supported them more for the ideology of the War and southern nationalism and slavery than for their stand on agrarian economics, which he did not support. William Smith (1797-1887) , of Prince Edward Co., had served in US House, had been governor of VA (1846-49), and was a gen. in CSA. William G. Bean notes: "As a young man, he had organized the mail service from Washington to Milledgeville, Georgia, so efficient [sic] that he was occasionally granted an extra payment by the Post Office authorities, hence the sobriquet, 'Extra Billy.'" Bean, notes.

[386] John Echols (1823-1896) was born in Lynchburg and studied at Washington College and Virginia Military Institute, both in Lexington, VA; and took a law degree from Harvard College before becoming an atty. and winning election as Commonwealth Atty. In War, he was a Brig. Gen. who served in T.J. Jackson's Valley campaign (1862-63) and in Jubal Anderson Early's Valley Campaign (1864). In summer of 1863 he was appointed to the official investigative committee that studied the loss of Vicksburg. After War, he made his home in Staunton, where he practiced law and developed railroad companies. Jeffrey D. Wert, "Echols," *Hist. Times.* John Daniel Imboden (1823-1895), from Staunton, attended Washington College, became a school teacher, and was such an ardent secessionist that he may have frightened some of his Valley neighbors too much to be elected to the secession convention for VA. In War, he served as a gen. in both Valley campaigns. Following War, Imboden moved to Apperson's adoptive highlands, living in Damascus (Washington Co., where he worked to promote and develop mineral and mining resources. Emory M. Thomas, "Imboden," ibid.. Walter Preston (1780?–1866) was part of a prominent landowning family in Washington Co. An atty. with major landholdings and business interests throughout southwestern VA, Preston made his home in Abingdon, where he made a reputation as an eloquent lawyer and an impressive political orator. Defeated for the office of VA Atty. Gen. before War, Preston during War won election to CSA congress, in the campaign of 1861 defeating Fayette McMullen, a fascinating and eccentric mountain character whom the diarist had met before the War in his travels as an assistant to Dr. William Faris. Summers, *Hist. of SW VA*, 759-60. Ran Tucker (John Randolph Tucker [1823-1887) was from the most famous family of jurists in VA and the South. A distinguished lawyer, Tucker did well both in practice before the bar and in his teaching of law, as had his ancestors. He was also successful in wartime and postbellum politics, winning election as state Atty. Gen. during War and as US congressman in US House, 1875-1887. "Tucker [family]," *Encyclopedia of Southern History.*

To-night our class [of would-be medical students] should have met again—it did not—it will be among the things that were—will be forgotten—The ladies have engrossed the attention of the Young Men and they are no longer Students of Medicine, but they are devotees to Cupid's shrine.

A tableau [see earlier note on thematic costume party] comes off at Mrs. T's [Frances Thornton] this evening.

A very large number of sick were received to-day.

[FIELD HOSPITAL NEAR GUINEY STATION DEPOT, CAROLINE CO.]

FRIDAY, MAY 29TH, 1863

This morning [news] from Vicksburg is better than it was Yester-day, though all of us are doubtful about [John Clifford] Pemberton's being able to sustain Himself. Joe [Joseph Eggleston] Johnston is coming up in the enemy's rear, and the hope is, will cause him [U.S. Grant] to turn and protect his flank and rear.

[Clement Laird] Vallandingham of Ohio[387] has been sent south.[388]

---

[387] Clement Laird Vallandigham (1820-1871) was from New Lisbon, Ohio and was the most famous, or infamous "Copperhead," or Peace Democrat of the North [some wore copper pennies on their vests or jackets to identify themselves; the term became opprobrious, connoting *traitor* more than *pacifist*]. He attended Jefferson College (PA) and taught school for some years while reading law on his own; he passed the Ohio bar in 1842. A successful attorney in New Lisbon, he eventually moved to Dayton, bought a newspaper, *Dayton Empire*, and ran for political office as a northern Democrat, successfully in state assembly elections, unsuccessfully for US Congress. After several tries, he was finally elected to US House in 1858, where he established himself as a "contentious conservative and state-rights advocate." War Democrats "gerrymandered" his original district to remove him from Congress in 1862, and state political leaders planned to block him from the gubernatorial nomination, which he sought. In 1863, Maj. Gen. Ambrose E. Burnside [identified earlier], by then commander of Dept. of Ohio, gave Gen. Order # 38, "forbidding expression of sympathy for the enemy." On 30 April 1863 in Columbus, Vallandingham deliberately provoked Burnside—and sought "sympathy" votes for himself for gov. with a speech derogatory of Lincoln's policies in war and peace. He was arrested, tried by military court at Burnside's hdq. in Cincinnati and denied a writ of *habeas corpus*. Sentenced to 2-years' confinement in a military prison, Vallandingham did not go to prison, because Lincoln commuted the sentence, provided that Vallandingham be "banished" to the Confederacy. John E. Stanchak, "Vallandingham," *Hist. Times*.

[388] As diarist notes, Vallandingham was "sent south" by troops who escorted him below the CSA lines in Murfressboro, TN. From there, he was escorted by CSA troops to Wilmington, NC, from whence he went to Bermuda and from there to Windsor, Ontario in Canda. From Windsor, he conducted his campaign for gov., being nominated ringingly by Ohio Democrats outraged at his treatment. "Lincoln interested himself in the election, endorsed Republican candidate John

To-day I wrote to Dr. Walls in regard to the "pic-nic"—He says the band will be down if nothing occurs to prevent it. He & Dr. [John Alexander] Straith sent 16$ to help us out.

Miss Mollie T[hornton] wrote me a note this morning stating that she was about leaving for home. She still is suffering with neuralgia. Mr. Catlett & the young Mr. Thornton was [sic] over this morning.

[FIELD HOSPITAL NEAR GUINEY STATION DEPOT, CAROLINE CO.]

SATURDAY, MAY 30, 1863

The wind and dust was [sic] very disagreeable all day—No news from Vicksburg. Dr. [William D.] Christian called on his return home—He states that the impression in the army is that Gen'l A[mbrose]. P[owell]. Hill will be put in command of a corps of the army—The two corps in army will be divided into three and be commanded respectively by [James] Longstreet, [Richard Stoddert] Ewell, and [Ambrose Powell] Hill. I expect it a good plan. [389] I [sic; diarist quit writing on this line].

Brough (1811-1865), downplayed the illegalties of a civilian's arrest and trial by military authorities, and claimed that a vote for the Democratic contender was 'a discredit to the country.'" On 13 October 1864, Brough defeated Vallandingham handily (288,000–187,000). Subsequently, Lincoln and the military chose to ignore Vallandingham, even when he returned to Ohio "in disguise" and even when he became active again in politics, attending the Democratic convention in Chicago and helping to write the "disastrous" peace plank in the platform for George B. McClellan [identified earlier], onetime commander of the Army of Potomac and Democratic nominee for president in 1864. After War, Ohio and national Democrats became embarrassed by him, limited his participation in 1866 convention in Philadelphia of "recently reconstructed Southern Democrats" and "old Federals," and refused to nominate him for state senate. Returning to the practice of law in Lebanon, Ohio, Vallandingham in 1871 shot himself fatally while attempting to demonstrate to other lawyers how an alleged victim may have shot himself in an incident for which he was the defending attorney. Note two things about Vallandingham: 1) the US Supreme Court, in *Ex parte Vallandingham,* ruled that the court should not have issued a writ of habeas corpus for a civilian in a military case; and 2) Edward Everett Hale (1822-1909), taken with the story and inspired by Vallandingham's remark that he did not want to live in a country presided over by Lincoln, wrote the remarkable short story, often dramatized, "The Man Without a Country," *Atlantic Monthly* (Dec. 1863); the Philip Nolan of the story was Vallandingham, and Hale made this clear after the War, to protect the contemporaneous Philip Nolan, who rose to prominence in later years. See Stanchak.

[389] The rumors were true; Longstreet became commander of Corps I, Ewell of Corps II, and A.P. Hill of Corps III. Apperson's judgment of the plan is only partially upheld by subsequent history. Lee came to trust Longstreet, especially his skill at "counterpunching" against an attack. The writer Shelby Foote gives Longstreet high marks, although other historians are critical, in particular of Longstreet's alleged slowness at Gettysburg (3-4 July 1863). Ewell was able to ride, if awkwardly, and he seemed to give good service generally, but suffered a bad fall at "Bloody Angle"

I wrote to brother Nat to-day—also to Miss Mollie T[hornton].

To-night I went to the [Guiney Station] Depot with Dr. Gilkerson to see a wounded man—He was a member of Co. "H" [original "Rockbridge Grays"] of 1 VA Batll [Battalion; 1st VA Bde] stabbed by Mr. [Thomas Coleman] Chandler [the physician who owned the home in which T.J. Jackson died of pneumonia] near the depot [of Guiney Station]. Several of the Batt'l—all ineb[rieated] went to Mr. [Thomas Coleman] Chandler's house and acted very badly. Mr. C[handler] in self defence opened one's abdomen [stabbed a man in the abdomen]. The wound was in the median line about an inch above the *Umbilicus* [navel; in the lumbar region; diarist's italics]. A large quantity of *Omentum*[390] protruded and was troublesome to reduce.

No class [of medical college aspirants] met again to-night. We will do nothing without a prompter.

[FIELD HOSPITAL NEAR GUINEY STATION DEPOT, CAROLINE CO.]

SUNDAY, MAY 30TH, 1863

We have seen another Sabbath.

With me I am sorry to say, I fear, that I have spent it unprofitably.[391] I read a few chapters in Proverbs, attended my daily duties, took a nap and Dr. Thomas and myself walked over to Mr. [Thomas?] Motley's. The evening, of course, passed off very agreeable. The Young Ladies were very entertaining.

News from Vicksburg is somewhat encouraging. It is reported that [Ulysses S.] Grant is falling back from the place and giving up the seige [sic].[392]

(Spotsylvania, 12 May 1864) and could not command in the field the final eleven months of the War. A.P. Hill receives the most critical judgments, being thought too slow and even reticent in one phase of Gettysburg and too aggressive and even careless in other phases. Some authorities even suggest that A.P. Hill may have suffered some psychosomatic or other emotional disorders that impaired his generalship. See, among many things, Shelby Foote, *Civil War; a Narrative*, 3 vols. (New York: Random House, 1958, 1974); many pieces by Edwin C. Bearss, but especially, "Hill," *Hist. Times.*

[390] "Omentum [L., a covering]. A double fold of peritoneum [membrane] attached to the stomach and connecting it with certain of the abdominal viscera [internal organs of the abdomen]...." *Taber's.* Italics are in diary.

[391] As noted, he uses p*rofit* in the Biblical sense of something redounding to the nonmonetary glory of God by improving a believer.

[392] Grant was only maneuvering to make a more effective siege. Lincoln, however, was deeply concerned about lack of progress in the siege. Long, 359-60.

[FIELD HOSPITAL NEAR GUINEY STATION DEPOT, CAROLINE CO.]

MONDAY, JUNE 1ST, 1863

Thus begins another month. Months now pass apparently as rapidly as days used to do. I wonder if time flies faster in one's imagination the older we get.

I rose early this morning and commenced working diligently with my monthly report—I regret very much that [there are] some items in the report that make it look badly. The deaths of several men who died [sic] were not reported to me 'till the present. Hence they are reported in this month when they should have been reported in [earlier] month reports.

I visited Mr. [Thomas?] Motley's again this evening in Company with Dr. Gilkerson—a Mr. Owens was there. I prescribed for a servant of the old Gentleman [Mr. Thomas Motley]. I rec'd a letter from Miss Mollie F.T. [Thornton].

[FIELD HOSPITAL NEAR GUINEY STATION DEPOT, CAROLINE CO.]

TUESDAY—JUNE 2D 1863

"Aunt K" [Keziah Shepherd] came up from Richmond to-day—Miss Mollie [Graves] was with her—She brought the articles for the pic-nic.

I have been very much confused to-day with my reports—The Ward Masters' reports and mine do not agree and some men who died in other months are reported in this.

[FIELD HOSPITAL NEAR GUINEY STATION DEPOT, CAROLINE CO.]

WEDNESDAY, JUNE 3D, [18]63

This morning I was up at work early, finished monthly reports and handed them in—I rec'd a letter from Cousin B[ettie] and one from "Mollie" [Mary Camden] in Richmond. Mr. S[amuel]. Mohler & myself walked over to Mrs. T's [Frances Thornton]. Were introduced to two Misses Taffy.

Miss Patsy Thornton was there and I was enjoying a lively conversation wth her when Dr. B. sent for us—The sick was pouring in—Some more of the army—I am writing at 3 Thursday morning—I have been writing [prescriptions, reports, and official correspondence] all night.—

[FIELD HOSPITAL NEAR GUINEY STATION DEPOT, CAROLINE CO.]

THURSDAY JUNE 4TH 1863

To-day has been one of my busiest days. Caravans of invalid were coming in during the day. Write, write write! All day long. In the afternoon I went down to the place selected for our pic-nic—A very nice crowd of ladies was there—only an 1/2 hour was allowed me and I could not enjoy myself much—Miss Mollie [Thornton] was there—I am writing at midnight[.] Dr. Syd[nor] has been ordered to report to Dr. [Hunter Holmes] McGuire [field medical director for Richard Stoddert Ewell's corps].

We are to move at 7—to-morrow.[393]

2 MILES ABOVE SPOTSYLVANIA C.H. [COURTHOUSE, SPOTSYLVANIA CO.]

FRIDAY, JUNE 5, 1863

This morning [sic] we did not get off until 2 P.M.

The young ladies were down to see us —. I had a very good time between work and chat —

Miss Mollie [Thornton] seemed very sad—Indeed she is a good girl who deserves that which I can not confer—What her feelings to-wards me is, I have taken no pains to learn more than my society [companionship] was as agreeable to her as any other which I did to enjoy also. I walked over to the widow's [Frances Thornton] with her and took my leave of Mrs. Thornton —She has always been kind to us and dispensed her hospitality with a willing hand. She wished for us good luck and expressed a hope that we might soon return.

When the wagons started, Dr. [W.W.] Drane and myself went over to Hillford and took leave of Mrs. Motley & family.[394] Mr. [Thomas?] Motley desired us to write him[.] Capt. [John] Glaize [QM of 2d Inf.] was there. We then passed Mr. Peter Catlett's and bid his family adieu [including Sue Catlett]. We did not overtake the Ambulance train until we reached the "telegraph road" 5 mi. from Guinea's [Guineys Station]. Capt. [John] Glaize's [forage] train is along with ours.

---

[393] R.E. Lee decided to take the first and second reorganized corps—Richard Stoddert Ewell's and James Longstreet's—and march north, "to take the War to the North." He left the 3rd reorganized corps under Ambrose Powell Hill as a counterweight to Joseph Hooker near Fredericksburg. Long, 361.

[394] William G. Bean identifies Dr. W.W. Drane as a surgeon assigned to field-hospital duty with 2nd Corps (reorganized) of ANV. Prof. Bean also identifies Hillford as the family home of the Motleys, apparently including Thomas, Sue, and Gwynn Motley. Bean, notes.

To us there are very many pleasing recollections from the acquaintances that we have made at Guineas Depot. There is no one but must feel somewhat saddened to leave a place that had [been] a home for 6 months.

Our orders are to move from Racoon Ford [on Rappahannock River]. I wish to go home [Wilderness in Orange Co.] to-morrow—

I have a presentiment that there is ahead of us an exciting and active campaign, & one perhaps very important. We camped 1 1/2 miles below Spotsylvania C.H. [Courthouse, Spotsylvania Co.]

Dr. Wright[395] is left in charge of the Hospt. at Guineas [Guineys Station Depot]. Asst. Surg[eon] Gilkeson is with him. Judge[sic] [John Henry] Noland was left also. Tents and stores and supplies were turned over to Dr. W[right]. This Hospt. will be known as Hospt. of 3d Corps [Ambrose Powell Hill's newly reorganized corps of ANV] commanded by Gen'l A.P. Hill. I have not yet learned what Divisions will comprise his Corps. The Small Pox Hospt. was left in charge of Dr. Gresham. Dr. Jamison[396] got permission of Dr. Black to go with us. Dr. "Syd" [Sydnor] returned to-day. "Aunt Kesey" [Keziah Shepherd] will remain with Dr. Wright until we get settled and can make her services available.

2 MIS. ABOVE SPOTSYLVANIA C.H. [SPOTSYLVANIA CO.]

SATURDAY, JUNE 6TH, 1863

We left Camp early but did not get very far before a Battalion of artillery impeded our progress, and here we have been standing for 6 long hours—when we shall move I know not—the army [2d Corps commanded now by Richard Stoddert Ewell] is a short distance ahead of us.

It is reported that the army has been crossing at Fredericksburg. Heavy firing has been heard there.[397] It is only a feint I guess. [J.E.B.] Stuart is fighting in Culpeper Co.[398]

---

[395] Possibly Augustus R. Wright, originally of Georgia. Cunningham, 24n.

[396] Possibly the Harvey Allen Jameson identified as hospital steward with 4th by Robertson, 58.

[397] Joseph Hooker's Army of the Potomac made reconnaissance at Franklin's Crossing on Rappahannock River near Fredericksburg, where they found Ambrose Powell Hill's 3rd Corps entrenched. There was skirmishing and shelling "for several days," but no real engagement, according to Long, 363.

[398] Actually, J.E.B. Stuart was on two different days putting on a spectacular dress parade of his cavalry at Brandy Station in Culpeper Co., with "high jocularity" between his cavalry and infantry units of the I and II Corps. Very real fighting would soon come, and Stuart and his cavalry, including the cavalry of his hard-charging Gen. William "Grumble" Jones were to be surprised by a Federal attack across the Rappahannock River on 9 June 1863. Long, 361-64.

In the afternoon a heavy rain fell—we were standing in the road about 2 mis. from the [Spotsylvania] C.H. [Courthouse] near Sunset. Then the train moved off and at White Hall Mines [Albemarle Co.] I left the train to cross the country to see my parents [in Locust Grove, Orange Co.]. It was one of the most tiresome trips I have had for a long time. I got lost twice on the trip. One time I took the wrong direction on striking a road and went back over the same road I had before traveled[.] [T]his was indeed discouraging[.] After reaching Parker's Old Store [on the Orange Plank Road] I aimed to follow my old path that I had before followed but it was overgrown very much with bushes. Thinking I had taken a wrong road I aimed to strike through the woods to the right one. In this I was mistaken and soon found myself buried in the depths of the forest[.] [T]he underwood was very thick and wet and I got very wet[.] When I found myself in a place I knew (it was Billy Higginson's Old Place) I had no more difficulty in reaching home. Reaching there I was almost "*gone up*".[399] I did not retire at all.

[LOCUST GROVE, ORANGE CO.]

SUNDAY, JUNE 7, 1863

After breakfast I lay down to snooze a while. Mr. H. Roach and Lady came over. I was glad to see them. I remained a while after dinner, took leave of all, and father took me up to near Palmyra Church where I overtook the train.

Mother gave me some things which I needed very much. I called to see Isabella who lives at Mr. Hatcher's.

The troops are all ahead of us—We crossed at Somerville's Ford [on Rapidan River in Culpeper Co.] and camped a short distance beyond. I desired very much to see my uncle's folks but could not.

The fields look green—grazing is very fine.

---

[399] Colloquialism a little hard to follow in context; usually it means "gone up to Heaven," or even "saved" in spiritual sense. Apparently, he was so relieved after the ordeal, that he considered himself close to salvation; although he may also mean to say that he was so tired that he was almost dead in strictly physical sense.

[ALONG RAPIDAN RIVER, CULPEPER CO.]

MONDAY, JUNE 8, 1863

I finished reading Victor Hugo's [illegible; possibly *La Legend des siecles*][400] to-day—am much pleased with the work. The delineations of the struggle between Duty and inclination are strongly and impressively drawn. [Illegible word] of conscience at the human breast is a good picture and truthful.

This morning we left camp early. In passing the house once occupied by my uncle where I lay very sick in the fall of '61 I could not help feeling again grateful to my kind relatives who nursed me through that dangerous spell.

We arrived at Culpeper C.H. about 1 P.M.—I rode with Capt. [John] Glaize—he is a model man.

Our camp for the night was on the Sperryville road near town. The troops are all in camp on that road—Many speculations as to what we will now do. I infer that we will go to the [Shennadoah] Valley and cross into Loudon [Co.] in the rear of the enemy. Many are predicting a Maryland campaign. A large body of cavalry has collected near here under Gen'l [J.E.B.] Stuart.[401]

I wrote to Miss Mollie Thornton to-day.

We rec'd 5 days' rations—including to-day—for 31 men [with field hospital crew].

[FIELD HOSPITAL ON THE SPERRYVILLE ROAD, CULPEPER CO.]

TUESDAY, JUNE 9, [18]63

This morning early we heard firing of canon [sic] and small arms in direction of Brandy Station [Culpeper Co]. About 10 o'clock wagons and straggling cavalry men were seen hurrying along toward the [Culpeper] Court

---

[400] Victor Marie Hugo (1802-1885) wrote a three-part epic, *La Legende des siecles* (Paris, 1859), the first installment of which was published while he was in exile in Guernsey from Napoleon III, and translated into English in the Civil War Era as *The Legend of the Ages.* The first part treats of "duty and inclination," starting with Eve in Paradise as she faces the possibilities of motherhood. Hugo's high romanticism, especially as translated into English, would likely appeal to the romanticism of the diarist. As J. Tracy Power notes in *Lee's Miserables* (Chapel Hill: University of North Carolina Press, 1995)—his study of the common soldiers of the Army of Northern Virginia—*the* book of Hugo's appealing to the majority of Confederate soldiers was the novel about the wrongly accused Jean Valjean, *Les Miserables* (Paris, 1862). Lee's foot soldiers called themselves sarcastically *Lee's Miserables.*

[401] Official reports estimate around 8,000 mounted soldiers with J.E.B. Stuart; although it should be noted that the Federals' Maj. Gen. Alfred Pleasonton (1824-1897) commanded a force of some 11,000 mounted soldiers also moving along the Rappahannock River. See Long, 359-63; Jeffrey D. Wert, "Brandy Station," *Hist. Times.*

House in a mass of confusion. A stampede had taken hold of them and they were looking for the rear.

When we learned the news it was to the effect that the Yankee cavalry [under Maj. Gen. Alfred Pleasanton] had crossed [the Rappahannock River] and fell upon [J.E.B.] Stuart so instantaneously that several of his regiments were surprised and thrown into disorder and he came near being routed. [William E. "Grumble"] Jones' & [Wade] Hampton's Brigades bore the brunt of the fight.—The 12th, 11th, 9th, 7th, 6th, and 4th and 2d Va Cavalry suffered considerably. Also the 2d N. Car. & 2d S. Car., Col. Williams of 2d N. Car. was killed & Lt. Col. [Frank] Hampton of same regiment killed.[402]

Some censure Gen. [J.E.B.] Stuart for carelessness—I have no doubt that he is too confident of success and feels a sense of security by relying upon the former [viz., timid cavalry] movements of the enemy for a precedent. This evening I learn that "Aunt Betsy" Robinson is in town [Culpeper Court House] at her daughter's, Mrs. Daniel. I intend calling on her to-morrow if we remain here—Gen. [Jubal A.] Early's Div. went toward Brandy [Station] this evening.

---

[402] The famous Battle of Brandy Station, 9 June 1863 was the largest cavalry engagement of the Civil War. It involved some 11,000 Federal cavalry forces and at least 8,000 CSA cavalry forces. Jeffrey D. Wert says, "Screened by an early morning mist, the Union troopers splashed across the [Rappahannock] river at about 4 o'clock. Brig. Gen. John Buford's [1826-1863] division, crossing at Beverly Ford [Culpeper Co.] surprised the pickets of Brig. Gen. William E. "Grumble" Jones [1824-1864] Confederate brigade, overrunning its camp and capturing 150 prisoners. Jones's startled troopers quickly regrouped and fiercely contested the ground as they withdrew toward Brandy Station. 4 mi. downstream at Kelly's Ford [Culpeper Co.], Brig. Gen. David M. Gregg's [1833-1916] Union cavalrymen pushed aside Brig. Gen. Bevery H. Robertson's [1827-1910] pickets and moved to connect with Buford. The 2nd Division, under Union Col. Alfred N.A. Duffie, was late, trailing Gregg's troopers." Eventually, Stuart was able to regroup and concentrate "his scattered brigades" in a successful engagement that drove Pleasanton's Federal cavalry from the field. The toll was high: Stuart lost 523 killed, wounded, or missing, including Frank Hampton, brother of the famous CSA general; Pleasanton lost 936, including a valued Brig. Gen., Benjamin "Grimes" Davis. Wert also quotes a fellow Confederate to the effect that Brandy Station "*made* the Federal cavalry." Always before, Stuart's cavalry had embarrassed the Federals, but in this case it was Stuart who was caught unawares with heavy losses and long moments of the confusion and disorientation described by the diarist. There were repercussions, as Wert also notes: "As the Confederates moved north, the flamboyant general eagerly sought to erase the stain; his attitude would have grave consequences for Lee at Gettysburg." Wert; Long, 363-64. Long notes that prior to this bloody engagement, infantrymen often jibed, "whoever saw a dead cavalryman?"

The movements of Gen. [R.E.] Lee are no doubt discovered to the enemy by the boldness of [George] Stoneman[403]—a thing very much to be regretted. Wrote to Cousin Bettie.

[FIELD HOSPITAL ON SPERRYVILLE ROAD, CULPEPER CO.]

WEDNESDAY, JUNE 10, [18]63

This morning Gen. [Jubal A.] Early returned to the Sperryville Road. I went to the village [Culpeper Court House] and saw Aunt Betsy and Mrs. Daniel's family. I then went to the [field] Hospital and found an acquaintance—Jerry Thompson—badly wounded[404]

Heard of several others. News from Vicksburg this evening is very cheering. O how I do hope no disaster will befall us there. I met Mrs. Dr. Quisenberry [wife of the neighborhood physician in Wilderness] on the street this evening. I was so glad to see her. She wishes my address for Dr. [Quisenberry]—he is in Richmond at [General] Hospt. no. 1. I called at Mrs. D's [Daniels's] after night and spent a few hours pleasantly. Saw [G.W.] Boteler to-day. Dr. [Joseph E.] Claggett has charge of the [field] Hospital at this place [outside Culpeper Court House, on the Sperryville Road].

We move to-morrow at 2 A.M.

Gen. [R.E.] Lee's dispatch to Richmond of the fight yesterday is encouraging. All of us expect Mail to-day but failed to get it.

[HOSPITAL CAMP, SPERRYVILLE, RAPPAHANNOCK CO.]

THURSDAY, JUNE 11, [18]63

Agreeable to orders last evening we were up and off. Taking the Sperryville Road [in Culpeper Co.], we passed through Woodville [Rappahannock] and camped at Sperryville. The army took the right hand road at Sperryville and has

---

[403] Stoneman (1822-1894), already identified, was by then removed to desk duty because of "lackluster leadership" at Chancellorsville; however, the diarist is correct that R.E. Lee's once mysterious rapid marches were now followed more closely and more accurately by the Federals, in this case because of Alfred Pleasanton's (1824-1897) boldness; and Joseph Hooker was able to report to Lincoln that R.E. Lee was leading a very large force of the ANV into the North on a major invasion. On Stoneman, see Robert D. Hoffsommer, "Stoneman," *Hist. Times.*; on Pleasanton, see Patrick M. McCoy, "Pleasanton," ibid.

[404] Jerry W. Thompson of Orange Co. and 7th VA Inf., age unknown, was listed as private by David F. Riggs, *7th VA Inf.*, 96; and by Scott, *Hist. of Orange Co.*, 271. Both describe Thompson as killed in action during War, but he must have survived this wound, since Riggs identifies the death date as 7 April 1865.

started in the direction of "Little Washington" [NW sector of Rappahannock Co]. None of us are told where we are bound yet—we are 31 miles from Warrenton [Faquier Co.] & 26 from Front Royal [Warren Co]. I have predicted that we would go to the Latter place and cross the Blue Ridge to Manassas and perhaps fight again in the already twice historic place.[405] Gen'l [George Edward] Pickett's Div.[406] arrived at Culpeper C.H. last evening. We have a fine force now.

The country from Culpeper C.H. [Clulpeper Co.] to Sperryville [Rappahannock Co.] is not very good. From Woodville to Sperryville it is better than from Culpeper to Woodville [viz., he thinks the countryside improves as one travels northwest in the Co]. I do like to see the mountains—How much like home [Smyth Co]. Woodville is quite small and Sperryville is less —

We pitched our tents and took a stroll through the village [Sperryville] looking at the fair young damsels as they stood at their doors and windows looking as inviting as a newly bloomed and beautiful rose. Supper over and we were ordered to move. Taking the road to Little Washington 6 miles distant. That point was reached about midnight. We passed through after dark and I could not see the place; but from the appearance in the distance I fancy it is quite a nice place, all the houses were surrounded by clumps of trees, and some had beautiful groves.

---

[405] Gen. Richard Stoddert Ewell, in command of the newly organized II Corps of ANV (which included Jackson's old Brigade) did cross the Blue Ridge toward Front Royal, much as his Brigade. had done before on the way to battles in the "twice historic" Manassas. The diarist predicted the route correctly but did not realize that Lee's plan was to strike north of the Mason-Dixon Line. Ewell's Corps was the first to advance north of the Potomac and the first to enter PA on Lee's aggressive northern offensive.

[406] George Edward Pickett (1825-1875), from Richmond, graduated from West Point, 1846, last in the class that included George Brinnan McClellan and Thomas Jonathan Jackson. Serving effectively in the Mexican War, he was breveted Capt. for service there. Thereafter he served in TX, VA, and Washington territory until 1861, earning regular promotions. Resigning his US commission, he joined the CSA as a Col. and soon became a Brig. Gen. He served under Gen. James Longstreet, Seven Days' Campaign (25 June–1 July 1862); and was wounded at Gaines Mill (27 June 1862). He commanded a Div. successfully at Fredericksburg and on this drive into PA led a Div. that included the Brigades of Brig. Gens. James Lawson Kemper (1823-1895), Richard Brooke Garnett (1817-1863), and Lewis Addison Armistead (1817-1863). Well-trained and on this occasion reported to be very confident, he was determined to do well in the planned northern campaign. John T. Hubbell, "Pickett," *Hist. Times*.

[HOSPITAL CAMP AT FRONT ROYAL, WARREN CO.]

FRIDAY, JUNE 12, 1863

This morning early we were on the road. I walked in company with Dr. Ellsberg some three or four miles. Gen [John Brown] Gordon's[407] (formerly [Alexander Robert] Lawton's Brigade) was thrown in rear to protect the [2d Corps supply wagon] trains.

At Gaincs X Roads thc army took thc lcft towards Flint Hill [Rappahannock Co.], the road to Fort Royal [Warren Co]. I was riding on horseback with a brother of Capt. [John] Glaize [Qm and chief of forage operations for Bde on this march] and had gotten far ahead of our train. Our horses were hungry and we turned aside to a field of grass and were allowing our horses to eat the clover when some man, perhaps an officer[,] rode up and asked us our names and where we belonged, and saying at the same time that he should report us to Gen'l [Richard Stoddert] Ewell's [2d Corps] HdQers and if a guard were near he would most assuredly turn us over to the guard. His reason was that we were grazing a man's field. The ideas was a very ridiculous one to us for that [sic; grazing is what] most of our horses are dependent upon. What orders may have been issued I know not and if a law was broken it was done in ignorance—We gave him our names—he ordered the fence to be replaced but as I did not pull it down I refused to put it up. I regret that I did not ask him who he was.

We reached Flint Hill a little village about noon—The country from Sperryville to Front Royal presents a very *run-down* [diarist's italics] appearance especially on the left towards the mountains. We reached Front Royal about dark and camped on the same ground, I think, it was the 14th of May of last year [during T.J. Jackson's Valley Campaign that established the reputation of the "foot cavalry"].

---

[407] John Brown Gordon (1832-1904) was a Georgian who had attended University of Georgia, but left it to read law and pass the bar, practicing law in Atlanta for a time. Immediately before War came, Gordon was in NW sector of GA, attempting to develop mines in the hills. He raised a co. of mountain men called the Racoon Roughs, whom he served originally as Capt. Showing himself to be a good organizer and courageous fighter, Gordon rose in rank quickly and was promoted to Brig. Gen. after Sharpsburg (1 November 1862). R.E. Lee was said to have trusted him quite a great deal, especially during and after this fateful northern thrust. James O. Hall, "Gordon," *Hist. Times.*

It is very evident now that we are after [Robert Huston] Milroy[408] at Winchester. [Gen. James] Longstreet has not come over [with 1st Corps]. He is watching [Gen. Joseph] Hooker, I guess

[HOSPITAL CAMP, FLINT HILL, RAPPAHANNOCK CO.]

SATURDAY, JUNE 13, 1863 —

This morning we moved off early. Near Ninevah [Warren] we stopped and remained 'till next morning. All the wagons of army are in camp here—Some little cannonading is heard in direction of Winchester [Frederick Co]. It is said that Road's [sic; Robert Emmett Rodes] Division is in the lead.

I wrote a letter to "Mollie" of Richmond [Mary Camden]. Some of our boys went out on guard to-night. Some seem to anticipate "Yankee Cavalry"—I do not.

Rained some to-day.

[TEMPORARY HOSPITAL CAMP NEAR WINCHESTER, FREDERICK CO.]

SUNDAY, JUNE 14, 1863

Cannon booming early this morning—about 9 o'clock we moved—at the toll gate above White Post [Clarke Co]. we went to the left to Newton [Clarke and Frederick Co]. By the time we arrived there the fight had opened in good earnest. Gen. [Richard Stoddert] Ewell had his [ANV 2d Corps] batteries in position and were [sic] throwing shell into the enemy's ranks [Robert Huston Milroy's cavalry] very rapidly. This continued 'till dusk—The place [Winchester] is entirely invested.[409] There is no escape for [Robert Huston] Milroy except the hazardous alternative of cutting his way through our [2d ANV Corps] lines.

---

[408] Robert Huston Milroy (1816-1890) was a native of Indiana and graduate of Norwich Military Academy in VT (1843). He led Indiana Volunteers in Mexican War, and afterward studied law at Indiana University, practicing before the bar and serving as a judge in his native state. When War came, he organized more Indiana volunteers and took them to western VA, distinguishing himself on the Federal side of Jackson's Valley Campaign in 1862 and rising to rank of Brig. Gen. A good leader, Milroy on this day set his troops to guard the northern (lower) entrance to the Shenandoah at Winchester (which changed hands some 70 times during Civil War). Ewell's II Corps overwhelmed Milroy and prevented the orderly retreat that he attempted on 15 June. Close observers then and now do not blame Milroy for the Federal disaster of 15 June 1863 at Winchester, but military authorities apparently did, for he never held major field command again. Jeffrey D. Wert, "Milroy," *Hist. Times.*

[409] "Invest." In military terms, "surrounded." From Latin for dressing or clothing. *OED.*

I met some ladies here and had a very pleasant walk—a Miss Shipley —

We [the hospital staff] slept in a clover field—I commenced a letter to Dr. W[illiam] Faris —

[TEMPORARY HOSPITAL CAMP NEAR WINCHESTER, FREDERICK CO.]

MONDAY, JUNE 15TH, 1863

Soon after we rose orders came for us to proceed right away to Winchester. The enemy [Robert Huston Milroy's horse troops] had succeeded in forcing his way through our lines and many had escaped. Gen. Johnston's Division [sic; Edward Johnson][410] met them at Stevenson's Depot [sic; Stephenson Depot, Frederick Co].

We were up and of[f] in a trice. Dr. B took possession of the York House for a [field] Hospital. The "Taylor Hotel" is the Yankee [field] Hosp't. I found several of our men there [Taylor Hotel] who had been taken prisoner a few evenings ago near Newton [Clarke and Frederick Cos.] in the Cavalry skirmish. The result of that skirmish was insignificant to the report concerning it [viz., the

---

[410] Edward Johnson (1816-1875). Maj. Gen. Johnson had taken over Thomas Jonathan Jackson's old Div. after Jackson's wounding at Chancellorsville (4 May 1863). Born in Salisbury [Saulsbury Furnace], Botetourt Co., Johnson graduated West Point, 1838, served in Seminole and Mexican wars, and on western border action, then New York City when War came. Capt. in Federal army, he resigned commission and formed 12th GA Inf. , but soon became Brig. Gen. on basis of friendships with James Longstreet, Richard Stoddert Ewell, R.E. Lee, and George E. Pickett. Known as "Allegheny Ed" and "Old Allegheny" for his prowess in mountain and valley campaigns in 1862 under Jackson, he was badly wounded in foot at McDowell (8 May 1862) and faced a slow convalescence of nearly a year. He carried an "outsized club" used daily as a walking cane, but also as a weapon in battle. He was captured at Spotsylvania (12 May 1864), despite using his club against would-be Federal captors after he lost his horse and was surrounded. An old Federal Army friend, Maj. Gen. Marsena Rudolph Patrick (1811-1888) intervened and saved him (and some other Federal troopers); imprisoned briefly, he was exchanged in May 1864 to serve with Army of Tennessee John Bell Hood's (1831-1880) Franklin and Nashville Campaign, working directly under Lt. Gen. Stephen Dill Lee (1833-1908). Captured again, at Nashville (15-22 December 1864), he was kept in Old Capitol Prison (on 1st Street in Washington, D.C., the temporary home of US Congress after Capitol was burned by British in War of 1812; other inmates included spies Bell Boyd and Rose O'Neal Greenhow and Andersonville Prison commandant Heinrich Wirz) until July 1865. After release and parole, he took up farming in Richmond area. John E. Stanchak says that "Old Allegheny" was "remembered as a gruff, badly dressed, voluble swearer, and as one of the Confederacy's best division commanders." Idem, "Johnson," *Hist. Times*.

CSA cavalry lost this skirmish in the process of winning the larger battle to recapture Winchester]. A company from Montgomery[411] was in it.

There is some excitement but none compared to what was when [Nathaniel Prentiss] Banks was driven off [24 May 1862].[412] The enemy [General Robert Huston Milroy's cavalry] left all his wagons and artillery. Prisoners are being brought in very rapidly. They are moved out to the fortifications. The boys are Collecting Captives [sic][413] . A large amount [of Captive supplies] is sent to Dr. Black—including notion that a Yankee notion vender could have—shoes, boots, trunks—medicines and confectionaries. Any quantity of medical & blank books,[414] paper and ink —

The captured Yankee mail was brought in and we oppened [sic] some of it—a very tedious job.

---

[411] Probably Baldwin's Squadron led by Capt. William Marshall Baldwin, the precursor to 22d Cav. that was formed in Oct. 1863. Most likely the Montgomery "mounted riflemen" were some of the men who fought under Baldwin in eastern KY and upper east TN, then fought in WV and later formed Co. K, 22d Cav. under Col. Henry S. Bowen. The entire Baldwin Squadron did not fight as a unit in the Winchester Campaign, as some were stationed in Saltville (Washington Co.) area guarding the CSA's salt mines. Jeffrey C. Weaver, *22nd VA Cav.*, Virginia Regimental Histories Series (Lynchburg, VA: H.E. Howard, 1991) 1-12. Other Montgomery troops in the Winchester battle were Co. E, the old Highlanders commanded by Capt. Charles A. Ronald in 4th VA Inf., but they were infantry forces. Robertson.

[412] Nathaniel Prentiss Banks (1816-1894) was a fervent antislavery activist from Waltham MA and a one-time Democrat who became Gov. of MA, 1858, after helping to start the new Republican Party in protest over the Kansas-Nebraska Act. A poor general, Banks had Abraham Lincoln's sponsorship and rose rapidly through the ranks to become Maj. Gen. Embarrassed twice in T.J. Jackson's Shenandoah Valley Campaign, including the loss of Winchester on 24 May 1862, Banks was several times saved in his military career by Lincoln, who moved him in 1863 to the Miss. River campaigns. Fighting very badly at Vicksburg, he was removed again to NW LA in 1864 to direct the Red River Campaign of that year; failing abysmally there, he could not be saved again, even by the president, and left the Army to win election as congressperson representing the Waltham area from 1865-1877. Michael T. Cochran, "Banks," *Hist. Times.*

[413] Capitalization is diarist's. William G. Bean says that Apperson uses a colloquialism to say that the soldiers are collecting booty, esp. guns and equipment, left by fleeing Federal soldiers. Bean, notes. Bean must be correct, for the Federal troops were long gone from this area and could not be "captured" by this time.

[414] Blank book was for keeping diaries and journals. These very entries were made in a blank book left behind by a Federal soldier in another campaign. Notes and photographs, Apperson collection.

[YORK HOUSE FIELD HOSPITAL NEAR WINCHESTER, FREDERICK CO.]

TUESDAY, JUNE 16, 1863

Yankee goods are everywhere in profusion—Orders to-day are that the sick and wounded be moved to Jordan Springs [Frederick Co]. There has been a very great deal of sickness here in town this summer and for hygenic reasons it is best to have our sick away—[415]

The captures this time is [sic] larger than from [Nathaniel Prentiss] Banks [May 1862]—about 5,500 prisoners are taken[416]—Old Milroy [Robert Huston Milroy] made his escape [to Federal garrison at Harper's Ferry in new state of WV]—I am glad he was not taken, but would have been glad to have heard of his death. Our government would have been under the necessity of pursuing a course towards him that would have given the enemy a pretext for more atrocities.

This is a most splendid victory[.] [I]ndeed it is a double one—One over [Robert Huston] Milroy and another over the Minds of our soldiers—showing them that Gen'l [Richard Stoddert] Ewell is Competent to manage the [2d ANV] Corps and is worthy of his predecessor [Thomas Jonathan Jackson; capitalizations are diarist's].

Our army is pushing on towards the Potomac and by this time I should not wonder if a part of it is over in Maryland.[417]

I finished a letter to Dr. W[illiam] Faris and wrote one home [to the Appersons in Orange Co].

Dr. Syd[Sydnor] went home to-day.

---

[415] Notice the slowly evolving concept of disease spread by agents of some kind that could be nurtured in filthy conditions; however, the germ theory is not yet formed. "Germ," *McGrew's.*; Cunningham.

[416] Estimates of this size are not confirmed in *Official Reports*, and diary entry seems very high; Long suggests that Federals suffered 95 deaths and had 348 wounded while Ewell's II Corps ANV suffered 48 killed, 219 wounded. Missing in action or captured for CSA Long estimates at 3 and for Milroy's Federal troops, 4000. Long also finds estimates of 23 guns, 300 loaded wagons, over 300 horses, and many QM stores, despite Milroy's efforts to destroy supplies that he could not take with him on retreat. R.E. Rode Report, R.S. Ewell Report, *OR*, 15 June 1863; Long, 366.

[417] Richard Stoddert Ewell's advance forces of II Corps ANV were crossing the Potomac into MD on 16 June 1863 according to *OR* and Long, 367.

[YORK HOUSE FIELD HOSPITAL NEAR WINCHESTER, FREDERICK CO.]

WEDNESDAY, JUNE 17 [18]63

Most of the habitues of the Hosp't were sent to the [Jordan] Springs [Frederick Co. west of Winchester] to-day. We shall close out and leave to-morrow—Dr. B's [field hospital] Corps will follow the Army.

A General Distribution of goods and chattels [horses and mules] were [sic] made to-day. I disposed of my old clothes and filled my portmanteau with new ones—Some of our illustrious collagues are very greedy —. The[y] select and secrete for more than themselves [that is, they intend to sell some of the Captures]—I would not have believed that some who have done so would have done it.

I have had a tedious time opening the Yankee Mail.

Several souvenirs were in the letters and some money. The money belongs to the Hosp't Dept.

The Med. Director of [Robert Huston] Milroy's army is a perfect dog. Dr. B & he do not get along well to-gether.

[YORK HOUSE FIELD HOSPITAL NEAR WINCHESTER, FREDERICK CO.]

THURSDAY, JUNE 18, 1863

To-day we made preparations to march ~~but did not get off~~ [diarist's strike-through]. I have made arrangements with Mr. Neil [418] to take charge of some things I have selected. It is forbidden that we take much baggage along [into the northern campaign] and it ought to be so too.

I leave some 4 shirts[,] 1 pr drawers, 1 flannel shirt[,] 1/2 ream of paper, several packages of envelopes, *Bennett's* Surgery, Bennett's Principles of Medicine[419] , and several other articles —. Mr. [Sagisimend] Neill proposes to

---

[418] Possibly Sagisimend Neill, born 1824, who owned a home and land in Berryville, Clarke Co. not far east of the York House in Frederick Co. There are no males with name *Neil* in Clarke or Frederick Co. in 1870 census. VA. Census, 1870. On next entry, diarist spells the name *Neill.*

[419] Diarist's italics. John Hughes Bennett (1812-1875) was a prominent Scottish surgeon who taught at the University of Edinburgh. He delivered lectures on surgery, esp. skin pathology, and these lectures were published originally in Edinburgh by Arthur and Charles Black Press and then in at least six editions in England and US and translated into French, Russian, and "Hindoo." The edition likely found by the diarist called "Bennett's Practice of Medicine" among the "Yankee captures" is *Clinical Lectures on the Principles and Practice of Medicine by John Hughes Bennett* (1858, 2nd American edition from 6th Scottish edition; New York: William Wood, 1863). The "Bennett's Surgery" in the "captures" is likely John Hughes Bennett, *Introduction to Clinical*

leave Winchester in a few months and go west. I gave him a letter of introduction to Mr. R[ichard J.] Venable in Marion[420]—He [Sagisimend Neill] is a Tinner by trade.

I think some of our boys will not need any more goods for a seige [sic].

~~Friday, June~~[421]

We left Winchester about noon—Took the Martinsburg [Berkeley Co., WV] road and camped about 2 miles above Bunker Hill [Berkeley Co., WV]. A heavy rain fell. I was very unwell.

All my baggage is in Dr. B's wagon. I have a valise[,] bed (blankets & bed sheets only)[,] 1 Box of stationery and 1 Desk.

Dr. Wilkerson & Dr. Hagy are at Jordan Springs [Frederick Co; field hospital for those who fell sick in Winchester on early part of the northern march]. Dr. Hagy is in charge. [Drs.] Jamison & Hacket were left there.

I sent a letter to Mr. Motley this morning. I have rec'd no mail since we left Guinea [Guineys Station Depot , Caroline Co]. J[ohn].M[McAllister]. Sexton,[422] "Smyth Blues" he [sic] gave me some aromatic sugar Mrs. Faris sent me. B[enjamin] P[atterson]. Walker [423] sent me a pair of socks, a present from Miss Mary F[aris].—the nicest pair of home-made socks I have ever seen.

[TEMPORARY FIELD HOSPITAL SOUTH OF KEARNEYSVILLE, JEFFERSON CO., WV]

FRIDAY, JUNE 19, 1863

Left camp [near Bunker Hill, Berkeley Co., WV] early—took the Charles Town [424] [Jefferson Co., WV] road to Smythfield [sic; Smithfield, Jefferson Co.,

---

Medicine; Six Lectures on the Method of Examining Patients, and the Means Necessary for Arriving at an Exact Diagnosis (3d ed.; Edinburgh: Arthur and Charles Black, 1857).

420 Richard J. Venable, born 1819, and his brother Robert operated a dry-goods store in Marion and often advertised in the *Marion Visitor.* Armstrong, *Hist. of Smyth*, 2:133; Wilson, *Smyth Co. Hist.*, 166; VA Census, 1870. Although Marion is southwest of Winchester, the diarist thinks of the highlands region as generally *west* of the Valley.

421 Diarist's strike-through; he apparently decided to write more for Thursday entry.

422 John McAllister Sexton, (1842-1864), was a mechanic from Smyth Co. assigned as clerk for Joseph C. Sexton in Co. A, original Smyth Blues; later assigned to Brigade Commissary; died 6 August 1864 from gunshot wound to thigh, and bur., Frederick, MD. Robertson, *4th VA Inf.*, 72.

423 Benjamin Patterson Walker (1837-1906) was a laborer from Smyth Co. who knew Apperson before secession. Walker joined Smyth Blues early, was wounded at Kernstown (23 March 1862), recovered and returned to Co. D, 4th VA Inf. In 1864 he was detailed as nurse at Emory General Hospital, Emory & Henry College, and continued to stay in touch with diarist. Robertson, 78. Bur. in Smyth Co., but not listed in Sturgill and Sturgill. Archives, EHC.

424 Charles Town is a small community in Jefferson Co. , WV, some 15–20 m iles northeast of Winchester. The capital of the State of WV (formed in 1862 and admitted to Union in 1863) was

WV] and there took the Shepherdstown [Jefferson Co., WV] Road. Dr. [W.W.] Drane & myself went to a Mrs. Cockrell's and got our dinner.—a really good vegetable dinner. Dr. Syd[nor] overtook us at night in camp below Kearneysville [Jefferson Co., WV].

We hear various rumours—[James] Longstreet [1st Corps of ANV] is at Upperville in Loudon Co. A[mbrose] P[owell] Hill [3d Corps of ANV] has drubbed [Joseph] Hooker [Army of Potomac]—[Joseph Eggleston] Johnston has whipped [Ulysses] Grant [at Vicksburg, MS] and [Braxton] Bragg has defeated [William Starke] Rosecrans [in middle TN].[425] Too much—I do not know that our Army is in Maryland at all. Yet, hardly think it is [Richard Stoddert Ewell's 2d Corps was entering MD].

There is no doubt but [John Daniel] Imboden is at Cumberland [Allegany Co., MD][426] and [Albert Gallatin] Jenkins[427] at Chambersburg [Franklin Co.] Penn: Rhodes [sic; Maj. Gen. Robert Emmett Rodes, already identified, was div. commander assigned to support flank of Jubal A. Early on the PA attack] is at

---

and still is Charleston in Kanawha Co. around 300 miles west of this area. State of WV, *Official WV Map*, 2000.

[425] It is true that James Longstreet's 1st Corps was moving through Loudon Co.; all other rumors are completely misguided. See Long, 360-70.

[426] John Daniel Imboden (1823-1895) was Brig. Gen. in 1863 and was functioning as an independent force acting separately from the 3 ANV corps marching north. The Staunton native, alumnus of Washington College, onetime school teacher and attorney, and former state delegate was in the midst of his "Imboden's Raid" that focused on destruction of Baltimore & Ohio RR lines in MD. The raid also captured "large numbers of livestock" from Federally controlled areas of WV and western VA. When the PA phase of Lee's coordinated drive north began, Imboden guarded the CSA left flank; it fell to his brigade to guard the retreat from Gettysburg, which he performed capably. In 1864 he worked with Jubal A. Early to coordinate a threatening strike at Washington, D.C. and he fought against Philip Henry Sheridan (1831-1888) in the Shenandoah Valley campaign led by Richard Stoddert Ewell. After War, he developed mineral and mining enterprises in Damascus, Washington Co., VA on the southern border of Smyth Co. where our diarist was developing his own New South business interests. Emory M. Thomas, "Imboden," *Hist. Times.*

[427] Albert Gallatin Jenkins (1830-1864) was Brig. Gen. commanding a brigade of cavalry that included home guards and guerillas. This brigade, new in August 1862, had made a successful 500-mile raid through western VA and Ohio. For the PA campaign, Jenkins Brigade led the advance for the three corps of ANV, in course of which he captured Chambersburg (Franklin Co., PA) and made a threatening raid toward PA state capital Harrisburg (Dauphin Co.). Prior to War, the Cabell City (Carroll Co., VA) native had graduated from Jefferson College in PA and Harvard Law School; practicing law in Charlestown [in what became Kanawha Co., WV], he served in US House of Representatives 1856-60. When War came he formed 8th VA Cav. and led raids in western VA but then served six months in CSA Congress (February 1862-August 1862). Wounded twice in battles in 1864, he died of complications of wound at Cloyd's Mountain (9 May 1864). Jeffrey D. Wert, "Jenkins," *Hist. Times.*

Hagerstown [Washington Co., MD] and [Edward] Johnson's Div. is near Sharpsburg [Washington Co. near Frederick Co., MD]. Capt. [Moorman B.] White of Cavalry [14th VA Cav.][428] at Point of Rocks [on Potomac River, Montgomery Co., MD] and captured 2 trains of cars and 53 prisoners.[429]

We stop for the night, perhaps longer. A shower of rain fell —

[TEMPORARY FIELD HOSPITAL CAMP SOUTH OF KEARNEYSVILLE, JEFFERSON CO., WV]

SATURDAY, JUNE 20TH, 1863

This morning it is cloudy—no move to-day. The [Potomac] river is said to be rising. If [Joseph] Hooker [still commanding Army of Potomac] should throw a force on Johnston [sic; Maj. Gen. Edward Johnson] while the river is up it might be bad.

The whole thing I think will be explained as soon as the defeat of [Robert Huston] Milroy is finished and by threatening Washington City [D.C.] and drain part of the [Federal] army from the west [Nashville, TN area and Vicksburg, MS]. Gen'l [Joseph] Hooker is evidently unable with his present force to cope with the Army [ANV] under Gen'l [R.E.] Lee. The Conscription Act [3 March 1863] in the North is proving a dangerous thing[430]—It is reported,

---

428 Moorman B. White (ca. 1828- 1874) was "a chivalric and brave soldier," who led co. A, 14th VA Cav. A hotelkeeper in Lewisburg, Greenbrier Co. [by 1863 in WV], he joined Cav. at age 32 and was apparently captured, 14 June 1863 on this very campaign. Driver, *14th VA Cav.*, 188.

429 This skirmish on 17 June 1863 was "won" by CSA Cav. Also participating may have been James H. White (1835-death date unknown), onetime Capt. of Co. I, 6th VA Cav., but not then "leading" any charge and perhaps not present at the engagement at all. See Musick, *6th VA Cav*, 168. The diarist may have known of James White's earlier role in 6th Cav. and misunderstood who was leading this skirmish. Official records do not confirm that the 6th Cav. or the 14th Cav. captured prisoners and supply wagons at Point of Rocks, but Richard Stoddert Ewell's 2nd Corps ANV crossing into MD did capture a number of prisoners, as did John Daniel Imboden on his independent raid . Also, Albert Gallatin Jenkins's cav. captured supply wagons in MD and PA as the three corps and the flanking forces moved north.

430 Actually, the CSA first passed a conscription act, 16 April 1862; and the Federal act for US followed 11 months later. Never popular as a concept, the conscription act allowed bounty to be paid for substitutes and included many exemptions that struck some as class-biased; the July conscription coming due as the diarist was writing proved particularly unpopular and there were draft riots, most notably in New York City in that month. Patricia L. Faust estimates that only about 6% of those conscripted for Federal service actually served. The act was widely avoided in CSA as well, but she also estimates that by 1864 between 25% and 33% of CSA troops fighting in VA and east were conscripts, a sign that by then few were volunteering or reenlisting. Generally "unpopular, unwieldy, and unfair" for both sides, "conscription raised more discontent than soldiers." Idem, "conscription," *Hist. Times.*

I do not believe it though, that Gov. [Andrew Gregg] Curtin[431] of Penn: has called on the President for protection but it is refused and he calls for 30,000 malitia [sic] to defend the state. With 30,000 raw malita [sic] now to organise and defend the State when part of it [Chambersburg and York] is already in our possession and if Gen'l [R.E.] Lee is inclined to do so he could overrun the State, Gov: [Andrew Gregg] Curtin's malitia [sic] to the contrary notwithstanding.

I have been reading to-day a speech by Fernando Wood of N.Y. before a Democratic mass meeting [on 3 June 1863 in New York City at Cooper Institute].[432] He calls loudly for peace and adds that unless some terms of peace are arrived at and speedily, the question will not be "will the North acknowledge

---

[431] The diarist does well to be skeptical. The PA governor was personally raising a remarkable number of enlistees from his state, and he was assured of personal and military support from his friend and ally Abraham Lincoln. Andrew Gregg Curtin (1817-1894) was called by some "the greatest of the Northern war governors" according to John E. Stanchak. Born in Bellefonte PA, he began political life as a Whig but was so fervently anti-secessionist that he was elected PA's first Republican office-holder when he became governor in 1860. Managing a massive state budget defict (equal to 1/2 the large Federal deficit) he was still able to raise even more money through appropriations and he personally recruited Federal soldiers. PA sent more than 427,000 enlistees during War. When public morale fell and Abraham Lincoln came under heavy political attack after Sharpsburg (14-16 September 1862), Curtin organized a Union Governors conference at Altoona PA to declare support for Lincoln and emancipation. A bitter enemy of fellow Republican the infamous Simon Cameron ("Czar of PA"), Curtin encouraged Lincoln to remove Cameron from cabinet, which finally happened in January 1862 when Cameron was sent as ambassador to Russia. However, Cameron returned to power in PA Republican Party, and in postbellum years prevented Curtin from holding office again, until Curtin finally switched parties and became a Democrat. Idem, "Curtin," *Hist. Times.*

[432] Wood was at this time former-governor, recently defeated for reelection because of his statements about a secessionist New York. Before War came, Fernando Wood (1812-1881), then Democratic Gov. of NY, had proposed on 6 January 1861 that New York could be a "free city," able to trade with CSA or USA during wartime. A native Philadelphian from a Quaker family, Wood was consistently anti-war, but he was also very politic and shrewd in his abilities to pick up popular trends in opinion and move with those trends. When War came, he at first cooperated with Lincoln, but reversed himself again after the Federal embarrassments at Fredericksburg and Chancellorsville. At this low point in Union morale, before the twin victories at Vicksburg and Gettysburg, Wood called often for peace and for letting the southern states form a separate nation. He helped Clement L. Vallandigham to found the Democratic Peace Party, but avoided the negative tag of "Copperhead" that attached to other conciliatory northern Democrats. Wood won election to US House of Representatives and served from 1863-1877, wielding some influence despite a general disdain among northern Democrats for leaders who had been conciliatory toward the CSA and antagonistic to the martyred Abraham Lincoln. His younger brother Benjamin Wood operated a very popular anti-war newspaper in New York City that stayed in trouble with Lincoln authorities; and this brother Benjamin also founded a popular and long-lived German-language newspaper in The City. Long, 22, 361.

the South["], but it will be "will the South acknowledge the North". He denounces the action of the [Lincoln] administration towards [Clement L.] Vallandigham [see earlier notes]. Vallandigham has been nominated by the Democratic convention of ~~N York~~ Ohio unanimously for Governor.

I have been reading a novel by Capt. [Frederick] Chamier entitled "Ben Brace"[.][433] Were it not for his sailor dialect I should like it.

[TEMPORARY FIELD HOSPITAL NEAR KEARNEYSVILLE, JEFFERSON CO., WV]

SUNDAY, JUNE 21, [18]63

Soon the clouds that had gathered last night passed away and the sun came out though not warm. I got in a writing humour to-day by some means or other ~~I got into~~ and wrote another letter to Miss Mollie Thornton. Why I write to her I cannot exactly tell. I like the young lady very much but to think of anything existing between us than a friendship I I [sic] cannot. I may never [be] in the vicinity of Guinea Station [Guineys Station Depot, Caroline Co.] again. Miss Mollie may think me importunate. She can think as she chooses. I am not dependant [sic] upon anyone.

I finished the story of "Ben Brace"—I think it does very well. The historical allusions of the work are highly interesting and I presume correct.

It has been a very pleasant day to us in camp—We move to-morrow at 5 a.m. We cross the Potomac [about five miles to northeast].

[TEMPORARY FIELD HOSPITAL NEAR SHARPSBURG, WASHINGTON CO., MD]

MONDAY, JUNE 22, [18]63

As was ordered last evening we moved this morning. At Shepperdstown [sic; Sheperdstown, Jefferson Co., WV] Dr. B sent me to Martinsburg [Berkeley Co., WV] on business for the Hospt Dept. I took 100$ up for the Med: Officer in chg. [charge] to buy supplies. Asst. Surg. Hadley is in charge. He seems to have

---

[433] Frederick Chamier, *Ben Brace: The Last of Nelson's Agamemnons* (London: Richard Bentley, 1836). The novel was widely reprinted in editions from 1836 to 1906 in US and England. It was also published with subtitle, *A Nautical Romance.* Chamier (1796-1870) had some naval experience, but made his name with this novel and with a companion novel featuring Ned Brace. Note that the diarist had been interested before in Admiral Horatio Nelson.

a hard time. A large number of sick and no appliances or food.[434] He says there are some fair ladies who have opened their homes very much.

My ride up was warm but pleasant to me. I love horseback exercise. When I returned I crossed at the ford [of the Potomac River in Jefferson Co., WV] and at Sharpsburg [Washington Co., MD] I found our [supply-wagon] trains. At this time last year [mid-September 1862] one of the most sanguinary conflicts of the War. We have a good shady grove.

I was at work at my old register to-day. I wish to get all my work done correctly.

I have been reading the "Iron Cross"[435]—it is a story that is pretty thick as the boys say—[colloquialism; hard to follow because of its thematic density]

I took a bath this evening.

[TEMPORARY FIELD HOSPITAL NEAR BUTTONTOWN, FRANKLIN CO., PA]

TUESDAY, JUNE 23D [1863]

This morning we moved off towards Hagerstown [Washington Co., MD]. The citizens of Sharpsburg [Washington Co., MD], are rabid unionist—not ever do they want peace with our independence.

Passing the battlefield of Sharpsburg, or Antietam, none of us failed to feel a sad Fate of this dreadful conflict [17 September 1862]. All over the field were lined groups of graves marked by name boards. The husbandman had been here since the dreadful day of fire and smoke & death rolled over this field, and now corn was growing. The fencing along the road was marked by thousands of [musket-] balls. We passed some few citizens who seemed to see us, but generally they were worse and showed that we were not welcome.

---

[434] According to Cunningham, passim, hospital supplies of all sorts were fully adequate for the CSA forces, esp. ANV, through this campaign of summer 1863; the privations from shortages did not come until after the defeats of this disastrous summer. He does note that sometimes supply wagon-trains, esp. ambulance wagons, were not moved to field hospitals as quickly as needed. The diarist also generally reports adequate supplies in the period 1861-summer 1863.

[435] Sylvanus Cobb, Jr., *The Iron Cross, or, The Countess of Errol; a Tale of High and Low Life* (New York: Samuel French, 1850, 1859). Cobb (1823-1887), born in Waterville ME, was son of a prominent Universalist reformist minister of same name. The senior Cobb led campaigns for antislavery and temperance. The junior Cobb often dramatized such themes as in this play. This play was later republished as a novelette, and the junior Cobb made his name with novelettes of social justice and high-Victorian morality. The diarist likely responded favorably to the temperance and high-morality in the play, but of course saw no evil in slavery.

We passed Tillman Town [sic; Tilghmanton, Washington Co., MD], or as some of the boys vulgarly said, "Dillberrytown".[436] This is a log-built village and presents a very common appearance.

We passed Hagerstown some 15 mi from Sharpsburg at 2 o'clock. Here some of the young ladies wore Secesh Badges—but as before the citizens wore an uninviting countenance. I think if those who have advocated a movement to wrest Maryland from the thrall [slavery or imprisonment] that surrounds her could see her people for a while they would cease to advocate much risk for her.

Our camp was in one mile of Buttontown [Franklin Co., PA] in Pennsylvania, where the line between Penn: and Maryland passes.

The crops through this country are fine. Fields of wheat and corn; Meadows with most Luxuriant grass which is now being mowed and placed away for Winter use. This looks so sweet to us. It brings back recollections of the days when we were at home and felt the gratification of peace and happiness. We camped on a meadow of beautiful clover and Timothy [a kind of grassy ground cover capitalized in 19th cent. style]. [437] Sent out and got some milk from an old farmer. Capt. Averick QM 33d Va Reg't [438] was killed to-day by some unknown person from the bushes.

[TEMPORARY FIELD HOSPITAL NEAR CHAMBERSBURG, FRANKLIN CO., PA]

WEDNESDAY, JUNE 24TH [1863]

Off again—Buttonsville [Franklin Co., PA] on the line is built of Logs, and the houses are very small. Here we put our foot for the first time in a Free State. The people on this side of the line seem as much towards accommodating us as on the other [MD]. No difficulties 'till we got to Greencastle [Franklin Co.] 10 1/2 mi[.] from Chambersburg. I was walking along the streets and a lady and a

---

[436] Although not common in American English, "dill" refered to an aromatic plant but also to a stupid and somewhat zany character; and a *dillberry* would be an offspring of a stupid and crazed character. *Dictionary of American Slang*, comp. and ed., Harold Wentworth and Stuart Berg Flexner (1960. 2d supp. ed.; New York: Thomas Y. Crowell, 1975).

[437] See "Timothy," secondary meanings, *OED*.

[438] Name is illegible. Dr. Bean believes that the name is Averick. I can find no Averick, or anyone whose name starts with the letter *A* who served as Capt. in 33d or in any rank at all who served with their ordnance or as their QM. The regimental history does not describe this incident, although it generally does describe deaths of officers. The diarist may have the name wrong, or the killing may have escaped official records. Reidenbaugh, *33d VA Inf*, Virginia Regimental Histories Series (Lynchburg, VA: H.E. Howard, 1987), passim; see esp. 67-70; 111.

captain were talking in somewhat an excited manner. I stopped to hear the argument and the officer turned off [turned away]—The woman, lady I will not call her, turned to me and said she liked for persons to tell the truth whether speaking of friends or foe. I asked her what the difference was[.] [S]he said he told things on Gen'l [Robert Huston] Milroy that could not have been correct—I said that from what I had seen and heard it was almost impossible to say anything mean about [Gen. Robert Huston] Milroy that would do him injustice. She soon turned upon me and for awhile the argument was very warm. She said our men came into their village [Greencastle, Franklin Co., PA] like demons, and forced the doors of some houses and fired others. I told her I did not advocate but rather deprecated any rash or harsh treatment, and all ungentlemanly manners, but that, in many instances, this was done without the knowledge of the officers in command. A young man of my acquaintance—rather rough at his expression—had been listening for some time. He says, "Give her a black bean [symbol of a terrible assignment or "detail" for a soldier][439] and let her alone" and dashed off down street. If a spark had fallen into a magazine the explosion would not have been more sudden and furious. I left while the crater of her fury was throwing its molten lava in all directions.

We camped a mile out from Chambersburg [Franklin Co]. The troops are camped in almost every direction.

The report to-day is that A[mbrose] P[owell] Hill [ANV 3d Corps] is at Sharpsburg [Frederick Co., MD some 40 miles southwest of Chambersburg] and Gen'l [James] Longstreet [ANV 1st Corps] at Berryville [Clarke Co., VA, some 55 miles southwest of Chambersburg]. I do not think it possible.

We got some mail—I got two letters—one from Sisters M[ary] and B[ettie] and one from Cousin Bettie.

Our camp was near the house of a Mr. Hade, a staunch old Penn: Farmer. His chickens, as did the chickens of other farmers along the route, filled the mess kettles of many a weary soldier and his garden was protected by great efforts by a guard.[440]

[439] "Black bean" was a CSA soldier's symbol for an unwelcome, even obnoxious, assignment or "detail." For explanation of colloquialism, see Valerius Cincinnatus Giles, *Rags and Hope; the Recollections of Val C. Giles, Four Years with Hood's Brigade, Fourth Texas Infantry, 1861-1865*, comp. and ed., Mary Lasswell (New York: Coward-McCann, 1961) 104.

[440] Dr. Bean considers this report to be a considerable exaggeration. Bean, the biographer of Alexander Swift [Sandie] Pendleton, finds no records of such abuses. In his notes, he writes:

I found he had some fine young horses and went to see him as regards to them. He said he had no horses to sell, and that all had been taken from him, but if I wanted the horse, and so forced the sale, why I must have him. This was touching my conscience very deep. I did not wish for him to think that I would force him to do a thing that would force him to take my money in exchange for his property merely because we were in an enemy's country.

He said I offered him enough so I took the horse at 150$.[441]

He is three years old in the fall and well grown—is an *Iron Gray* [diarist's italics].

[TEMPORARY FIELD HOSPITAL NEAR CHAMBERSBURG, FRANKLIN CO., PA]

THURSDAY, JUNE 25, [18]63

This morning Dr. B ordered some of the boys to town to assist in the distribution of some Medical Stores, which had been taken from the Druggists.

I went and was engaged all day. The stores taken was [sic] very small indeed. Not so much as a country practitioner [such as Dr. William Faris] would keep.

> In the invasion of Pennsylvania Lee issued an order on June 27, 1863, exhorting the troops to abstain from private pillaging and plundering; and directed all officers to arrest and punish summarily all offenders. Doubtless there were individual offenses but few recorded instances of vandalism. The soldier could buy any property, generally paying in Confederate money. But since the army was living on the country, it seized supplies—such as food, forage, and medicine—paying for them. Lieutenant Colonel Sandie Pendleton, Ewell's chief of staff, stated "at the rate of a dollar, CSA, to a gold dollar; if not we give them a certificate to be honored at the end of the war. As private personages, we pay them what they ask, 3 CSA dollars for one greenback."

Bean, notes.

> CSA dollars in PA were accepted by PA merchants at 15 CSA dollars to 1 gold dollar; CSA dollars in PA were accepted by PA merchants at 3 CSA dollars to 1 greenback [Civil War US dollars not "backed" by gold, and transferable for gold only at market rates, then trading at about 5:1 for gold dollars] . The official rate, 1 CSA dollar for 1 gold dollar, was of course hopelessly overvalued; and the records show that CSA troops then adjusted to prevailing markets, certificates showing 3 CSA dollars for 1 greenback.

In his biography, Bean quotes Pendleteon speaking with even more emphasis:

> [T]hanks to Southern Chivalry and rigid discipline there has been the most perfect order. Not the slightest indignity has been offered to any one, even the meanest woman nor will be, I am sure.

William Gleason Bean, *Stonewall's Man: Sandie Pendleton* (Chapel Hill: University of North Carolina Press, 1959) 135.

[441] 150 CSA dollars were worth 50 US greenbacks or 10 gold dollars in PA at this time. Remember that the diarist is earning 21 CSA dollars per month, or 252 CSA dollars per year; if the horse was a good one, then the price, a bit more than seven months' pay, seems appropriate.

Miller & Hinsby, JS Nixon, and Hyser were the Druggists from whom we took articles. The most valuable articles seem not to be visible[.] Only 1 1/2 oz. Quinine & 1 dram of Morphine were among the captures. These stores are taken and duplicate Bills and made out with receipts attached and the cash paid for them.

In the first place when our troops came no town officers could be found. A council of citizens were [sic] held and the requisition of the [CSA] government laid before this Council. The quantity of each article called for was so large that the citizens at once said it could not be filled—It was then agreed that they should render in [quantities] of what they had. Some did so. Judge Kimble presided at the meeting of the citizens. He seems to be a very prominent character among the citizens of the burg [Chambersburg, Franklin Co., PA].[442]

Near night Dr. B received orders to search for Tea & Mustard. Many of the merchants refused to open their doors. A guard was brought into requisition [a force of soldiers was "detailed" to go with Dr. Harvey Black and the diarist to buy tea and mustard] and then we had but little difficulty. If the proprietor was not at his house two of the citizens were called and informed what was required.

Nearly all of these seemed churlish and out of humour. One, [Jacob] Hoke, a grocer seemed to take all things easy. He is evidently a better or no worse man than many of his neighbors.[443]

---

[442] In other places, Apperson identifies this judge as Alexander K. McClure (1828-1909), a political and personal friend of Abraham Lincoln. Bean considers the identification in the diary to be wrong, and suggests that Apperson's record in "Reminiscences" is right. Cf. Bean, notes.

[443] Jacob Hoke (1825-1893) was a merchant in Chambersburg PA who kept records of the invasion by the Army of Northern Virginia (ANV). Long after R.E. Lee's failure at Gettysburg and subsequent retreat, the Town of Chambersburg suffered a second invasion the following summer of 1864 when Brig. Gen. John McCausland (1836-1927) was ordered by ANV 2d Corps Commander Jubal Anderson Early to cut railroad lines, but also to seek monetary damages from Chambersburg citizens because of the extreme damage done by Gen. David Hunter (1802-1866) to citizens in the Shenandoah Valley and the piedmont in VA. McCausland's men burned much of Chambersburg, including some homes where citizens had paid the money requested. The incident in Chambersburg shows how much had changed in a year, and Hoke notes the differences carefully as he assesses Confederate army conduct in July 1863 and July 1864. His account of Lee's invasion includes his own judgments of Gen. Daniel Edgar Sickles (1819-1914), who brought his troops into an exposed position in front of Gen. James Longstreet's 1st Corps and later blamed his commanding officer Maj. Gen. George Gordon Meade (1815-1872) for the ensuing debacle; descriptions of Lee's retreat; and an appendix with accounts of the 1864 burning of his town and some of his personal merchant's papers from both episodes of CSA invasion. He published his account, and apparently seven copies still exist, one in Special Coll., Library of Davidson College, Davidson, NC. Jacob Hoke, *The Great Invasion of 1863, or General Lee in Pennsylvania...and Other Valuable Historic Papers of Jacob Hoke* (Dayton, OH: W.J. Shuey, 1888).

I had no dinner to-day—The citizens gave many of the boys dinner, I understand.

Dr. Drane & myself had a fine mess of oysters which we bought in our round [of visits to patients in campsites].

Rain has been falling very hard all day. The weather is cool.

Chambersburg is a fine town. The streets are too narrow, but the houses well built and mostly of brick. The Court House is a very fine building—erected in 1802 at cost $44,543—The Town Hall is a large building, too. The citizens give us the Cold Shoulder some. The doors are closed and the windows shut. [F]rom the windows above, often peering through the blinds we see pretty faces staring at the rebels. I wonder if they have seen any horned ones.

[TEMPORARY FIELD HOSPITAL NEAR CHAMBERSBURG, FRANKLIN CO., PA]

FRIDAY, JUNE 26, [18]63

Still raining this morning. Dr. B. requested me to accompany him—He is unwell. Soon after reaching the town the troops ([Edward] Johnson's Div.) marched through. Moses Gibson[444] was sent to Winchester [Frederick Co.] with some packages of Medicine. Dr. [J . William] Walls 5th Va. Infty is placed in charge of Hosp't at this place very much against his wishes.[445] Here the want of a strong force in Dr B's Department is felt.

The room we occupy was Judge Kimbles Law office. His papers and books we [put] in desks and drawers, but were not interrupted 'till Maj. [Joseph McClung] Paxton QM[446] left, and the 25 Va. Reg't was quartered in the town

---

[444] Moses Gibson born in Darkesville [later WV] enlisted in Co. G of 2d VA Inf. on 5 July 1861 and transfered to Co. D, old Smyth Blues, 1 March 1862. He became a clerk to Surg. Hunter Holmes McGuire; promoted to hosp. steward on 30 April 1863 before this northern invasion. Death date unknown, but still living in 1906 according to Frye. Frye, *2d VA Inf.*, 100; Robertson, *4th VA Inf.*, 52.

[445] J. William Walls (1837-1881), according to Lee A. Wallace, Jr., "taught at Winchester Medical School. Assigned to Harpers Ferry as Assistant Surgeon, May 16, 1861. Assigned to duty with [Joseph Eggleston] Johnston's Army of the Potomac, and appointed from Tenn., Nov. 16, 1861, as Surgeon, 10th Regt. Ala. Inf.; relieved June 16, 1862. Served as Surgeon, 5th Regt. Va. Inf., Nov. 1862 to Dece. 1864, when assigned to 10th Regt. Ala. Inf. Paroled April 20, 1865 at Mt. Jackson [Shenandoah Co]. Died in Philadelphia, May 19, 1881. Bur. Mt. Hebron Cem., Winchester." Idem, *5th VA Inf.*, Virginia Military Regimental Histories Series (Lynchburg VA: H.E. Howard, 1988) 167. May not be the Dr. Walls referenced earlier.

[446] Possibly Joseph McClung Paxton (1844-1884), a farmer from Smyth Co. who served in QM corps with 4th and later with QM post in Lynchburg. He was wounded several times and captured several times and was much respected in the 4th. However, Paxton was not an officer, apparently reaching rank no higher than Sgt. Robertson, *4th VA Inf.*, 67.

Hall & C.H. came in and soon the papers were strewn in every direction. The Judge is a strong Union Man, and came in with the longest physiognomy[447] I ever saw. He evidently feels the force of reality, and finds that War spoken of and War read about is far different than War at his own door.[448]

A gentleman on the sidewalklooking at the soldiery [Edward Johnson's division, comprising the infantry of the 1st VA Bde] as it passed remarked "poor fellers! they known not what awaits them ahead, there are too many for them." I remarked to him not to commiserate our condition, it was as good as his own, that our leader know [sic] where he was going and what he was doing.

[Joseph M.] Thomas[449] was left with Surg. [J. William] Walls. Dr. B. rode in an ambulance —. & I rode his horse. Met some of the old members of the 4th in Jenkins Cavalry.

We passed through Green Village [about 5 miles NE of Chambersburg], and several smaller villages—or I suppose they were called vilages [sic].

This is a most magnificent country. The dwelling houses are small and yards & gardens are seemingly contracted; But there are splendid Barns all along.

We camped near Shippensburg [Cumberland Co., about 20 miles NW of Gettysburg, Adams Co]. All wet.

---

[447] "Physiognomy" in first meaning was the "divination" or other "understanding" of character or personality from the outward appearance of the face. Secondary meaning, "often humorous" and attributed to novelist Nathaniel Hawthorne, was a sour face or countenance. *Webster's International Dict.*, 2nd ed. The diarist often picks up and uses phrases peculiar to the writers he is reading, whether the poet Byron or the novelist Hawthorne (1804-1864).

[448] In his "Reminiscences," Apperson describes how his own father Alfred's chickens were taken by both CSA and Federal troops who marched through Th e Wilderness. "Reminiscences." Bean, Notes.

[449] Capt. Joseph M. Thomas, born 1838 in Smyth Co., was 3rd generation Scottish-American and was a farmer before the war, then developed lumber business in Smyth Co. after War. Before the war, he had served on squire's court in a case involving a freed black woman Tabitha, whom he and the others on the court decided to allow to keep her freedom and her residence in Smyth Co. in an interesting landmark case. *Smyth Co.*, ed., Presgraves, 41; Armstrong, *Hist. of Smyth*, vol. 2, 16.

[TEMPORARY FIELD HOSPITAL CAMP ON CO. LINE, CUMBERLAND AND FRANKLIN CO., PA]

SATURDAY, JUNE 27 [1863][450]

Off early. Shippensburg is another pretty place but O Lord they do dispise [sic] us so much. They are sure to count the Yankee ambulances and turn up their mouths in a scornful manner.[451]

It know it hurts but it cant [sic] be helped. The unchanging fate of War has thrown us over here and they must submit.

Q. Master & Commissaries are overrunning the Country and gathering up everything that will be necessary for our use.

I have been highly pleased all along this trip to see so little destruction of property by our soldiers and grateful to find that the men had behaved themselves. One store in the road had been robbed of every thing nearly. Some of the boys in our train were as bad as any. Some said he saw a soldier with a clock under his arms. He was plodding along. I wonder what he wanted with it. [O]thers had pitchers and chamber[pots]. Such is War.

I have conversed with several men to-day. They claim to be [John Cabell] Breckinridge Democrats[452] and friends to the peace party [founded by Fernando

---

[450] On this date, Joseph Hooker, the failed commander of the Army of the Potomac was replaced by the competent and astute George Gordon Meade, one who understood entrenchments, tactical placement on high ground, and otherwise marshaling forces defensively against the aggressive R.E. Lee. Most authorities consider the change fortuitous, rather than part of any long-range plan; Hooker even forced the issue of resignation in an argument concerning whether to abandon Harpers Ferry. Whether Lincoln and his strategist then-general-in chief Henry Wager Halleck (1815-1872) were prescient, blessed, or lucky, Meade was far better prepared than Hooker to meet the unprecedented artillery barrage and the huge infantry charges that Lee was preparing in this invasion. See Long, 373.

[451] Bean notes, and Robertson confirms, that on this march the ANV had captured many Federal ambulance and ordnance wagons, which were in the train of their long march. Pennsylvanians were offended that CSA forces would so use captured ambulance wagons. Bean, notes; Robertson, *4th VA Inf.*, 26.

[452] It seems highly unlikely that Pennsylvanians would at this late date be admitting to support for Breckinridge, especially when most of the citizenry encountered by the diarist were enraged by the CSA invasion. Support for the peace party of Wood and Vallandigham may have been evident, however. John Cabell Breckinridge (1821-1875) of KY had run as the candidate for president nominated by the southern wing of the Democratic Party in 1860. Never himself an extremist secessionist, he allowed his name to be put forward as part of a strategy to find a compromise national candidate more moderate than Stephen Arnold Douglas (1813-1861), the eventual nominee of the northern wing of the Democratic Party. Breckinridge had risen to political power rapidly, and was the youngest man to serve as Vice President of the US, 1857-1861 with President James Buchanan (1791-1868) of PA (in fact, of Mercersburg in Franklin Co].

Wood and Clement Laird Vallandigham]. I asked them if they were willing that the South should go and let the War close. At this some seemed inclined to hang their heads and say that secession was a dangerous doctrine, others said peace in any way. I can gather but little that seems to be the common sentiment of the people. It seems though that they are full of regret that the War should commence and dispair [sic] now of whipping us back.

All are expecting a fight at Harrisburg [Dauphin Co., state capital]. It is reported that McClelland [sic; George Brinton McClellan] is in command in Harrisburg but the citizens spurn the idea. He may be poltroon enough to take command of a state force. But what has he to count upon?[453]

A tender [a caisson] in 3 Richmond Howitzer Co. exploded in the road to-day but without injury to anyone.

We are in camp to-night some 4 or 5 miles of Carlisle [Cumberland Co., PA, some 25 miles north of Gettysburg]. To-morrow Dr. B takes part of his force to town [Carlisle] for some purpose.

We got a [sic] mail this morning—Nothing for myself.

[TEMPORARY FIELD HOSPITAL CAMP NEAR CARLISLE, CUMBERLAND CO., PA]

SUNDAY, JUNE 28TH [1863]

This morning we went to town. Carlisle is the prettiest inland town I have ever seen. I was horseback with Dr. B. We went out to the barracks. Here Gen'l [Richard Stoddert] Ewell had his HdQtrs [for ANV 2d Corps].

Because extremist secessionists did support him, he became persona non grata in the nation's capital after secession by SC, and a warrant was issued for his arrest, although he had himself not committed, nor advocated the commission of, any treasonable act. Fleeing to the newly formed CSA, he became a high ranking general, albeit one who never expected the CSA to win its independence by political or military means. In final months of War, February through April, he worked to negotiate a surrender to end the bloodshed and destruction that he had tried to prevent in the first place. William C. (Jack) Davis, "Breckinridge," *Hist. Times.*

[453] The diarist is hearing pure rumor. McClellan was on inactive military duty and getting himself ready to enter politics, to run as Democratic nominee for president in 1864. He was not in charge of state defenses in PA, and Lee was not heading to Harrisburg in any case. Edward G. Longacre, "McClellan," *Hist. Times.*; Long, 373-76. *Poltroon* is a Flemish-dialect French word meaning "coward"; it connotes also laziness, and is related to a Flemish word for *bed* or *cushion. OED.* In the context, the diarist seems to mean to say something about foolhardiness rather than cowardliness, and may have chosen the wrong word; however, plenty of military authorities , not least commander-in-chief Lincoln, would use the word *poltroon* in correct sense to describe "Little Mac."

A requisition was made on the people of Carlisle for Stores. The[y] responded that they had nothing to give. That portion belonging to the Med. Dep't was filled very well by Messrs Elliot[,] Haverstick & Balstone. Mr Elliott has been a druggist in Carlisle for a long time. He is small in size, has an insinuating eye, very loquacious, and has the air of a sharp trader—a rank Republican.[454] Haverstick is a fine looking man—seems to love property, and was willing to rely upon Elliot's sagacity to trade for him. Balstone is a weakly looking man—both mentally & physically. He yielded entirely to the others. Having to give up the med: stores was a trial for them.

Dickinson College is at this place [Carlisle]. Many of young men that have been educated here are now in our ranks.[455] The people of this section are more agreeable to us than at Chambersburg. The churches were opened and divine services held. Mr. Bliss, a Presbyterian preached. I did not hear him—several of our officers were walking with the ladies of this place.

I spent the day at the C.H. where Dr. B. and others were stipulating for [bargaining for][456] medicines.

[TEMPORARY FIELD HOSPITAL CAMP IN ADAMS CO. NEAR GETTYSBURG, PA]

MONDAY, JUNE 29TH [1863]

This morning we were to go to town again—Very little business was done. We went for the purpose of taking the Chemical Apparatus from the College [Dickinson College], but for some reason it was forbidden.

The troops marched at noon—The course of our march was on the back tracks. Orders were that we were going to protect the captured Stores.[457] The

---

[454] Apperson is transfering southern stereotypes about sharp-trading northern businessmen to the entire Republican Party. On such image-making, see William Robert Taylor, *Cavalier and Yankee: The Old South and American National Character* (1961. Reprint ed.; New York: Oxford University Press, 1993).

[455] Dickinson College is a fine private liberal arts institution associated with the Methodist Church. A number of Virginians attended the school in the antebellum years, but I cannot find any in the 4th or 7th regiments, and do not know whom the diarist is talking about; he must be speaking more broadly about Dickinson College graduates serving in the ANV.

[456] "Stipulate for" means to make an agreement about or establish a covenant with; and in the 19th cent. is used in exactly this sense to describe trade agreements. *OED.*

[457] The three corps of the ANV were dispersed broadly through Franklin, Adams, and Cumberland Counties in southern PA, and R.E. Lee was awaiting news from his "eyes," Gen. J.E.B. Stuart, who was to tell him about the movements of the Army of the Potomac. Meanwhile, part of R.S. Ewell's 2nd Corps, with Dr. Black's hospital corps, was marching from Carlisle, while Longstreet's 1st Corps and A.P. Hill's 3rd Corps were at Chambersburg. Stuart, in maneuvers that

people seemed delighted at our going back [they were now marching southward] and a few went so far as to jeer us. The sentiments of a good many were expressed in the words of one man. He was asked if he could have peace in letting the South go what would he do? "I would let you'uns go" said he. I can say that they are not allowed to speak truly and unreservedly.

We camped in a barren field—no clover or grass or any sort.

The whole train has a horse (I mean the men) They go out and in the name of the [CSA] government they take possession of the horses and pay any price they choose.—From 50 to 100$ is all they pay[458] Dr. B got a very fine horse for 100$—I do not advocate such conduct.[459]

[TEMPORARY FIELD HOSPITAL ON FREDERICK CITY ROAD NEAR SCOTLAND, FRANKLIN CO., PA]

TUESDAY, JUNE 30TH [1863]

This morning we marched to Green Village [Franklin Co. SW of Carlisle and NW of Gettysburg] and turned left [south] to Scotland [Franklin Co. E of Chambersburg and NW of Gettysburg]] and went into Camp. The citizens army whom we have been traveling [sic] are as bitter enemies as they can be.[460] One woman struck Dr. Ellsberg twice with a broom handle and ordered all the

---

remain subject of controversy today, made no report on the day expected; he was at Rockville [Montgomery Co. just above the Potomac River], MD, with the Army of the Potomac between him and Lee's three corps. Apparently R.E. Lee learned of George Gordon Meade's appointment as commander of the Army of the Potomac on this evening of 29 June. Lee, not knowing where the Federal forces actually were, worried that Meade was threatening his line of communications with VA; and he ordered all three corps to concentrate force and mass at Gettysburg and Cashtown in Adams Co., PA. Stuart, misunderstanding Lee's admittedly ambiguous orders, thought he was expected to "ride around" the Army of the Potomac as he had done before; and thus he did not arrive at the battlesite until 2 July. His absence cost Lee troops at a crucial time; and his lack of communication kept Lee uninformed in timely fashion about the movements of the Army of the Potomac. See Long, "2-4 July 1863."

[458] For good horses, judging by Apperson's own recent transactions, the "discount" or forced-sale underpayment would seem to be between 50% and 67%.

[459] Dr. Harvey Black was generally a very upright Calvinist who often had to call down his young charge Apperson, and roles are oddly reversed here, with the occasionally fun-loving steward "scolding" his strict supervisor in the privacy of this diary—though we can assume that the diarist did not actually say anything to his supervisor, benefactor, and occasional nemesis.

[460] Bean says that the diarist refers to women living along the road; where the men in the area traded and sometimes conversed with the traveling CSA forces, the women were often hostile and sometimes extremely vocal, according to other diaries, soldiers' reminiscences, and Apperson's own "Reminiscences." Power, *Lee's Miserables*; and Bean, *Sandie Pendleton.*

rebels out of the yard. They are Tartars [Russian soldiers known for fierce resistance in battle].

It is now positively known that [James] Longstreet [1st Corps] & A.P. Hill [3d Corps] are in the neighborhood. We are on the Frederick City Road. I got a letter from Miss Mollie F. Thornton to-day —.

Raining to-day. I wrote, or commenced, a letter to Dr. Faris. Have been riding my horse for two days —like him.

[TEMPORARY FIELD HOSPITAL NEAR GETTYSBURG ON CARLISLE PIKE, ADAMS CO., PA]

MONDAY, JULY 1ST [18]63

This morning we marched early. Passed [John Bell] Hood's Division near Fayetteville [Franklin Co., PA]. [James] Longstreet's [1st] Corps are on the road. Entered the Mountain at the gap where the Iron works of Thaddeus Stevens stood.[461] They are now in ruins. The gap [Black Gap] is low, but the road rough. My little horse travels very well. When we reached the top of the mountain cannon were heard in direction of Gettysburg very distinctly. A fight was evidently progressing;—At the foot of the [South] mountain is Middleburg [Adams Co]. Here we saw Dr. Wright in charge of the Field Infirmary of A.P. Hill's [3d] Corps.

We stopped for a short time and then moved on. We soon came to the battle ground. Passing through Gettysburg skirmishers were firing on the right. We turned to the left [northward] and camped on the Carlisle Pike. [Jubal A.] Early's & [Robert Emmett] Rode's Divisions did the bulk of the fighting. Gen'l. [John Fulton] Reynolds commanding the 11th Army Corps of Yankees was killed. This 11th Corps was badly used up.[462] [Reynolds was commanding the

---

[461] Thaddeus Stevens (1792-1868) was US Representative from PA and one of the most powerful congresspersons of the era, chairing the Ways and Means Commitee. A onetime Whig, he did have business interests, such as this ironworks, but he is best remembered for his avowedly Radical Republicanism, pushing for uncompensated emancipation, black troops, black voting, a Freedman's Bureau, and a Civil Rights Act, all of which eventually came to be. Patricia L. Faust says, "The indefatigable egalitarian once remarked bitterly that he would never see 'merit balance the crime of color,' and he did not. Southerners hated him for his vindictiveness and many colleagues resented the biting sarcasm he used against them on the House floor. But when he died in Washington, D.C., 11 Aug. 1868, many acknowledged him admiringly as the 'Great Commoner.'" Idem, "Stevens," *Hist. Times.*

[462] John Fulton Reynolds (1820-1863) was a native Pennsylvanian, graduate of West Point, and universally loved and respected. Decorated in the Mexican War, he then taught tactics and served as commandant of West Point, where he was when War came. Rapidly promoted, he

1st Corps, General Oliver O. Howard the 11th; it was the 11th Corps that was damaged, and those men fled to town, after which the 1 corps, unsupported and alone, was overwhelmed].

[TEMPORARY FIELD HOSPITAL NEAR GETTYSBURG ON CASHTOWN ROAD, ADAMS CO., PA]

THURSDAY, JULY 2D, [18]63

This morning early Dr. [Hunter Holmes] McGuire [chief of surgeons in field] came and asked Dr. B. to ride with him. I was told to go along. We went to Gettysburg. I have never seen so many wounded at any place as I saw wounded Yankees here.[463] Our Ambulance train was put to hauling the wounded of the enemy from the field to the [field] Hospital.

We selected a base near the Mummatown [Mummasburg, Adams Co.] road for a Hosp't. but did not remain there long. There were about 3000 prisoners taken yester-day. Gen. [Alfred] Iverson (N.Carolinian)[464] lost nearly his whole brigade. [John Brown] Gordon's[465] Brigade of [Jubal A.] Early's Div. [in R.S.

---

became Brig. Gen., was briefly captured but exchanged, and performed superbly at Antietam (September 1862) and Fredericksburg (13 December 1862) and at Chancellorsville (1-4 May 1863), winning promotion to Maj. Gen. and was offered command of the Army of Potomac to replace Joseph Hooker. "Regarding politicians with deep suspicion," according to Jeffrey D. Wert, he declined because he feared undue and unwise interference from the president. It thus fell to George Gordon Meade to command the Federal troops in this fight, and on the first day of fighting, Reynolds was killed while moving troops forward to replace Union cavalry. Wert, "Reynolds," *Hist. Times.*

[463] It is hard to disaggregate the figures day by day, but CSA and Federal troops all told suffered more than 51,000 casualties for the three days fighting; of the 14,529 Federal troops wounded and the 3,155 killed in the battle, it is likely that the greatest suffering for the Federals happened on this first day. No battle of such magnitude had been seen by anyone, not just the diarist; he was surely looking at several thousand wounded men "at any place." *OR*, 5 July 1863; figures estimated by Long are slightly lower but still "staggering." Long, 375-76.

[464] Leading these "N. Carolinians" was Alfred Iverson, Jr. (1829-1877), a Georgian and son of a US Senator who fought in Mexican War leading GA volunteers, then returned home in 1848 to practice law, and then in 1855 became a professional soldier, a cavalry officer. When War came, he raised an army of North Carolinians and fought successfully , esp. at Gaines Mill (27 June 1862). Promoted to Brig. Gen., he did well at Chancellorsville (1-4 May 1863), but here his Brigade was "savaged...partly through errors made by its leader," according to Edward G. Longacre. He is said to have been unnerved by the magnitude of the suffering that he saw, and his reputation was certainly hurt almost beyond repairing. He did recoup his reputation somewhat in cavalry campaigns in 1864. Idem, "Iverson," *Hist. Times.*

[465] John Brown Gordon (1832-1904) was identified earlier; promoted after a serious wound at Sharpsburg (17 September 1862), he became Brig. Gen. and a particularly trusted officer of Gen.

Ewell's 2d Corps] lost most men, I guess—it seemed to have borne the brunt of the fight.

The enemy took position on a very elevated ground [in a line stretched from Culp's Hill to Cemetary Hill along Cemetary Ridge to the base of Little Round Top] and from appearances there will be work to drive him from it. The fight commenced about 2 o'clock and raged fearfully 'till night. [Richard Stoddert] Ewell [2d Corps] had the left [at Culp's Hill and Cemetary Hill], A.P. Hill the center [3d Corps in front of Seminary Ridge] & [James] Longstreet the right [1st Corps in front of Big Round Top and Little Round Top. Longstreet struck at Gen. George G. Meade's left at the Round Tops, but Meade moved troops from right to left and counterattacked. With fierce losses on both sides, Meade secured Little Round Top. Lee then sent A.P. Hill's 3d Corps toward Cemetary Hill; and Hill did not have enough troops to make the assault, although two of his Bdes. actually held positions on Cemetary Hill until Federal reinforcements pushed them back. Lastly, Ewell's 2d Corps made a charge at Culp's Hill, the second such attempted; and Ewell too was repulsed with bloody results on both sides. The day ended with the Federals strongly entrenched but battered, with Meade gambling that Lee would on 3 July attack the Federal center at Cemetary Ridge, which he reinforced and dug in. Meade rejected some counsel to retreat due to the extremely heavy losses already suffered. Meanwhile Lee held his own counsels, also rejected suggestions of a retreat, and planned a crushing assault on the Cemetary Ridge in the Federal Center; Lee also intended to use J.E.B. Stuart, who had at last appeared, to strike the Federal rear with his notorious cavalry while a fresh division led by Maj. Gen. George E. Pickett would lead the huge assault from the woods in Seminary Ridge across a field and up onto Cemetary Ridge. While Stuart was to ride in from the rear and Pickett's men charged frontally, Lee also intended to launch one of the world's greatest artillery barrages, featuring more than 140 pieces that would fire for more than two hours before the planned charge].

We move [sic] our Hosp't near the Cashtown road. We had to remove the wounded from Early's Division [of 2d Corps] and consequently took but very few from any other part of the [Ewell's] Corps. We had no medical force anyway.

R.E. Lee, eventually a Maj. Gen. by 14 May 1964; at War's end he was commanding the 2nd Corps of the ANV. James O. Hall, "Gordon," *Hist. Times.*

The fighting ceased about night—very little advantage gained on our side—the right and left wings gave way somewhat, but the center remained permanent [on Cemetary Ridge].

[TEMPORARY FIELD HOSPITAL NEAR GETTYSBURG ON CASHTOWN ROAD, ADAMS CO., PA]

FRIDAY, JULY 3RD, 1863

This morning early the fight was renewed. At one o'clock [P.M.] the firing of artillery exceeded anything I have ever heard.[466] Dr. [Hunter Holmes] McGuire sent me out to find a suitable place for Hosp't. I found water very scarce wherever I went. After making the selection and reporting I was sent by Dr. B to select a road leading to it. The wounded commenced coming in from Stonewall Brigade [1st VA Bde, including Smyth Blues, Smyth Grays, Grayson Daredevils]—They were sent to the Barn I had selected. Drs. Snidow and [Samuel B.] Morrison came over from Charlottesville [general hospital directed by J.L. Cabell] and were sent by Dr. B. to the Barn. Dr. [J. William] Walls [of 5th VA Inf.] came & Dr. McGuire sent him out to take charge—He and I rode some distance in search of more commodious Quarters. One house was found deserted—The furniture scattered over the house—clothing torn up and in confusion on the floor.

Orders came about Mid-night for the sick to be moved to the rear of Fairfield road [Adams Co. road through a gap in South Mountain]—I was sent to inform Dr. [J. William] Walls and give him instructions what to do.

---

[466] It exceeded anything anybody had heard, at least in the US, and possibly anywhere in the world to that date in 1863. One hundred and forty pieces commanded by then–Col. Edward Porter Alexander (1835-1910) lay metal on Federal positions on Cemetary Ridge for around two hours preparatory to Lee's climactic 3d day charge. Porter Alexander, from Washington, GA, had graduated 3rd in his class from West Point, had served in Utah Territory, had taught at West Point, and with Albert J. Myer had developed the "Wigwag" semaphore communications process that set a standard for artillery communications in the era. Many authorities believe that no army had ever before concentrated as many as 140 pieces of artillery in a single battle aimed at one site, but the Federal forces withstood the assault and replied with fire from their own implacements, numbering perhaps 100. Although Alexander was well-supplied, he did run out of ammunition, while the Federals had plenty of rounds left to shoot into the oncoming "Pickett's Charge." John E. Stanchak, "Alexander," *Hist. Times.*; Jeffrey D. Wert, "Gettysburg Battle," ibid..; Long, 377. Long believes that the Federals had only 80 pieces, not 100.

[ON THE MARCH FROM GETTYSBURG, PA TO WILLIAMSPORT, WASHINGTON CO., MD; NO CAMP ESTABLISHED DURING THE DAY OF 4 JULY 1863]

SATURDAY, JULY 4, '63

Rain is falling—All the transportation we can procure is sent on with wounded—We moved in the direction [west on Chambersburg Road and then south through edge of Adams Co. to MD] as instructed.[467] About mid-way to Fairfield [SW corner of Adams Co., PA] we stopped but had not gotten our things fixed before orders came for us to move on. Our army has fallen back—abandoned the prospect of taking the position held by the enemy. We were much later starting than we should have been but our ambulance train could not get up with the second load any sooner.

Rain fell very rapidly. We moved on—and reached Fairfield just a short while before night. A few moments to stop and feed—Two Regiments of our cavalry started out, it being reported that the Yankees were upon us. One went to the left on the Emmitsburg Pike [Emmitsburg is in Frederick Co., MD]—the road we were to take...[diarist's elipses] before they reached the summit of the Gap firing could be seen very distinctly. This compelled us to take [a] right [turn] through Manson's Gap, and the old Furnace road was a very "hard road to travel". [Gen. Imboden reports that he left the main road, Emmitsburg Pike, and took the "near cut" through South Mountain toward Greencastle in Franklin Co]. Night came on, the rain poured down—The road was very narrow, and in a very narrow pass. A stream dashed along, first on one side then

---

[467] This march of the ambulance trains of wounded was led by Gen. John Daniel Imboden (1823-1895), whose cavalry had not been used extensively in the three days of battle. Later a businessperson in Damascus in Washington Co. near Apperson's adoptive Smyth Co., Imboden wrote a moving account of this march in the popular turn-of-the-century series, *Battles and Leaders.* Among other things, Imboden relates how the train extended for seventeen miles, and how he marched the ambulances bearing wounded without major stops westward to Fairfield [across the South Mountain in southwestern corner of Adams Co.] and then west across the northwestern tier of MD to Williamsport [Washington Co., MD] on the Potomac River across from WV. Imboden says that he commanded a force of some 3,000 soldiers, counting 700 wagoneers and several hundred wounded ordnance men who were well enough to carry a gun. On the retreat there was an attack by Federal troops including some 7000 effectives, and Imboden's cavalry officers and the armed wounded protected themselves successfully. After a brief night's sleep at Williamsport, Imboden led the wagon train of wounded [perhaps numbering 5,000 or more wounded persons!] on into Winchester to safety and treatment at that general hospital. John Daniel Imboden, "The Confederate Retreat from Gettysburg," *Battles and Leaders of the Civil War*, vol. 3 (ca. 1880. Reprint ed.; New York: Thomas Yoseloff, 1956) 420-29.

on the other[.] Our train was loaded with wounded who shrieked often from the jolting of the vehicles.

It soon became so dark that no man could see an inch from his nose. The cry of "halt!" from the drivers were [sic] sent along the lines, continuously almost which told "that something had broke"[.] We overtook the rear of the train about mid-night and about two or three miles from the junction of the road we were on another Emmitsburg road. Here it became very evident that the enemy was at work on the train. The cannon was firing still on our left. *Screamed* orders [diarist's italics] could be heard ahead. Wagon Drivers came back with their trains—the [18th] Cavalry was wandering and skulking through the darkness and like the drivers were making for the rear. I heard Gen. [Alfred] Iverson[468] say that nothing could be done until daylight. The remnant of his Brigade was sent up to protect the train. Finally we could go no further [sic] for the wagons had blocked the roads. When the train stopped I dismounted and took a seat on a large stone to wait the issue. Everything grew quiet except the rain that beat upon the trees [illegible word].

Morning came. I was very cold and with the aid of some matches I carried I made a fire. All the Hospital men had gone back about two miles. I was alone with 4 ambulances, and some two or three nurses. I mounted my horse and rode back past the train to get breakfast. Gen. [Ambrose Ransom] Wright[469] with his Brigade came up and we were soon on the road again. My horse's feet were very sore, and it was with much difficulty that I could get him along.

---

* *Note—At this point the diarist ceased his writing until 25 January 1864. As Gen. Imboden records it, the long day's march to Williamsport on the Potomac and then across to the relative safety of Winchester, was a harrowing story of Federal attacks, unremitting rain, and the awful cries of the suffering thousands—perhaps 5,000—in the ambulance train:*

---

[468] Alfred J. Iverson, Jr. (1829-1911), already identified. Edward G. Longacre says that Iverson acquitted himself of grievous tactical errors on the Gettysburg battlefield during this march, but other authorities say that he was so traumatized by the overwhelming defeat of his men that he was of no use on this retreat and of little use thereafter in the war. Idem, "Iverson," *Hist. Times.*

[469] Ambrose Ransom Wright (1826-1872) was a Georgia attorney and aspiring political leader in the CSA. "Rans" Wright was originally a Col. with the 3rd GA Regiment in NC, but was promoted to Brig. Gen. in spring 1862 and transfered to ANV. He led them bravely and effectively at the major VA battles and at Gettysburg on 3 July 1863, his GA troops had come all the way across the valley and temporarily lodged themselves on Cemetary Ridge before being repulsed. Jeffrey D. Wert, "Wright," *Hist. Times.*

Some were simply moaning; some were praying, and others uttering the most fearful oaths and execrations that despair and agony could wring from them ....During this one night I realized more of the horrors of war than I had in all the two preceding years.[470]

As the diarist marks it in his reminiscences, and as is reaffirmed by the tone of his diary after the new year of 1864, Apperson too had seen more of the horrors of war on this engagement than he could have imagined as an enthusiastic volunteer with the Smyth Blues. His anxiousness to attend the Medical College of Virginia and his dissatisfaction with Dr. Harvey Black, both emotions severe by April of 1863, were now aggravated to a new level. His old 4th VA Regiment was much reduced in size, and it was under the guidance of "Old Baldy" Richard Stoddert Ewell, who led the mountain soldiers through yet another Valley campaign and into yet another pitched battle in Apperson's native Wilderness. Now pessimistic about the future of the CSA but even more upset with Abraham Lincoln and northern Republicans than before, Apperson begins to note shortages of medical supplies as well as shortages in ordnance and even ammunition for the fighting troops. Aware of his own advancing years, he aches to complete his official training as a physician, but his education is delayed by two irresistible forces: His sponsor Dr. Harvey Black is not going to grant him leave to study medicine in Richmond, and without Dr. Black's approval, he cannot attend the lectures; and he now knows too much about field surgery and emergency treatments to be spared from those duties as the casualties increase. The once-ardent secessionist is now compelled to serve the Confederacy by the two patron physicians, Dr. William Faris and Dr. Harvey Black, who were always skeptical of the claims of the "Cause" and never hopeful of the outcome of the War. Each commands him to repair the march of Mars, *because that repair is* what doctors do, *regardless of the government or other cause being served. Such repair will have two meanings, the primary one from Latin being the* patching-up *and otherwise* tending *the wounds of the soldiers of both armies on these long and hard marches ; but the second ary meaning—from Old French—will be in effect too, viz.,* to go to *or* to go with *the march of the most terrifying of the old pagan gods.*[471]

---

[470] Imboden, 424.

[471] Apperson, "Reminiscences"; "repair," *OED.*

1864 JOURNAL

ORANGE C.H. [ORANGE CO.]

JANY 25, [18]64

I commenced again to keep a journal while here at Orange C.H. Va. My last writing was a long while ago, and a wide gap exists between this and where I stopped before. Much has passed, many lessons have been learned and very few applied as they should have been.

The [field] Hosp't of 2d Corps has been here since August [1863] having left twice since to follow the army.[472] We are now living a life similar to that of of [sic] the frozen reptiles—no variations. The weather heretofore has been bad, and exceedingly Cold, but to-day is a lovely day. Sun shines brightly and the air is as still as a summer morn.

I am situated in a tent opposite Mr. [James] Chapman[']s dwelling in a tent—very snugly fixed.[473]

The day has been more busy than usual. The Ex[amining]. Board convened and decided on giving several furloughs. These were written and sent up.

---

[472] Dr. Bean notes that the ANV of R.E. Lee and the Army of the Potomac of G.G. Meade maneuvered in the fall of 1863, producing skirmishes at Bristoe Station on 18 August, 12 September, 24 September, and 18 October in 1863. Bean, notes. E.B. Long writes that Meade, pushed by President Lincoln, tried hard to turn R.E. Lee's right flank by crossing the Rapidan in November and engaging the ANV at Mine Run, where Lee was well-entrenched. Other skirmishing took place along the Rapidan River at Raccoon Ford and Morton's Ford. While President Lincoln was chagrined that Meade could not mount a successful offensive, Long says, "the Federals could not find a spot for a major assault. It was already becoming clear that Lee had halted the Union offensive before it really started." Following these skirmishes and still more maneuvering, Lee established the ANV on the south bank of the Rappahannock River near Orange Court House and Meade established the Army of the Potomac on the north bank of the same river facing his adversary as a bitter winter set in. Long, 440. Thus, Dr. Black's field hospital could re-establish itself at Orange Court House after "going mobile" for the fall when the diarist found little opportunity and apparently less will to write.

[473] Dr. Bean identifies James Chapman as a prominent citizen of Orange Court House who had a brick building on Main Street and owned a vacant lot in front of that building; Apperson's tent apparently was pitched on the lot facing Chapman's building. Bean, notes. This Chapman is possibly the James Chapman, born 1820, who was living in Bedford VA in 1870 according to census. VA Census, 1870.

The health of the army is very good. Not more than ten men are rec'd [admitted into field hospital] per day. The mortality however is very heavy. I finished a letter to Dr. Q[uisenberry] this morning.

The 4th Va Regt came in town to-day to relieve 1 Va Battl [1st Battalion], but there was some mistake about the order and it returned. It is Court day—many of the old fogy are in the place .

A member of 14 N Ca. Regt rec'd an injury at a saw mill which resulted in the loss of his left foot. Dr. Black performed Chopart's operation.[474]

We had some very sweet Music to-night from a band with Capt. Yarber. It is very remarkable that I have such a desire for music and yet cannot perform or sing. I sometimes think I am fit for nothing except an abode in *hoosierdom* [diarist's italics].[475]

I recd the Marion paper this morning—I noticed the obituary of the death of Lt. McReady by Miss Campbell. She did well.[476]

I fully intended to write a long letter to-night but it is too late now.

ORANGE C.H. [ORANGE CO.] VA.

[THURSDAY] JAN. 26TH [18]64

Sunday—This is another bright warm day. The ground is becoming quite dry, the streets are passable.

---

[474] Francois Chopart (1743-1795) was a French surgeon, already identified, who developed a technique for amputating the foot at the juncture of the "two rows of bones that make up the tarsus [broad and flat part of the foot]." "Charpot's amputation," *Taber's.*

[475] Indiana was nicknamed the Hoosier State, and for some reason the diarist regards Indiana as a place peopled strictly by the untalented and lazy. Many Virginians had migrated to Indiana and Illinois, including the family of Abraham Lincoln, and perhaps a certain resentment of the president attaches to this contempt.

[476] *The Marion Visitor* was founded in 1858 by George J. Curtis and James W. Kennedy; Apperson himself sometimes wrote for it. The newspaper did not survive the War, and apparently no copies of it remain. The subscription agent, E.S. Watson, sometimes appears in the pages of the diary as a visitor to camp who brings messages and materials from Smyth Co. Wilson, *Smyth Co. Hist.*, 164-67. Henry H. McCready (1842-1863) was a farmer from Smyth Co. who joined Co. D [Smyth Blues] in 4th, rose through ranks of enlisted men through 1st Sgt. and then was commissioned 3rd Lt. in May, 1863; wounded at Chancellorsville (3 May 1863), he was killed at Payne's Farm (27 November 1863). Robertson, *4th VA Inf.*, 62. Said to be buried in Smyth Co., he is not listed in Sturgill and Sturgill. This McCready is not related to the Edward H. McCready (1841-1861), a farmer and Pvt. also in Co. D of 4th who was killed at !st Manassass and was 1st Smyth Co. casualty of War. Armstrong, *Hist. of Smyth Co.*, 112. I cannot identify Mrs. Campbell; but she may be the wife of Dr. Jerome B. Campbell, a physician in Marion, Armstrong, 37, 49.

I ballanced [sic] the [field] Hosp't-book to-day and Dr. B. examined provisions received for month of December. The Hosp't fund is not sufficient now for the use of Hosp't. That [which] we accumulated heretofore is now nigh exhausted. The price of all articles of provisions have lately commanded such high prices that $1.25—is not sufficient to meet the wants.[477]

I have the semi-annual Returns of Property to make out for the last half-year.

To-morrow it must be done.

The newspapers contain very little news of any importance. There are notices of several Brigades in the Western Army reenlisting in a body. This is laudable. Gold in New York is 158 & 9—a very favorable omen.[478]

I shall commence a letter to my friend Mollie "T-" [Thornton] now[.]

---

[477] $1.25 in CSA dollars was allotted daily for a patient by law enacted 1 May 1863; at approximately 7 cents in gold—and falling quickly in 1864—such an amount probably was woefully inadequate to needs as well as wants. On 15 February, the CSA congress doubled this subsistence allotment, but Cunningham reports that run-away inflation—ten-dollar watermelons and three-dollar -a dozen onions—overwhelmed the new allowance. The Subsistence Dept. attempted unsuccessfully to regulate prices in the final year of the War, and Cunningham also reports that all hospitals faced critical shortages of food for their patients because of inflated prices and severely depleted supplies. Cunningham, 80-82.

[478] In New York markets, the gold dollar—not used for currency in the War , but rather exchanged for greenback dollars at market rates—was quoted at $1.58 and $1.59 in greenback dollars. This indicated an inflation rate of some 58% for the four- year period, or an annual rate of 12% for American greenback currency. Apperson sees this as a good sign, or omen, that the economy in the Northeast was in trouble. As noted earlier, however, inflation for CSA currency was running at almost immeasurable rates [but likely at least 50% per annum], and thus in comparative context the news is not very good. Another thing pointed out by Sharkey, passim, is that US inflation with greenbacks occurred in the context of a rapidly growing economy whose very expansion may have caused some inflation; but the CSA economy, especially by 1864, was a shrinking one, and the inflation was most likely caused primarily by monetary forces [an oversupply of CSA currency in relationship to the value of the products and services created in a given year]. In all of this, note that he is quoting New York market rates for one day and not an accurate record for the actual four-year trend of inflation. Davis Rich Dewey computes the actual four-year trend for the US greenback to be an average increase of some 12% per annum, and a total increase over the War of some 46 - 48%—and he notes that the rate was falling in April 1865. Idem, *Financial History of the United States* (New York: Longman's, Green, 1934), 267, 299, 329-30. For the CSA, Richard C. Todd uses the compilations of Richmond banking firm of William B. Isaacs to compute an early inflation rate of 12% per annum, an 1863 rate of some 100% per annum; and an ending rate of between 2000% and 6000%. Idem, *Confederate Finance* (Athens: University of Georgia Press, 1954), 84, 110-20, 156, 174, 194.

[FIELD HOSPITAL, ORANGE COURT HOUSE, ORANGE CO.]

[WEDNESDAY] JAN. 27TH [18]64

Wednesday—Another lovely day. I have not been very busy. One of the worst things to me is the manner in which I am squandering the very prime of my life. I am growing less competent every day to concentrate my mind upon anything useful. I study how to dissipate the hours rather than invest them and lay up that wealth that will stay with me when friends and gold have long gone. I wish most fervently that I was situated so that I would be compelled in some way to improve my time [use of time]. I have a dull routine to follow. I look out upon many of my acquaintances and see them rising[.] [S]till I am doing nothing. I must rise and shake off this lethargic monster that has fastened upon me. There are some of my friends that I know have not favoured me as they ought.

I finished my letter to Miss M[ollie Thornton] to-day.

This morning Dr. B. sent me a long list of orders for the government [operating procedures] of [field] Hospt. [in Orange Co]. I am not affected by but one. He requires the lights to be extinquished by 9 o'clock—it is that now I presume and I must stop.

[FIELD HOSPITAL, ORANGE COURT HOUSE] ORANGE CO., VA.

[THURSDAY] JAN. 28 [18]64

Thursday—Another fine day—warm enough to have no fire. Have been very busy with Semi-Annual Returns of Property.

This evening I met Mr. Jas [James] L. Robinson and he informed me that Uncle Joe [Joseph Apperson] was in town, and walked with me to see him—It is the first time I have seen him since I was sick in [18]'61.[479]

I was glad to hear from him but am fearful that the people are having a very sad time.[480]

He came up after salt for his family.[481] I ought to have insisted on his staying with me to-night but I am not situated to do much better for him than he can

---

[479] Probably James L. Robinson, born 1811, who owned a farm in Orange Court House, Orange Co.; his uncle Joseph Apperson, born in 1810, had a farm in Orange Court House, Orange Co. VA Census, 1870.

[480] In "Reminscences," Apperson reports that the US Army seized the livestock of his father Alfred Apperson and took from his farm chickens, hogs, sheep; and also stripped him of his corn and wheat.

do for himself. This are some things that make me almost miserable in meeting some of them who[m] I ought to love better than I do.

I wrote a letter home (to father) and will give it to Uncle [Joseph Apperson] to-morrow.

I am sad and lonely to-night.

ORANGE C[OURT] H[OUSE] [ORANGE CO.], VA.

[FRIDAY] JANUARY 29TH, [18]64

Friday. This morning early I walked around the depot to see my uncle [Joseph Apperson] and gave him the letter I had written. He tells me that father paid 80$ per barrel for corn for his family. This is hard indeed. All he had taken from him by the enemy and now 80$ per barrel to keep him & his family from starvation. My God where is the charity—the Christian feeling that has been the boast of our people! O Avarice! There is no help for us. Damn! Damn! We go to misery, ruin and degradation!

I made off weekly Statements for this week to-day. 96 men rec'd and 17 died. The mortality is very heavy—worse than ever before. Mostly among North Carolinians. There are few men in the Corps that are being taken sick, but the grade of disease is very grave.

I have been reading [James Finlay Weir] Johnston's "Chemistry of Human Life".[482] Had a short conversation with Miss Mary Chapman—[483]

---

[481] Saltworks in regions of the CSA produced salt for citizens and military. The most important saltworks were in Saltville, VA, on the border between Smyth and Washington Cos. The town was listed by Hummel in Washington Co. during War, but the saltworks themselves were located in Smyth Co. *VA List*, ed., Hummel. There were quotas of salt set aside for citizens of different regions of the CSA, and there were also some efforts to set price limits. See advertisements and notices, *Abingdon Virginian*, 1862-1864, esp. December issue of 1863, Archives, EHC; Wilson, *Smyth Co.*, 193-95.

[482] James Finlay Weir Johnston, *Chemistry of Common Life*, 2 vols. (Edinburgh: Blackwood, 1855). Johnston (1796-1855) was a prominent Scottish chemist who sought to make practical applications of chemical engineering to agriculture in Great Britain. A native of Scotland, he received college training and a master's degree at University of Glasgow despite lacking public school background. He established a university at Durham, where he studied agricultural chemistry and taught it; he became chemist to the Agricultural Society of Scotland and a Fellow of Royal Societies of London. He published much, including a series on agricultural reform through chemical engineering in *Blackwood* magazines. He visited the US in 1849-50 and made important observations that he included in these two volumes, his last and generally most respected book, kept in print until 1879.

[483] Apparently the daughter of James Chapman, whose lot is where Apperson pitched his tent.

Dr. Newton [possibly Newman][484] called and gassed for an hour or so. Clouds are hovering over us. I infer rain or snow.

ORANGE C.H. [ORANGE CO., VA]

[SATURDAY] JAN. 30 1864

Saturday. Very cloudy this morning and the air growing colder.

I have spent almost a useless day. Worked part of the day on reports of Property—Sat around and gassed a good deal.

D[rury].W. Venable [carpenter from Smyth. Co. and ambulance driver of Co. D, 4th VA already identified] was in town—Loan[ed] him my overcoat. Had an oyster supper at "Aunt Kesey's" room [this could not be Keziah Shepherd]. Have spent about four dollars to-day in eatables.

There is at this time a very diversified state of sentiment on the Condition of the Country. Some men are very despondent and others are quite hopeful. The despondent look only to the awful condition of our country, the scarcity of provisions and the reported large number of desertions from our Army: While the hopeful look at the promptness [with] which our men are reenlisting, the apparent growing disaffection at the North, the upward tendency in specie market, and the reluctance and high bribes paid for recruits in the Federal army.[485]

---

[484] I cannot locate a Dr. Newton. If the handwriting says *Newman*, there was a George S. Newman, surgeon from Orange Co. listed as practicing in Orange Co. and serving with Orange Rangers, 6th VA Cav. according to W.W. Scott, *Hist. of Orange Co.*, 275; but this Dr. George S. Newman is not listed by Musick, *6th VA Cav.*, passim.

[485] Long estimates 4-year total desertions for CSA at more than 104,000, and Gov. Zebulon Baird Vance formally discussed the problem with President Jefferson Davis in summer of 1863 during the seige of Vicksburg and before the battle of Gettysburg. On the other hand, reenlistment was high for the CSA even in winter of 1864. By "bribes," the diarist refers to bounties paid for reenlistment in Federal army, worth about $300 from the Army, but there were also some local and state bounties paid reenlistees. Long, 714-15. On draft riots, esp. in New York City and other protests even after spectacular Federal successes in Gettysburg and Vicksburg, see Maury Klein, "Draft Riots," *Hist. Times.* On specie markets and the downturn in greenbacks (but also the even more devastating devaluation of the CSA dollar), see ff 773 and also Sharkey, passim.

ORANGE C.H. [ORANGE CO., VA]

[SUNDAY] JAN. 31ST 1864

Sunday. To-day closes the first month of the New Year. How rapidly time flies! How soon we shall look at this as an old year! How little good too we are at putting up to balance the great account with God.

I attended Church to-day (Presbyterian). Rev. A.P. Neil preached from Romans 8th Chapter & 28 verse. Gen. [R.E.] Lee was one of the Congregation.[486] Mr. N. is Chaplain to our [field] Hospt.[487] A very worthy young man, but not a very edifying or brilliant minister yet. He will doubtless improve very much. The Episcopal Congregation is a large one.[488] The Presbyterian Small. The Methodist and Baptist churches are used as Hospitals. Mr. Neil is Methodist in his persuasion [though unable to preach in his Methodist church, since it was then a hospital].

I have read a poem this evening on Capt. [John] Smith and Pocahontas by Martin.[489] I am not very much taken with it.

The day is bad—cloudy, hazy, and muddy.

I rec'd a letter from cousin Bettie and answered it.

I wish very much to go down there but cannot. I rec'd my paper, the "Sentinel," from Marion.[490]

---

[486] "And we know that all things work together for good to them that love God, to them who are the called according to *his* purpose." Rom. 8:28, (KJV). The very Calvinist line suits Lee's theology as explained by Freedman, *R.E. Lee*, passim; it also fits well with the theology of Dr. Harvey Black, and by his mature postbellum years, of Apperson himself, "Reminiscences." Pitts notes that Presbyterians formed the Presbyterian Church of the South early in the War largely out of conviction of a calling and a destiny, and the theme of God calling a select group to lead the South out of the Union and into War was sounded often, Pitts, op. cit. chapt. 3, but esp. 26. I cannot locate this particular minister A.P. Neil. Three organized Presbyterian churches were listed for Orange Co. in 1864, Scott, 172.

[487] He is not listed so under Robertson, *4th VA Inf.*, passim; and is not so listed under Pitts, or in Cunningham. However, chaplains for hospitals served on fairly irregular basis and easily slipped through such records.

[488] St. Thomas' Episcopal Church at Orange Court House was the largest of four Episcopal churches, and R.E. Lee often attended it, as did other CSA officers, according to Scott, 49.

[489] I cannot locate such a poem by any poet named Martin. There are a gracious plenty of such themes in poems, as noted in Marcella M. Bush, "From Mythic History to Historic Myth: Captain John Smith and Pocahontas in Popular History," Ph.D. diss., Bowling Green State University, 1997.

[490] The newspaper in Marion before and during the War was *The Visitor*, published and edited by Maj. Albert Gallatin Pendleton of Co. D. Neither Armstrong nor Wilson discusses any other newspaper in Marion or anywhere else in Smyth Co. for the era, and Scott does not list a

ORANGE C.H. [ORANGE CO.] VA.

[MONDAY] FEB'Y 1ST 1864

Monday—To-day has been a dark murky day. I have been drawing up a requisition for medicines, and working on Monthly report. Walked down the Street but but [sic] found the trip very disagreeable. The mud is as red as paint and as tenacious as putty.

While standing in front of my tent I was called by Miss M.C. [Mary Chapman] On going over she pretended to inquire after my conduct a few evenings ago when I was sitting with her on her father's porch and left her very abruptly. I did not intend to arouse any curiosity but it seems that I did and if she knows me much longer she will find out other odd traits.

She loaned me the well-known novel "Children of the Abbey".[491] Her sister was on the porch also, and to me looked as obdurate as War.

To-day's paper shows that an amendment has been made to the bill in Congress that repealed the substitute law. As the amendment is, if properly carried out, I have no doubt good will come, but I fear it will be abused. It exempts a certain class of planters.[492] It may not give satisfaction to the soldier at

---

newspaper named *Sentinel* for Orange Co. Possibly it is some kind of religious tract, not published in Marion, but received there by the Farises and sent along to him. Armstrong, Wilson, Scott.

[491] Regina Maria Dalton Roche, *Children of the Abbey*, 4 vols. (Belfast, Ireland: J. Smyth, 1835). Roche (1764?-1845) wrote this immensely successful series of novels concerning two girls raised by nuns, and the works stayed in print for decades. David James O'Donoghue says it is "a story abounding in sentimentality" and was probably among the top two sellers among British novels in the 19th cent. Idem, "Roche," *Dictionary of National Biography*.

[492] Several conscription acts from 1862 to 1864 enforced the draft on white southerners. The first exemptions had to do with age and occupation, but over the years, the age boundaries of the eligible conscripts were expanded from the very young to the very old, and the exempted occupations were narrowed considerably. The 2nd conscription act exempted planters who had at least 20 slaves, apparently because of fear that such planters must stay home to prevent slave uprising; but this exemption, as Apperson notes, was bitterly resented by "plain folk" and "middling" footsoldiers. The suspicion then, as now, lurked that the power and prestige of planters kept them out of the War unless they volunteered. Lewis Cecil Gray in his monumental study of slavery in the South takes this exemption as a useful categorical device; according to Gray, ownership of 20 slaves made one a major slaveholder, or large planter. Gray operated on the hypothesis that the CSA above all political entities would know how to define the categories of slaveholding. Idem, *History of Agriculture in the Southern United States to 1860*, 2 vols., Carnegie Institute Contributions to Economic History (ca. 1930. Reprint ed.; New York: Peter Smith, 1980). The several acts signed into law on 28 December 1863, to which Apperson refers in Richmond newspapers, did not create these exemptions, but only reaffirmed them. What they did do was to eliminate the practice of substitution, that is, paying a substitute to fight for one. As the diarist feared, the practice could not be eliminated just because a law was imposed. See Long, "conscription," but esp. 449.

present, but the producing interests of the Country [viz., the planters who controlled most of the exportable cotton that could be sold for weapons] must be husbanded or we will "starve out". The question of supplies is one of vital importance and deserves the most profound legislation. This bill will no doubt shield some who ought to be in service, but nothing can pass that will not be objectionable. The provisions of the bill renders it [objectionable] no doubt.

ORANGE C.H. [ORANGE CO.] VA.

[TUESDAY] FEBRUARY 2ND [18]64

This morning I went to work on monthly report and finished it and [finished the] returns [requisition orders] for medical officers.

Orders have been issued from the War department in Richmond forbidding the issue of rations to Hosp's attendants, or so it reads. At any rate The Commissary of the Army has refused to issue [rations to attendants]. This seems the most ridiculous and absurd thing that has been issued. How can a man be confined to a post of duty for the government—under its control absolutely and *critically* [diarist's italics], and yet not [be] furnished with rations? One dollar and twenty five cents.[493] are furnished as commutation but what will this purchase, even of the O.C.S. dept.? [Official Commissary Service]—and how can we buy in the country and attend our duties also? Well may Mr. [Henry Stuart] Foote throw an odium on the Heads of Departments at Richmond.[494]

But the Order cannot surely mean what it reads! Time will show however.—Those whose duty it is to comply have so construed it, and once it is

---

[493] By this date in 1864, Davis Rich Dewey estimates that $1.25 CSA currency was worth about six cents in gold, at a time when all prices, esp. for food, were escalating rapidly. Dewey, 329-30.

[494] Henry Stuart Foote (1804-1880) was a Virginian who practiced law in Richmond for a time and then gained considerable fame as criminal law attorney in MS; elected to US Senate in 1847, he feuded with Jefferson Davis, MS other Senator, over the issue of state rights and the possibility of secession, both of which Foote opposed. Foote was elected Gov. of MS in 1853, but he left the state for CA because it was growing increasingly pro-states rights and secessionist. Returning east in 1858, he settled in Nashville, and became prominent in TN politics as an outspoken Unionist. Somehow, he was elected to CSA Congress, where he campaigned against war measures and constantly attacked the CSA heads of departments, esp. the Commissary. In February 1865 he actually opened his own peace negotiations with President Lincoln, but was arrested by CSA forces before he could get to D.C. The CSA Senate voted censure, but did not expel him, and he attempted to go to D.C. again, but Lincoln would not see him. Consequently, he traveled to Europe. Late in life, he made friends with President Ulysses S. Grant, who appointed him superintendent of US Mint in New Orleans. Patricia L. Faust, "Foote," *Hist. Times.*

decided by high authority it must be obeyed by subs. [subordinates] To-morrow a protest will be sent up in form to Gen'l [Richard Stoddert] Ewell.

This evening Dr. Ellsberg & myself visited Mr. [James] Chapmans[sic]. Capt. Boykin, the intended of Miss Emma [Chapman, sister of Mary and daughter of James] was present, Also "Dr. Boteler" [.][495] With the young ladies we had a very pleasant game of whist. Left about 10 o'clock.

When I returned I found a letter from my [friend] Dr. Quisenberry.

ORANGE C.H. [ORANGE CO.] VA.

[WEDNESDAY] FEBY 3 1864

Wednesday Having returned late last night I rose early this morning. Much earlier indeed than I supposed it was. I read "Children of the Abbey" till nearly day when I became exceeding tired and dozed a short while. Having to go on business to Gen. [Richard Stoddert] Ewell's Hd Qrs[496] I had breakfast early and was upon the road a short while after sunrise. The air was quite pleasant when I arose but soon the wind raised and the atmosphere became disagreeably cold.

Leaving the old pike at Dr. Terryle's [possibly Dr. Uriel Terrell] I passed Pisgah Church and arrived at the end of my trip in that direction about 10 o'clock.[497] Transacted [sic] my business, I returned. Called to see Col. [Robert H.] Dungan but his Regt was on picket duty and I failed. The troops have very

---

[495] Probably Alexander R. Boteler, Jr., who was not a doctor, and thus the diarist has put that title in quotes, as he did before for another clerk of his acquaintance. Boteler (born1843?, death date and postwar occupation unknown), was a clerk from Jefferson Co., VA [later WV] who joined Co. B, 2d VA Inf., was discharged from 2d Inf. but apparently reenlisted, by unofficial records, in Rockbridge Artillery and then served, officially, in commissary (OCS) with Hokee's Brigade, Jubal Anderson Early's Div., 2d Corps, commanded by Richard Stoddert Ewell, which assignment would put him here with the diarist. Frye, *2d VA Inf.*, 85.

[496] Professor Bean says that R.S. Ewell's 2d Corps headquarters were at Morton Hall on the Rapidan River near Raccoon Ford, NE from Orange Court House. Bean, notes. W.W. Scott affirms the identification, and notes that it is a pre-Revolutionary structure built by Charles Bruce and passed along through in-laws by marriages to Dr. George Morton, who left it to Judge James Morton. The handsome structure itself, generally called Soldiers Home, was burned down in 1857, and Ewell's headquarters are thus on the grounds of the Morton Hall. Scott, 211-12, with sketch.

[497] Possibly Chesnut Hill, the onetime home of Dr. Uriel Terrell. Scott says that Chenut Hill was "famous in old days as a favorite hostelry of Henry Clay and other statesmen." The Terrell home was later bought by W.G. Crenshaw, Jr. and generally called Chesnut Hill but sometimes Dr. Terrell's. Scott, 214-15.

excellent winter tenements. Stopped at Gen. [R.E.] Lee's HQ[498] to complete my work. I came on [home to quarters at Chapman's lot] about 4 o'clock—Soon as I procured something to eat I became sleepy—took a nap and have [been] reading "Children of the Abbey" since.

The object of my visit to the army was to get some light on Gen. Order No. 8 A[ssistant] A[djutant] Gen[eral's] Office requiring rations to be commuted to Hospt Attendants, and not allow them to be drawn of the Commissary. Gen. [R.E.] Lee orders the Commissary to issue as usual [viz., what the diarist wanted to happen]. Mr. Neil, our Chaplain left to-day.

On my trip to-day I passed the spot where Mr Geo[rge] A. Sleet once lived.[499]

In the days when prosperity smiled and he had all heart could wish around him he owned a large tract of land here. Riches often take to themselves wings & fly away is a trite saying and when the sun of his prosperity was declining and the shades of adversity begun [sic] to lower, I had the honour of living with him, or working for him for one month. 'Twas a merry party that worked in clay making brick for a house he was building. The debris of the Old Kiln was left. I remember all the boys—where are they now?—gone, gone gone—the cruel hand of death has taken them away. I am perhaps one of the few who have felt that the days I spent there were indeed *halcyon* days [diarist's italics].

ORANGE C.H. [ORANGE CO.]

THURSDAY FEBY 4 [18]64

A medical examining board composed of Surgeons [Harvey] Black [E.C.] Higginbotham & Claggett[500] was convened here to-day by order of Surgeon L[afayette] Guild for the purpose of examining invalid soldiers who may become unable for service from wounds or sickness. The board meets Mondays & Thursdays. Surgeon H[igginbotham] was unwell and did not attend.[501]

---

[498] Professor Bean states that R.E. Lee's ANV headquarters for February 1864 "were off the Orange Court House-Fredericksburg turnpike (now Route 20), a few miles east from Orange Court House." Bean, notes. Scott does not address the issue specifically, 210-15.

[499] George A. Sleet was not in Orange Co. by 1870, as diarist seems to indicate. There is an Elizabeth Sleet, a widow born in 1830, who may be his widow; she had a home in Orange Court House in 1870. VA Census, 1870.

[500] Professor Bean supplies the initials for Dr. E.G. Higginbotham. I cannot identify either Dr. Higginbotham or Dr. Claggett.

[501] According to Cunningham, the surgeon E.G. Higginbotham's attendance or absence may not have mattered much, for by1864 the CSA was attempting to keep its "invalid" men in the ranks, if at all possible. By orders of 23 February 1863: "'general debility,' 'slight deformity,' partial deafness, speech impediment—'unless of a very aggravated character,' functional heart

I have been working on Semi Annual returns. Did not do much—Surgeon Walls spent the day with us —

I wrote a letter to broth[er] N ["Nat," or Cincinnatus Apperson]—finished "Children of the Abbey"—I have no praise for the book I fear—too much color. I see a bill has been proposed in Congress by a gentleman from Ga. to offer to the federal government the proposition of sending delegates to some point to come to some terms of an adjustment of the civil difficulties now enshrouding us.[502]

[ORANGE C.H., ORANGE CO.]

FRIDAY, FEB: 5 [18]64

This morning I was loth [sic; loath] to rise—the air was cool. I finished Semi Annual Returns and we sent them off. Mr. Janell[503] called to inquire for his son who died of S. Pox at Guiney's [Station, Caroline Co.] last March. Poor Old Man the wounds occasioned by the death of his boy bleed yet. I was touched with his manner.

The news in to-day's paper is good. Gen. [George Edward] Pickett has made a capture of a small number of Yankees near Newbern, N.Ca.[504] A Yankee

---

trouble, muscular rheumatism, epilepsy—unless clearly proved, varicocele—'unless excessive,' myopia, hemorrhoids—'unless excessive,' 'opacity of one cornea, or the loss of one eye,' ' loss of one or two fingers,' and 'single reducible hernia' were 'not deemed sufficient and satisfactory for exemption." Even these loose screenings of the enlisted who were wounded or sick were altered on 10 December 1863 by this interesting language quoted in Cunningham: "When a conscript is found equal to, or in the performance of the active duties of the various occupations of civil life, he is able to discharge the duties of a soldier." Cunningham, 164-65.

[502] According to Warren Akin, CSA congressman from GA, his fellow representative August R. Wright on 3 February 1864 introduced a resolution proposing a peace negotiation for a reunited US government acknowledging certain rights of states. Akin notes that no action was taken, and notes further that Wright left Richmond suddenly, possibly out of fear of being expelled from the House and perhaps otherwise disciplined. Warren Akin, *Letters of Warren Akin, Confederate Congressman*, ed., Bell Irvin Wiley (Athens: University of Georgia Press, 1959) 27.

[503] Possibly Willis Janell, born 1805, who had a home in Stanardsville Township, Greene Co., and who may have lost a son in the campaigns of 1863. VA census, 1870.

[504] Then spelled New Berne, NC, this town by 1864 was an important Federal base near the Neuse River. On 1 and 2 February 1864 George Edward Pickett led troops from Kinston and attempted to capture the base guarded by Brig. Gen. I.N. Palmer, while CSA navy forces attacked the US gunboat *Underwriter* in the Neuse River. Pickett's attack succeeded briefly, and the *Underwriter* was destroyed, but both CSA army and navy forces had to withdraw by the end of 2 February 1864. See Long, 459-460.

gunboat [*Underwriter*] is taken, and the English government has concluded to release the Alexandria.[505]

I rec'd a letter from Mollie T[hornton] to-night. Am writing one to Dr. Faris.

ORANGE C.H. [ORANGE CO.]

SATURDAY FEB: 6 [18]64

This morning I was agreeable surprised by a call from Col: [Robert Henry] Dungan [of Marion and 4th Inf. VA]. He is going home on a leave of 24 days. There is much enjoyment in store for him there I know. He merits all he can get too. It may be that I overrate him; but I have ever esteemed him, and admired his noble efforts to rise in the world. If he is spared to see peace in our country we may safe [sic] predict for him a bright and useful future. Come what may such men as he will not slumber in the dust of oblivion. We may blur the light of the sun from its shining place on high: but need not hope to quench the light glory has kindled in the soul of man.

I finished my letter to Dr. F. and mailed it. Made out Monthly Statement of sick and wounded.

Maj. [Wells] Hawks [commissary of 2d Corps, R.S. Ewell's corps of ANV] was at my quarters to-night and brings the intelligence that the enemy was making demonstration at Morton's Ford [a ford of Rapidan River partly in Orange and partly in Culpeper Counties][506]—that firing had been kept up all day. This is a diversion by the enemy.

Part of their army has been moving towards N. Ca. and this demonstration is done with a view of stopping a further movement on our part.

I was at [Harvey Allen] Jameson's Room [Jameson, already identified, was a farmer from Smyth Co. who also served as hospital steward in 2d Corps]; had a party at Euker [euchre].[507] Ellsberg, Drane, and Thomas were at Mrs. [James]

---

[505] On 6 April 1863 the CSA *Alexandria* was in the harbor at Liverpool, "fitting out" for sea with war munitions. The British government seized *Alexandria* and held it almost ten months, then releasing it with the statement that proof was lacking that the ship was armed for war purposes. The mere seizure did damage to CSA materially and spiritually, and marked a radical departure from earlier British sympathy for free trade and an even earlier flirtation with recognition of the CSA. Long, 335.

[506] There was a skirmish on 6 February 1864, a demonstration much as diarist surmises. *OR*, 1:33:113-43.

[507] Euchre was a card game in which seven was the lowest card; winner had to take three of five tricks; jokers were often added, and there were some tricks in the counting of the totals. The

Chapman's I got a letter from Mrs. F. and Laura to-night. Mrs. F informs me that Willie [son of Dr. and Mrs. William Faris] and is improving very rapidly which I am pleased to hear—I heard he was not doing well, and wrote Dr. concerning it.

Sent off duplicate property returns; and financial weekly to Surgeon [Hunter Holmes] McGuire [chief surgeon of 2nd corps ANV].

[FIELD] HOSPT. 2ND CORPS ANV ORANGE C.H. [ORANGE CO.] VA.

SUNDAY [FEBRUARY 7, 1864]

This morning the first intelligible sound we heard was the loud reverberation of artillery on the [Rapidan] river towards Barnett's Ford.[508] Some small arms were very distinctly heard at intervals and irregular. The artillery at first seemed very close, owing perhaps to the condition of the air transmitting the sound. [I]t soon began to recede, however, and by noon ceased. The explanation seems to be that Kilpatrick's, [the so-called *Kilcavalry* of Hugh Judson Kilpatrick (1836-1881)] from some prompting and for some cause moved across Robinson river and attacked our pickets near Locust Grove [Orange Co., and the Apperson's home]. [Lunsford Lindsay] Lomax's Brigade[509] engaged him, and at last account he was falling back, and Gen. "Jeb" [J.E.B. Stuart] was trying to cut part of his force off by moving around with two brigades of Infantry and one of Cavalry. This of course he will fail to do.[510] If Mr. Kilpatrick [Gen. Hugh Judson Kilpatrick] started a raid he has been equally foiled. It seems that the whole

---

game was usually lively, as in the party here, and involved much deception and trickery, so that the expression *euchred*, grew out of the game and came to mean to be deceived by a trick. *Webster's 3d International.*

[508] Barnett's Ford was on the Rapidan River, and it was in both Madison and Orange Cos. This demonstration became a skirmish recorded as such, 6 February 1864, *OR*, 1:33:113-43.

[509] Lunsford Lindsay Lomax (1835-1913) was a cavalry officer who slowly won the respect of the men who had served under the much-beloved Turner Ashby. A native of Newport, RI, Lomax was son of a VA artillery captain, and he grew up in New England "with an abiding affection for his Southern heritage." West Point graduate and classmate and friend of Gen. Fitzhugh Lee, Lomax rose rapidly through ranks, and eventually heard praise even from notoriously demanding cavalry Gen. William E. "Grumble" Jones. Lomax performed well with his cavalry in these maneuvers noted by the diarist, and eventually was promoted again, to Maj. Gen. At Appomattox Court House, Lomax refused to surrender but instead went to NC, where he eventually surrendered alongside Joseph Eggleston Johnston at Greensborough. After the War, Lomax served as president of the institution that became Virginia Polytechnic Institute and State University at Blacksburg. Edward G. Longacre, "Lomax," *Hist. Times..*

[510] Actually, the federal troops were compelled to withdraw back across the Rapidan and move northward after the evening of 6 February 1864. Long, 461-62.

arrangement is a diversion to obscure some movement of their men. It may be that an advance will be made on Gen. [Jubal Anderson] Early in the Valley [Early was operating largely in the Valley, using strategies similar to those of T.J. Jackson], or the intention of the whole thing may have been to prevent Gen. [R.E.] Lee sending any portion of his army away. The Stonewall Brigade lost some men at Morton's Ford yesterday—wounded and prisoners.[511]

Our friend F.D. Hill of the Ambulance train left us to-day—He goes to the Cavalry Corps for duty in the A[djutant] Gen's office.[512]

I attended church to-night. Mr. [Beverly T.] Lacy preached from Hebrews 13 c[hapter] & 8 v[erse]. "Jesus Christ, the same yester-day, to-day and forever."[513] He treated the text as presenting to the mind two essential attributes of Christ—immutability of nature and eternity of existance [sic]. As he was yesterday so he is to-day and will be through the illimitable and endless future. [Illegible word] by the ideas presented in the parallel expressions "yester-day" and "forever" that Christ had been the same through all the Eternity of the Past. But applying the text more impressively to the present time—said he: "it is more important for you to know how he is now, and what are the attributes, and what he will do to save men from the awful end to which they are hasting." He said He had laid aside His Amen until seated in heaven and taken on flesh and blood, and came to our side that he might save us, and if we were ever saved from the pains of hell and handed to the pearly gates of heaven it would be by the saving hand of Christ. Speaking of his kindness to men he saith of the miracles he worked, how he wept over the fate of Jerusalem, and His words to the thief on the Cross, and then assured his Congregation that 'twas the same being who now called us to Him, who still strove with Man, and loved his soul, and interceded with His father to spare us yet a little longer, that we might be made holier, happier, and better. And now that the most horrible calamities that ever befel [sic] a nation were upon us, O how much we stand in need of such a friend as that of Mary Martha & Lazarus had. And if we survived the War

[511] Morton's Ford was the site of the attempted advance and the retreat by Gen. Kilpatrick on 6 February.

[512] I cannot locate an F.D. Hill in 4th Inf., but often ambulance personnel are not so listed. I cannot find him subsequently in 22d, 6th, or 14th Cav.

[513] Beverly T. Lacy was the chaplain for the 2d Corps and a close friend of R.E. Lee. Heb. 13:8 : "Jesus Christ the same yesterday, and today, and for ever." Epistle attributed to St. Paul warns against "divers and strange doctrines" [Heb. 13 : 9] and reminds believers that Jesus Christ is unchanging even if the world is changing, a theme often preached by Lacy, Pitts, 62.

still that friend was needed—the trials danger and snares of the world still beseet the faith of every man.

The sermon was a good one—

[FIELD HOSPITAL, ORANGE COURT HOUSE, ORANGE CO.]

MONDAY, FEB'Y 8TH, 1864

To-day nothing passed that is worthy of notice. While looking over some papers I find a mistake in some Annual Returns of Property ending 31 Dec., '63 of 44 pillows, drawn from Surgeon Hagy and receipted for but were not placed in Returns. Wrote to Surge[on] Gen. [Lafayette Guild] asking him to have them added.

We learn to-day that some 20 prisoners were lost from "Stonewall" Brig[ade] in the skirmish at Morton's Ford. The enemy came over [the Rapidan River] and captured our men in rifle pits. Lt. Anders[514] of Co. F, 4 Regt was in command of the post when the enemy came over. He was taken. 17 Yankees were killed and about 40 captured. Mr. F.D. Hill left to-day. I regretted to see him leave. He is ordered to report for duty in the A[ssistant] A[djutant] Gen'l office of cavalry.

"Aunt K" [Keziah Shepherd of hostess and matronly fame] came up from Richmond to-day—Capt. Rogers was with her—he is a great case.

Ellsberg & *Judge* [Nolan; diarist's italics] were at my tent 'till late with their violins—the music was very sweet.

[FIELD HOSPITAL, ORANGE COURT HOUSE, ORANGE CO.]

TUESDAY, FEB. 9TH [1864]

This morning was very cold.

The numbers of men coming to [Field] Hospt for admittance are very small. I have very little to do. It would be better though if I had more. I am wasting my time shamefully.

---

[514] The diarist always refers to the 4th VA Inf. in more familiar terms than used here. There is no Lt. Anders listed in 4th VA, and I cannot understand what unit he is talking about. The 4th Cav. , whose F Company was from Goochland, was active in this campaign and was in this area protecting the Rapidan and the Rappahannock throughout the winter of 1864, but there is no Lt. Anders listed with 4th Cav. Kenneth L. Stiles, *4th VA Cav.*, VA Regimental Histories Series (Lynchburg, VA: H.E. Howard, 1985).

Drs. [Z.B.] Herndon and Straith were in town. Dr. H. is preparing for a heavy bird hunt to-morrow—Dr. S[traith] to see his fiancee.

I went birding with Master Richardson, had some sport, and killed 4 birds. I did not display any great marksmanship.

I have a headache to-night.

[FIELD HOSPITAL, ORANGE COURT HOUSE, ORANGE CO.]

WEDNESDAY, FEB. 10TH [18]64

To-day is Ash Wednesday—the day celebrated in the Roman Catholic Church in olden times by sprinkling ashes over the penitents thereby fitting them to begin the fasting of Lent with meekness and submission. The Episcopal Congregation [of St. Thomas's in Orange Court House] met to-day. I did not attend, and those who did were far from manifesting the spirit of those who used to commemorate this 40 days fasting & prayer.

This evening Drs. Ellsberg, Thomas, and myself went to the daguero[type] gallery and had our shadows fixed on metal. I am not sure that it is not all a fancy, but some of my friends request it and a small sacrifice will suffice their desire.

Dr. E[llsberg] & myself visited Mr. C's [James Chapman family]—Found the young ladies in the parlour. We had been there but a short time when surgeon Straith came. Miss E.C. [Emma Chapman], who is soon to be wedded had retired—two ladies [were] left and three gentlemen. I resigned any chance I may have had, from being first, and occupied a neutral ground, no doubt to the gratification of at least one lady [he probably means Mary Chapman, daughter of James].

Surgeon S[traith] rose to retire and I followed.

To me it is a matter of almost perfect indifference whether I am esteemed or disliked, except that I prefer to have the good will of every animated creature—even a dog. And when I find that I may be thrown among indifferent, no act can be regarded more friendly than that which informs me that my society is not pleasant and agreeable. Candor in such matters is seldom found because few can work their courage up to the point necessary to speak plainly and calmly their sentiments to another, lest it give offence, but with me, nothing can give me a higher opinion of the person than to find so high a regard for the feelings of another as well as their own high character. I feel that I have not met such here [at James Chapman's], and do not think I shall mar the pleasure of their evenings with my presence. Often I know very well that I am not proposing [sic] or entertaining, and in the language of a gifted but perhaps misguided poet I will say:

> "Yet, though denied this pitiful resource,
> With no reproach thy sign shall be paid;
> It is, my genius I accuse, the source
> Of all my ill. _____."

and when they turn from me with a cold demeanour and darkened brow, they turn from one who is too proud to acknowledge any superiority in position further than that given by character alone. Poverty and humility must not bow to pride and fortune or the condescension will be ignominious.[515]

I wrote to my friend Mollie [Thornton] when I returned. The air is cool —.

[FIELD HOSPITAL, ORANGE COURT HOUSE, ORANGE CO.]

THURSDAY, FEB: 11 [18]64

This was one of the coldest mornings. The sky is clear. Nothing of interest passed to-day. My father came up to see me. Since his misfortune by the Yankees he is very sad and wishes to revive his farming elsewhere. I am altogether unable to give him proper advice. I think it best for him to stay at home. There is surely more happiness for him, though he will run some risks and perhaps loose [sic] much of what he has already and have a very hard time to live, but where will he go that he will be safe and will not have a labor? He is paying 80$ per barrel for corn and expects to pay more when he buys again. The picture is too sad for me to dwell upon —

He paid me 60$ for balance on [the] saddle —

I rec'd a letter from Cousin Bettie—She has had a love-scrape.

[FIELD HOSPITAL, ORANGE COURT HOUSE, ORANGE CO.]

FRIDAY, FEBRUARY 12, [18]64

My father left this morning. He is very much dejected.

---

[515] Prof. Bean writes, "Although Apperson had visited the [James] Chapman home several times, he finally decided that they were too aristocratic for his comfort and ease. He ceased the visitations." Bean, notes.

This morning we forwarded a requisition to the Surg. Gen. of the State of N.Ca. [P.E. Hines][516] for a small quantity of Med & Hospt supplies for the troops from that state. Gov: [Zebulon Baird] Vance has procured clothing and need: by blockade [sic; blockading] enemy steamers and in that way doing very much for the benefit of the army.[517]

It is worthy of a very high encomium.[518] While there is some dissatisfaction among the people of the Old North State, her governor has struck boldly for the honour and good name of his State and when this trouble is over no one can throw any aspersion on the executive of the State—he has done his duty. Surg'n Grisham, the Asst. Surge'n Gen'l[519] is on official business to the Army now.

I got a letter from Mrs. [Mary] Tomlin to-day. I was at Ellsberg's room—had a very boisterous time with some of the pleasure-seeking young girls: returned about 11 o'clock.

[FIELD HOSPITAL, ORANGE COURT HOUSE, ORANGE CO.]

SATURDAY FEB 13 [18]64

To-day has been a very busy one to me—weekly report to make off—requisition & c[etera] to draw up—we rec'd a bill of med: from Z.B. Herndon, Med[ical] Pur[veyors], Richmond:

Uncle Tommy came in to see me for a short while—got a letter from Willie F[aris]—and a comic sketch from Richmond—Valentine[.]

---

[516] Hines identified, Cunningham, 285.

[517] Zebulon Baird Vance (1830-1894) was an often cantankerous foe of Jefferson Davis, but as Les D. Jensen notes, he "in fact supported the Confederacy strongly. He worked to maintain North Carolina's fighting spirit and helped the state maintain and expand its considerable munitions and clothing factories. His state supplied more troops to the Confederacy than any other, and they were maintained largely at state expense, thus relieving the Confederate government of the burden. Vance initiated his own overseas supply purchases and often shared state supplies with Confederate troops of other states." Idem, "Vance," *Hist. Times.* Apperson may be talking about Vance's blockade-runners.

[518] "Encomium…warm or high praise. . . in Eastern Orthodox Church service, a celebration of praise for the passion of Jesus Christ." *Webster's 3d Int'l.*

[519] No Grisham—and no Gresham—is listed by Robertson in the 4th VA Inf.; and no Grisham—or Gresham—is listed by Cunningham.

[FIELD HOSPITAL, ORANGE COURT HOUSE, ORANGE CO.]

SUNDAY, FEB. 14TH [18]64

This is a most lovely morning. The sun shines beautifully and the wind blows as calmly as it is wont to do in mid-summer—Later it blew harder.

Many *billet doux*[520] [diarist's italics] have been sent around to-day—the young and sentimental can disgorge themselves of flattery & frivolity.

I attended church [possibly at St. Thomas' in Orange Court House]. Rev. Mr. [Beverly T.] Lacy preached upon the Crucifixion of Christ. The leading points in his remarks were upon the promises of that great event. "The most important event in the history of time and the annals of eternity." He argued that all history centers upon that event—the past [,] present and future.

Then his main purpose as expressed by himself was that the "witnesses of the Crucifixion were the representatives of the race." For every individual now living a prototype was an eyewitness of the death of Christ, whether good or bad, virtuous or depraved. He drew analogies between many of the beholders of that event, and many now in existance [sic]. There lives now the roman ruler [viz., Pontius Pilate, who "found no fault in this man" but agreed to the crucifixion], the priest and pontiff [the high priest and the official of the Sanhedrin who arrested Jesus], the centurion and soldier [who asked forgiveness and sought grace through Jesus' blessing during the passion], the thief of both conditions [the one who mocked and the one who asked forgiveness and sought grace during the crucifixion], the sorrow[ing] follower [on Good Friday], the meek and lowly deciple [sic; disciple], the weeping and prayerful Mother all stand now in His awful presence[.][521] There were the exponents of fallse [sic; false] religion the enemies of true religion—just as now—The Congregation was a good one—and the sermon was listened to with much interest.

He preaches again to-night.

EVENING—

Mr. [Bevery T.] Lacy preached from Job 42 chapter & 5th & 6th verses—

"I have heard of thee, by the hearing of the ear, but now mine eye seeth thee.

"Wherefore I abhor myself and repent in dust and ashes."[522]

He glanced over the life of this good man, and held up his virtues. I have never looked at the history of Job with so much interest as I shall do hereafter.

---

520 "Billet-doux—Fr., Love letter." *Webster's 3d Intl.*.

521 Lk 23 (KJV).

522 Jb 42:5-6 (KJV). punctuated slightly differently.

His fidelity to God is truly a noble theme. The temptations of Satan, how strong! How wisely God used him as an instrument of Grace in the soul of man. He did not persecute Job because He knew not how deep and fine the faith He had poured into his heart, but that he might prove that His ways were Mighty and would prevail[.] When the flocks and herds of this Oriental prince [Job of Uz] were carried away by the robbers, his servants slain, and his children by the very hand of nature torn from his earthly presence at one stroke he exclaimed "God gaveth and He can take and I will praise His name"[523] Satan seeing all came[,] then said that as his person was safe he would for selfish reasons still cling to God for favour—Then came that loathesome disease, his friends importuned him to give up his believe [sic] in God, his wife urged him to curse God and die,[524] still he cried "Though God slay me yet will I trust in His name"[.][525] And when God was finally revealed to him—as expressed in the text—when his eyes beheld Him, though to us kind, yet he *abhorred himself* [diarist's italics].[526] The minister said to know God was the highest knowledge and for man to know himself was next—The remaining portion of his text was on our knowledge of ourselves and our knowledge of God. How despised, how poluted [sic; polluted] and depraved we are when seen as Job saw himself. When the light of knowledge has thrown its rays into our hearts and illuminated the crevasses[527] and recesses of that abode of sin how terrible will be the realisation of such a habitation. But sooner or later we must know ourselves and feel in our hearts that we are depraved and despicable in the sight of God.

[FIELD HOSPITAL, ORANGE COURT HOUSE, ORANGE CO.]

MONDAY FEB 15 [18]64

This morning snow is falling. The Examining board met. I acted in the capacity of Secretary. If some of smart satirical writers had the opportunity they

---

[523] Job 1:21: "And said, Naked came I out of my mother's womb, and naked shall I return thither: the Lord gave, and the Lord hath taken away; blessed be the name of the Lord." (KJV).

[524] Job 2:9.

[525] Job 13:15: "Though he slay me, yet will I trust in him: but I will maintain mine own ways before him." (KJV).

[526] Job 42:5-6 :"I have heard of thee by the hearing of the ear: but now mine eye seeth thee. Wherefore I abhor *myself*, and repent in dust and ashes." (KJV).

[527] Apperson uses the correct French word for the English *crevice*.

would make a good thing out of it—. There is a large amount of humbuggery in these boards[528] —

I got a letter from [brother] Nat [Cincinnatus Apperson] to-night and wrote one to Dr. Quisenberry.

Had a game of whist.

My tent fellow [Dr.] Sydnor left this morning on a leave of 15 days.

[FIELD HOSPITAL, ORANGE COURT HOUSE, ORANGE CO.]

TUESDAY, FEB. 16 [18]64

To-day has been a very cold day. Nothing of any importance transpired. I have been reading Shakespeare—"The Tempest"[529]

[FIELD HOSPITAL, ORANGE COURT HOUSE, ORANGE CO.]

WEDNESDAY, FEB. 17, [18]64

Still cold. Colder perhaps than at any other time this winter. To-night Dr. Ellsberg & myself went out. I am not in the habit of going where I am ashamed to be seen but in this instance I am not sure I would have felt pleasant to have [been] caught. I can only say how terrible the depravity of the human race.

[FIELD HOSPITAL, ORANGE COURT HOUSE, ORANGE CO.]

THURSDAY, FEB. 18TH [1864]

The weather is still terrible.

To-day the papers announce the military bill and the tax bill.—The latter is too complex for my narrow mind. One thing I am satisfied of however—one third of the Confederate money will be repudiated after the first of April virtually—. This bill will fall like an earthquake upon some, but it is a stern, pressing necessity.[530]

---

[528] Cunningham agrees with the assessment, especially by 1864; and he quotes R.E. Lee to the effect that the examining boards were bringing men into the army who were too sick to fight and who became "burdensome rather than advantageous." Idem, 163-65

[529] William Shakespeare, *The Tempest* (ca. 1611); probably performed for the court in 16ll shortly after it was written; according to Edmund Kerchever Chambers, "Sylvester Jourdan's *A Discovery of Bermuda*, containing an account of the shipwreck of Sir George Somers in 1609, was published about 1610, and that or some contemporary narrative of Virginia colonisation probably furnished the hint of the plot." Idem, "Shakespeare," *Encyclopedia Brittanica.*

[530] As noted earlier, the military conscription bill for the CSA greatly expanded the ages and classes of men eligible for forced draft into the army. The diarist exaggerates in talking about 1/3

I have been saving some money but it seems useless to do so.

[FIELD HOSPITAL, ORANGE COURT HOUSE, ORANGE CO.]

FRIDAY, FEB. 19TH [18]64

No change in the weather for better.

The wise address from Congress prepared by Mr. [Jabez Lamar Monroe] Curry of Ala. is out to-day—It is worthy of our Cause. [531]

---

of CSA money being "repudiated"; however, its value in gold dollars did drop by approximately 70%. The tax bill reaffirmed an income tax and also "forced people to exchange their paper money, above the denomination of five dollars, for long-term four percent interest-bearing bonds.... The purpose of the tax bill was to check inflation," but it failed as noted earlier, by Todd, op. cit.: $1 gold dollar = $34-49 CSA dollars by December 1864, while at end of 1863, $1 gold dollar = $20 CSA dollars. Clement Eaton, *A History of the Southern Confederacy* (New York: Macmillan, 1954), 258. The penalty for not exchanging the paper money for the bonds was forced reduction of old currency by one-third. The idea was sound enough, viz., remove paper money from circulation by selling bonds, but CSA bonds had little market value, and the CSA had little way to enforce its will on its citizens. The supply of money continued to increase much more rapidly than the supply of goods and services, and inflation worsened, reaching close to 70% increase in prices measured between beginning of 1864 and beginning of 1865, according to Todd, op. cit. For Smyth Co., here are prices recorded in 1863-1864:

wheat$10 bushelfactory jeans$3.00
bacon $1.50 lbcommon jeans$10.00
calico $8.00 ydflour$50 barrel
grain $5.00 bushelhorse$1,500

Source: Armstrong, *Hist. of Smyth*, 141.

While not precise, because we have no base line for Smyth Co. in 1862, these prices suggest an inflation rate of between 50% and 70% for the year 1863 compared to the year 1862.

[531] Jabez Lamar Monroe Curry (1825-1903) was one of Jefferson Davis's few staunch supporters, and was surely the most capable of those loyal to the beleagured president. Born in Lincoln City, GA, Curry was raised in AL, was educated at Franklin College (IN) and took a law degree after study at Harvard College Law School. He practiced law in Talladega, served as a Texas Ranger in the Mexican War, served in AL general assembly, as federal elector for 1856 for James Buchanan, and in US House, 1856-1861. In CSA House, he served on Committee on Commerce, monitoring CSA finances. Loyalty to the unpopular Davis cost him reelection in 1864, after which time he served in the army, as Lt. Col. and aide-de-camp to gens. Joseph Eggleston Johnston and Joseph Wheeler. After the War, Curry became an ordained Baptist minister and in fact is most noted for his postbellum activities on behalf of education. President of Howard College for freedmen in D.C. [now Howard University], he also served as professor at Richmond College [now University of Richmond]. Most importantly, he raised money from private sources to help build and improve schools, especially for African Americans, all over the South; he worked effectively both for the Peabody Fund and the Slater Fund. See Patricia L. Faust, "Curry," *Hist Times.*

This particular resolution was written by Curry on behalf of a joint commitee of the CSA houses; it ringingly reaffirmed the CSA and the policies of its president, and spoke against several

The boys have a subject for dissection. I was engaged with it but a short while this evening. Had an excellent Oyster Supper and some good smoking material. Dr. Ed. Newton, Maj. Capers[532] and several others were at my tent. Had some good music.

I wrote a letter to Cousin Bettie.

[FIELD HOSPITAL, ORANGE COURT HOUSE, ORANGE CO.]

SATURDAY, FEB. 20TH [1864]

The weather is better.

I was at the dissecting room nearly all day—I am not sure I learned much.

Have been reading Shakespeare [*The Tempest*] some. Wrote a letter to Willie Faris.

[FIELD HOSPITAL, ORANGE COURT HOUSE, ORANGE CO.]

SUNDAY, FEB: 21ST [1864]

I have heard two sermons to-day. The first in the forenoon by Rev: Mr. Clark, of the Methodist church and the other in the evening by the Rev: Mr. Smith of the presbyterian [sic].[533]

Mr. C[lark] preached from the first five verses of Pslams [sic][534] His sermon was rather a tiresome one to most persons.

---

independently organized peace movements in the southern regions. The resolution was issued as the CSA congress concluded a session, and the next session would not include Curry and others who had supported Davis. Jessie Pearl Rice, *J.L.M. Curry, Southerner, Statesman, and Educator* (New York: King's Crown Press, 1949) 238.

[532] Maj. Capers, the fiance of a local lady, is not listed in 4th or 7th regiments, nor in other VA infantry and cavalry regiments. I cannot find a Dr. Edward or Edmund Newton in Cunningham, or in any of the VA infantry or cav. regiments. There is a Dr. George S. Newman listed by W.W. Scott as serving in field hospital in Orange Co. and neighboring cos. Scott, 275.

[533] Scott does not list either name as a minister in Orange Co. Pitts lists two missionaries [viz., not attached as chaplain to a particular regiment], no first names known, who served in the era : Clark of the Army of Tenn. and Smith of Jackson's Brigade. The Clarks are likely different men, but Smith, a Presbyterian missionary , could well be this preacher. Scott, passim; Pitts, 141; 153-54.

[534] If the diarist means the first five psalms, then the Rev. Clark was preaching about psalms then generally attributed to King David; all emphasize perseverance through travail and the hope of salvation for the faithful; if he means the first 5 verses of the 6-vv Psalm 1, that psalm emphasizes punishment for the ungodly and unfaithful and the recognition by God that faithful believers often must suffer at the hands of the unfaithful. (KJV). Ps 2, which begins memorably in Jacobean trans. "Why do the heathen rage, and the people imagine a vain thing?" was a standard with wartime ministers, according to Pitts, 110.

The adaptation of air and water and vegetation to our wants was the principal topic of his discourses.[535]

Mr. S[mith]. preach[ed] from the text in the prophet Jeremiah "What have I done?" His discourse showed man in [sic] as a rebellious creature in ignoring God, disowning his authority, breaking His laws, committing sin knowingly—and treating the Spirit with utter diffidence.[536]

I[n] the course of his sermon he said the future is judged of by the past. That we judge what is to take place by comparing the past with the future—That voices of the future are echoes of the past—the songs of childhood live on in the heart of man like the song when the minister has gone. —

In regard to cloaking of sin he said it was like damping the fire down by throwing wood upon it—it may be hid for a limited time but would finally break out and be but the larger for being hid.

Of the Striving of the Spirit with man he said [it] reminded him of everything like a long passage through which the children of mortality were

---

[535] Ps 1:3-4: "[3] And he shall be like a tree planted by the rivers of water, that bringeth forth his fruit in his season; his leaf also shall not wither; and whatsoever he doeth shall prosper.[4] The ungodly are not so; but are like the chaff which the wind driveth away." (KJV).

[536] Quote seems a little off the mark, cf. Jer 2 : 18: "And now what hast thou to do...?" (KJV). There follow a series of repetitive and rhythmic answers, arranged in so-styled "poetic material" that is "interspersed" with prosaic material over the first 25 chapters of Jeremiah; the answers all reflect the rebellious nature of people, especially the Judeans of Jeremiah's time, their ignoring God, their denying and disavowing God's authority, their breaking God's law, and their infidelity to the covenant between Yahweh and Abraham, all the things catalogued by the Rev. Smith in this sermon. Robert Davidson discusses the poetic material as response to the call from Yahweh, idem, "Jeremiah," *Oxford Campanion to the Bible*, ed., Bruce Metzger and Michael D. Coogan (New York: Oxford University Press, 1993). The specific language of *diffidence*—doubting and lacking confidence in God's abilities and powers—is not Jacobean, but rather from John Donne, according to connotations explained in *Webster's 3rd International Dictionary* and *OED*, this verse:

> That affliction grew heavy upon me;
> and weighed me down
> Even to a diffidence of God's mercy
> John Donne, quoted, loc. cit.

Donne's sermons, whether re-set as poetry or treated as prose sermons, were important to ministers of this era; and it is interesting that the diarist here picks up and makes his own the poetic and non-biblical word, *diffidence*, while apparently missing the prophet Jeremiah's Biblical phrase—unless the minister the Rev. Smith himself missed the Biblical line; if the latter is the case, it is uncharacteristic of the diarist not to look up the line in his own Bible and then note the minister's error. In any case, in this instance, Apperson seems more interested in the language of poetry derived from the Bible than in the words and theology of the Bible.

passed from life into death. On either side of this pass were the boundless domain of safety and happiness. Leading from this passage were doors in the walls standing open. The pilgrim entered and instead of turning into the first or second door he came to as directed by the placard on the side he pulls the door and shoves it fast, the 2d he locks and the 3d also and so on—the doors become farther apart as he passes on.—presently he comes to the last one. Just before he steps in his grave, he deliberately extends his arm and closes that—he is lost. The figure is a fine one.

One part of his sermon I am not satisfied with altogether. He makes the heedless churchgoer, whatever his moral character may be, vastly more sinful than he that hears not a sermon in a month. If, then, it is more sinful to visit Church than it is to remain at home then I fear we are unpardonable sinners.

I wrote a letter to Laura F—[Faris]

[FIELD HOSPITAL, ORANGE COURT HOUSE, ORANGE CO.]

MONDAY, FEB. 22D 1864

To-day has been one of the busiest for a long time. The Ex[amining] Board met and I was engaged 'till night preparing the papers. The weather has been fine. I rec'd a ticket to Miss E.C.'s [Emma Chapman's] wedding for the 25th. I acknowledge I was somewhat surprised.[537]

[FIELD HOSPITAL, ORANGE COURT HOUSE, ORANGE CO.]

TUESDAY, FEBY 23 [18]64

The day passed off as usual. I was at the [railway] Depot [in Gordonsville, about nine miles south from the courthouse][538] this morning to see some of our boys [4th Va Inf.] going home. This evening a concert was given at the C.H. [Orange Court House] & Mr. Baker preached at the Presbt [Presbyterian]

---

537 Part of the surprise is that he considered the Chapman family too aristocratic for his company and thought them disdainful of him. The bridegroom was Maj. Hardy of QM corps for 2nd Corps of ANV. Bean, notes.

538 Gordonsville, on the Louisa Co. line, was the western terminus for the Louisa Road turnpike as well as the western terminus for the Louisa Railroad, which became the Chesapeake and Ohio Railroad. The depot also served as major terminus for the Orange and Alexandria Railroad, which later became the Southern Railroad, and as the major terminus for the Charlottesville and Rapidan Railroad. The turnpike and the three rail lines were all completed in the decade before the War. Another line, the Richmond and Narrow Gauge, which became the Potomac, Fredericksburg, and Piedmont, was set to come through the same depot, but construction was delayed until twelve years after the War ended. Scott, 131-32.

Church—[539] Like a fool I chose the former and was almost disgusted—Everything was burlesque. Something over two hundred persons were present—the Actors were habited like Negroes and played and sang in Negro style. Most of the audience seemed to enjoy it—I did not.[540]

I am reminded of what I heard a minister say, not long since. It is as follows. In the great, populous and fashionable city of Paris lived an eminent Doctor of Medicine. The afflicted from far and near came to him for medical advice. The[re] came to him one day a man on whose brow the cares of the world seemed to rest with a leaden weight. He told the learned Doctor of this ailment—almost entirely of the mind. He was so far convicted [sic] of the probability of some coming trouble that he was in reality suffering bodily. At the time there was a commedian [sic] entertaining large audiences nightly at the theatre with his great display of talent, brilliancy of wit, and affableness of humour and gayety [sic; gaiety]. The learned Doctor advised this poor sick man to rouse himself up and throw off this *ennui* [diarist's italics]—go and hear this great player and jester—attend his *commedies* [sic] and it will all pass away.

Alas! said he I am that Commedian [sic] himself—How true the words.

If every man's *internal* cares were written on his brow How many would be written there. The[y] need our pity now.

I rec'd a letter from Dr. Quisenberry—.

---

[539] This church, built in colonial era, was called the Church of the Blind Preacher, or Belle Grove. The Blind Preacher was James Waddel, a Presbyterian minister blind since birth in Ireland (1739) who was so popular that the Episcopalians of St. Thomas' Episcopal Church also licensed him and paid him to preach for them as well. The Rev. Baker is probably Clay Baker, who bought the Hopewell home of the Rev. Waddel and arranged to have the exhumed remains of the Blind Preacher re-buried at Belle Grove. The Church of the Blind Preacher "stood on the north side of the Orange highway, about a half mile northeast of Gordonsville." William Wirt in his story "The British Spy" memorialized the Rev. Waddel preaching in the church, reprinted in full, 198-201 in Scott; see also ibid., 47-48, 197-200, picture, 204.

[540] Standard entertainment in the antebellum era, continued through the War, was *Jim Crow* singing, in which white men in "black face," or "blacked up," performed in burlesque style as African Americans. Some songs were performed well, but generally the effect was deliberately funny, wickedly deprecatory, and pointedly racist. *Jim Crow* was later memorably applied as a term to the laws segregating public facilities and also to the disfranchisement ploys adopted by southern states in the early 20th cent. Comer Vann Woodward, *The Strange Career of Jim Crow* (1954, rev. ed.; New York: Oxford University Press, 1974). Apperson is often racist in his expressions and declarations, and it seems unlikely that he was here offended by the racism in the humor, but he clearly disavowed anything humorous in the presentation. One interesting thing is that Apperson, unlike anyone else I have read in the era, generally capitalizes *Negro*.

[FIELD HOSPITAL, ORANGE COURT HOUSE, ORANGE CO.]

WEDNESDAY, FEBY. 24 1864

This has been a fine day. I wrote to Mrs. [Mary] Tomlin. This evening I went to the Hotel[541] to see a poor man who is very ill—a Mr. Foster. His life has been that of dissipation. He has followed for a living itenerant gaming and is I suppose about thirty years of age. Dissipation brought on debility and dropsy ensued.[542] A few days ago an opening was made and about 2 gallons of water taken from him. He is now to all appearances beyond the hope of recovery—a few more days and he will be ushered into the presence of his Maker. He is now almost uncared for. The friends that once swarmed around him have found nothing more to bind them to one whom money or other worldly ties connected before and now they leave him to die without even the kindness of a call from those who knew him in better days. It is so true that in prosperity friends crowd our way thick and fast, and in adversity leave us like we were afflicted with a loathsome disease.

I met Mr. Ja[mes M.] Brown but did not recognise him 'till he made his name known.[543]

---

[541] Orange Court House featured several *Ordinaries*, viz., places where a traveler could hire out a bed and pay for board, especially during court sessions; but *hotel* often designated a place with formal dining hall, perhaps ballroom, and meeting room, as well as living areas rented out for weeks or even years. The Hotel so noted may be Orange Springs, built by James Coleman as a tavern and originally called Healing Springs. Originally a center for "gaming," Orange Springs became by wartime a more reputable place for travelers and for townspeople to take meals. It was often center of important meetings, like the Continental in Marion; and was a social center for parties and celebrations. The diarist's notes suggest that the Hotel, if Orange Springs, may have remained a center for gaming during the War despite Scott's claims that the place had been reformed. Scott, 124-25.

[542] *Dropsy* is the nineteenth century term for generalized *edema* [from Greek for swelling], that is, a condition in which circulatory problems, pulmonary problems, lymphatic obstructions, renal complications, or inflammation or organs or tissues. Although drinking may exacerbate edema, or dropsy, the condition can also arise from congenital problems or bad diet. Mr. Foster may have been a rounder, but his edema or dropsy could well have been caused by conditions over which he had no control at all. The treatment in the era was bloodletting, which Apperson describes here, and that treatment seldom cured, usually weakened, and occasionally killed. Experiments in modern applied chemistry eventually developed drugs that could treat edema, and understanding of diet—primarily the reduction of salt intake and the increase of water intake—could save the lives of the afflicted and often provide a normal style of life. Definitions and etymology of words, "dropsy" and "edema," *Taber's.*; chemical history and blood pathologies, *McGrew's*, 79, 309, 310.

[543] James M. Brown (birth date unknown - death date unknown, but living in Rappahannock Co. in 1927) was probably a farmer. He enlisted in Co. B of 7th VA Inf., the northern central piedmont regiment that included many of Apperson's Orange Co. neighbors and some relatives. Wounded at Gettysburg (3 July 1863), he was on the rolls in October 1864. Riggs, 65.

[FIELD HOSPITAL, ORANGE COURT HOUSE, ORANGE CO.]

THURSDAY, FEB. 25, [18]64

The Med: Ex[amining] Board met to-day. Surg'n Higginbotham was not present. Ten cases were acted upon.

To-night the wedding came off—a very brilliant affair. I went but was *de trop* [superfluous]. Too many greater lights shone there for "small fry" to be seen—. I am very well aware that I got an invitation more from the prompting of Courtesy than desire for my Company. I went too more to show regard for the honour than to find enjoyment. I very well know that I am deficient in the particulars that make one noticeable on such occasions, and when I go am satisfide [sic] with less than I ought to be. I feel too much respect for truth and candor to assume a place that might throw a stigma on my name afterwards.

For the party I must say it did honour to the family. The pride & chivalry of the ~~Confederate~~ A.N.V. were well represented. A finer looking set of gentlemen, prettier girls, and a livelier party perhaps will not be assembled soon again. Among the distinguished characters were Maj. Gen'ls [James Ewell Brown] Stuart & [Robert Emmett] Rhodes [sic; Rodes] and Brig: Gen'ls [Robert Hall] Chilton & [Edward Aylesworth] Perry.[544] Then staff officers of all

---

[544] James Ewell Brown Stuart and Robert Emmett Rodes have already been identified. Robert Hall Chilton (1815-1879) was from Loudon City, VA. and was educated at West Point Academy (1837). He served in Indian wars along frontier of KS and TX, and then was breveted Maj. for bravery in Mexican War, when he saved the wounded Jefferson Davis by carrying the MS officer to safety under heavy fire at Buena Vista. After Mexican War, he served in army staff officer corps, and he so served in ANV. Unpopular with CSA Senate, he was denied line generalships, despite R.E.Lee's firm support, and he instead served as Inspector Gen. In his only combat service in the line, he led a VA inf. unit with some cavalry support in defense of Richmond (10 May 1864). Serving with distinction, he exonerated himself in the face of the Richmond politician critics, but as soon as the campaign was over, he returned to staff duties. After War, he ran a manufacturing firm in Columbus, GA. E.G. Longacre, "Chilton," *Hist. Times*. Edward Aylesworth Perry (1831-1889) was born in Richmond, MA and grew up in New England. Attending Yale University for one year, he left school and traveled south, studying law and teaching in AL. In 1857 he moved to FL, where he passed the bar and began practicing law. Passionate on behalf of states rights, he closed his law offices and formed Co. A, 2d FL Inf., which he served as Capt. Promoted to Col. and commander of FL regiment, he was later called by Gen. James Longstreet to join the 2nd Corps of ANV. According to Prof. Bean, his was the only FL regiment in the ANV. Wounded at White Oak Swamp of Seven Days' Battle (30 June 1862), he was promoted to Brig. Gen. At Gettysburg, as Fred L. Schultz notes, "he and his men broke through the Union lines in a brilliant but unsupported advance. His brigade and two others consequently withdrew, with his command sustaining some of the heaviest losses of the battle." Wounded again at the Wilderness (6 May 1864), he was removed to the rear for convalescence and limited duty the remainder of the War.

grades—Surgeons and Q.M.'s . The bride was very lovely indeed—I do not flatter myself to be any favorite with her [Emma Chapman] but overcame my embarrassment enough to offer my Congratulations—'twas coldly rec'd. I had the honour of being introduced to a few young ladies but having the impression that other and gayer Company was preferable to them I did not occupy their time very long. The supper was a magnificent one—Dr. Drane and myself were on an equality and left about mid-night. The dance was kept up 'till about 4 o'clock in the morning.

May the two whom God has made one have a long and happy life.

When I returned to my tent I found a letter from my friend Mollie [Thornton]. To read one letter from her is worth all the gayety that Mr. C[James Chapman] could have at his house in a month. I know I am reading the mind of a true woman.

[FIELD HOSPITAL, ORANGE COURT HOUSE, ORANGE CO.]

FRIDAY, FEBY 26TH [1864]

To-day the bridal party went to Richmond. May peace & happiness attend them and may they never be called to view any but the roseate hues of life. They have my blessing.

The weather is fine—the day passed away without anything unusual.

I called on Miss M[ollie] Graves and had a game of whist.

[FIELD HOSPITAL, ORANGE COURT HOUSE, ORANGE CO.]

SATURDAY, FEB 27TH [1864]

The letter I rec'd of Dr. Q[uisenberry] a few days ago offered me a chance to be transferred to a [general] Hospital near Richmond. I had a conversation with Dr. B. this evening. He said if it is referred to him he will disapprove it. This I expected. He of course could not be expected to approve transfer while he is asking for more appointments [viz., that is more stewards to help him because his general hospital was short-handed]. I have no desire to leave the place I hold except that I think it will [be] better for me. I have been in the Medical Department of the Army for three years and am no better posted now than when I came in, in the sort of knowledge that I desire most. I have been kept in the writing department and thereby see but very little of the sick. I hate to leave

---

After the War, he moved to Pensacola, where he distinguished himself as a lawyer, and became prominent politically, winning election as governor in 1884. Idem, "Perry," *Hist. Times.*

the field—The [general] Hospt Service may have some very distasteful things to me but by going there I may have an opportunity of getting to Richmond to attend a course of lectures [at Medical College of Virginia in Richmond] next ~~Spring~~ Winter. Then I shall be with Dr. Q[uisenberry] my old friend which by the way is a very important item. If I go I may be thrown out upon some of the quicksand but if so I am prepared to battle with them. It is to me a very important item to have something to stimulate me. I must have it; while here I have not. My life here is one of dull monotony, a sameness from morning 'til night. I do not know, or have no assurance, that I have made Dr. B a friend after all the diligence I have endeavored to practice. My mind is unsettled on the point. Dr. B will not advise me and I would not ask him to do so.

I wrote to Mollie F.T. [Thornton]

[FIELD HOSPITAL, ORANGE COURT HOUSE, ORANGE CO.]

SUNDAY, FEB. 28TH [18]64

This morning I went to Church. Mr. Martin preached from Titus 2.8. "For the grace of God that bringeth salvation hath appeared to all men."[sic][545]

I failed to gather anything from his sermon that I can remember. My mind seems to be cramped somehow or other—I have no recollection at all.

I walked out with Surg'n Hagy this evening and he advised me to go to Richmond. I came back to my tent and wrote to Dr. Q[uisenberry] a letter telling him I would come.

I went again to the Presbyterian Church and was asked out of my seat for a lady, so I left, being unable to find another.

Maj. [Lt. Col. John Singleton] Mosby sent in 72 prisoners to-day. He had a fight near Leesburg [Loudon Co.], and left 28 of the enemy on the field and brought these away with him. A very gallant affair.[546]

---

[545] The verse is Titus 2:11. I cannot locate a Presbyterian preacher named Martin in Orange Court House in this era, Scott, 172; there is a post chaplain, Joseph E. Martin, who may be the preacher in question, Pitts, 149.

[546] John Singleton Mosby (1833-1916), already identified, had formed Mosby's Rangers, the 43rd VA Cav. and developed quick-strike forces in this period. This skirmish took place at Dranesville (Fairfax Co.) as Mosby's Rangers intercepted a battalion of Californians commanded by a captain unidentified in the official records. The Californians had come from Vienna (Fairfax Co.) and were supposed to be scouting and perhaps raiding Leesburg, some 25 miles northwest from their base. According to Mosby's report, his surprise attack, featuring wild rebel yells, "surprised and confounded...the unsuspecting Yankees...with no time to form...leaving on the field at least 15 killed and a considerable number wounded, besides 70 prisoners in our hands, with all their horses, arms, and equipments." The Dranesville skirmish was related to a larger

There are rumours afloat in Camp to-day that the enemy is concentrating at Culpeper C.H. for a move upon us.[547]

[FIELD HOSPITAL, ORANGE COURT HOUSE, ORANGE CO.]

MONDAY, FEB 29 [18]64

To-day the Med: Ex Board met—The no. of men examined were smaller than usual.

I rec'd a letter from Cousin Bettie.

The weather is cloudy and betokens rain—God has sent the rain for our good, I doubt not. The rumour of movements of the enemy are true. The movements to-day have been with some activity. Gen. [R.E.] Lee came up on the Cars to-day—he looked like a hero as he is.

To-night I attended a lecture by the Rev. [Beverly T.] Lacy [chaplain- at-large of the ANV] on the the [sic] "Moral Character and religious influence of Gen. T.J. Jackson." I cannot express any thing but an admiration of the deeds of that truly great man. The recital of the great struggles of this army [the VA Bde] seemed to have produced the effect in my mind that made me live over again the glories of the past. Oh! I feel now only a small degree of the enthusiasm that must be felt in after days of the glory that fills the hearts of all who followed him in his superlative acts to repell [sic] the base invader. No pen will ever do justice to his name —

"How sleep the brave who sink to rest

---

affair involving Mosby and 2d MA Cav. and 16th NY Cav., both under command of Capt. J.S. Reed of 2d MA, who was killed. Mosby's report was accepted, and the Rangers' leader officially commended by Asst. Adjutant Gen. Maj. H.B. McClellan, by Gen. J.E.B. Stuart, and by Gen. R.E. Lee. The CSA officers also commended Capt. Reed of the Federals, Rept. No. 2, 21-22 February 1864, *OR* 33:159-60.

[547] Rumors were accurate. Federal "Kilcavalry" of some 3500 horsemen commanded by Gen. Hugh Judson Kilpatrick (1836-1881; already identified) were moving eastward from Culpeper, attempting a raid into Richmond, which was weakly held, to rescue Federal prisoners. A diversionary raid under Brig. Gen. George Armstrong Custer (1839-1876) started on the same day when he rode into Albemarle Co. Long, 469-70. Custer, born in Harrison City, Ohio, graduated last in his class from West Point three days prior to 1st Manassas (21 July 1861). "Headstrong, contemptuous of army regulations, and ever thirsty for glory," Custer made enemies in the ranks but won publicity and some respect from important leaders, especially Philip Sheridan, already identified. After War, Custer was courtmarialed for misconduct in Kansas during Indian fighting, but was reinstated by his sponsor Sheridan; in 1876, Custer's blundering tactics against the Sioux caused his own death and the devastation of his forces at the Battle of Little Big Horn. Dean E. Smith, "Custer," *Hist. Times.*

By all their country's wishes blest"[548]

I allmost [sic] regret now, and I know I shall bitterly, that I have ever consented to leave the field—Though in a position that is insignificant yet the mental satisfaction of seeing the glory and feeling the order and enthusiasm of being where danger raises excitement is preferable to being in a position of [illegible; sense is, inactivity of a job behind the front lines]

[FIELD HOSPITAL, ORANGE COURT HOUSE, ORANGE CO.]

TEUSDAY [SIC] ~~FEB~~MCH 1ST [1864]

This morning before I arose the the [sic] streets were alive with the marching columns of [Brig. Gen. Richard Heron] Anderson[549] and Heaths [sic; Henry Heth] Divisions.[550] Part of [Robert Emmett] Rode's [551] passed on too after eight [o'clock]. Rain is falling and the streets are muddy.

---

[548] I cannot find the author of this epitaph; it appears for a number of soldiers in War.

[549] Richard Heron Anderson (1821-1879) was born in Sumter, SC, grandson of a Revolutionary War hero of same name. Graduating from West Point in 1842, he also attended cavalry school in Carlisle, PA; he served in border wars and was brevetted 1st Lt. "for gallant and meritorious conduct" in Mexican War. When War came, he resigned Fed. commission and became Col. of 1st SC Inf. Veteran of defense of Pensacola, he also served in Peninsula Campaign (March-August 1862), 2nd Manassas [26 August-1 September 1862], Sharpsburg [17 September 1862], Fredericksburg [13 December 1862], Chancellorsville [3-4 May 1863], and Gettysburg (3-4 July 1863), winning accolades from R.E. Lee and James Longstreet and eventual promotion to Lt. Gen. His command was scattered after Sayler's Creek (6 April 1865), and he passed postbellum years in poverty in Beaufort, SC. Peggy Robbins, "Anderson," *Hist. Times.*

[550] Henry Heth (1825-1899) was already identified. In this action, the context is that he "remained embarrassed by his precipitate action" at Gettysburg (3 July 1863), which had cost heavy casualties in his division. In this phase of fighting, he showed competence as well as courage, and he later acquitted himself well at Bristow Station (Prince William Co., 14 October 1863), The Wilderness (5-7 May 1864), and in defense of Petersburg and surrounding area in final year of War. After War, he attempted a New South business career, "with indifferent success," and then served as an agent in Office of Indian Affairs. Resisting great illness and debility, he was able to complete his memoirs before his death in 1899, and these were published in 1974. John T. Hubbell, "Heth," *Hist. Times.*

[551] Robert Emmett Rodes (1829-1864) was a native of Lynchburg and a graduate of Virginia Military Institute (VMI). Like Heth, he was embarrassed by his own poor reconnoitering at Gettysburg (3 July 1863), and like Heth, his errors there cost his own division heavily. Prior to Gettysburg, he had been promoted to Maj. Gen. because of boldness and effectiveness at Chancellorsville (1-4 May 1863) and in other action; and after Gettysburg, he performed capably. A scholarly and often "modest" fellow, quiet until the moment of battle, Rodes had taught at VMI after a 9-year career as engineer for an Alabama railroad. "Modest, soldierly, an inspiring leader in

It seems to be true that the enemy ["kilcavalry" of Hugh Judson Kilpatrick] is moving—it is regarded a raid. Last evening a body of Cavalry [led by George Armstrong Custer] was near Charlottesville, but did not get possession of the place. Another party seemed to have crossed below Germanna [ford in Orange Co; this was likely Col. Ulric Dahlgren, 1842-1864, who was pressing toward Richmond]. The R. Road at Fredericksburg was broken [viz., the defenses of the line were broken and the line disrupted; this episode is not recorded in *Official Records*].

The day is a horrible one, unfit for marching.

I finished the story of (Mustang Gray) by Jerry Clemens [sic].[552] The pictures are deeply drawn sometimes and the book is very exciting. Those border ruffians live a [illegible adjective] life —.

[ORANGE COURT HOUSE, ORANGE CO.]

WENESDAY, MARCH 2ND [1864]

We have been striving all day to gather some news, but can't get any that can be reliable. One report says the enemy [Col. Ulric Dahlgren] has attacked the fortifications of Richmond—. ~~The~~ the departmental clerks met him and successfully protecting [sic] the place.[553] The troops that yesterday marched toward Liberty Mills [Orange Co.] returned to camp to-day.

---

attack, Rodes has been overshadowed by more colorful, but not more capable figures. Robert D. Hoffsommer , "Rodes," ibid..

[552] Diarist's punctuation. Jeremiah Clemens (1814-1865) of Huntsville, AL, was an eminent attorney, prominent politician who reversed himself more than once on the issues of southern secession and independence, and the author of at least four novels, each of which was reissused a number of times. Graduate of University of Alabama and the law school at Transylvania (KY) College, Clemens served in US Army in TX and then entered politics, holding local and state office in AL and then becoming US Senator. Also a newspaper publisher and editor in Memphis, Clemens was an elected member of AL secession convention, but he protested its action of secession. Reversing himself when War came, he accepted the chance to serve in CSA political offices and for three years supported the war effort; reversing again, in 1864 he abandoned CSA and supported Abraham Lincoln for reelection in presidential campaign of that year. During his hectic and controversial political career, he also wrote novels, including *Mustang Gray* (1857), a story of frontier action that was reissued during War and widely read. "Clemens," *Appleton's Cyclopaedia of American Biography*, vol. 1, eds., James Grant Wilson and John Fiske (New York: D. Appleton, 1888).

[553] The diarist is heavy with sarcasm, aimed both at Federal cav. , whom he despised, and at officials in Richmond, whom he resented. Richmond was then poorly defended, though not literally by "departmental clerks." The diarist consistently regards personnel of urban general-hospitals as privileged and even pampered; and he consistently regards staff officers and other

The enemy captured the Courts Martial at Fredericks Hall [Louisa Co.; on main rail line southeast of the field hospital].[554] There is but very little anticipation of apprehending the raiders —

I rec'd a letter from W.F. Faris [his Smyth Co. patron Dr. William F. Faris] to-night.

The day has been fine.

[ORANGE COURT HOUSE, ORANGE CO.]

THURSDAY, MCH 3D [1864]

The Ex: Board meet to-day.

The number of men were fewer than usual. Having but few men gave the illustrious members time to discuss the cases before them. There is a wide difference in the character of the two members from the other Hospital. [555] One gives his decision with an air of importance that would make you believe that it was final, absolute, and unrepeatable, the other makes it known by the most unostentatious manner—if you do not watch him or should be inattentive you would fail to get it without a direct question: the one passes his opinion with or arrives at his conclusion in a dogmatical way, while the other speaks as tenderly as a woman, and seems to conclude by weighing, impartially in his mind the merits of the case.

Col. [Robert Henry] Dungan called to-day of [sic] his return from home. He had but a very short while to stay. I had but a short Conversation with him.

---

clerical personnel working in Richmond and city centers as noncombatant "departmental clerks." In any case, Hugh Judson Kilpatrick had failed to mount the coordinated attack he wanted to bring off, and Col. Dahlgren was killed near Richmond in his largely unsupported part of that unsuccessful attack. Confederate troops examining Dahlgren's body found papers, evidently written by the col., suggesting a bold plan to assassinate Jefferson Davis and other CSA leaders as well as to free Federal prisoners in the capital. The authenticity of the papers remains in question, as does the amount of discretionary power and authorization that Dahlgren actually possessed . Long, 471; Patricia L. Faust, "Dahlgren Papers," *Hist. Times.*

[554] *Court martial* is usually an occasion, that is, the trial of a military person for allegedly violating army or navy law in wartime. The term, as used by diarist here, is more formally a *place* where such trials were held, specifically the courtroom for special courts martial involving at least three officers serving as judges. Long.; see also *Webster's 3d International Dict.*.

[555] Probably the general hospital in Gordonsville [also Orange Co.], superintended by Dr. B.M. Lebby. Gordonsville was on the main rail line [that became Chesapeake and Ohio R.R. line], and its general hospital was situated about ten miles southwest of the Orange Court House field hospital and very near the Louisa Co. line. Cunningham, 286; Scott, 115.

This evening I repaired to the [Orange Court House railroad] depot to hear from the enemy [troops and citizens went to the railroad depot to hear official news dispatches and also to hear rumors from the train crews taking a break and any soldier passengers at table]. But failed to hear any thing authentic. Everybody is grasping for rumour, and the most erroneous are seized upon with avidity and scattered like thistle-down before the wind. One report had it that the raiders were within 7 or 8 miles of the C.H. [Courthouse] and that our infantry were closing in upon them. The truth of the matter is about as follows:

The Yankees under [Gen. Hugh Judson] Kilpatrick made a demonstration at Richmond and were repulsed by the departmental Battl [battalion], and afterwards attacked by Gen: W[ade] Hampton, who captured nearly 200 of their numbers. After leaving Richmond, the peninsula was the next point to gain, where probably the whole Yankee force is now safely resting. Indications here seem good however for a movement of some kind. Heath's [Henry Heth] Div: is off on the [railroad] Cars somewhere.[556]

We hear that four of the department clerks were killed, and 15 wounded. Among the killed is Mr. Elroy, the chief clk [clerk] of Treas[ury] Dept. [557]

---

[556] By 1 March Hugh Judson Kilpatrick had not gotten close enough to Richmond to coordinate his planned attack with Col. Ulric Dahlgren; thus Kilpatrick never attacked, and moved toward the peninsula, as the diarist had heard. On the following day, 2 March, Col. Dahlgren was trapped in an ambush at Mantapike Hill (King and Queen Co.] between the courthouses of King and Queen Co. and King William Co. His ambushers were from Fitzhugh Lee's Cav., and were commanded in the field by Capt. E.C. Fox and Lt. James Pollard. General Wade Hampton did catch up with and attack and capture some of the Dahlgren troops on their retreat; Hampton's official estimate for the engagement of 2 March 7 miles outside of Richmond is that he captured 75 men. Henry Heth's troops were ordered to ride to Richmond on horseback, not railroad, and Gen. R.E. Lee sent word, "halt them if not needed" [as they were not; they were halted and returned to Orange Co]. Official records put the men captured at "more than 100," but not 200, and Long finds evidence that the figure of 100 is accurate; the main casualty was Col. Dahlgren himself, something not known to President Lincoln until the col.'s father, Admiral John A. Dahlgren inquired after his son's remains in order to arrange a proper military burial. Long also notes that the Gen. Kilpatrick's attack, despite the fear and loathing inspired by his "kilcavalry," essentially "sputtered out...through lack of surprise, lack of force, and, finally, lack of drive to see it through." In nearby Albemarle Co., seat of Mr. Jefferson's university, Col. George Armstrong Custer's raids were "fairly successful," and, as the diarist noted, Custer's raiders escaped largely unscathed. Gen. R.E. Lee reported movement of Fed. cav., and prepared himself for what became the Battle of the Wilderness. O.R., Ser. I, 33:1188-1255; Long, 471-72.

[557] I cannot confirm the name or rank of anyone named Elroy killed in defense of Richmond. I have looked in the VA. regimental histories and in the O.R.

[ORANGE COURT HOUSE, ORANGE CO.]

FRIDAY, MCH. 4 [18]64

This has been a lovely day.

News came this evening that the Yankee Brig. Gen. Dhalgreen [sic][558] was killed below Richmond [and] a large number of his force killed by Gen. Fitz Lee. [Railroad] Cars [of troops called up temporarily for defense of capital] are expected up from Richmond this evening.

L.Y. Cooper returned from sick leave.[559]

There is a great dearth of news.

I completed and sent up Monthly report of sick & wounded, and Return of Med: Officers. It shows 254 rec'd and 23 deaths.

[ORANGE COURT HOUSE, ORANGE CO.]

SATURDAY, MCH. 5[18]64

This evening the [railroad] cars came through from Richmond. Crowded with soldiers returning to the Army. The papers give a full account of the late raid and confirm the report that the enemy had been attacked in Prince William Co. and routed. It was Col. [Ulric][560] and [not] Gen. [sic; Admiral John Adolph

---

[558] John Adolph Bernard Dahlgren (1809-1870) was not a Brig. Gen., but an Admiral. Son of Swedish consul to US in Philadelphia, Dahlgren grew up in Philadelphia, joined navy without commission and then was commissioned in 1842. He served 15 years at Washington Naval Yard as director of ordnance. He invented and developed several ordnance pieces, most notably the Dahlgren Gun, a howitzer used by both sides during Civil War. When War came, he volunteered for sea duty and his son Ulric Dahlgren (1842-1864) joined staff of Maj. Gen. Franz Sigl, Army of Potomac. Admiral Dahlgren commanded South Atlantic Blockade and was chiefly involved in efforts to seal the harbors of Charleston and Savannah. After War, he served in Pacific and then returned to his old command at Washington Navy Yard. Emory M. Thomas, "Dahlgren," *Hist. Times.*

[559] L.Y. Cooper (b. 1830; death date unknown) was apparently from Washington Co., occupation unknown. At age 32 he enlisted at Goodson (present-day Bristol) for three years in Co. A, Goodson Rifle Guards under command of John F. Terry. Historian Thomas M. Rankin says: "6'0", blue eyes, black hair, fair complex [sic]." Sick at hospital in April 1862, he returned to duty the following month until 2 January 1863, at which time he joined 2nd Corps ANV field hospital as nurse, thus serving with Apperson at Orange Court House until end of December 1864. His sick furlough 2 February—4 March 1864 is confirmed by Rankin. No further records after December 1864. Idem, *37th VA Inf.*, Virginia Regimental Histories Series, ed. Harold E. Howard (Lynchburg: H.E. Howard, 1987), 106.

[560] Ulric Dahlgren (1842-1864), son of the admiral, was born in Neshaminy, PA and studied law and civil engineering. When War came he joined the staff of XI Corps of Army of Potomac, and he also served in staff of Maj. Gens. Ambrose E. Burnside, Joseph Hooker, and George C. Meade. However, he prefered line duty, especially with quick-strike cavalry, and according to

Bernard] Dahlgren that was killed. Upon his person were found some papers disclosing the force and the atrocious intent of the raid. Also, his orders to his men, the manner of proceeding and his plan of operation. The City of Richmond was to be burned, the prisoners liberated, and the President [Jefferson Davis] and the Cabinet killed. Well Dhalgren [sic] has issued his last orders.

Many rumours of andvance [sic; advance] of the enemy.

Dr. Sydnor returned to-day.

A carpet bag belonging to a bro[ther] of Lt. [John] Bishop[561] [Smyth Blues] was handed me at the depot to-dlay by a member of Co. [D?] to be kept 'till called for.

We had a very interesting case of diptheria in hosp't to-day. The patient came in yester-day. His throat eventually showed some enlargement. To-day the organs of respiration seemed to be impeded in their action so much so as to require an operation to prevent asphyxia.[562]

Dr. Wilkerson opened the trachea[563] but there was not life or sensibility enough in the parts to produce any evidence that it would be of any use. No

---

Edwarrd G. Longacre "often volunteered for hazardous duty." The plan to raid Richmond in 1864 was not his first such proposal, as he had tried unsuccessfully to get Maj. Gen. Hooker to let him attempt a cavalry raid of the CSA capital in May 1863. It was he who captured a CSA courier in summer of 1863 and learned that R.E. Lee could expect no reinforcements for the invasion of PA, intelligence that "supposedly stiffened Meade's resolve to remain at Gettysburg instead of falling back into Maryland." Joining the "Kilcavalry," his quick-strike raid remains enigmatic, shrouded in confusion and controversy, since he had earlier attempted and failed to gain official sanction for such a raid. The Dahlgren Papers may have been his own invention, or perhaps an invention of CSA troops—or they may have been authentic. The CSA considered them authentic, and he was buried in an unmarked grave, with the southern press labeling him a war criminal. Richmond-area Unionists later unearthed his body and re-interred him in Philadelphia. Edward G. Longacre, "Dahlgren," and Patricia L. Faust, "Dahlgren Papers," in *Hist. Times*.

561 John J. Bishop (birth date unknown, died 30 October 1862) was a cooper from Smyth Co. who joined the original Smyth Blues, which became Co. D, 4th VA Inf. "Ordnance Sgt. at muster; promoted to 2nd Lt., Apr. 15 1962, and to 1st Lt., Aug. 29, 1862; wounded and captured, Aug. 30, 1862, at Second Manassas; exchanged Oct. 8, 1862; died Oct. 30 1862 at Aldie [Loudon Co. field hospital] from effects of wound." Robertson, *4th VA. Inf.*, 40. There are several Smyth Co. soldiers named Bishop who served, but this is the only officer confirmed also by Smyth, *Smyth Co.*, ed. Presgraves.

562 "Asphyxia....condition caused by insufficient intake of oxygen." *Taber's*.

563 "Trachea (from Gk. *tracheia*, rough)...A cylindrical cartilaginous tube, 4 1/2 in. (11.3 cm) long, from the larynx to the bronchial tubes. It extends from the 6th cervical to the 5th dorsal vertebra, where it divides at a point called the carina into two bronchi, one leading to each lung...Syn: *windpipe*." Cutting into trachea could restore breathing in asphyxia in extreme cases,

coughing symptoms of irritation was produced. Something prevented a free impress [old style, *intake*] and express of wind. The patient died in a few hours afterwards. Post mort[em] revealed the posterior nares and soft palate, Larynx and appurtenant of the trachea entirely covered with pseudo membrane. The mucous membrane was whitish with red blotches.[564]

I got a letter from Dr. Faris by to-day's Mail.

[ORANGE COURT HOUSE, ORANGE CO.]

SUNDAY, MARCH 6TH, [18]64

This morning I attend[ed] divine service at the presbyterian church. Rev: Dr [Beverly T.] Lacy [chaplain of ANV 2d Corps] preached from the parable of the rich man and Lazarus. It was I think one of the best sermons I ever heard him preach. Delineating the character of the rich man as possessing every thing the craving heart of man could wish and the poor man as having nothing but a Christian fortitude and hope. He drew a beautiful picture of the life of both and ask [sic]: which will you choose?—then turning away and directing the attention of the audience to the end—Lazarus dying, his body left to be thrown in a receptacle for the pauper whose life is extinct, his soul is bourne away by angels on willing wings to the bosom of Abraham, the rich man died and *was buried*, all the pageantry of wealth and nobility followed his spiritless body to the grave but look beyond—he Cries [sic] for one drop of water to cool his parched lips.

In the outset of his discourse he said of the grandeur of these parables that they surpassed everything that has been written, this was the grandest, the highest of all—As a biography it was complete—in one short passage a picture of life is drawn that surpassed what volume[s] had striven to do. Not only was

---

and cutting in could also be exploratory to see if repair work could be done on carina or bronchi. *Taber's.* The damage here obviously reached the limits of 19th cent. hospital surgery.

564 "Tracheitis...An inflammation of the trachea. It may be acute or chronic and may be associated with bronchitis and laryngitis." Note also "acute airway obstruction...due to presence of copious, thick, and purulent secretions. Administer humidifed oxygen as prescribed and suction as necessary to remove secretions. Administer prescribed antibiotic therapy. Be prepared for emergency endotracheal intubation or tracheostomy if airway obstruction persists...." *Taber's.* As Cunningham notes, such procedures as antibiotic treatment, humidified oxygen, suction, and endotracheal intubation were not then available among surgeon's techniques in Civil War. Cunningham, 218-46.

the existance [sic] here given, but the veil was thrown back and we could behold in the future the glory or misery of eternity.[565]

He said in the course of his sermon that there were but three chances that the passions of man led him—wealth, power, and luxury—The course of earthly ambition—To hoard the silver dross of earth, to wield the scepter and hold sway over the suppliant, or please the taste with viands of luxury—were the highest of earth's aspirations.

But it availeth nothing,—Wealth cannot purchase exemption from the hand of death, power cannot repel it, and the halls of luxury are ever open to his entrance.

The Rev. Dr. [J.L.] Burrows preaches to-night.[566]

I was at the depot [Orange Court House railway station][567] and was told by Mr. [James] Chapman [onetime landlord to the diarist and occasional host to

---

565 Text is Luke 16:19-31, a parable told by Jesus. Unlike other parables told by Jesus, there is a specific name attached to a character, viz., *Lazarus.* Because it seems to be the only parable Jesus told in which a real name is given one of the characters, "there was an idea in early times that it [was] a story from real life," according to Lockyear, "Lazarus," *All the Men of the Bible.* However, 20th century biblical scholars follow Alexander Jones's flat statement, "[the Lazarus] parable [is] a story form without reference to a historical personage," idem, ed., *The Jerusalem Bible,* 121 ff. For the famous chaplain Beverly T. Lacy, a minister of the 19th century, Lazarus probably was a historical personage actually known to Jesus, and that appears to be the way that he handled this discussion. The story of Lazarus the poor man and his treatment in Heaven compared to that of a haughty rich man was then popular in Virginia among Protestant ministers, and interpretations were often available in tracts. Although Lacy was Presbyterian, it is possible that this service was conducted at St. Thomas' Episcopal Church in Orange Court House, for historian W.W. Scott, a CSA veteran of the 13th VA Inf.[Co. A, originally Montpelier Guards], describes that church as being used most frequently for services for the CSA officers, including the late Gen. T.J. Jackson, famously a Presbyterian. If not St. Thomas' Church, then the site was probably the builidng one-half mile northeast of Gordonsville called Presbyterian Church of the Blind Preacher (James Waddel). Scott, 47, 172, appendices. Pitts notes that the CSA commanders, especially R.E. Lee, did not approve narrowly sectarian services and often arranged for ministers of different sects to serve together in worship services, in his example, a Baptist and a Methodist officiating before a Presbyterian preached a sermon in an Episcopal church. On the sermon, see Pitts, who notes that CSA preachers often treated of the theme of salvation predicated on humility to accept grace—and the great difficulties of the wealthy so to humble themselves, idem, 91-119.

566 This preaching was likely in the St. Thomas' Church building; although evening preaching and singing sometimes occurred in log cabins built at campsites, Scott, 47, 172; Pitts, 109. Dr. W.G. Bean identifies him as "eminent pastor of the First Baptist Church, Richmond, Virginia." Bean, notes. He is identified by Pitts as "Evangelist" chaplain, ANV, 140. Given the evangelical nature of Baptists in that era, and Rev. Burrows's relationship both with Professor Lewis Minor Coleman and with the artillery of ANV, The Rev. Dr. J.L. Burrows, pastor of First Baptist Church, Richmond, VA, and the Rev. Dr. J.L. Burrows, Evangelist Chaplain of ANV, seems to be one and the ilk.

him] that he had news from Richmond that Beast Butler had been removed and prisoners were being exchanged—good.[568]

I attended services [conducted by the Rev. Dr. J.L. Burrows] at night. The house was filled to overflowing, and I must say to the honour of the Church going portion of our army I have never seen a more attentive or interested an audience [his phrasing].

The text was Job 20–11; "His bones are full of the sin of his youth."[569]

It is not our fortune to hear many such sermons in the course of our lives, ever.

The discourse was principally for the youth of the country.

In the commencement [introductory part of sermon] he [Burrows] selected two characters and by comparison he held them up to his hearers—one had led a temperate, correct and useful life and when he became aged in years he was a man in every part—form erect, step steady, eye undimmed, will clear, and intellect perfect —

The other[,] a debauche [sic], had run his race and was bowed down by the infirmities of [old age and degenerative illnesses] by the time [he] arrived at the age of 30:

Then he discussed, "The evil Consequences of misspent Youth"—physically, mentally[,] socially and spiritually. Physically the drunkard and reveller were pictured in the most forcible language.

Mentally—the drone and careless—In this connection he said "there were men who had not mind enough to regret their own deficiencies".

Socially—the man who lost sight of those finer feelings of our nature and only courted the company of the gay and vicious, spent their time rioting and

---

[567] The depot was built by Charlottesville and Rapidan Railroad Co. and leased by the Chesapeake and Ohio Railroad. Scott, 132.

[568] Benjamin Franklin Butler (1818-1893), already identified, was called "Beast" because of the alleged harshness of his military rule over New Orleans as military governor of LA, May - December 1862; his ruling that southern women who insulted northern troops were to be treated as prostitutes was especially resented. He was also called "Spoons" because of alleged theft of civilian property. From January 1863 to November 1864, Butler served as Gen. of the Army of the James, and briefly permitted exchanges of prisoners; but Maj. Gen. US Grant subsequently stopped all exchanges. See John D. Kallman, "Butler," *Hist. Times.*; Long, sv. Lincoln and Grant both understood that tending to Federal prisoners would sap CSA resources and make one more economic reason for the CSA to surrender. The diarist seems to imply that it was Beast Butler's fault that prisoners were not exchanged; actually he permitted and even encouraged such exchanges; the policy was Lincoln's, implemented by Grant.

[569] Job 20:11: "His bones are full of the sin of his youth, which shall lie down with him in the dust." (KJV).

debauching: and the young lady who was peevish, morose, and slatternly in her manner, and for the want of finer cultivation in youth neglected the growth of these qualities was illy[570] fitted for the companion, wife, and mother —

Then Spiritually of course we cannot go [depart] from the preordaining. He said the habits must be formed in youth or the chance against safety grew daily. If the susceptibility of the heart becomes dormant, hard will it be to resuscitate it. Habits formed and the future career of man is marked out and his destiny is plain—Can the Ethiopian change his skin or the leopard his spots? —

He closed by an allusion to the responsibility of the position held by the Youth of our country—They are the prop and stay of our course—by them it must be debased or aggrandised.

Dr. [J.L.] Burrows delivered an address on the life and character of Col. [Lewis Minor] Coleman[571] who died near Guiney [Depot Station in field hospital of Caroline Co.] last winter from a wound rec'd at Fredericksburg—a prof. [of Latin] at University of Va.

[FIELD HOSPITAL, ORANGE COURT HOUSE, ORANGE CO.]

MONDAY, MCH 7TH 1864

Nothing outside of the meeting of the Med: Ex: Bd. More men were before it than usual.

I wrote to Miss Mollie [Thornton] —

[FIELD HOSPITAL, ORANGE COURT HOUSE, ORANGE CO.]

TUESDAY, MCH. 8, 1864

This morning is very dark and rainy.

---

570 This adverb form of ill is actually correct, according to *Fowler's*, "-ly," s.v.

571 Lewis Minor Coleman (1827-1863) was Lt. Col. of artillery in charge of 1st VA Arty. at Battle of Fredericksburg. Born in Hanover Co., he married Mary Amber Coleman, and they had three children. Graduating from University of Virginia in 1846, he became Prof. of Latin there and also Principal of Hanover Academy. When War came, he enrolled as Capt. of Arty. for Morris Battery at Centreville [Fairfax Co.]. Sick two mos. in fall 1861, when he returned to unit, he was not elected officer in reorganized battery. He became in 1862 Maj. of Arty. , line position, 1st Arty., and then was promoted to Lt. Col. of Arty. as Battle of Fredericksburg began (13 December 1862). Gregory J. Macaluso, *Morris, Orange, and King William Artillery*, VA Regimental Histories Ser. (Lynchburg: H.E. Howard, 1991) 83. Wounded severely while moving howitzer guns in to position at Fredericksburg, he was commended by both Gen. T.J. Jackson and Gen. R.E. Lee: Lee, "Report on Fredericksburg," *OR*, Ser. 1, 21:556; Jackson, "Report on Fredericksburg," *OR*, Ser. 1, 21:633. He never recovered, and died in field hospital at Caroline Co., 21 March 1863.

This evening I attended the Lecture of Dr. [J.L.] Burrows. As is everything that comes from him it was very fine. The Character of Col: Lewis Minor Coleman was truly an admirable one. Graduating at the University of Virginia with the highest honours of his class at the age of 17, he went home with his mind well stuffed with knowledge from the Store-house of Wisdom, he sought forgiveness of his sins and united himself with the Church. He then turned his attention to teaching—first in a school in Hanover Co., then a professor at [University of Virginia] Charlottesville. When the war broke out he raised a Company of Artillery [Morris Batty] and was afterward made Lt. Col. [of 1st VA Arty] at Fred~ [Fredericksburg] on the 13th day of Apl [1863] he rec'd a wound in the leg from which he died [sic; he was wounded on 13 December 1862 and died in hospital in March of 1863].

Having lived a pure, ordered, Christian life, he passed from Earth away with a perfect victory over the grave. I could but think it was sweet to die with such a Christian fortitude and religious hope—so sure of the Crown beyond the grave. His death was the greatest victory of life: Had death been denied him, he would have lived in vain.

The only thing I could propose as an objection to the lecture was His deeds were all good deeds and in thinking of them they make us incredulous.

[FIELD HOSPITAL, ORANGE COURT HOUSE, ORANGE CO.]

WENDESDAY [SIC] MCH 9 [18]64

This is a beautiful morning.

To-day I had the pleasure of meeting apparently, a very excellent lady—a Mrs Walker, from Ala., whose son is sick in this [field] Hosp't. I showed her wehre her son was and withdrew—Afterward I went back, offered her my services, and went to Mr. Hiden's[572] with her. She thanked me most kindly. Afterwards I had conversation with her—she is intelligent, amiable, and a fine conversationist [sic]. She found her son doing well—will stay a few days and return.

---

[572] Possibly James C. Hiden, a minister who had a farm and a home in nearby Gordonsville; he often wrote for the *Gordonsville Gazette*, and was prominent socially. He also served as chaplain for the army post at University of Virginia. Scott, 129, 276; Pitts, 146.

To-night I met Jno. F. Payne [John Foster Payne][573] on the Street and asked him to call at my office which he did. Old distastes in my memory are growing dim. He seemed to enjoy himself while he staid.

[FIELD HOSPITAL, ORANGE COURT HOUSE, ORANGE CO.]

THURSDAY, MCH: 10 [18]64

The day has been a very stormy one. Rain falling in torrents and the wind sweeping in gusts. The examining board met. A large no. of Cases were disposed of. I have been reading to-day Shakespeare's "Much ado about nothing."[574] Spent the evening at "Aunt K" [Keziah Shepherd, still serving as hostess for such evenings in Orange Court House]—Dr. Hagy & Dr. Wilk[erson] "Seth" & my self at euchre[575]

[FIELD HOSPITAL, ORANGE COURT HOUSE, ORANGE CO.]

FRIDAY, MCH. 11— [1864]

Nothing to-day —

[FIELD HOSPITAL, ORANGE COURT HOUSE, ORANGE CO.]

SATURDAY, MCH. 12: [1864]

Mrs. Walker's son is worse—she moved him up to Mr. [the Rev. Dr. James C.] Hiden's. I dressed to visit some ladies at Maj. [Welles Joseph] Hawks'[576] but did not go—Got 2 letters by Mail—One from my friend Mrs. [Mary] Tomlin,

---

[573] John Foster Payne [no data on birth or death dates] was probably from Gordonsville [Orange Co]. He enlisted late in April 1862 as Pvt. infantryman in Gordonsville with Fort Loudon Guards, who became, with a Winchester unit, Co. H of 13th VA Inf., which was mostly Orange Co. soldiers. Hospitalized often, he could have met Apperson in a field hospital in Spotsylvania, where the "old distastes" may have started. Not long after this diary entry, he was captured and imprisoned in Elmira, NY at Point Lookout, until transfered for exchange 22 March 1865; weak and ill on dismissal from Federal prison, he was hospitalized in Richmond; and then there are no further records. Riggs, *13th VA Inf.*, 133.

[574] William Shakespeare. *Much Ado about Nothing.* 1598 but "stayed"; widely performed from 1607. Catalogue, *Ency. Brittan.*

[575] See earlier description of game of chance.

[576] Hawks, already identified, was here acting as sustenance commissary for ANV 2d Corps. See R.E. Lee, report, O.R., Ser. 1, vol. 33, 1111. On this tour, Maj. Hawks was trying to buy dairy cattle from VA farmers in Valley, and there were great difficulties in getting the farmers to accept CSA money, or even to admit that they in fact owned some dairy cattle.

another from Miss Mollie [Thornton]. Both were interesting—the latter particularly so.

[FIELD HOSPITAL, ORANGE COURTHOUSE, ORANGE CO.]

SUNDAY, MCH 13, [18]64

This morning I attended church at the Episcopalian Church [St. Thomas's]. Bishop [John] Johns preach[ed] from the Prov: 14-32: "The ~~Righteous~~ Wicked is driven away by his wickedness, but the righteous hath hope in his death".[576]

After dinner I distributed quite a number of religious papers in the wards—Mr. [Beverly T.] Lacy sent them over this morning—this evening I

---

[576] Proverbs 14:32: "The wicked is driven away in his wickedness: but the righteous hath hope in his death." King James trans. The Rt. Rev. John Johns, bishop of the Episcopal Church in VA already identified, was here taking an important step in his career. Always "low church," that is, relatively uninterested in traditional Anglican rituals, he was evangelical, that is, vigorously engaged in spreading a message of salvation by grace on an individual basis; and he was pietistic, that is, emphasizing a very personal spiritual relationship between God manifest in Jesus Christ and the believer. The VA Protestant Episcopal Church in the tidewater, southside, and older areas of the piedmont—such as Orange Court House—tended toward "high church," that is, emphasizing traditional Anglican rituals and a much more formalistic approach to collective salvation based on sacraments administered through appointed priests in a hierarchy. The highlands and valley Episcopal churches, fewer in number, smaller in size, and possessing less wealth in land and slaves, tended toward the evangelical and pietistic, and Bishop Johns was popular with them. The diarist, reflecting his adoptive highlands culture more than his native settled-piedmont culture, is pietistic and evangelical; and he seems to respond to Bishop Johns with some interest and enthusiasm. These issues of dispute inside the Episcopal Church were carried over into the ANV, where for instance the Rev. William Nelson Pendleton, an ordained minister but also an officer in charge of artillery, represented vigorously the high church and ritualistic patterns of old Anglicanism and was very opposed to Bishop Johns' s evangelism and pietism. Around 1864, Bishop Johns introduced a new element of controversy, when he began preaching vigorously against slavery and also began preaching that the CSA cause, to the extent that it was involved in slavery, was morally wrong. These high church/low church disputes were thus complicated by the overwhelming moral issue of slavery and sudden doubts about the righteousness of the CSA effort. The diarist, always enthusiastic about states rights and slavery, is hearing on this occasion one of Bishop Johns's sermons that indicts slavery is unrighteous and wicked. It is among other things interesting that the diarist seems to accept the message. See Jon W. Wakelyn, "Episcopal Church," *Encyclopedia of the Confederacy*, ed., Richard N. Current (New York: Simon & Schuster, ca. 1993).; see also Susan Pendleton Lee, *Memoirs of William Nelson Pendleton* (1893. Reprint ed.; Harrisonburg, VA: Sprinke, 1991); and R. Miller and J. Wakelyn, ed., *Catholics in the Old South: Essays on Church and Culture* (Macon, GA: Mercer University Press, 1999).

attended the Episcopal church again and heard from: "Without God in this world" [.] A colection [sic] was taken up by the [St. Thomas] church for a contribution for the benefit in the lower end of the [Orange] Co.[577]

[Maj. John Singleton] Mosby sent in some 20 prisoners to-day.

Furloughs have been suspended—We may look for moving very soon —

~~Attended church this evening—did not think much of the sermon~~[578]

[FIELD HOSPITAL, ORANGE COURT HOUSE, ORANGE CO.]

~~TUESDAY~~ MONDAY, MCH 14 [1864]

Ex: Board met to-day. Had a larger number of cases than usual, mostly for furlough.

No news—Attended church in afternoon

[FIELD HOSPITAL, ORANGE COURT HOUSE, ORANGE CO.]

~~WEDNESDAY~~ TUESDAY MCH 15 [1864]

I rode down to Gen. [Richard Stoddert] Ewell's HdQers [of 2d Corps, ANV] to-day on business for Dr. [Hunter Holmes] McGuire. Called at Col. [Robert Henry] Dungan's quarters and took dinner with him. I enjoy[ed] the call very much. He is a meritorious man. I returned after dark while very tired and cold. Got a letter from Dr. Quisenberry.

[FIELD HOSPITAL, ORANGE COURT HOUSE, ORANGE CO.]

WEDNESDAY, MCH 16 [1864]

To-day I and Dr. Sid [Sydnor] called on the young ladies at Capt. [John] Glaize's quarters [QM for 2nd VA. Inf.]. Found them very interesting. Miss Schultz is tall, spare-made lady[.] Miss [Margaret] Miller is less in stature by

---

577 The War was bringing hardship to the lower end of Orange Co. The original Orange Humane Society, an eleemosinary institution started with private funds and maintained by a public levy, once funded schools and otherwise helped the poor; but by this phase of the War, the funds were depleted, and churches were feeding and clothing and sheltering the indigent. Scott, 138-43.

578 The diarist has scratched through the entry: This sermon of the evening, of which he "did not think much," was *not* delivered by Bishop Johns; usually the diarist states his objection to sermons he dislikes, but unfortunately for us does not do so here.

[sic; but] more fleshy—dark complexion[,] black hair and eyes[579] From what I could judge from her [Margaret Miller's] disposition, I took her to be a splendid young lady. Miss [Elizabeth] Baylor I did not see enough of to pass any opinion. I am supposed to ride with her to-morrow.

It is at some sacrifice too that I do so. I have no horse and the examining board meets. I sent an application to Surgn. Gen. [LaFayette Guild] for transfer [to Richmond][580]

[FIELD HOSPITAL, ORANGE COURT HOUSE, ORANGE CO.]

THURSDAY, MCH 17– [1864]

I engaged Dr. Drane to write [Apperson's official reports to Examining Board] for me to-day and borrowed Dr. Wilkerson's horse, found Miss [Elizabeth] Baylor at the [Orange Court House] depot [built by Charlottesville and Rapidan Railroad and leased by Chesapeake and Ohio Railroad]. Was introduced to Mrs. Hall—a beautiful lady. The ride with Miss B. was an interesting one. Perhaps because of the many compliments that passed—I must say that I am suspicious of her being quite a coquette [diarist's italics], and for once I have feigned a perfect resignation to her fascinations. She may fool me.

I returned home about noon. Wrote to Miss Mollie T[hornton].

[FIELD HOSPITAL, ORANGE COURT HOUSE, ORANGE CO.]

FRIDAY, MCH 18– [1864]

This morning I rec'd a note from Miss Lizze Baylor inviting me to go to Montpelier to-day.[581] I answered by saying that I was not positive about going;

---

[579] Although otherwise unidentified, Schultz and Margaret [Maggie] Miller are said by Prof. W.G. Bean to be "ladies whom Apperson had previously met in Orange Court House." Bean, notes.

[580] He is still attempting to attend lectures at Medical College of Virginia; and he is still attempting to escape the hardships of field hospital line-work in Richard Stoddert Ewell's Valley Campaign. Note that his immediate supervisor Dr. Harvey Black still does not offer his support for the transfer; and note also that the diarist has had no furlough of significant length since the 2d Corps was reorganized more than a year ago.

[581] This mansion, "[a]bout four miles from Orange Court House," was once home of James Madison. The original structure dates to 1760, and its "plain rectangular structure, with a hall running through the centre having two rooms on each side...has been so merged in the grander house that it can not now be differentiated from it. The chief enlargements were made in 1809, after designs by William Thornton, architect of the Capitol at Washington; and [Benjamin] Latrobe lent his assistance in further improvements, which included the addition of the wings.... The beautifully terraced garden laid out in the form of a horseshoe was Madison's own plan." It

but soon fixed up matters and started. The wind blew furiously; and I did not think the ladies would go. When I arrived I found a house full. The ladies seemed inclined to go and away we started—Surgn. Hinkle was escort to Miss Maggie Miller and myself to Miss [Elizabeth] Baylor. The wind howled and whistled and swept the hills about us but on we went. We visited the classic place—the last resting place of one [James Madison] who ruled when peace and prosperity were the pride of the western continent. But now the spot he once trod bears the impress of armed men gathered to battle for the freedom that was the boast in the days of Madison.

After visiting the cemetary and graves we returned—The wind had lulled and only now and then a gust played around us.

My ride this evening [afternoon] is one I still remember. The impressions made are not to be easily obliterated. It is seldom—very seldom—I give way to what I regard a whimsical notion of yielding to the flattery of women, but I must admit I did so to-day, and perhaps engaged in it more or less myself—'twas unavoidable on my part.

I returned about 7 o'clock and retired.

[FIELD HOSPITAL, ORANGE COURT HOUSE, ORANGE CO.]

SATURDAY, MCH 19– [1864]

Nothing to-day—The weather is good—I called on Mrs. Walker this evening—Her son has been very ill—Got a letter from Dr. [William] Faris asking me to do something for a young man—I fear I cannot help him

Called on Miss Mollie Graves and spent an hour.

[FIELD HOSPITAL, ORANGE COURT HOUSE, ORANGE CO.]

SUNDAY, MCH. 20– [1864]

Went to church this morning [probably at St Thomas]. Mr. [Richard Terrell] Davis, a Methodist [sic] elder, preached, but I cannot eulogize the sermon.[582]

---

stands on what once were some five thousand acres "patented by Ambrose Madison and Thomas Chew in 1723." Scott, 208-9.

[582] The preacher is surely not Methodist, but the Episcopalian Richard Terrell Davis, chaplain to 6th VA Cav. and then stationed at Orange Court House with the rest of 2nd Corps of ANV. Davis (1830-1892) was born in Charlottesville and attended University of Virginia, attaining master's degree; he then earned divinity degree at Virginia Theological Seminary and was ordained Episopal priest. He was appointed chaplain to 6th Cav, an outfit that included

When I returned to my Qtrs, I found Col. Beck of 44th GA. Regt. After dinner we called on Miss [Mollie] Graves and spent an hour. Col. B is a very interesting man, intelligent and refined. He spent the evening with me. When we parted he asked me to write him, which I think I shall do. I did not go to church at night.

[FIELD HOSPITAL, ORANGE COURT HOUSE, ORANGE CO.]

MONDAY, MCH 21– [1864]

The examining Bd. met but very little business was done, owing to orders issued from the HdQters of the army.

R. Roads in East N.C. are so much crowded that no travel is allowed.

The board went over to see the Med. Director [Hunter Holmes McGuire].

I visited Capt. [John] Galize and had a very delightful time with the girls. Miss [Margaret] Miller is really a sweet girl. Miss [Elizabeth] Baylor is truly fantastic; and Miss Schultz I think is competent to rule as she will.

[FIELD HOSPITAL, ORANGE COURT HOUSE, ORANGE CO.]

TUESDAY, MCH 22 [18]64

The board met again to-day.

Portion of the order was not applicable to the action of this Board. [583] Been snowing some.

I wrote a note to Mrs. F[aris]. Also one to Dr. F[aris] in answer to one I got from him in regard [to] young [John F.] Bonham. I am sorry I cannot now get a place in a Camp for [Bonham]. He may [italics] think I have not tried. [584]

---

companies stretching from Wise Co. in far southwest highlands to Loudon Co. in northern central piedmont. He was absent on surgeon's certificate for sick leave for 30 days at end of 1863. He served the entire War on horseback alongside his brother Eugene Davis (1822-1894) and was said by John L. Ogle to be "at the head of the regiment in every battle." After War, he became rector of St. James Episcopal Church, Leesburg (Loudon Co.), from 1866-1892. Doctor of Divinity, possibly honorary, from Washington & Lee College, 1877. Buried in Union Cem., Leesburg. Musick, *6th VA Cav.*, 109; Pitts, 142.

[583] There were several efforts in 1863, 1864, and 1865 to bring in more soldiers for the CSA—and to keep currently enlisted soldiers in the CSA—by making it very hard to leave despite illness or injury and by making it very hard to be exempt for those reasons. The diarist probably refers to this order of 10 December 1863 that eliminated many diseases as grounds for medical exemption or dismissal under a new general principle: When a conscript is found equal to, or in the performance of the active duties of the various occupations of civil life, he is able to discharge the duties of a soldier." Quoted, Cunningham, 163-65.

[FIELD HOSPITAL, ORANGE COURT HOUSE, ORANGE CO.]

WEDNESDAY, MCH 23 [18]64

Snow fell last night about 12 inches or more. To-day we had some rare fun balling [throwing snow balls]. Surgn. Newton caught it on himself at the hands of a big burly Paddy [Irishman].

I called on Miss [Mary Camden] Allen and find her very interesting.

The ladies were in this morning. I wrote a letter to Nat. [brother Cincinnatus of 7th VA Inf.]—and one to Cousin Bettie.

[FIELD HOSPITAL, ORANGE COURT HOUSE, ORANGE CO.]

THURSDAY MCH: 24 [1864]

This morning the sun shone out and by evening the snow had nearly melted. I hope the weather will be fine.

The Ex. Board met and disposed of some cases.

I rode out to see the young ladies at Capt. G's [John Glaize]—They had went [sic] out—returned about night enjoying themselves very much over a frolic with the soldiers. Some officers had escorted them to the "Stonewall" Brigade [1st VA Bde including 4th Inf. from Smyth Co.], and were chatting very animatedly when a party attacked them with snow balls, drove them off and took charge of the ladies. One young man in his endeavours to regain his place was severely injured about the eyes.

I had only a partially pleasant time—there being none but myself to occupy the time —

The wind blew cold on my return. Got a letter from Laura [Faris]

---

[584] Evidently Dr. William Faris asked the diarist to find a place in the field hospital, perhaps as steward, for John F. Bonham (1842-1881) , a soldier from a family politically prominent in Smyth Co. John Bonham was serving in B. Co. of 48th VA Inf., alongside his brother Oscar L. Bonham (1832-1863), who was killed at Gettysburg (4 July 1863). Dr. Faris probably thought that field hospital service was far less dangerous than infantry service, and that one casualty in his friends' family was enough. John Bonham was not transfered to field hospital service, but he was given some sick furlough and then transfered to another infantry co., E, in 48th. He did survive the War. Smyth, *Smyth Co.*, ed., Presgraves, 26; confirmation of birth and death dates, service, and occupation, Chapla, *48th VA Inf.*, 110.

[FIELD HOSPITAL, ORANGE COURT HOUSE, ORANGE CO.]

FRIDAY, 25TH MCH [1864]

Slight indication this morning that "falling weather" will come soon. I commenced some unfinished work this morning—what I ought to have done yester-day but was soon interrupted by a call from "Miss B" [Elizabeth Baylor] and Capt G [John Glaize]—It seems that Miss B anticipated a visit to a portion of the army to see some friends and expected another escort at the village [585] while Cap't G. proposes tending some business. Capt. offers me his horse to go with her which of course I readily consented to. The ride was a very cold one. Snow, rain and hail commenced falling and when we returned 'twas really disagreeable.

I must say that to-day's experience has taught me something more of the weakness of human nature. I may be harsh—too much so perhaps but I cannot help it. There only needs a proper phase in affairs of all mankind to see frailties. There are some so much so than others. I met a lady [Elizabeth Baylor]—was highly pleased with her entertainment, felt well under her little compliments and indulged to some extent myself. I thought her proud and dignified—To-night I wonder, was I right? She may leave for home to-morrow.

When I returned Srgn. Walls was at my tent. He and I called on the Misses [Mollie] Graves & [Mary Camden] Allen. I am well pleased with her [Mary Camden] so far. Will it last? She has a strong will.

After supper there were quite a crowd. Rain falling rapidly.

---

26 March–4 May 1864

Without explanation, the diarist stops recording his observations for this period of time. Previously, when he leaves off several weeks, he summarizes what happens in a paragraph or two; but not this time. On 6 April, he does note delivery of bales of hay and sacks of corn, barley, and oats to the different regiments of the 2nd Corps of the Army of Northern Virginia.

---

[585] I do not know which villlage he means to describe in Orange Co.

The Last Year

5 MAY1864—15 APRIL 1865

There had been a long period of inactivity in the eastern theatres, E.B. Long noting that no major battle had occurred since fall 1863. Apperson's brothers and old-time friends and neighbors form Locust Grove were in eastern North Carolina with the 7th VA Inf. fighting to regain New Berne [as then spelled] on the coast. This mission failed.

Gen. James Longstreet, in command of reorganized 1st Corps of the Army of Northern Virginia, was brought back from eastern TN, where his corps had been since the Battle of Chickamauga (19-21 September 1863). R.E. Lee's ANV was now restored to full strength, and he began maneuvering in front of Gen. George Gordon Meade and the Army of the Potomac, which was encamped at Culpeper Court House (Culpeper Co. immediately north of Orange Co.). Ulysses S. Grant, newly promoted to Lt. Gen. for his successes in the Mississippi River Valley—especially the capture of Vicksburg and the sealing off of the most important river highway of the CSA—had joined Meade in Culpeper Court House. The Army of the Potomac also included a new cavalry commander, Gen. Philip Henry Sheridan (1831-1888), who had become almost a legend in western fighting. Thus, a reinforced and still legendary Army of Northern Virginia faced off against a huge and reinvigorated Army of the Potomac. As the diarist had noted in March, it seemed likely that someone would have to move soon, and that more fighting on a large scale would have to come—and once again in the area of his field hospital and on sites where he had grown up.

E.B. Long catches the mood in Virginia but also in much of the country in April:

[E]yes turned anxiously toward Virginia—when would it again become the focal point for the struggle?[586]

[Field Hospital, Locust Grove, Orange Co.]

Thursday, May 5 [1864]

ILLEGIBLE: Sentence of some fourteen words.

---

[586] Long, 480.

This was the first day of the Battle of the Wilderness, in which Ulysses S. Grant began the relentless campaign that would end the War in Old Virginia. He would fight his way southward toward Richmond through the thick woods of the Wilderness; enduring terrible losses along the route. Pushing through the Wilderness campaign, he would then order a long and painful siege of Petersburg, finally taking it and then press on inexorably to the Confederate capital and victory in Virginia. During this same beautiful May season, Gen. William Tecumseh Sherman began the long and equally painful march through Georgia and the Carolinas that would end the War in the South Atlantic.

Particularly bloody fighting took place in the neighborhood where the diarist grew up, in fields in front of the church where he was baptized, and in fields in front of the Old Field School where he studied as well as on fields and farms and churches where his family and friends still lived. Some of his entries, brief as they are, were written within sight of the home where he grew up; and in the midst of the carnage, he was able to visit his father. His field hospital was set up in Locust Grove itself.

More than 100,000 Federal troops struggled through the Wilderness, and an incredible 2,246 were killed there; 12,037 were wounded; and 3,383 were missing. CSA numbers were never reliably compiled: A much smaller force of some 60,000 troops apparently suffered casualties—killed, wounded, and missing—totaling more than 7,500.[587] *A safe estimate is that the diarist was in the presence of at least 3,000 fatalities for both armies, and was on the scene for the treatment of some 5,000 CSA troops—and all of this at his birthplace and boyhood home.*

[FIELD HOSPITAL, LOCUST GROVE, ORANGE CO.]

FRIDAY, MAY 6, 1864

I rec'd from Father $85 in old Currency. [barely 4 gold dollars; 17 US greenback dollars][588]

---

[587] Estimates given, *OR*, Ser. I:36, pt. 1; interpreted by E.B. Long, 494.

[588] The CSA issued new currency and withdrew old currency, attempting to halt inflation by reducing the supply of money. For a few months, including these days in May, it worked and the rate of inflation halted in the summer of 1864, that is, prices stopped rising. The new currency was stabilized for this season at 20 CSA dollars for one gold dollar and some 4 CSA dollars for one US greenback dollar. Note that even this improvement shows an increase in prices of some 33% since April 1861. In the late fall, however, it is going to become uncontrollable, and these summer days of relative price stability will come to seem almost halcyon. Source is Richmond banking firm of William B. Isaacs and Co., James Henry Hammond Papers, 1864, South Caroliniana

[FIELD HOSPITAL, LOCUST GROVE, ORANGE CO.]

SATURDAY, MAY 7, 1864

Loan Dr. Thomas $20 in old currency. [about 80 cents in gold; 4 US greenback dollars]

[FIELD HOSPITAL, LOCUST GROVE, ORANGE CO.]

SUNDAY, MAY 8, 1864

Paid $40 for a silver watch. [about 1.6 gold dollars; 8 US greenback dollars]

On this day most of the fighting shifted to Spotsylvania Court House in neighboring Spotsylvania Co. to the diarist's east and south. Both Gen. James Longstreet and Gen. Ambrose Powell Hill were incapacitated during this part of the fighting, and thus Gen. R.E. Lee had to rely on new commanders for two of his three ANV corps. Casualties were still coming to Locust Grove field hospital, both from previous action in Orange Co. and from new action in Spotsylvania Co.

[FIELD HOSPITAL, LOCUST GROVE, ORANGE CO.]

[MONDAY] MAY 9TH [1864]

Borrowed from Dr. Hagy 150$ in New Currency. [7.5 gold dollars; 37.5 US greenback dollars]

[FIELD HOSPITAL, LOCUST GROVE, ORANGE CO.]

[TUESDAY] MAY 10– [1864]

Met Surgn Edwin Phillips, 6 Ver[mont Inf.] [589] at Wilderness [illegible name of city] Vermont. Asst. Surgn. Tompkins, 77 NY [Inf.] [590]

Library, University of South Carolina, Columbia, SC. Calculations are by Richard C. Todd, op. cit.

589 6th Vt. Inf. was commanded by Col. Elisha Barney, and with four other Vt Inf. companies, was part of 2nd brigade [Col. Lewis A. Grant], 2nd Div. [Brig. Gen. George W. Getty], 6th Army Corps [Maj. Gen. John Sedgwick], Army of Potomac, commanded by Gen. George Gordon Meade and directed by Lt. Gen. Ulysses S. Grant. *OR*, Ser. I, 36:1, 112.

590 77th NY Inf. was commanded by Maj. Nathan S. Babcock and with New England and PA . companies was part of 3rd brigade {Brig. Gen. Thomas H. Neill], 2nd divisino. [Gen. Getty], 6th Army Corps [Gen. Sedgwick], Army of Potomac [Gen. Meade], directed by Gen. Grant. Ibid.

[ON ROAD FROM LOCUST GROVE TO MINE RUN, ORANGE CO.]

[WEDNESDAY] MAY 11– [1864]

On picnic last night, and on security to-day.
Left Locust Grove and camped at Mine Run Church

[FIELD HOSPITAL, OLD SPOTSYLVANIA COURT HOUSE, SPOTSYLVANIA CO.]

[THURSDAY] MAY 12– [1864]

Had a fight to-day. Established our hospt. near Spotsylvania Old C.H. [Court House]—
Recd a large number of wounded[591] —
[Gen. Edward] Johnson's[592] Division used up.

[FIELD HOSPITAL, OLD SPOTSYLVANIA COURT HOUSE, SPOTSYLVANIA CO.]

[FRIDAY] MAY 13 [1864]

Attending wounded —
Rainy—Roads very muddy.

[FIELD HOSPITAL, OLD SPOTSYLVANIA COURT HOUSE, SPOTSYLANIA CO.]

[SATURDAY] MAY 14 : [1864]

Attending wounded —
Still Rainy.

---

[591] Even the diarist's adjective *large* is an understatement. For this *one* day—"one of the most murderous days of the war"—*OR*, Ser. I, 33:1, 12 May 1864. estimates Federal casualties at 6800 and CSA casualties at 5000, confirmed by Long. Long also says, "[t]wo great armies had fought, and only rather unimportant bits of ground changed hands. Yet attrition was more serious for the Confederates. Where were the replacements to come from?" Long, 500.

[592] "Allegheny Ed" Johnson (1816-1873) already identified. Gen. Grant sent Federal troops under Gen. Winfield Scott Hancock (1824-1886) at the salient known forevermore as Bloody Angle. Gen. Richard Stoddert Ewell's Inf. forces of 2nd Corps ANV were not protected by artillery, which had been withdrawn; Ewell's Inf. forces moved back to a second line of defense and stiffened and held their ground. The Bloody Angle included "only a few hundred yards of entrenchments" at Spotsylvania, but was charged by more than twenty Federal Bdes. *OR*, Ser. 1. 33:1, 11 May 1864; Long, 499. Gen. Johnson and his men were trapped and overwhelmed and captured at Bloody Angle, and John E. Stanchak says: "As a result of his old foot wound, Johnson carried an outsized club into battle, using it as a cane in daily life. He used it to club several of his captors before an old army friend, Union Maj. Gen. Marsena R. Patrick (1811-1888), recognized Johnson, realized his embarrassment at being captured, and saw to his kind treatment." Idem, "Johnson," *Hist. Times.*

[FIELD HOSPITAL, OLD SPOTSYLVANIA COURT HOUSE, SPOTSYLVANIA CO.]

[SUNDAY] MAY 15– [1864]

Receiving, attending and sending off wounded [probably to general hospital in Gordonsville, Orange Co.; others to hospitals in Richmond].

[FIELD HOSPITAL, OLD SPOTSYLVANIA COURT HOUSE, SPOTSYLVANIA CO.]

[MONDAY] MAY 16– [1864]

Surgns [Samuel Rush] Sayers[593] & Love assigned to Surg. [Harvey] Black —

Brigades of [Gen. Edward] Johnsons Division thrown to-gether.

The enemy reputively to be withdrawing on the left and moving to the right.[594]

[FIELD HOSPITAL, OLD SPOTSYLVANIA COURT HOUSE, SPOTSYLANIA CO.]

[TUESDAY] MAY 17– [1864]

Fair to-day —

Sending off wounded to Milford [field hospital in Caroline Co.] and Louisa C.H. [field hospital in Court House, Louisa Co]. A "Permanent Hospt." [but not a general hospital] is also being established—All cases that cannot be moved a distance with safety are sent there [Milford, Caroline Co.]— It is on the southside of Po River, near the "Stuart House"[595]

Preparing to Move —

---

[593] Samuel Rush Sayers (1833-1914) was a physician from Smyth Co. who was mustered into 4th VA inf. as staff surgeon; he was transfered to 27th VA. Inf. , was wounded and captured at Gettysburg (4 July 1863); released from prison, he was returned to 27th Inf. until 18 January 1864 when he rejoined 4th Inf. as field surgeon. He survived War and returned to practice medicine, eventually in Wythe Co., and is buried in Wytheville. Robertson, *4th VA. Inf.*, 71; Reidenbaugh, *27th VA. Inf.*, 173.

[594] Diarist is correct; Federal troops moved east and south, to their right, not retreating, even tactically, but only realigning themselves for another engagement. Long, 502.

[595] Po River joins Ni River and Mat River and Ta River to form Mattaponi River that flows into York River; Mattaponi are Native Americans who hold land and fishing rights at mouth of York by king's charter predating establishment of Commonwealth of VA. The Millford "permanent" field hospital was located on rail line for Richmond, Fredericksburg, and Petersburg Railroad.

[FIELD HOSPITAL, OLD SPOTSYLVANIA COURT HOUSE, SPOTSYLVANIA CO.]

[WEDNESDAY] MAY 18TH [1864]

Sending off wounded. News from Richmond is good—[Gen. Pierre Gustave Touissant] Beauregard has repulsed [Gen. Benjamin Franklin] Butler.[596]

[FIELD HOSPITAL, STUART HOUSE, MILFORD, CAROLINE CO.]

[THURSDAY] MAY 19TH [1864]

Moved to near "Stuart House" and pitched tents—Received a number of wounded—began a Register of Cases but soon stopped—

The enemy reported moving to the right to-wards Guiney's [Guiney Station, Caroline Co.]

Surg. Taylor is in chg. of Permanent Hospt [Milford]—Dr. [Harvey] Black Req. [made requisition] on Capt. Lock for 500$ Hospt. funds—and turned it over to Srg. B[ushrod]. Taylor for use of the sick & wounded in Permanent Hospt.[597]

[FIELD HOSPITAL, STUART HOUSE, MILFORD, CAROLINE CO.]

[FRIDAY] MAY 20– [1864]

Gen. [Richard Stoddert] Ewell [commander of 2d Corps ANV] had a fight yesterday evening beyond the Spotsylvania C.H. [Court House] Wounded are coming in this morning.[598]

---

[596] Not Richmond, but the southern and eastern angle of attack on Petersburg along the James River at Drewry's Bluff, or Fort Darling (Chesterfield Co). Long and other authorities believe that Gen. Butler (already identified) fell back needlessly, and could have pressed on to victory, leaving Petersburg open to successful attack, and perhaps even Richmond. Long actually says, "[i]neptness in top Union command was never more evident than in this campaign." Long, 503.

[597] Bushrod Taylor, no birth and death data, was surgeon in 48th VA Inf. commended for bravery after Gettysburg. Promoted to chief medical officer of 2nd brigade, 2nd Corps of ANV. Chapla, *48th VA Inf.*, 156.

[598] Long declares that the Battle of Spotsylvania Court House was ended on 19 May, but notes that skirmishing and other action continued, as R.E. Lee moved his forces to block George Gordon Meade's next move and Winfield Scott Hancock's next move, both ordered by Grant. Federal casualties, killed, wounded, and missing for Spotsylvania are listed as 17,500; some of these the diariest tended, and the fighting he certainly saw. CSA casualties are not reliably given, but certainly killed, wounded, and missing from CSA forces at Spotsylvania are beyond 5,000 and perhaps 10,000. The diarist may have tended to as many as 10% of those CSA wounded. Federal casualties came frorm a base of more than 100,000 troops, constantly replenished for Grant. CSA casualties came from a base of some 50,000, almost none of whom could be replaced readily. O.R., Ser. 1, vol. 36, Reports, 20 May 1864. See also Long, 505-06.

Made requisition on Capt. [J.T.] Lock [commissary of sustenance for 2d Corps] for $1000 and turned over to Henry Earhart [agent for hospital supplies for 4th VA Inf.][599] to purchase supplies. Some 400 or 500 mostly wounded, have been sent in to-day. The trip yester-day was costly. Sending men off in wagons. Guiney Station is reported burned. This I regret deeply.[600]

[FIELD HOSPITAL, STUART HOUSE, MILFORD, CAROLINE CO.]

[SATURDAY] MAY 21– [1864]

Army [Gen. R.S. Ewell's 2d Corps, temporarily led by Gen. Jubal Anderson Early because Ewell was traveling in a wagon and suffering from severe diarrhea] moving to-ward the right. Large number of sick and wounded sent in to-day. Sending them off to Chesterfield [Chesterfield Co. south of Richmond; field hospital thought to be safely removed from maneuvering around Richmond and other maneuvering south of James River].

[TEMPORARY HOSPITAL, ON MOVE, BEAVER DAM DEPOT, HANOVER CO.]

[SUNDAY] MAY 22– [1864]

Moved this morning. Changed our course three times. Yankees on our left. Camped near North Anna River, opposite Beaver Dam.

---

[599] Henry Earhart (1836-1892) was from Montgomery Co., Blacksburg section, occupation unknown. He joined Co. L, which had no nickname, in 4th VA Inf. In 1862 he was detailed as agent for hospital supplies and worked directly with stewards and surgeons in 2nd Corps ANV. He returned to Blacksburg after War, and is buried there. Robertson, *4th VA Inf.*, 48.

[600] Winfield Scott Hancock's cavalry led the advance ordered by Grant, and attacked the station depot on 20 May. More serious fighting ensued; the station apparently was destroyed in the fighting, as was much else among those who had for long periods hosted the diarist. Hancock filed his report very late, complaining about "almost total failure" of his subordinates to send in written reports of their actions. He lists flags captured, and claims to have some 400 CSA prisoners from Guiney's Station action. He does not mention burning the station, but offers few details. Hancock, Report, *OR*, Ser. 1, 36:340-42; Gen. James Longstreet forwarded a report of terrible damage to buildings at Guiney Station, ibid., 1054-60.

[ON THE ROAD, BEAVER DAM TO HANOVER JUNCTION, HANOVER CO.]

[MONDAY] MAY 23– [1864]

Moved past Beaver Dam. The ruins of the [Beaver Dam railroad] depot [for Chesapeake & Ohio Rail Road] show that the enemy had been there. About 6 miles from Hanover Junction there was much excitement about the enemy in front and very near. The [wagon] train was turned off to the right [southerly direction], crossed Little River at Widow Cooks [sic],[601] and camped on the premises of Widow Coleman [602] near Hanover Academy. The Yankees got two ambulances and a blacksmith forge and fixtures from us to-day.

We stopped at the [Little] River [near] Dr. [Horrace] Stringfellow's[603] to get some water. They are surely models of kindness. I did not make myself known. The army is at Hanover Junction [town with depot for Chesapeake & Ohio Railroad].

[TEMPORARY HOSPITAL CAMP, TAYLORSVILLE, HANOVER CO.]

[TUESDAY] MAY 24 [1864]

We moved to Taylorsville Va [Hanover Co. on Taylors Creek River] and camped to await orders. Heavy firing is heard on the left.[604] [Gen. Richard Stoddert] Ewell's [2d corps ANV] is in the centre, [Gen. Ambrose Powell] Hill's [3d corps ANV] on the left and [Gen. James] Longstreet's Corps on the right.

---

[601] There is no white woman named Cook listed in Hanover Co. census, 1870; however, there is Edmonia Cooke, born 1802, who lived in Hewlett district of Hanover Co. and owned land; she is perhaps the Widow Cooke. VA, *Census*, Hanover, 1870.

[602] Apparently Matilda Coleman, born 1790, who owned land in the same Hewlett distrrict of Hanover Co. The Colemans held a number of slaves, and at least five black farmers working land in 1870 in the Hewlett disrtrict were apparently once their slaves. VA, *Census*, Hanover, 1870.

[603] Horrace Stringfellow, born 1800, owned land and slaves in Hewlett district of Hanover Co. At least five black farmers operating farm land in the Co. in 1870 were apparently once his slaves. The diarist's family may have known Dr. Stringfellow; hence his oblique reference, "I did not make myself known." VA, *Census*, Hanover, 1870.

[604] The fight the diarist heard to his left was at Ox Ford of the North Anna River; the ford is at junction of Caroline and Hanover Co. Gen. R.E. Lee interposed the ANV between two parts of the Army of the Potomac, which was crossing the North Anna River on this day. Lee's configured forces, in an "apex," fit snugly inside the bend of the river where the Army of Potomac was attempting to cross in three waves, each wave separated by the features of the river, and all reinforced by Philip Sheridan's cavalry. There was sharp fighting and skirmishing on 24 May at Ox Ford, and the ANV held its "strong position" and thus slowed the progress of Gens. Winfield Scott Hancock, Horatio Gouverneur Wright (1820-1899), and Gouvernor Kemble Warren (183-1882), Long, 508

All the odds and ends of the army are congregated at this place. I saw Gen. [John C.] Breckinridge and part of his command.[605]

[CAMP HOSPITAL, TAYLORSVILLE, HANOVER CO.]

[WEDNESDAY] MAY 25- [1864]

In camp to-day—The enemy moving to our left [still maneuvering around North Anna River crossings]. Dr. Sutton reported for duty.

[CAMP HOSPITAL, TAYLORSVILLE, HANOVER CO.]

[THURSDAY] MAY 26TH [1864]

In camp. Enemy operation appears to be changing his course to our right. Firing on the left.[606] Weather shining and sultry.

[CAMP HOSPITAL, MERRY OAKS, HANOVER CO.]

[FRIDAY] MAY 27TH [1864]

Moved from Taylorsville this morning. Stopped at Ashland about 1/2 hour and was ordered on. Fell in with wagons of [Richard Stoddert] Ewell's [2d Corps]. Saw the remnants of [Gen. "Allegheny" Edward] Johnson's Division [which comprised the remnants of the Stonewall Bde]. Larger than I expected—Saw the [Smyth Co.] "Blues" [4th VA Inf.] & Col. [Robert Henry] Dungan. The enemy moving towards the Peninsular [sic].

Camped at "Merry Oaks." Loan C.W.Sydnor 10$ in old issue [less than fifty cents in gold; about two US greenback dollars].

---

[605] John Cabell Breckinridge (1821-1875), already identified, had returned from the Battle of New Market [Shenandoah Co.], 15 May 1864, which William C. Davis calls "the most important small battle of the War." Idem, "Breckinridge," *Hist. Times*. Breckinridge's KY forces were joined by 247 cadets from Virginia Military Institute to halt the advance of Gen. Franz Sigel up the Valley and drive him back to Strasburg in same Co. In sharp fighting, the *OR* lists 831 US casualties from a force of 5,500, and 577 CSA casualties from a force of 5,000. As Long notes, "The sharp defeat proved somewhat humiliating for the Federals; the pressure eased momentarily [sic] in the Shenandoah Valley. The courage of the cadets has made New Market a legend, though they were a small part of the victorious Southern force." Davis, 502.

[606] Gen. U.S. Grant moved all forces northward back across the North Anna River, ending the Battle of North Anna, the firing that the diarist records. *OR*, Ser. 1, 36:26, May 1864. Grant then ordered Phillip Sheridan's cavalry to lead the way far to the right of the ANV to cross the Pamunkey River; all infantry and other forces followed, creating the "new course" that the diarist sees. Long, 508.

[FIELD HOSPITAL, MECHANICSVILLE, HANOVER CO.]

[SATURDAY] MAY 28– [1864]

Left camp early—Passed Atlee's [illegible word; name of community is Atlee's Station, Hanover Co.], and stopped at Mechanicsville [on Chickahominy River]. Every house is deserted: The army in position near Old Church [apparently Aenon Church]. Cavalry fighting. [607] I was very unwell this evening.

[FIELD HOSPITAL, MECHANICSVILLE, HANOVER CO.]

[SUNDAY] MAY 29– [1864]

I lay in bed till noon—All quiet to-day [Army of Potomac was advancing across Pamunkey toward south of Richmond, and Gen. Lee ordered ANV to lie in wait and prepare their lines].

Dr. Love and Thomas[608] returned from Spotsylvania [Spotsylvania Co.]C.H. No Yankees in that neighborhood.

[FIELD HOSPITAL, MECHANICSVILLE, HANOVER CO.]

[MONDAY] MAY 30TH [1864]

Went to Richmond to procure supplies for the month; failed to get them—back for them to-morrow. Called at Capt Rogers. Rev. Dr. [Bevery T.] Lacy came out in the ambulance [to counsel and comfort wounded men].

Went upon Cary Street—was not much edified. [diarist's italics]

[Brig. Gen. Matthew Calbraith] Butler's Brig. was stampeded [sic].[609] Fugitives report a hard fight 7 miles below [Haw's Shop]. [Gen. Robert

---

[607] Gen. R.E. Lee again positioned himself in front of Army of Potomac, which was crossing Pamunkey near Hanovertown. The diarist hears cavalry fighting at five sites and along Totopotomy River, especially Aenon Church. Gen. P.G.T. Beauregard was maneuvering south of Richmond in strong defenses, but Lee reported to President Jefferson Davis that Beauregard's forces were outnumbered two to one. *OR*, Ser. 1, 36:1, 1188; *A Register of Military Events in VA, 1861-1865*, comp., N.E. Warriner (Richmond: VA Civil War Commission, 1959) 50, hereinafter *A Register*, comp., Warriner.

[608] Thomas may also be a doctor; I cannot find a doctor by that name in 2nd Corps ANV. I cannot fully identify Love, a surgeon attached to 2nd Corps ANV on this occasion.

[609] Actually, Butler's forces held the line, and were not "stampeded." Maj. Gen. Matthew Calbraith Butler (1836-1909) was in charge of reorganized SC Cav. divi. comprising many green horse troops. Butler, born in Greenville, SC and raised in Edgefield, SC by his uncle Sen. Andrew P. Butler, was also nephew of naval figures Oliver Hazard and Matthew Calbraith Perry, and a veteran of Indian territory wars. He attended South Carolina College, was admitted to SC bar, and

Emmett] Rode's Division had a hard fight this evening [probably Armstrong's Farm]. Sent back near 200 wounded.[610] At work 'till 3 o'clock at night.

I spent about 10$ [new issue; about one-half gold dollars; about 2.5 U.S. greenback dollars] for nothing to-day.

[FIELD HOSPITAL, MECHANICSVILLE, HANOVER CO.]

[TUESDAY] MAY 31ST [1864]

Rec'd and sent to Richmond a number of wounded, mostly of [Gen. Robert Emmett] Rodes' Division, [Brig. Gen. George Pierce Doles leading GA forces], [Brig. Gen. Junius] Daniels [NC forces formerly under Daniels; he was slain on 12 May in Mule Shoe Campaign and passed on 13 May], [Brig. Gen. Goode] Bryan's [16th GA] of Rodes' and [Brig. Gen. John] Pegram [leading VA infantry] of [Gen. Jubal Anderson] Early's [2d Corps ANV][611] did the fighting. [Maj. Gen. Robert Frederick] Hoke's Division arrived to-day.[612] Col. Beck reported sick. Rec'd supplies from Med. Purveyor.[613]

---

married daughter of SC gov. Francis Pickens. He served in CSA state gen. assembly in SC, but resigned to command 2nd SC Cav. Distinguished at Brandy Station (9 June 1863), Butler had lost a foot to a wound, but recovered and used crutches and could still ride a horse in command. He was commended for bravery and for stopping the Federal advance at Haw's Shop. *OR*, ser. 1, 36: 1188; *A Register*, comp. Warriner, 61. See also Edward G. Longacre, "Butler," *Hist. Times.*

[610] Surg. Gen. Lafayette Guild's official records for Gen. Robert Emmett Rode's division on the Wilderness Campaign was 1,534 wounded, so that this one day of fighting constituted a major portion of his wounded. *OR*, ser. 1, 36:1075.

[611] Richard Stoddert Ewell was traveling in ambulance for part of fight; Jubal Anderson Early took his place, and has been criticized for poor reconaissance, possibly causing severe losses for 2nd Corps and for Rode's division. Long, 511-12. George Pierce Doles (1830-1864) was from Milledgeville, GA, survived this terrible day, but was killed on 2 June at Cold H arbor in later phase of this long campaign. Junius Daniel (1828-1864) was from Halifax NC and was rated"excellent combat officer" by Jeffrey D. Wert, who noted his accomplishments at Wilderness (5-6 May) and at Spotsylvania (12 May), where he was killed and his NC troops were given to other leaders. Goode Bryan (1811-1885) was from Hancock City, GA, and a West Point graduate who fought well on this occasion in leading his GA troops, but ran out of ammunition. Bryan would become severely ill in September 1864 during the continuing Rapidan to James River Campaign and resign his commission, becoming yet another casualty of this series of battles. John Pegram (1832-1865) was from Petersburg, VA, and from a distinguished VA military family. Also a West Pointer, Pegram survived these fights, married famously to Hetty Cary in the "gala social event of the year in Richmond," and perished a few days later at Hatcher's Run [6 February 1865). See James I. Robertson, "Pegram," *Hist Times.*; Jeffrey D. Wert, "Doles," and "Daniel," ibid.; and John E. Stanchak, "Bryan," ibid.

[612] Robert Frederick Hoke was from Lincolnton, NC, and was son of a cotton mill operator. He advanced rapidly in War, was commended for bravery in taking a Federal garrison at

[FIELD HOSPITAL, DR. WILLIAM LUMPKIN'S GROVE, HANOVER CO.]

[WEDNESDAY] JUNE 1– [1864]

Moved across the road to the grove in rear of Dr. [William] Lumpkin's dwelling.[614] The dust is almost intolerable. Began a Register of names. Sending patients to Richmond.

[FIELD HOSPITAL, DR. WILLIAM LUMPKIN'S GROVE, HANOVER CO.]

[THURSDAY] JUNE 2ND [1864]

[Richard Stoddert] Ewell's Corps [2nd ANV] made an advance on the enemy this evening, and gained an advantage. The firing was considerable for a while. Not many wounded.[615] Dr. [H.P.] MacGruder returned.

[FIELD HOSPITAL, DR. WILLIAM LUMPKIN'S GROVE, HANOVER CO.]

[FRIDAY] JUNE 3– [1864]

Firing along the whole line, musketry, and artillery. From the noise a most desperate fight is going on.

Reports in the evening are that the enemy made repeated assaults on our lines and were repulsed at every point. Our loss small. [616]

Plymouth, NC, and on this occasion was serving with Gen. P.G.T. Beauregard in defense of Richmond and Petersburg. Edward G. Longacre, "Hoke."

[613] Note that even in this hard campaign of spring and summer 1864 with Richmond and Petersburg under siege, it is *logistical* problems of *delivery* for medical supplies rather than lack of medical supplies that bedevils the steward and his field hospital supervisors, a point emphasized by Cunningham.

[614] Probably Dr. William Lumpkin, born 1808, who practiced medicine and had land in Hewlett section of Hanover Co. VA, Census, 1870.

[615] Jubal Anderson Early was leading Ewell's 2d Corps. This attack was described by Long as "abortive." There were few casualties because the attack did little good. Grant was maneuvering along the Chicahominy River, and Lee was positioning his 3 corps of ANV in front of the Army of Potomac, stretching his defenses from the Chicakahominy northward to swampland along the Totopotomy ; the ANV was well entrenched, and there were reinforcements. Long adds, "The stage was set on the flat lowlands along the Chickahominy for one of the bloodiest battles of history." Long, 513.

[616] The charge by Army of Potomac at Cold Harbor was repulsed "at every point." This was Lee's last major success in an "all-out" engagement. Long offers judgment with the significant caveat that "it was a great victory for Lee—if the stemming of a tide by a human wall can be called victory." Grant expressed regret at attempting the all-out assault in the way that he did. Federal losses of their 50,000 forces numbered around 12,000—an incredible 7,000 fell in less than one

Sent Dr. Hagy by mail some letters.
Sending wounded to Stone's farm.

[4-6 JUNE, SAME SITE, BUT NO ENTRIES]

[FIELD HOSPITAL, DR. WILLIAM LUMPKIN'S GROVE, HANOVER CO.]

[TUESDAY] JUNE 7 [1864]

Sent letters to [Drs.] Hagy & [H.P.] MacG[ruder].

[FIELD HOSPITAL, DR. WILLIAM LUMPKIN'S GROVE, HANOVER CO.]

[FRIDAY] JUNE 8 [1864]

Sent to Capt. Lock statement of sick and wounded for the mo[nth] of May.

[FIELD HOSPITAL, DR. WILLIAM LUMPKIN'S GROVE, HANOVER CO.]

[THURSDAY] JUNE 9– [1864]

Finished monthly reports.
[On pass to Richmond]

[FRIDAY] JUNE 10 [1864]

In Richmond to-day. Saw several lady friends. One particular lady. *Not much disappointment.*[617]

[FIELD HOSPITAL, DR. WILLIAM LUMPKIN'S GROVE, HANOVER CO.]

[FRIDAY] JUNE 11 [1864]

Sent duplicate receipts for medicines for Surgn. [Peter E.] Hines[618] and Surgn. Straith.

[*no entry for 12 June 1864*]

---

hour while the diarist treated casualties. CSA forces were around 25,000, adequate for a well entrenched force; numbers of CSA casualties were not "small," but perhaps around 1,500. Long quoted, 513; *OR*, ser. 1, 36:1, 2 June 1864.

617 This was likely Mary Camden, the "Mrs. Allen" and "Mrs. A" and also the "Other Molly" of previous entries. In "Reminiscences," the diarist speaks of foolishness and "carryings on" in his youth in this period, and seems to refer to Mary Camden, although not by name. Dr. Bean also concluded that the "particular lady" was Mary Camden. Bean, notes.

618 Peter E. Hines was surgeon and medical director of NC general hospitals in Richmond according to Cunningham, 215.

[FIELD HOSPITAL, ABOVE GOODALL'S TAVERN, HANOVER CO.]

[MONDAY] JUNE 13– [1864]

Unexpectedly ordered last night to move this morning. Destination uncertain.[619]

Made a large requisition on Med. Purveyor [Peter E.] Hines.

Handed Dr. [Hunter Holmes] McGuire reports for May.

Left Camp on the Meadow Bridge Road at 8 o'clock.

Camped three miles above Goodall's Tavern.

Weather cool.

Yankees moving towards Lynchburg from Staunton. Troops pleased with the idea of going to their old *range* [*another campaign up and down the Valley; note the contrast with the diarist's skepticism when it was Thomas Jonathan Jackson leading the troops up and down the "old range"*].

[FIELD HOSPITAL, ABOVE LOUISA COURT HOUSE, LOUISA CO.]

[TUESDAY] JUNE 14– [1864]

Moved early. Crossed the river at a Mill.

Camped within 14 miles of Louisa C.H. The day was amiable to a tramp [viz., hike].

I walked most of the day—tired at night.

Got a letter from M. [Mary Camden]. Sad story hers. Med. Supplies arrived.

[FIELD HOSPITAL, GREEN SPRING VALLEY, LOUISA CO.]

[WEDNESDAY] JUNE 15– [1864]

Left Camp at 6 1/2 A.M. Passed Louisa C.H. about 3. Henry Earhart came to us with supplies.

The day very hot—roads dusty.

Above Louisa CH. we came to that part of the R. Road torn up by [Gen. Philip] Sheridan [commander of all cavalry of Army of Potomac][620] The damage is very slight. Can be repaired in a very short time.

---

[619] Jubal Anderson Early began his own Valley campaign, and the diarist will be traveling with the 2nd Corps much as he did before with Thomas Jonathan Jackson.

[620] This part of track was probably Trevilian Station, where Sheridan was repulsed. Other track was irreparably destroyed, as were telegraph lines to Richmond.

The outrages of the enemy on inoffensive citizens are without doubt unparalleled in the history of civilised nations. The garments of children and tableware of families are destroyed.[621]

Camped in Green Spring Valley near Dr. [James L.] Wills.[622]

[ON THE ROAD FROM GREEN SPRING DEPOT, LOUISA CO. TO CHARLOTTESVILLE, ALBEMARLE CO.]

[THURSDAY] JUNE 16– [1864]

Left Camp later than usual.

Made Req[uisition]. for five days.

[TEMPORARY ENCAMPMENT, NORTH GARDEN DEPOT, ALBEMARLE CO.]

[FRIDAY] JUNE 17– [1864]

Marched to Charlottesville and took Lynchburg road. Troops on the train. I walked to the [Southern Railroad Depot between forks of Hardware River] depot above North Garden and slept 'till morning.

Saw [Harvey Allen] Jameson [hospital steward from Smyth Co.] at Charlottesville.

Loan Dr. [W.W.] Drane 10$ and [Harvey Allen] Jameson 10$ [about 1/2 a gold dollar; about 2 US greenback dollars]. Spent 71[cents; about 3.5 cents in gold currency; about 14 cents in US greenback currency] for ice cream.

The road is very rough. Dudley's Mountain [Albemarle Co.] stands out boldly. Have some old memories of that ridge.[623]

---

[621] John D. Kallman and Jeffrey D. Wert regard Philip Sheridan as indomitable and relentless and powerful rather than especially cruel. They do note that his destruction of supply lines and his destruction of stores in the "breadbasket" of the Valley was remarkable—also something ordered by Ulysses S. Grant and fully approved by President Abraham Lincoln. They do not disagree with the diarist's contention that civilian property, including tableware, was confiscated and/or destroyed. Kallman, "Sheridan;" Wert, "Sheridan's Richond Raid," *Hist. Times.*

[622] Probably James L. Wills of Trevilian Station, Louisa Co. Born in 1828, he had property there; but I do not know if he was a physician. VA Census, 1870.

[623] Dudley's Mountain is in central Albemarle Co. according to Green Peyton's Map of Albemarle Co., cited and displayed, VA Place Name Society, *Occasional Papers* (1961), No. 14. Terrible fighting in Albemarle Co. and Hanover Co. from 28 May to 3 June 1864, often called Cold Harbor (Hanover Co.), was strung along ridges and creeks in Albemarle and Hanover Cos. included action at Aenon's Church, Haw's Shop, Crump's Creek, Jones' Farm, Totopotomy Creek, Armstrong's Farm, Matadequin Creek, Shady Grove, Mechump's Creek, and Bethesda Church. *Register*, comp. Warriner. He had stopped there in February of 1859 on his original trip west. "Diary," 1859, Archives, VPSI, Blacksburg.

[ON THE ROAD BETWEEN LOVINGSTON, NELSON CO., AND LYNCHBURG, CAMPBELL CO.]

[SATURDAY] JUNE 18– [1864]

Overtook wagon trains about 7 miles from Lovingston [Nelson Co., northwest of Lynchburg]. When we reached that place [Dr. W.W.] Drane & myself procured some bread and milk at the house of the overseer of Col. Dillard.[624] The wagons moved three miles on the Amherst C.H. Road and halted that the teams might feed awhile on the luxurious clover.

Citizens represent that cannonading [comes] in direction of Lynchburg [Campbell Co].[625]

Started on the road at 7 o'clock and traveled to the summit of a hill ~~before~~ after crossing Tye River[626] Orders came for the [ambulance wagon] train to be in Lynchburg to-morrow.

I spent 2$ [about 10 cents in gold; about .4 greenbacks] for dinner to-day.

---

[624] Probably at Massie's Mill, a township in Nelson Co. on the wagon road between Lovingston and Amherst Court House, and about seven miles from Lovingston. In that township are two landowners named Dillard who owned slaves, Walker W. Dillard (born 1825) and Oregon D. Dillard (born 1816). VA Census, 1870.

[625] Federal cavalry Gen. David Hunter (1802-1866) was in command of Army of West Virginia and was sweeping through the Shenandoah Valley. He won a battle at Piedmont (Augusta Co.) on 5 June, cut railroad lines, cut supply lines, and destroyed many stores of goods, some of which were civilian. His name became synonymous with the hardness of modern war in the Valley and he is to this day roundly hated by descendants of the resident civilians. On 18 June 1864 Hunter attacked Jubal A. Early's corps at Lynchburg, and was defeated and retreated. He retreated so far into WVA that he left Early a path "down the valley" [northward] into Washington, D.C. Early took what remained of Stonewall Bde. and others on a wild drive down the valley and toward Washington, thrilling southerners and terrifying northern politicians, but ultimately losing the campaign and retreating back up the valley. Hunter was encouraged to resign on 8 August 1864 after meeting with Philip Sheridan and U.S. Grant to discuss his strange decision to retreat so far that Early's corps would find the roadways to Washington, D.C. lightly defended.

Hunter was born in D.C., graduated from West Point, and served posts in the northwestern frontier territories before The War. After Lincoln's assassination, Hunter was president of the commission that tried the conspirators who had killed the president; he then retired as brevet Maj. Gen. in his native city. Kimberly A. Keefer, "Hunter," *Hist. Times.* Long, 525.

[626] Tye River is in the James River Basin. It rises in western Nelson Co. and runs across the edge of Amherst Co., then joins Buffalo River and eventually the James River. There is a railroad depot on the county line between Amherst and Nelson Co., and the summit where the diarist camped must be in Amherst Co. *A List*, ed., Hummel.

[On the road from Lynchburg, Campbell Co. to Salem, Roanoke Co.]

[Sunday] June 19– [1864]

Moved at 3 this morning. Most of the baggage left to follow in the ambulance [wagon] train as rapidly as possible.

Weather intollerably [sic] hot and the air filled with dust. I do not think I was ever so dirty.

Reached Lynchburg at 1/2 past 2 [P.M.]. Had good news from Richmond. [627] The fight on yester-day [at Lynchburg] resulted in the repulse of the enemy. [David] Hunter is said to be moving towards Salem [Roanoke Co].

We are near the battlefield, at the house of a Mr. [Thomas L.] Bocock.[628]

Moved at 8 [A.M.]—and travelled 'till [illegible, possibly dusk]: Made about 12 miles above Lynchburg [moving westward and southward up the Valley]

Loan [Dr.] Ellsberg 10$ [fifty cents in gold currency; two greenback dollars].

The enemy moving up the Va. and Tenn. R.R. [toward Kanawha Valley of West Virginia; this will leave the Shenandoah Valley's downward slope open to Gen. Jubal Early's corps].

[ON ROAD IN CAMPBELL CO. MOVING WEST AND SOUTH]

[MONDAY] JUNE 20– [1864]

Left camp at 6—[A.M.] travelled 'till we cooked rations and camped at Mrs. [Hanna] Campbell's at 10 [A.M.]. [629] The enemy have crossed the Mountains [the Blue Ridge]. [George Pierce] Dole's [sic; Doles's] Brigade [of Georgians] had a skirmish at Liberty [Bedford Co.] [630] yester-day—22 dead left on the field.

---

[627] That is, news from the capital of the CSA about the progress of The War. Long says, "On land the two major Federal offensives seemed stalled, facing defiant Confederate defenders. Grant's army gots its breath on the Petersburg lines, while Lee's army dug in. In Georgia Sherman's Federals discovered [Joseph Eggleston] Johnston had moved into a new line." Long, 526.

[628] Thomas L. Bocock, born 1819, owned land in Eastern Division of Campbell Co. VA Census, 1870.

[629] Probably Hanna Campbell, born 1807, who owned land and slaves at Brookville Township, Campbell Co. VA Census, 1870.

[630] George Pierce Doles (born 1830) as identified earlier; he was killed 2 June 1864 at Cold Harbor; this is the remnants of his GA brigades. The GA regiments won this engagement in part of the Lynchburg Campaign; it was one of the factors causing David Hunter to retreat to Kanawha Valley. *A Register*, comp. Warriner, 63.

[CAMP, NEAR BIG LICK, ROANOKE CO.][631]

[TUESDAY] JUNE 21– [1864]

Marched at 6. [A.M.] and camped about 8 [miles] west of Salem on the road to Hanging Rock from Big Lick [Roanoke Co]. The cavalry succeeded in cutting off a portion of the enemy [General David Hunter] in the gap of the [Catawba] mountain on the New Castle Road and caused him to destroy 6 pieces of artillery and leave three more—also destroyed some wagons.

The country through which we have passed is as fine as any I have ever seen. Crops are luxuriant. The enemy has not injured the country near so much as I have seen it. The R.Road bridges and depot are burned but the track is unhurt. A large woolen factory at Bonsack [Roanoke Co.] was reduced to ruins.

[CAMP NEAR BIG LICK, ROANOKE CO.]

[WEDNESDAY] JUNE 22– [1864]

Contrary to expectations we have the very desirable privilege of remaining in camp to-day.

We stopped in a wood near Mr. [John W.] Day's [632] about a mile from Botetourt's Springs.

I had a good bath and feel better. The enemy [David Hunter's cavalry] resting to-day also I learn.

[William] Mohler[633] came up with the baggage wagons left on the 19th. Dr. [Harvey] Black went home. Dr. Sutton[634] relieved of duty at this hospt. and ordered to report to 21 N.C. Infantry.

Wrote to M[ollie] T[hornton].

Rev. Dr. [Bevery T.] Lacy makes himself an agreeable companion for camp by his anecdotes to each of which he gives a "local habitation & name."[635]

Loan Dr. Hamilton 10$ [2 greenbacks; 50 cents in gold currency]

---

[631] Big Lick later became a railroad center and was renamed Roanoke. *A List*, ed., Hummel, 26.

[632] John W. Day, born in 1817, owned land in Big Lick Township. VA Census, 1870.

[633] Samuel Mohler, identified earlier, was killed at Lynchburg on 18 June 1864. William H. Mohler (1833-1912) came from Kerr's Creek in Rockbridge Co. and was 5th Sgt. with Co. G, Kerr's Company of 58th VA Inf. He was captured often, and occasionally unaccounted for, but was likely in the area during Lynchburg Campaign and the Valley skirmishes between David Hunter and Jubal A. Early. Driver, *58th VA Inf.*, 123.

[634] I cannot locate a physician named Sutton in 4th or 7th VA brigades, or in Cunningham.

[635] Lacy, already identified, was a very popular preacher. He was employing an old parson's trick, setting a Biblical lesson in a local area by renaming the characters for local people and identifying the area as the locality. See Pitts, 108-19.

[CAMP AT JOHNSON FARM NEAR BUCHANAN, BOTETORT CO.]

[THURSDAY] JUNE 23 [1864]

Moved this morning. Walked around the grounds at this Spring [possibly Springwood where a spring feeds James River in Buchanan Co]. Nice place. The unfinished Female College is a large commodious building.

I am surprised to see so many troops—more than I had any idea of are here.[636] Camped just below a splendid farm owned by the Widow Johnson 6 mis.[637] from Buchanan. We sent to Buchanan this morning about 20 sick.

[CAMP NEAR NATURAL BRIDGE, ROCKBRIDGE CO.]

[FRIDAY] JUNE 24– [1864]

Moved at day—At Buchanan the Ambulance [wagon] Train was sent to the 1st Lock on the canal [on James River] below to send sick to Lynchburg [Campbell Co.] Va. This necessitated us to walk.

Five miles below Buchanan [Botetourt Co.] [William] Mohler & myself turned across the mountain to Col. Richard Burke[638] and were well-treated by the family to buttermilk & c. Leaving there we visited Natural Bridge[639]—the center of army admiration at this time—The army is in camp in the neighborhood. Our train on Cedar Creek about 1/2 mile above the bridge.

The day has been very hot. Made order on Capt. Lock for 50 lb. Bacon & 25 of salt. —

---

[636] The old Virginia Bde or Stonewall Bde was almost gone, but these forces from the mountains were combined with other troops, and Jubal Anderson Early was commanding a corps of some 14,000 men. *OR*, ser. 1, vol. 36, 23 June 1864, "Report of Jubal A. Early." This date marked the beginning of Early's march down the Shenandoah Valley to the Federal capital.

[637] Possibly Elizabeth Johnson, born 1790, who owned a large farm in Amsterdam Township, some six miles from Buchanan. There are a number, at least a baker's dozen, of black and mulatto people who were once slaves on this land who are in the census in Buchanan Township. VA Census, 1870; Hummel, *A List*, 20.

[638] There was no Richard Burke living in Botetort or Rockbridge Cos. in 1870; however, there was a Richard W. Burke, born 1813, who was living in Stonewall Township of Rappahannock Co. He appears to have had some military experience, and may be the Col. Burke of this note. VA Census, 1870.

[639] This remarkable rock formation makes a bridge across a tributary of the James River in southwestern Rockbridge Co. and has always attracted the curious. The formation gives the name to the county of Rockbridge, which was formed in 1778 from a part of Augusta Co. *The Hornbook of Virginia History*, 4th ed. , ed., Emily J. Salmon and Edward D.C. Campbell, Jr. (Richmond: Library of Virginia, 1994) 169.

[CAMP NEAR LEXINGTON, ROCKBRIDGE CO.]

[SATURDAY] JUNE 25TH [1864]

The wagons left camp later than usual. I walked forward and reached Lexington about noon. The sun is boiling hot, the fields as hard as a pavement, and the roads shoe-mouth deep in dust. The ambulance train has not come up to the time of writing —

At Lexington the sad spectacle of the gloating destruction of the enemy is seen. The bare walls of V.M.I. call for a stern and unflinching position. I see writing on the pedestal from which the brass statue of [George] Washington was taken[.][640] [A]n avowal by the first Md. Cav. [CSA unit] to burn a college & gubernatorial mansion. May they kept [sic] it.

Lexington is a sweet place.

[CAMP NEAR GREENSVILLE, AUGUSTA CO.]

[SUNDAY] JUNE 26– [1864]

Left camp at 3 [A.M.]—ambulance train has not yet arrived. Started on foot—Breakfast at Widow [Nancy] Lyle five miles from Fairfield [Rockbridge Co].[641] This is an odd looking ancient village: Being Sabbath the doors and porches were filled with ladies, decked in their tidy apparel and looking as fresh "dew besprinkled roses" just opening at noon.[642] Here we waited 'till the ambulance train arrived. It passed 1/2 mile from the village [Fairfield] and remained 'till 3—then overtook the wagon train below Greenville [Greensville, Augusta Co], 11 miles from Staunton [Augusta Co]. Dr. Hagy came up with us.

---

[640] William Couper, historian of Virginia Military Institute, says that David Hunter burned the college buildings of V.M.I. and the home of wartime governor John Letcher (1833-1888), who had recently been defeated in a contest for CSA House of Representatives. The statue of George Washington was apparently of bronze, not brass, and it was removed to Wheeling, WV. Prof. Bean also notes that the wooden statue of George Washington atop the main building of Washington College (today's Washington and Lee University) was also removed by Hunter. Both statues were returned to the Lexington colleges after the War, but ex-governor Letcher was financially ruined by the experiences. Couper, *One Hundred Years at V.M.I.,* 4 vols. (Richmond, VA: Private printing, 1939) 3:23-39; W.G. Bean, Notes; Patricia L. Faust, "Letcher," *Hist. Times.*

[641] Prof Bean says that the Lyle mansion was still standing on Valley Pike, state Hwy 11 in 1970, situated about five miles from Lexington and five miles from Fairfield. Prof. Bean, Notes. Nancy Lyle (born 1800) was listed as holding land in Lexington, Rockbridge Co. in this area. VA Census, 1870.

[642] The diarist seems to be quoting from a song, but I cannot find it.

Dr. [Harvey] Black also came up. Slight shower fell this afternoon, but not sufficient to lay the dust to any extent.

[CAMP SOUTH OF STAUNTON, AUGUSTA CO.]

[MONDAY] JUNE 27 [1864]

Moved at sunrise—Stopped the train at Staunton a few hours, then moved three miles below on the Port Republic Road. There is great diversity of opinion as to our destination. All agreed that we will go down [northward] the Valley or back to Richmond. I am inclined to believe the first supposition.

I visited Miss L.T.[643] —spent a pleasant evening. Got to camp sometime after dark.

Sgt. [John] Thomas[644] paid me 4$ [one-fifth gold dollar; 4/5 U.S. greenback dollar] for articles bought for him at Richmond, VA.

I paid Lt. [James W.] Brown[645] 30$ [1.5 gold dollars, 6 U.S. greenback dollars] for a leather haversack—I learned baggage will be reduced to-morrow—The proposition often repeated that nought from nought, nought remains, will prove correct in many instances.

Rec'd a letter from my brother [Nat, or Cincinnatus Apperson], he is not a prisoner as was reported.

[CAMP BELOW STAUNTON, AUGUSTA CO.]

[TUESDAY] JUNE 28– [1864]

In camp to-day. Wrote letters to Cousin Bettie, Willie & Laura [children of Dr. William Faris] & Mrs. [Mary] Tomlin.

The army is surely moving down [northward] the Valley.

---

643 Prof. Bean identifies L.T. as Lizzie Taylor, "whom Apperson first met at Orange Court House." Prof. Bean, Notes.

644 Probably John F. Thomas (1837?-death date unknown]. Thomas, from Madison Co., had enlisted in Co. A, Richardson Guards, of 7th VA Inf, which outfit included the diarist's brother and friends from Orange Co. A farmer, Thomas, is listed in regimental history as corporal, but this seems to be him, given the context and his friendships. He was detailed guarding baggage. After War, he moved to Richmond, and lived out his final days in Soldiers' Home in capital city, being buried at Hollywood Cem. Riggs, *7th VA Inf.*, 96.

645 James W. Brown (1838?-death date unknown) was a carpenter who enlisted at Woodville (Rappahannock Co.) in Co. G (Rappahannock Guard), was soon promoted to corporal and in 1863 became officer. Wounded at Gettysburg (4 July 1863) soon after promotion, he recovered but was either wounded or became sick again, and when War ended was paroled in Stuart Hospital, Richmond. Riggs, 65.

Loan [William] Mohler 10$ [one-half gold dollar; 2 U.S. greenback dollars] & [Herbert M.] Nash 10$.[646] Dr. B. paid me out of Hosp't Fund 30$ [1.5 gold dollars; 6 U.S. greenback dollars] for Haversack [because he was required to lighten his load, and he was afraid he would never get it back, and thus lose a fair sum of money unfairly]. Dr. B paid 20 cents [about a penny on gold standard; about four cents on U.S. greenback standard] on public letter to Surg. Gen. [Lafayette Guild].

Our camp is near Maj Jno Harmon's.[647]

We move early to-morrow. Left some blankets with Mrs. J. Airs[648] at Staunton [not the well-known city, but the township in Bedford Co].

[Camp above Harrisonburg, Rockingham Co.]

[Wednesday] June 29 [1864]

Move at 3:45 this morning down [northward] the Valley Pike. Left the cows at Mr. Bell's.[649] Grazed the teams four miles from Harrisonburg at noon and camped 2 mis. above. It is worthy of perhaps [sic] to remark that the wheat crop in the Valley and all along our route is the finest I think I have ever seen. It is just ripening.

[Camp near New Market, Shenandoah Co.]

[Thursday] June 30– [1864]

Moved at 4 [A.M.]—The day is cool—our ambulance train (37 ambs) is engaged picking up straglers [sic]. [Maj. Gen. John Cabell] Breckinridge's men do not know how to march.[650]

---

[646] Probably Herbert M. Nash, no birth and death date, no occupation data, who was assistant surgeon with 9th VA Inf., Benjamin H. Trask, *9th VA Inf.*, VA Military Regimental History Series, ed. Howard (Lynchburg, VA: H.E. Howard, 1984) 83.

[647] Prof. Bean says, "John A. Harmon of Augusta County, Virginia, was quartermaster of [Jubal Anderson] Early's Valley arm; he was one of Stonewall [Thomas Jonathan] Jackson's staff members." Bean, notes.

[648] Prof. Bean thinks that the family name is *Ayers*, Bean, notes. If so, this could be the wife of John W.J. Ayers, born 1831, who had a home in Staunton Township, Bedford Co. VA Census, 1870.

[649] Two possibilities among landowning men named *Bell* in Rockingham County: James Bell, born 1800, had a farm in Franklin Twp; John Bell, born 1805, had a farm in Ashby Twp., VA Census, 1870. Prof. Bean says: "The cows, which belonged to Dr. Black, were taken along for the sick and wounded." Bean, notes.

[650] John Cabell Breckinridge (1821-1875), already identified. According to William C. [Jack] Davis, Breckinridge's men *did* know how to march, and of course they had just distinguished

We camped one mile below New Market [Shenandoah Co.]—Part of the army is far in advance. Two divisions moved parallell [sic], with us on the Luray Road.[651]

Received letters from Nat, Cousin Bettie & Dr. Quisenberry.

[CAMP AT WOODSTOCK, SHENANDOAH CO.]

[FRIDAY] JULY 1– [1864]

Later moving than usual. The day is very warm—men stragling [sic] very much.

Camped at Woodstock.

Drew rations for 5 days.

[CAMP NEAR MILLVILLE, CLARKE CO.]

[SATURDAY] JULY 2 [1864]

Moved down [northward] the [Valley] Pike & camped at Millville, one mile from Winchester [Clarke Co]. Passed [Stephen Dodson] Ramseur's [652] &: [John Cabell] Breckinridge's Divisions.

---

themselves famously at the Battle of New Market (15 May 1864). Idem, "Breckinridge," *Hist. Times.* However, the diarist is a keen observer, and the standard of comparison is the Old VA Brigade, the "two-legged horses" and "cavalry on foot" trained by Thomas Jonathan Jackson. If there are many stragglers, enough for the ambulances to pick them up, then something seems wrong with the march, for there are not recorded instances of the VA Brigade leaving many stragglers on such a march.

651 The road connects New Market in Shenandoah Co. with Luray in Page Co. by crossing Massanutten Mountain.

652 Stephen Dodson Ramseur (1837-1864) was born in Lincolndton, NC, graduated 14th in class from West Point in 1860, and was serving as 2nd Lt in Arty when War came. Wounded many times, he distinguished himself early in artillery and later in coordinating cavalry and infantry. Lee had promoted him to Maj. Gen. in June of 1864 and assigned him to this Valley March led by Jubal Anderson Early. Jeffry D. Wert says: "At 27, the youngest West Pointer to attain the rank of major general in the Confederate army, he possessed a reputation for battlefield prowess rivaled by few other generals in the Army of Northern Virginia. Amid the staggering confusion and the nearly impossible coordination of offensive combat, Ramseur excelled." Idem, "Ramseur," *Hist. Times.*

[CAMP AT SMITHFIELD, JEFFERSON CO, WV]

[SUNDAY] JULY 3 [1864]

Entered Winchester[Clarke.] Was sent to Dr. [Hunter Holmes] McGuire [surgeon general for Early's Corps, ANV] for orders. He directed Dr. B [illegible word] at York House. The building is very bare, been much abused. Dr. Hagy left in charge. Drs. [S.B.] Morrison & [C.W.] Walker, his assistants. Blacknall, [steward Harvey Allen]Jameson and Thomas with a number of nurses left.[653] A small supply of medicines and Hospital appliances turned over. 149 sick had been rec'd before we left, which was about noon.

The army is moving on towards Martinsburg [Berkeley Co., WV]. We took the Charleston [Jefferson Co., WV] Road at Bunker Hill [Jefferson Co., WV] and camped at Smithfield [Jefferson Co., WV]. Two divisions go to Martinsburg and two on this road.

I met Miss Maggie Walker this evening but could not call on Miss Kate S[chultz]. Much to my regret.[654]

[CAMP NEAR HALLTOWN, JEFFERSON CO., WV][655]

[MONDAY] JULY 4 [1864]

To-day [Lt. Gen. Ulysses S.] Grant was to be in Richmond. His intention is doubtless a failure.[656] We passed through Charleston under almost a perfect ovation of ladies. The people were supprised [sic] to see us. I met with a very liberal company below the village—a Miss Severs of Baltimore. Should I pass that way again, I'll call.[657]

---

[653] Thomas may be John Thomas (1836?; death date unknown) of 7th VA Inf, an enlisted man originally with Co. K of 7th VA Inf., Rigss, 95. Prof. Bean supplies initials for doctors Morrison and Walker, whom I cannot find in any directory or VA regimental history, Bean, notes. Harvey Allen Jameson of 4th was already identified; Robertson, op. cit. I cannot find anyone named Blacknall in VA regimental histories.

[654] These were Clarke Co. friends also mentioned in Apperson, "Reminiscences." Prof. Bean supplies the name *Schultz*, Bean, Notes.

[655] Halltown (also Hallton) is near Harper's Ferry, Shetler, *WV Civil War Literature*, 318, 817.

[656] Ulysses S. Grant was "investing" Petersburg and had settled in for a long and painful siege; Grant never announced any timetable for taking the CSA capital. As for Jubal Anderson Early's march down the Valley toward the U.S. capital, Long notes of contemporaneous sources that the sporadic skirmishes, none of which slowed Early's Corps, frightened MD and DC citizens: "Citizens north of the Potomac were in an uproar and even Washington was apprehensive. Was it only a raid or a serious invasion?" Long, 530; 532.

[657] Severs is not identified more fully. In Apperson's "Reminiscences," he notes some "youthful foolishness," of which he was ashamed, and specifies Mary Camden [Mollie A., Mrs.

Our train stopped near Halltown [Jefferson Co., WV]. There is cannonading at Harper's Ferry. From a hill near Halltown we could see distinctly all the batteries. The enemy has gone to Maryland Heights and will probably stay there. The capture of that place will not justify the loss of life that would ensue.[658]

[CAMP AT FLAG'S MILL, JEFFERSON CO., WV]

[TUESDAY] JULY 5TH [1864]

This morning I was sent with Surgn [Samuel Rush] Sayers [attached to 4th VA Inf.] to Martinsburg [Berkeley Co., WV] to call for medical supplies at that place. Took a wagon and Ambulance. I got to Martinsburg about 1 P.M. but our trip did not pay. The capture here was large, but the soldiers had pillaged everything. After hard work a small quantity of stores was gathered & sent to Dr. Hagy at Winchester. Maj. Garber is commanding the Post but is incapable of doing anything sober.[659]

We were kindly treated by the family of Mr. D.[660]

After finishing our mission as near as it could be I went out and camped near Mr. Flag's Mill. Mr. [James M.] Eads was with me.[661]

A.], but otherwise mentions no names. A woman for whom he had some regard, he usually calls *lady*, and gives a name and description. "Liberal company" is a bit wry and even smarmy, suggesting looseness. Idem, "Reminiscences," 564

[658] Lt. Gen. Jubal Anderson Early had by now determined to attack the Federal capital itself. He found the area around Harper's Ferry (Jefferson Co., WV) to be too well-defended, and so turned to Shepherdstown, MD, as his point of departure for crossing the Potomac River. Apparently Maryland Heights itself was not assaulted; the diarist may have heard the firing on two bridges, South Branch Bridge, WV and Patterson's Creek Bridge WVA. More fighting occurred during the week in MD at Keedysville, Noland's Ferry, Point of Rocks, and Solomon's Gap. The official reports note that a desperate call was put out for 24,000 militia volunteers from NY and PA to meet the emergency caused by Early's advance. *OR*, ser. 1, 37:169 table.

[659] I cannot locate a field grade officer named Garber in VA regimental military series histories or in *OR*.

[660] I have been unable to identify this person.

[661] James M. Eads (1834-death date unknown) was merchant from Smyth Co. He joined Rockbridge Grays, which became Co. H of 4th Virginia Infantry. Later he became brigade postmaster. Robertson, *4th VA Inf.*, 48.

[CAMP AT FLAG'S MILL, JEFFERSON CO., WV]

[WEDNESDAY] JULY 6– [1864]

This morning we took breakfast at Mr. Flag's. His daughters seem to be nice ladies. The people here are very much censured for Union proclivities, but I have never seen more generosity anywhere than among those who are favorable to our cause. There are a larger number of these too than many will admit.

The troops from the [Harper's] Ferry have moved to Shepherdstown [WV], and are crossing the [Potomac] River. At the crossroads I was stopped by an old lady to see a young man named [Alexander H.] Kite from Lovingston [Nelson Co.] who was severely wounded. I found some of the bones of the pelvis broken. He is evidently dangerous [that is, dangerously wounded].[662]

Found the Ambulance train near Shepperdstown [sic]. Last night the A.Q.M. [assistant quartermaster] of the army went into the [Harper's] Ferry and brought out a large quantity of shirts. The forage there and at Martinsburg [Berkeley Co.] is large, over any captures we have made.

Wrote to Dr. Q[uisenberry] & Dr. F[aris].

[ON THE ROAD NEAR SHARPSBURG, MD]

[THURSDAY] JULY 7– [1864][663]

Moved across the Potomac at Shepherdstown [WV]. I bought a hat for which I paid $2.50 cts. in gold [fifty CSA dollars; twelve US greenback dollars]—a very common hat too.

---

[662] Apparently this young soldier survived this ordeal. He is probably Alexander H. Kite (no birth and death data, no occupation data) who enlisted at New Market in Co. E (Culpeper) of 13th VA Inf., a regiment that included Nelson Co. enlistees. "Light complexion, hazel eyes, light hair." He is then listed as captured, POW, at Petersburg, 2 April 1865 and imprisoned at Point Lookout, with release and pardon, 28 June 1865. Riggs, 124. No person named *Kite* is listed among soldiers killed by official reports, 1 May–3 August 1864, *OR*, ser. 1, vol. 37, pts. 1 and 2.

[663] On the previous day, Jubal Anderson Early's troops had captured Hagerstown, MD. Gen. John McCausland (1836-1927) led Early's cavalry into Chambersburg and demanded $20,000 [apparently in US gold dollars, about $100,000 in US greenback dollars, and more than 400,000 CSA dollars] from the people in that town because of Gen. David Hunter's depredations in the Valley. When merchants refused to pay, McCausland torched the business district after evacuating 300 residents. He was apparently not reprimanded by R.E. Lee or other leaders for this action, and in fact he was well-respected by his superiors. Northern presses refered to the incident as "McCausland's atrocity," and he hid out in Europe some years after The War, then lived in "self-imposed isolation" in Mason City, WV. Son of Irish immigrants, McCausland had gained entry into VMI, and graduated at the head of his class in 1857. James I. Robertson, "McCausland," *Hist. Times.*

At Sharpsburg I stopped at Mr. Hebe's[664] to deliver a letter. The day is very hot.

The army is demonstrating on Harpers Ferry from the Maryland side.

Saw Charles St. John.[665]

[ON THE ROAD NEAR MIDDLETOWN, MD]

[FRIDAY] JULY 8– [1864]

This morning we moved to Middletown 8 mis. from Frederick City. The towns along the road are sure sacked. Many of stores are a confused mass of trash. Men run over goods and conclude there is nothing they want. At Boonesboro [MD] Dr. B. went into the Dry Store of Hoofman and Smith and selected a bill of $207 and paid cash [apparently $10.33 in gold or $41.40 in US greenbacks]. He is acting Med. Purveyor *I believe* [diarist's emphasis]. [Herbert M.] Nash [surgeon][666] will do the work *I think* [sic].

I am not satisfied here and am determined to avail myself of the first opportunity to be transferred—don't care where.

[CAMP AT FEDERAL GENERAL HOSPITAL, FREDERICK, MD]

[SATURDAY] JULY 9TH [1864]

This morning we entered the Town [Frederick, MD]. The sum of $200,000 [apparently CSA dollars and thus $100,000 in US greenbacks and $10,000 in gold] was levied on the Corporation [the incorporated Town of Frederick] and paid by the Mayor into the hands of Maj. Braithwaite A.Q.M. [assistant quartermaster].[667] The stores were overharried [overly plundered][668] and such

---

[664] I cannot identify this citizen.

[665] There is no Charles St. John listed in 4th VA Inf. or 7th VA Inf. and none for any VA regiments that I can find. C.B. St. John of Smyth Co. is listed as a freeholder in the Co. who was paid a sum of money because of losses by his family, according to Armstrong, *Hist. of Smyth*, 128. There are several soldiers named St. John in Orange Artillery; none named Charles, but possibly related. Macaluso, *Morris, Orange Arty.*

[666] Herbert M. Nash (no birth or death data, no occupational data) was assistant surgeon originally with 9th VA Inf, and probably from southside or the tidewater. He was commissioned in fall of 1861. Benjamin H. Trask, *9th VA Inf.*, VA Regimental Histories Series, ed. Howard (Lynchburg: H.E. Howard, 1984), 83.

[667] The only Braithwaite that I can find is an enlisted man in 14th VA CAV, Joseph C. Braithwaite; but this seems highly unlikely as the identification. Driver, 104.

[668] "Harry [M.E.]...to afflict with an army...plunder." *Webster's.* The prefix *over* seems peculiar to the diarist, since the verb carries a definition of extreme affliction and even plundering.

things as the army needed were bought and paid for out of the funds levied [that is, from the $200,000 collected from the Mayor of Frederick]. A large amount of Med[ical] Supplies were captured at the [US general] Hospital. These were not much [possibly, *narcotics*]. Several large boxes were procured from the Drug Stores in town. I was at none but Shy's or Schley's, and Johnson; the first [Shy] a strong union man, the other [Johnson] professed to be southern in his views. From the Drug Store we went to the Hospt and found a large supply of Med. Stores. Enough to have filled our wagons. The Hosp't here is neatly arranged. Surgn Wills in charge.[669]

I was engaged 'till near midnight, then went to camp about a mile from town.

A considerable fight ensued at Monocacy River this evening [afternoon]. The enemy was a part of the 6th Corps from [Lt. Gen. U.S.] Grant's army and were driven off with considerable loss. [Maj. Gen. John B.] Gordon's Division did the fighting. [Brig. Gen. Clement Anselm] Evans' GA Brig. have most of the loss. He was slightly wounded—I think from evidence apparent that there is a strong feeling of sympathy here for the South.[670]

---

[669] I cannot find a surgeon named Wills. One possibility is John A. Wills (no birth or death data, no occupation data), who was a driver in ordnance wagons for 4th VA Inf. and who would have been on this march. His job would have entailed gathering and disbursing such stores. Robertson, *4th VA Inf.*, 81.

[670] This fight at the Monocacy River on 9 and 10 July near Frederick, MD, was a fight won by Jubal Anderson Early's forces in a campaign won by the Federals. Among US leaders, only Gen. Lewis Wallace (1827-1905) organized himself to set up resistance to some 20,000 men commanded by Early at Frederick; apparently Lt. Gen. U.S. Grant was unsure until this day that Early's men were not still in Petersburg vicinity. Wallace's forces were not joined until late by the 6th Corps commanded by Maj. Gen. James Brewerton Ricketts (1817-1887). The forces of Wallace and Ricketts put up a brave fight, losing and being dispersed, "In disorder" according to official report filed by Wallace; but the fighting slowed Early's advance toward the capital "for one vital day." Jeffrey D. Wert goes so far as to say that "the Battle of Monocacy perhaps saved the Northern capital." Idem., "Monocacy," *Hist Times.*; *OR*, ser. 1, 10 July 1864, Edwin M. Stanton to Maj. Gen. Dix, 190. Evans (1833-1911), a very capable leader, was so moved by this and other battles that after The War he took orders and became a Methodist minister. He was wounded more severely on this (and four other occasions) than the diarist understood; but he did return to lead the GA division, replacing Gordon at Petersburg and continuing until surrender at Appomattox Court House. Wert, "Evans". John Brown Gordon (1832-1904) was already identified. No military or other authorities that I can find suggest southern sympathies here; and the diarist's testimony is singular, and even peculiar, in this regard.

[ON THE ROAD TO WASHINGTON, D.C. ON GEORGETOWN PIKE, MD]

[SUNDAY] JULY 10TH [1864]

Moved on the Georgetown Pike [Frederick Co., MD]. Most of our wounded (some 250) were left. The enemy is said to have gone into Frederick soon after we left.

I have never seen so much dust. At times it was impossible to see more than 30 or 60 yards ahead. No prospect for rain. The earth is baked like a brick. We made a march of over 20 miles.

[ON THE ROAD TO WASHINGTON, D.C., NEAR SILVER SPRING, MD]

[MONDAY] JULY 11– [1864]

We have been expecting to cross the [Potomac] River but at Rockville, we took the Washington City Road and camped within 2 mis. of the line of the D.C. To the surprise of all Gen. [Jubal Anderson] Early commenced knocking at the door of Washington. What force is there we cannot of course tell and the result of the move is too uncertain to be commented upon. Dust from the wagon train rose like a cloud along the road.

*[ON THE ROAD BELOW SILVER SPRING, MD
OUTSIDE THE CITY LIMITS OF WASHINGTON, D.C.]*

[TUESDAY] JULY 12TH [1864]

This morning we moved about 1/2 mile nearer the City and halted. Gen. [Jubal Anderson] Early in his shrewdness sent his inspectors around to make examination of his wagon trains to ascertain what amount of stores, Private & Public, had been taken along. Startling were the revealings — Statements of the Quartermasters were in full blast—some had a sufficiency of dry goods to commence business. Our department was not interfered with. There is a spirited skirmish fire going on and some desultory cannonading. I don't think & have not thought that we would do more than demonstrate. We are ordered to move to-night at sundown. The house of Montgomery Blair, Post Master General of the U.S. is in our lines and soon after dark a large fire was seen in the neighborhood of where the house stood. I suppose that is lex talionis [diarist's italics].[671]

---

[671] *Lex talionis* is law of retaliation, and the diarist is here saying that J.A. Early was justified in burning the Blair house in Silver Spring, MD because of Gen. David Hunter's depreadations in

[ON THE ROAD FROM SILVER SPRING, MD TO LEESBURG [LOUDON CO., VA]

[WEDNESDAY] JULY 13– [1864]

Last night we moved all night. Stopped at Dawsonville [MD] to rest the trains. I went to Poolsville [MD] and bought goods. The feeling in that place seems to be Southern. I cannot call names but I hope one man will not be interrupted.[672] Our train moves at sundown and I shall await its arrival. A party of men, soon after [John Cabell] Breckinridge's[673] army passed broke open a store. I never saw goods disappear so rapidly. I was in the street on the opposite side and saw the proceedings through the window. men mounted the shelves and with both hands threw goods backward like excited animals. They seemed not to want anything but still persisted in searching. One man after throwing down hundreds of dollars worth walked out with an armful of axe handles.[674]

About mid-night the train passed—crossed the [Potomac] River at Edward's Ferry and at Leesburg [both in Loudon Co.] by noon we camped in a sweet

---

the Valley. As for Early himself, however, the CSA gen. always insisted that he had never ordered this burning. The house in Silver Spring was actually built by the paterfamilias Francis Preston Blair (1791-1876), a Kentuckian and old Andrew Jackson protege and newspaper editor who formerly owned slaves but had joined the Republican Party and become antislavery though not by any means a friend of the Radical Republicans. One son, Francis Preston Blair, Jr. (1821-1875) was a prominent US gen. well-respected by U.S. Grant and W.T. Sherman, who were generally critical of so-styled political promotions in the US military. The other son, Montgomery Blair (1813-1883) was Postmaster General and as such responsible for modernizing the US postal services. All three of the Blairs were good friends of Abraham Lincoln, but were despised by the Radical Republicans, and Montgomery Blair was maneuvered out of the Cabinet not long after Gen. Early's troops torched the Blair family house. David Lindsey, "Montgomery Blair," *Hist. Times.* Long joins others in suggesting that J.A. Early must have approved of the Blair house burning, and likely ordered it. Long, 537. Official US Army reports filed by C.A. Dana to U.S. Grant indicate that the Federal offices always considered that J.A. Early had deliberately burned these and other homes and indeed "the damage to private property done by the invaders is almost beyond calculation." C.A. Dana, "Report," 11 July 1864, *OR*, ser. 1, 37:194. The diarist's vigorous defense of Early's actions in all these regards reads as a somewhat naive verification that Early ordered the Blair home burned as retaliation for Hunter's actions in the Valley.

672 Prof. Bean says that the connotation of *interrupted* here means *molested.* Bean, notes.

673 John Cabell Breckinridge (1821-1875) was already identified. His services in this raid and in the subsequent campaigns in Shenandoah Valley were highly praised. J.A. Early, "Report," 1 August 1864, *OR*, ser. 1, 37:602-06.

674 This and many other notations by the diarist suggest that the CSA troops on this campaign behaved much as had Federal troops in the service of Gen. David Hunter in the Valley. *Lex talionis* seems strained as justification for the looting and pillaging just described.

grove near Mr. Sanders [possibly Henry Saunders][675] . A rest of a day or so seems probable and then a move—but where.

[William] Mohler paid me 10$ [CSA; about fifty cents in gold; about two US greenback dollars] he borrowed some time ago.

[CAMP NEAR RODES OR RHODES FARM, LEESBURG, LOUDON CO.]

[THURSDAY] JULY 14– [1864]

Traveled from midnight [.] Crossed the river [possibly North Fork of Potomac in Loudon Co.] about 10 o'clock. Gen. [Jubal Anderson] Early was present watching the wagons pass over. Reached Leesburg about noon. Our camp is near Mr. Rode's [possibly Toulemiah Rhodes][676] in a beautiful cool grove. I wrote letters to Dr. F, M.J.C. [Mary Camden] & Cousin Bettie.

I forgot to State in yester-day's memorandum that I borrowed 30$ [about 1.5 gold dollars; about 6 US greenback dollars] from Dr. [John Alexander] Straith & 20 $ [about 1 gold dollar; about 4 US greenback dollars] from Dr. Black.

[CAMP NEAR RODES OR RHODES FARM, LEESBURG, LOUDON CO.]

[FRIDAY] JULY 15– [1864]

Sent the ambulance train and some med. Stores under charge of Surgn. Love to Winchester. Nearly all the attendants in Hospt. were sent.

We remained in camp. Drew on Capt. Lock yester-day evening for 1000$ hospt funds [about 50 gold dollars; about 200 US greenback dollars].

Dr. B turned over to Dr. Love 500$ hosp't funds.

[William] Mohler & I took tea at Mr. Rode's [sic].

---

675 No one named *Sanders* is listed in census for Loudon Co. in 1870; there is Henry Saunders, born 1789, who owned a farm in this vicinity. VA Census, 1870.

676 No one named *Rodes* is listed in census for Loudon Co. in 1870; there is Toulemiah Rhodes, who owned a farm in this vicinity. VA Census, 1870.

[CAMP NEAR SNICKER'S GAP OUTSIDE SNICKERSVILLE, LOUDON CO.]

[SATURDAY] JULY 16– [1864]

Dr. B turned over to Dr. Mott, private physician at Leesburg,[677] 25$ in federal funds [that is, 125 CSA dollars; 6.25 gold dollars] for use of sick and wounded left there.

Left camp at 7 o'clock, fell in rear of [Gen. John B.] Gordon's Division train. The day has been extremely hot and the road dusty. There seems to be no evidence of rain. The sky seems like a vast sheet of steel, not a drop of rain seems probable.

Dr. [Samuel Rush] Sayers & I took dinner at a private house.

The enemy is pressing us.[678]

Reported to have captured [Gen. John] McCausland wagon train.[679] I do not regret it. His men are scattered over the country and do nothing. Camped at the crossing at [Snicker's Gap] Snickersville Gap.

We passed through Hamiltonsville and Snickersville [western Loudon Co.].

[CAMP, HOLLINGSWORTH MILLS, CLARKE CO.]

[SUNDAY] JULY 17– [1864]

The army moved a short distance and halted. We came with the remainder of our Hospt. Train to Winchester. Everything there in confusion. Our wagons camped at Hollingsworth Mills.

Bathed changed my clothes and called on Miss Kate Schultz. Was introduced to her maiden sister, the latter a good looking, amiable girl. Had the pleasure of escorting Miss Kate to church. Mr. [J.Marsdin] Grandin[680] preached. Dr. B will not take immediate charge of the Hospital here but have a general supervision.

---

677 Probably Dr. David Mott, born 1830, who lived in Eastern District, Leesburg, Loudon Co., VA Census, 1870.

678 The enemy is Col. Charles Russell Lowell (1835- 1864), a Bostonian who had graduated 1st in his class from Harvard, and a nephew of poet James Russell Lowell. Col. Lowell was commanding Independent 22nd Cav. Bde. Jeffrey D. Wert, "Lowell," *Hist. Times.*

679 Col. Lowell was reported to have captured some fifty of McCausland's troops, but there is no official report of capturing wagons. Lowell's own men were in some distress and effected a cleverly masked retreat: "His retreat was favored by the dust which covered his flanks and prevented McCausland from seeing his weakness." C.A. Dana, "Report," 13 July 1864, *OR*, ser. 1, vol. 37, pt. 2:260.

680 Chaplain J. Marsdin Grandin, 33rd VA Inf., was a Clarke Co. native serving in a Shenandoah unit. He had been imprisoned in Gettysburg, was exchanged and returned, and would resign from chaplaincy in Sept. Pitts, 144. Lowell Reidenbaugh writes: "Chaplain of regiment as early as Jan. 1862. POW at Gettsyburg (4 July 1863). Exchanged from Johnson's

[TEMPORARY FIELD HOSPITAL, NEAR HOLLINGSWORTH MILLS, CLARKE CO.]

[MONDAY] JULY 18TH [1864]

To-day spent in the confusion attending the establishment of an [sic] hospital where there are several more patients than beds or room for them. All our Hospital attendants are on duty with Dr. Love in charge of the York House.

[OFFICES, TOWN OF WINCHESTER, CLARKE CO.]

[TUESDAY] JULY 19TH [1864]

To-day I moved into town. Office next door to Mrs. ____ [diarist's punctuation].

About 300 wounded were sent in from an engagement at Snickersville Ferry yester-day.[681]

The ladies of the place have been all attention. I have never seen such devotion. They are dining the men all the while. Young Walker of Ala. was brought—I know how much concered his Ma will be.

Orders this evening are significant. The wounded and sick are to be sent forthwith to Mt. Jackson [Shenandoah Co.].[682] There was some excitement in town to-day occasioned by the appearance of some 5 or 6000 enemy a few miles below Winchester. Our wounded and sick are suffering for the appliances to make them comfortable.[683]

Island 1863-64. Relieved from duty 9/1/64. Records are sadly lacking here." Idem, *33d VA Inf.*, VA Regimental Hist Ser. , ed., Howard (Lynchburg, VA: H.E. Howard, 1987), 123.

[681] No engagement is recorded at Snickersville or Snickers Ford on this day. There is a "sharp engagement" at Berry's Ford, Clarke Co., as Long notes, 542, and as recorded with some casualties for Jubal Anderson Early's men, Early, "Report," 19 July 1864, *OR*, ser. 1, vol. 37, pt. 1, 321-22. See also A Register, comp. Warrinner, 19 July 1864, "Berry's Ford," "Snickersville," s.v.

[682] Prof. Bean notes that "there were several hospitals in Mt. Jackson in the Valley," Bean, notes. Cunningham lists no general hospitals in Mt. Jackson, and thus these hospitals are likely field hospitals, but perhaps located in homes or office buildings or churches rather than tents or barns. Cunningham, appendices.

[683] In traditional nineteenth century conventions, "suffering from the appliances" means that the appliances are needed. Note that it is still likely a problem of logistics and transportation, rather than the poverty of the CSA or the peculations of speculators or the conspiratorial manipulations of traitors; Cunningham reports that there were supplies of all sorts and conditions located in Richmond, and that these supplies were more than sufficient for the CSA medical officers , but that there were increasing difficulties in getting the supplies out to the stewards and doctors in the field because of shortage of wagons, problems with railroad trains, torn-up rail lines, and dangerous and badly kept wagon roads. Generally, the diarist's notes seem to affirm

Dr. B paid over to Dr. [Hunter Holmes] McGuire 300 dollars in Maryland money [approximately the same as US greenbacks, and thus 1,200 CSA dollars or 60 gold dollars].

I called on the Misses Miller[;] had a pleasant evening indeed. The youngest is pretty, the middle one is talkative, and Miss Maggie is an excellent lady.

[FIELD HOSPITAL, DAVID MILLER'S FARM, OPEQUON TOWNSHIP, FREDERICK CO.]

[WEDNESDAY] JULY 20– [1864]

All is bustle and confusion.

We will leave to-day. The sick and wounded had all started by a little after noon.

I called on the Misses Miller to bid them adieu and left town with our Hd Qters wagon about 5 o'clock. The other wagons of our train had preceded us about three or four hours. I stopped opposite Mr. David Miller's at Middletown [Opequon Township, Frederick Co].[684]

Dr. Black came about 11 o'clock and I had to go on an errand to find Capt. [John Montgomery] Preston.[685]

Gen. [Stephen Dodson] Ramseur had an engagement with the enemy [Col. Benjamin Franklin Coates] in which [sic] lost nearly the whole of [John] Pegram's Brigade. The affair is considered by many of us to have been a very disgraceful affair.[686]

Cunningham on this point. Idem, 156-62. Early was retreating toward Winchester, and the diarist is hearing the fighting at Stephenson's Depot [Frederick Co] between Ohio infantry and NC infantry under Stephen Dodson Ramseur. Col. Benjamin Franklin Coates, "Report," *OR*, ser. 1, vol. 37 (20 July 1864) 314.

[684] David Miller, born 1816, owned a farm in Opequon Township, Middletown, Frederick Co. VA Census, 1870. By context, he seems to be no relationship to the Miller ladies who lived in the Town of Winchester, Clarke Co.

[685] John Montgomery Preston, born 1838 in Washington Co. was son and namesake of Washington Co. planter who later moved to Albemarle Co., where this Capt. Preston grew up. He joined as officer of 48th VA Inf., rising to Capt., and survived War, moving to Smyth Co. to establish a home and farm and other businesses on Upper Fork of Holston River, with business mailing address at Seven Mile Ford. Smyth, *Smyth Co. Families*, ed. Presgraves, 36-37.

[686] According to the account of Douglas Southall Freeman in *Lee's Lieutenants*, it was the Bde of Robert Frederick Hoke (1837-1912) that broke and ran at crucial point, dooming many to casualties and the Jubal Anderson Early forces to defeat at Stephenson's Depot. John Pegram (1832-1865) apparently did not let his forces break and run, but his brigade did suffer terribly, suffering some casualties; and many of Pegram's Bde were captured. Federals report capturing 250 CSA troops, with unclear report of wounded and killed, perhaps a dozen. See B.F. Coates, "Report," *OR*. Cf. Freeman, *Lee's Lieutenants*, 3:570. Long, surveying the controversies, notes

[FIELD HOSPITAL NEAR DAVID MILLER'S, OPEQUON TOWNSHIP, MIDDLETOWN, FREDERICK CO.]

[THURSDAY] JULY 21– [1864]

Went to Gen. [Jubal Anderson] Early's Hd quarters with Dr. Black and back to camp—then to Mt. Jackson [field hospitals]. Had my horse shod. I was very tired and sleepy when I arrived there. The sick are being sent off as rapidly as possible. At Strasburg [Frederick Co.] I dressed the wound of Gen. [William Gaston] Lewis.[687]

[FIELD HOSPITAL IN CHURCH YARD, FISHER'S HILL, SHENANDOAH CO.]

[FRIDAY] JULY 22– [1864]

Cooler to-day than usual. Smokey, but still very dry.

Our quarters are in a church yard. The army is at Fisher's Hill above Strasburg [Shenandoah Co]. Gen. [Jubal Anderson] Early presents quite an imposing front there. Perhaps he may fight.

Reported that [Lt. Gen. Ulysses Simpson] Grant is dead. No one believes it.

---

cautiously: "Federal infantry and [William Woods] Averell's cavalry defeated a Confederate division under Stephen D. Ramseur in a milling fight around the little red brick depot. A Confederate brigade broke, and over 250 Confederates were captured. The main body of Early's troops continued to withdraw southward toward Strasburg [Shenandoah Co]." Idem, 543. William Woods Averell (1832-1900) was an able West Point graduate with cavalry experience in Southwestern Indian fights during which 1861 wounds delayed his entry into Federal service in the War. Decorated for leadership of PA cavalry troops in Peninsula Campaign, he often fell afoul of more aggressive Federal officers, esp. Gen. Philip Sheridan, because of "dilatoriousness," and he was relocated after Chancellorsville to WVA, where he engaged successfully in this fight. In time, Sheridan removed Averell from all command, but his record does show some successes, as on this occasion. Edward G. Longacre, "Averell," *Hist. Times.*

[687] William Gaston Lewis (1835-1901) was descended of Revolutionary War veterans in NC and grew up in eastern NC, graduating with honors from University of North Carolina before becoming a school teacher and then a managing and planning engineer for main NC railroads on coast. Originally with NC 43rd, he rose in ranks and became regimental commander; on this occasion he was in temporary command of Hoke's Bde after the fiasco at Stephenson's Depot. Lewis apparently performed well in this fighting despite his wound and was later promoted to Col. He was later cited again for bravery, and was wounded severely near the end of the War on 7 April 1865 at Battle of Farmville. Idem, "Lewis," *Hist. Times.*

Surgn. Davis of Richmond is placed in charge of the [field] Hospital [at Strasburg]. A good man, I expect.[688]

[ON THE VALLEY PIKE TO KERNSTOWN [FREDERICK CO.]

[SATURDAY] JULY 23 [1864]

To-day we overhauled the papers pertaining to the purchases of supplies purchased [sic] in Maryland and the funds turned over to Dr. B in Maryland money.

The account nearly balanced. Memorandums [sic] were made. I have one, and Dr. B the other.

We have orders to move in the vicinity of the army [2d Corps of ANV maneuvering preparatory to Second Battle of Kernstown].

[ON MANEUVERS NEAR WOODSTOCK, SHENANDOAH CO.]

[SUNDAY] JULY 24– [1864]

Went to church. Rev. Mr. Clyrie, Lutheran preached.[689] Had washing done, 3$ for it [CSA currency; 75 cents in US greenbacks; 15 cents in gold dollars]. Packing up to move. I sent my bundles of sundries to Mr. Fuller in Staunton by W. Paramore,[690] ambulance driver.

The bundle contains

---

[688] I cannot identify a Dr. Davis, surgeon from Richmond. Since this is not a general hospital, and since Dr. Davis apparently held no high rank among medical corps officers, he is not listed by Cunningham, nor in biographical sources.

[689] I cannot find a minister named Clyrie. Since he was not a chaplain, he is not listed in Pitts, nor in regimental histories. There is nobody with name *Clyrie* in VA census of 1870, and thus this minister must have passed on, or perhaps relocated to some other state, between summer 1864 and the census of 1870.

[690] Prof. Bean opines that the "bundle of sundries" was "presumably purchases in Maryland"; and this supposition seems reasonable, for the list below is consumer items, some relatively rare; Bean, notes. I cannot find a soldier named *Parramore* in the regimental histories; there is a large landholding and slaveholding family named *Parramore* on the peninsula of Accomack Co., and many slaves were named *Parramore* by this family. It is possible that a slave or even a freed black is employed as an ambulance driver, and that he performs some odd jobs for a fee, much as did James Cooley. Also, sometimes medical personnel are not listed in regimental histories because they are attached to different regiments during a career—and sometimes they are attached to an entire corps, such as ANV, 2nd, as Apperson is in this section of diary, and thus such people are not listed as part of a given regiment. Fuller could be one of two landholding men named Fuller who had large holdings in the Staunton district of Augusta Co.: Frank Fuller, born 1796; and George Fuller, born 1804, both with business addresses in the City of Staunton. VA Census, 1870.

7 yds cassimere[691]
8 yds cambric [692]
2 yds cottonade [693]
4 prs India Rubber shoes
2 prs Leather Do [ditto; that is, shoes]
1 pr Ladies Do
3 yds cotton cloth
7 sheep skins dressed

We moved at 3 o'clock to Woodstock [Shenandoah Co.]—camped 2 mis. below Woodstock. I laid down on my horse's hay expecting to rest awhile and retire. Soon the quiet slumber was broken by drops of rain falling in my face. I rose and spread my blanket and went to sleep again, only to be aroused again. I then caught a wagon but found after about 2 hours sleep that there was no hay in or covering on the (forage) wagon while the rain was pouring through on me.

[FIELD HOSPITAL, HOLLINGSWORTH MILLS, CLARKE CO.]

[MONDAY] JULY 25 [1864]

We started to Strasburg [Shenandoah Co]. Rain fell in torrents. I had on a gum 'coat but it did not suffice. At Strasburg we met Qmaster Montgomery who informed us that Gen. [Jubal Anderson] Early had attacked the Yankees in the preceding evening and drove them hellbent towards Martinsburg [Berkeley Co., WVA]. We doubted the report at first but found it true. At Winchester [Clarke Co.] we found all our wounded and sick undisturbed [at their field hospital]. The Yankee Gen. [sic; Col. James Adelbert] Mulligan was severely wounded—We lost about 300 killed and wounded—The Yankees about the same number.[694]

---

691 "from an old form of Kashmire…a medium-weight woolen cloth of soft texture." *Webster's*, 2nd rev. ed.

692 "a fine, thin, closely woven white fabric made of linen…from Cambrai, a city of France formerly of Flanders…." Ibid.

693 "any of certain cotton fabrics made so as to resemble wool." Ibid.

694 The diarist's statistics are usually conservative, especially if he is personally involved in collecting the data and tending the wounded. Thus, something seems amiss in the records. Official statistics from the Second Battle of Kernstown list more than 1200 Federal casualties and suggest that some casualties may be unlisted; official records for CSA losses at Kernstown do not exist, but casualties were said to be "light." On this day, Early's forces pursued Gen. George Crook (1828-1890) out of Winchester toward Bunker Hill in a heavy rainstorm, and casualties are experienced, but nowhere near 300 CSA casualties. It seems then that CSA records and Federal records have missed a significant group of CSA casualties in the battles fought in late July around

The army moved at 3 o'clock. Rec'd mail—nothing for me. Called on Miss Schultz—Train encamped at Hollingsworth's Mills [Clarke Co. near Town of Winchester].

Dr. B sent Dr. [John Alexander] Straith yester-day 20$ in Federal money [80 CSA dollars; 4 gold dollars].

[ON THE MARTINSBURG ROAD NEAR BIG SPRING, CLARKE CO.]

[TUESDAY] JULY 26 [1864]

The rain yester-day made the air very pleasant. Our train moved on the Martinsburg Road.

Dr. B, Dr. [John Alexander] Straith, myself, were invited to dine at Mr. Schultz's to-day[695]—The dinner was an excellent one indeed—Kind people.

Left Winchester about 4 o'clock and found our train at Big Spring [Clarke Co]. The troops are in camp near the town [Winchester, Frederick Co].

[CAMP NEAR BIG SPRING, CLARKE CO.;
FIELD HOSPITAL, WINCHESTER, FREDERICK CO.]

[WEDNESDAY] JULY 27– [1864]

In camp to-day.

I rode into town this evening and called on Miss Doll. Dr. [William] Taylor has been appointed Medical Purveyor[696] and all medicines have been turned

---

Winchester. Cf *OR*, ser. 1, vol. 37, pt. 1 (23-25 July 1864) 310-350. James Adelbert Mulligan (1830-1864) was an Irish-American political general who was sometimes victim and sometimes beneficiary of northern politics in War. Politically active among Chicago Democrats, he raised the Irish Brigade that became the 23rd Illinois, for which he served initially as Capt.; this group was assigned to defend Lexington MO early in War, were defeated, and Capt. Mulligan was captured. Later exchanged, his Bde was disbanded by abolitionist Gen. John Charles Fremont (identified earlier; 1813-1890), and Mulligan himself lost his commission. Without authorization, he re-formed the Irish Bde, and Gen. George Brinton McClellan [identified earlier;1826-1885], himself a very active Democratic politician, restored Mulligan to command and set the Irish Bde in charge of a prison camp, with Mulligan commandant and Col. Still later reassigned when Gen. McClellan fell from favor, Col. Mulligan was sent to WVA, where he held a number of posts. He was Col. in command of 3d Division at 2nd Kernstown (23 July 1864), where he was wounded as diarist notes. He did not survive the wounds, and was buried on 26 July 1864. Posthumously he was brevetted Brig. Gen. Stewart Sifakis, "Mulligan," *Who Was Who in the Civil War* (New York: Facts on File, 1988). On ranks, *OR*, ser. 1, vol. 37, pt. 1., but esp. 663.

695 Possibly John W. Schultz, born 1826, who had land and a home in Stonewall Township of Frederick Co. near Winchester. VA Census, 1870.

696 Records are not clear on this score, and Cunningham does not show the appointment. Idem, appendices; however, there is a Dr. William Taylor (1827-1891) from Berryville [Clarke

over to him. There will be some confusion in regard to the papers to be made out.

Dr. B. was appointed when we went into Md. and made the purchases. Dr. [H.P.] Magruder and Dr. Morrison[697] made issues and I very much fear Dr. B will be required to make a return as Med: Purveyor.

[CAMP NEAR BIG SPRING, CLARKE CO.; FIELD HOSPITAL, WINCHESTER, FREDERICK CO.]

[THURSDAY] JULY 28– [1864]

Have been engaged with papers of the Med: Purveying Department to-day.

I have been too indulgent in eating to-day—We get as much milk as we wish here and apples.

The weather is very warm.

[CAMP NEAR BIG SPRING, CLARKE CO.; FIELD HOSPITAL, WINCHESTER, FREDERICK CO.]

[FRIDAY] JULY 29– [1864]

On the same work to-day as yester-day.

Part of our troops moved towards Williamsport [MD] to-day. Cavalry will go over I infer.

[ON THE ROAD TO WINCHESTER; NEAR COUNTY LINES OF CLARKE AND FREDERICK CO.]

[SATURDAY] JULY 30 [1864]

We moved camp a short distance. Dr. [Hunter Holmes] McGuire came and ordered us to Winchester [Frederick Co]. The day was very hot—Started at 2 o'clock.

Dr. [William] Taylor & myself got away from the train and went to a Mr. Severs to take supper. He is an uncle of Miss Severs spoken of on the 4th [July].

Co.] who signed with Co. D of 6th VA Cav. Later he was ranked Capt. in subsistence department and still later became Maj. in same dept. Buried in Grace Episcopal Church of Berryville, "[h]e may be the man of this name," according to 6th Cav. historian Michael P. Musick, 158.

697 W.W. Scott says "from personal memory" that Dr. H.P. Magruder of Orange Co. served as surgeon, sometimes attached to Orange Rangers, 6th VA Cav., and sometimes serving with field hospital of ANV, 2nd Corps. He is not listed by Musick, but Scott is generally accurate about those people whom he personally knew. Scott, *Hist. of Orange Co.*, 265. I cannot locate a Dr. Morrison.

He is an old bachelor[698]– We were undecided what to do—Our train behind, no feed for our horses, 6 mis. to Winchester and no feed there. Passing the Misses Stephensons we were hailed by the ladies for the news.[699] Finding out our forlorn condition a chamber was offered us and a stable for our steeds which we accepted. In the parlour we found evidence of affluence and prosperity in days gone by. A Miss Simpson from Balt. entertained us with some elegant music and Miss [Annie?] Stephenson gave us a very entertaining history of their suffering at the hands of the enemy—I was struck with the pride and confidence she manifested. Such a spirit can never be subdued. We retired about 1 o'clock very much pleased—Neither of the ladies seem to have any curiosity for our name, and we did [not] impose them upon them.

[CAMP ON HOLLINGSWORTH MILLS,
CLARKE CO. NEAR WINCHESTER, FREDERICK CO.]

[SUNDAY] JULY 31– [1864]

We reached Winchester and went out with our train to Hollingsworth Mills about 11 o'clock. We were much chagrined at finding our camp occupied by the Yankee prisoners. Mrs. H[ollingsworth] said we must take our camp. We compromised by squatting on another piece of ground near the house.

Surgn [Samuel Rush] Sayers sent to Mt. Jackson [Shenandoah] to take charge of [field] Hospitals. Surgn [Robert Frederick] Baldwin[700] ordered to Winchester.

I went to town and to church with Miss Maggie at 4 o'clock and 7 [P.M.]—She is a sweet lady.[701]

---

[698] The Miss Severs was from Baltimore, and was described as "liberal," with connotations of looseness. Her uncle may have been Thomas Severs, born 1795, who had a farm and land in Frederick Co. in 1870. VA Census, 1870.

[699] One of the Misses Stephensons may have been Annie Stephenson, born 1813, who still maintained a home in Opequon Township in Frederick Co. in 1870. VA Census, 1870.

[700] Robert Frederick Baldwin (1829-1875) was from Winchester, where he was serving as physician when War came. A graduate of University of Virginia, he held medical degree from University of Pennsylvania. Commissioned Col. of 31st Regular Militia, Frederick Co., he later became physician with Gen. Thomas Jonathan Jackson's Old VA Bde, and was captured at Romney (14 February 1862) and imprisoned, then exchanged in 1863. Regimental historian Lee A. Wallace, Jr. says: "Although in poor health he accepted an appointment as Surgeon; assd to 5th Regt. VA Inf. Unable to continue field service, he was given charge of the hospital at Staunton, where he spent the remainder of the war. Resumed practice in Winchester after the war. Apptd. Supt., VA State Hosp. for the Insane at Staunton. Died Nov. 15, 1875. Bur. Mt. Hebron Cem., Winchester." Idem, *5th VA Inf.*, Virgina Regimental Histories Series, ed. H.E. Howard (Lynchburg, VA: H.E. Howard, 1988) 93.

I hope we will be permitted to stay here awhile.

[OFFICES, TOWN OF WINCHESTER, FREDERICK CO.]

[MONDAY] AUG 1– [1864]

Moved into town to-day and took the office next door to Mr. Kelley's.

I shall begin to make up my papers now.

Rec'd three letters—one from MJC [Mary Camden] & one from Mollie T[hornton] & one from Cousin B[ettie].

I called on Misses Schultz. They were not at home—Came but others were there and I left.

Mr. [John Nelson] Gibson[702] paid me 20$ [1 gold dollar; 4 US greenback dollars] borrowed some months ago.

[OFFICES, TOWN OF WINCHESTER, FREDERICK CO.]

[TUESDAY] AUG 2ND [1864]

To-day I did but little work. Was invited to visit Mr. [James H.] Kemp's this evening and take tea.[703] I went with a party and had a very pleasant evening. Miss Maggie [Margaret Doll?] was my companion. Was introduced to the Misses Wolf—had for a time an adventure—something after the fashion of Major Jones of Georgia.

Called at Mr. Wolf's on my return. Had some excellent music.

Capt. Hardy[704] is at my quarters.

I sent Surg. [Samuel Rush] Sayers bed & valise to him by Capt. Waller [Redd] Preston.[705]

---

[701] This may be Margaret Doll, since he also speaks earlier of visiting Miss Doll. The Doll family lived in neighboring Shenandoah Co. in 1870. VA Census, 1870.

[702] John Nelson Gibson (1835-1889) was with commissary of ANV, 2nd Corps after some time in 6th VA CAV. Possibly from Faquier Co., he is buried in Ivy Hill Cem., Upperville (Faquier Co.). Musick, 117.

[703] James H. Kemp, born 1801, is listed in census as owning land and a home in Winchester. VA Census, 1870.

[704] Prof Bean writes: "Major Hardy was quartermaster of Early's Valley army." Bean, notes. I cannot find Maj. or Capt. Hardy in Robertson, *4th VA Inf.* or in idem, *Stonewall Jackson*, or in *OR*.

[705] Waller Redd Preston (1841-1872) was Asst. Adjutant General with 14th VA Cav. and then with staff of Gen. John Echols (1823-1896; already identified). Native of "Smithfield" in Montgomery Co., he attended University of Virginia, but left in 1861 to join Co. G of 4th VA Inf. Tranfered and promoted to Capt. in 14th Cav., he was transfered and promoted again, to Maj. sometime in late 1862. According to Robert J. Driver, Jr., "Served to end of war. Murdered in

Dr. B. is arranging our hospital at Mr. [Angus] McDonald's[706] near Four Springs [Frederick Co]. The Hospitals in town [Winchester] are in a bad condition. Very offensive and dangerous to sick and wounded as well as disagreeable to visitors and attendants.

[OFFICES, TOWN OF WINCHESTER, FREDERICK CO.]

[WEDNESDAY] AUG 3– [1864]

To-day the air has been more pleasant. I have done but little work. Too many fair forms are ever tripping by my window. The gentle wind moves the light trappings and reveals to our vision the most exquisitely formed ankles—the sight of which propels the imagination with blissful fancy. There is no remedy though. I suffer from their charms.

This evening orders came for the Infirmary Corps to move at daylight to-morrow morning.

I have packed up my goods and wrote a letter to Dr. F[aris]. The move is toward the river [Potomac]. Dr. [J.W.] Davis[707] is placed in charge of the [field] hospitals at this place and Mt. Jackson. The Hospt. at Twin Springs will be in chg. of Surg'n [Robert Frederick] Baldwin.

[ON THE ROAD NORTH OF POTOMAC RIVER NEAR SHEPHERDSTOWN, WVA]

[THURSDAY] AUG: 4– [1864]

This morning I went to Kernstown [Frederick Co.] with orders for Surg'n Love & Breedlove.[708] Surg'n D. [J.W. Davis] is sick.

Texas 8/1/72." Idem, *14th VA CAV*, Virginia Regimental Histories Series, ed. Howard (Lynchburg, VA: H.E. Howard, 1989) 167.

[706] Probably not the home of Angus McDonald, but the home of the Rev. William D. McElwee. Angus McDonald, born 1830, was a refugee from Scotland who was guest and beneficiary of the Rev. McElwee, and his family's refugee experiences in the Shenandoah have been chronicled. Prof. Bean writes: "The Angus McDonald family had refugeed to Lexington in late 1864 and were the guests of the Reverend William McElwee—a minister of the Associated Reform Presbyterian Church." Bean, notes. He cites Cecilia Peake McDonald, *A Diary with Reminiscences of War and Refugee Life in the Shenandoah Valley, 1860-1865* (Nashville, TN: no publisher, 1934) 187-256. In 1870, the Rev. McElwee was listed in Clarke Co., Angus McDonald and family listed in Bath Co. VA Census, 1870.

[707] Prof. Bean supplies the initials for Dr. Davis. Bean, notes. I cannot find Dr. J.W. Davis in Cunningham, *OR*, or regimental histories for VA.

[708] Dr. Love may be Robert V. Love (ca. 1843-1916) of 14th VA Cav. who enlisted at Churchville (Augusta Co.) as cavalryman, and was then detailed to work with horses and then human patients in quartermaster department of ANV, 2nd Corps. Apparently he was trained, as

Called at Misses Miller on my return—I rather hate to leave Winchester on some accounts.

I left Winchester in Company with Surg'n James McGuire.[709]

At Misses Stephenson [one is possibly Annie Stephenson] I called a few minutes. They remembered me but had not found out our names.

Overtook the trains near Shepherdstown [WVA]—very tired.

[ON THE ROAD NEAR SHARPSBURG, MD]

[FRIDAY] AUG. 5– [1864]

Moved at daylight—crossed the river [Potomac].

At Sharpsburg [MD] a skirmish ensued between our and the enemy's cavalry.[710] The Yankees moved towards Harper's Ferry, by way of the mountains. This evidently caused some change in the progression. We had passed the village [Sharpsburg], but returned to the opposite side and camped.

---

some of Apperson's colleagues were, for his reassignment came "on surgeon's recommendation." No further record after this time. Later resided, and was buried in California. Driver, 148. Dr. Breedlove may be J.W. Breedlove, listed as medical inspector for Western Virginia in field in 1864 according to Cunningham, 285.

[709] I cannot identify Dr. James McGuire. Prof. Bean says, "Presumably one of Dr. Hunter McGuire's relatives." Bean, notes. However, I cannot confirm this from the *Cyclopedia of VA Biography.*, which does list relatives. Also, I cannot confirm any relationship in the regimental histories of 2nd VA Inf. and 2nd Rockbridge Arty, in both of which Hunter Holmes McGuire had relatives. In Census, there is no James McGuire in 1870 living in Winchester, from whence the McGuires hailed, or Richmond, where the famous surgeon went after War in order to establish medical school at University of Richmond.

[710] The fighting of 5 August 1864 was actually at Keedysville, near Sharpsburg; there had been an earlier skirmish between same cavalry forces on 4 August 1864 at New Creek, WVA. Gen. William Woods Averell (already identified; 1832-1900) led Ohio, WVA, and other federal forces in skirmishes against Gen. John McCausland (already identified; 1836-1927). Gen. Averell's losses were approximately 9 killed, and 25 wounded at New Creek; Gen. McCausland lost 25 dead, but carried his wounded with him—there was no official count of his wounded from either records. The following day, Gen. Averell lost 7 men, and Gen. McCausland approximately twelve, but again CSA records are unclear and federal records do not enlighten. Most interesting is the report by CSA Brig. Gen. Bradley Tyler Johnson (1829-1903), concerning the "outrageous" conduct of Gen. McCausland and his troops in Chambersburg, PA and then in Keedysville: "Every crime n the catalogue of infamy has been committed, I believe, except murder and rape. Highway robbery of watches and pocket-books was of ordinary occurrence; the taking of breast-pins, finger-rings, and earrings frequently happened. Pillage and sack of private dwellings took place hourly. A soldier of an advance guard robbed of his gold watch the Catholic clergyman of Hancock on his way from church...." Johnson listed many other abuses, and called for an investigation of McCausland. An investigation was conducted, but he was not reprimanded. Bradley T. Johnson, "Report," 10 August 1864, *OR*, ser. 1, vol. 43, pt. 1, 1-6.

I was somewhat tired to-day. The horse I am riding belongs to a citizen of the place. His wife ask [sic] me as I passed to please ride him in the lot. It is hard and hurts I know but must be borne.

[ON THE ROAD NEAR FALLING WATERS, MD]

[SATURDAY] AUG. 6TH [1864]

Moved this morning in a hard rain towards Hagerstown [MD]—At Jims X-roads the army took the Williamsport Road, recrossed the [Potomac] river, and camped between the ford and Falling Waters.

The move is inexplicable. The Med. Purveyor [Dr. William Taylor] is gathering up stimulants.

Our camp is near Haynesville [MD].

I have read the "Baltimore American" of the 3d. It says 265 houses were burned by [Gen. John] McCausland in Chambersburg. They are rampant over it.[711]

A fine rain fell to-day.

[ON THE ROAD NEAR BUNKER HILL, FREDERICK CO.]

[SUNDAY] AUG 7– [1864]

This morning I was sent on rather an unpleasant trip. The Med: Div: is collecting stimulants for Gen. Lee's Army at Richmond and hearing a lot of whiskey was at or near Haynesville [MD] I was sent up to get it. After going through a process similar to that of our underground RR[712] I procured three barrells.

In the meantime I got a good breakfast. The army I found moving on my return—At Martinsburg [WVA] I found [George T.] Richardson[713] waiting with

---

[711] Notice that the diarist does not protest the account. See Bradley Tyler Johnson's official report, as noted earlier. The diarist's response, plus Gen. Johnson's, suggest that John McCausland was indeed responsible for "outrageous" behavior.

[712] The diarist is uncharacteristically sarcastic. The Underground Railroad was the system whereby abolitionist sympathizers arranged for runaway slaves to stay in white homes and barns while "stealing away" toward the "drinking gourd" of freedom above the Mason-Dixon line. He hates the use of liquor, and here equates his efforts to acquire it for medicinal purposes [fairly common practice in absence of other painkillers, such as morphine and opium, which were equally problematical, see *McGrew's* and *Taber's*] to the efforts of slaves to run to freedom, which effort of course the diarist also opposes.

[713] George T. Richardson (1839-death date unknown, but buried in Mt. Jackson, Shenandoah Co., VA] was a farmer, possibly from Smyth Co., who had joined 4th VA Inf. and served a year;

directions for me. I called to see my friends Misses D.[714] had a few moments pleasant communication and left—I met Dr. [Edmund Starchan] Pendleton[715] on my way up.

I got to Camp near Bunker Hill [Frederick Co.] before night very tired—horse nearly broken down.

I paid out of Surg'n [William] Taylor's funds for the whiskey $402.50 —federal money [1610 CSA dollars; 80.5 in gold dollars]

[OFFICES, TOWN OF WINCHESTER, FREDERICK CO.]

[MONDAY] AUG. 8– [1864]

This morning we came to Winchester and began again.

I got letters from my friends ~~Mollie T[hornton] & M.J.C. [Mary Camden] &~~ Mrs. T [Mary Tomlin] & Lizzie.[716]

This evening I was invited to take tea at Misses Miller—had a very elegant evening—Met Miss Sherry—a natural poetess. She has a poem in view now—another on the war in Winchester. I have been very busy writing.

Rec'd a letter from Dr. Q[uisenberry].

The weather is very warm. Almost intollerably [sic] so. Dr. B sent Ellsberg back to Richmond.

[OFFICES, TOWN OF WINCHESTER, FREDERICK CO.]

[TUESDAY] AUG 9– [1864]

Loan [Dr.] Drane $10 & [Dr.] Sydnor $10 [50 cents in gold dollars; 2.5 US greenback dollars]—

---

then re-enlisted in 4th after some months away. Wounded in hip at Payne's Farm (17 November 1863), he served at least throug this August part of Jubal Anderson Early's Valley campaign. James I. Robertson, Jr. says, "dark eyes, hair, and complexion." Idem, *4th VA Inf.*, 70.

714 Possibly Margaret "Maggie" Doll, of Doll family in Shenandoah Co.

715 Edmund Starchan Pendleton (1833-1909) was a physician from Iron Gate (Allegheny Co). He enlisted with Co. F of 4th VA Cav. as 1st Sgt., and was sent recruiting for one year, but was transfered in 1862 to medical corps and became Assistant Surgeon. Returned to Iron Gate, and is buried there. Kenneth L. Stiles, *4th VA Cav.*, VA Regimental Histories Series, ed. Howard (Lynchburg, VA: H.E. Howard, 1985), 130.

716 I think that he received letters from Mary Camden and Mollie Thornton, and chose to strike their names from the diary. Prof. Bean suggests that Lizzie may be Ellizabeth Baylor of Staunton. Bean, notes.

Paid 50 cents [2.5 cents in gold; 12.5 cents in US greenback dollars] for washing. Wrote a letter to Mrs. Thornton in regard to the paper she left with me. Also one to Maj. Palmer,[717] asking him to send it to her.

I then wrote to Dr. Q[uisenberry]. —

[Dr.] Drane went to Mt. Jackson [Frederick Co. field hospital] to get up Muster Roll.

The movements of the army are indicative.

Rumor says that [Gen. John] McCausland and [Gen. Bradley Tyler] Johnson were surprised near Moorefield [Hardy Co., WVA] and cut to pieces. I fear there is truth in this.[718]

[OFFICES, TOWN OF WINCHESTER, FREDERICK CO.]

[WEDNESDAY] AUG. 10– [1864]

Hotter to-day than usual. I have been writing nearly all day. This evening things became rather restless. Preparation is being made to remove the sick—Stores are being sent out now. After the train was loaded with invalids it was ordered to wait for orders.

There is a wedding in town [Winchester] to-night. Dr. Simms to Miss Burgess.[719] Dr. Black went. How impressive the impression presented—by this incident. To-night the great issue of battle seems to be pending. A mighty consume[720] [sic] of men are restless and swayed from flank to centre holding at

---

[717] I cannot find a Maj. Palmer in the VA regimental histories series.

[718] *OR* considers the engagement to have occurred in "Old Fields, at and near Moorefield"; but the rumors were accurate: For CSA, newspaper reporter J.H. Wartman filed this report on 9 August 1864 to *Richmond Whig*, and CSA staff accepted it and confirmed it in their records: "Our forces under Generals B.T. Johnson and McCausland suffered defeat near Moorefield, Hardy County, on Sunday morning last about daylight. They were surprised, attacked by forces under Averell, and stampeded and routed, the enemy capturing and killing 300 or 400 of Johnson's men, four pieces of artillery, and 800 or 900 horses. It was a perfect rout, our men scattering in wild disorder and confusion and running in different directions." *OR*, ser. 1, vol. 43, 991. Federal *OR* reports from William Woods Averell cite the same CSA casualties and speak of one federal officer killed and no more than 5 wounded or otherwise missing. Averell, " Report," 18 October 1864, *OR*, ser. 1, 43:500-01. Because Averell was slow to follow up and exploit his advantage by attacking Winchester aggressively, he was removed from command and ordered to Wheeling, WVA; Philip H. Sheridan (already identified) took command of reorganzied Middle Military Division, and Col. William H. Powell was given command of 2nd Cav. Div. of WVA. Special Orders No. 41, 23 September 1864, Sheridan per Charles Kingsbury, Jr., Ibid., 505

[719] I cannot locate a Dr. Simms in Cunningham, or in regimental histories series.

[720] Diarist appears to write the word *consume*, treating it as a noun that means a group or an organized force. I cannot find such usage in OED for mid-19th cent. *OED.*

bay a desperate foe. Here Cupid at the same time has finished one of his thousands of victims —

"Love will do what love dare attempt."[721]

I called on Miss Kate [Schultz] or rather met her on the street and saw her home.

I regret leaving Winchester as much as any place I have ever been at. There is so much interest on the part of the Citizens. They would be willing to live with us on half rations and that divided 'till it was nought than to see us leave. Such people merit the loudest praises of their fibre [viz., about their character]

[ON THE ROAD NEAR STRASBURG, SHENANDOAH CO.]

[THURSDAY] AUG 11– [1864]

We left town very hurriedly. I barely had time to bid the Misses Miller good bye. The weather is very warm—We traveled a back road to Strasburg [Shenandoah Co]. Stopped at Mrs. Sydnor's—Capt. Workman shared my couch.[722]

[CAMP WEST OF WOODSTOCK, SHENANDOAH CO.]

[FRIDAY] AUG 12– [1864]

Moved on to Woodstock [Shenandoah Co]. I was placed in charge of a number of *walking* cases [diarist's italics; viz., those sick or wounded but able to march]. Stoped [sic] at the Brook[723] and cooked rations for them. Our camp is in a grove 1/2 mile west of Woodstock [Shenandoah Co]. The army is falling back slowly. It is stated that reinforcements are at Culpepper C.H. [sic; Culpeper Court House, Culpeper Co., about 40 miles southwest of Woodstock camp] for Gen. [Jubal Anderson] Early. This time I expect it is correct.

---

[721] Possibly a very loose rendition of Plato, "Love will make men dare to die for their beloved...." Idem, *The Symposium*, sec. 179.

[722] Mrs. Sydnor may be the mother or other relative of the Dr. Sydnor, although I cannot locate a Dr. Sydnor in the VA regimental histories or in the Census for Shenandoah Co. Capt. Workman, I cannot identify. He is not listed in VA regimental histories, and must be an officer from another state. I also cannot find him in the *OR*.

[723] Probably Tom's Brook, Shenandoah Co. The village, also called Tom's Creek, is on the Baltimore & Ohio rail line; the brook feeds the North Fork of the Shenandoah River. The village lies about seven miles northeast of Woodstock. Hummel, *A List*.

Reported also that the enemy is leaving Richmond.[724] Capt. Lock paid Dr. B amt. borrowed of him.

[CAMP WEST OF WOODSTOCK, SHENANDOAH CO.]

[SATURDAY] 13– AUG. [1864]

In camp all day—[725]

[CAMP WEST OF WOODSTOCK, SHENANDOAH CO.]

[SUNDAY] AUG 14– [1864]

At church in the village [Woodstock, Shenandoah Co.] Dr. [Bevery T.] Lacy preached—A son of Dr. Converse was present and made a few remarks on behalf of the distribution of religious reading in the army—A contribution was taken up.[726]

At 5 P.M. Mr. Converse preached at our Camp—a large number of ladies were present. I was introduced to Misses Chipley, same them home and went again to church. Dr. [Beverly T.] Lacy preached on the influence of pious generals in the Army. T.J. Jackson & R.E. Lee were cited as models.[727] His lecture was of unpardonable length. Audience large.

---

[724] False rumor. Lt. Gen. U.S. Grant continued the siege of Petersburg and his large forces there were an obvious threat to Richmond. E.B. Long reports political unhappiness with Grant's siege, and calls for him to come back north, esp. after Jubal Anderson Early threatened the Federal capital. Early himself was maneuvering to set up intrenchments and defense at Cedarville, a Warren Co. village on the Cedar Creek, which comes from the North Mountain in Shenandoah Co. and flows into Frederick Co. and Warren Co. Philip Sheridan and a large force was moving up [south] the Shenandoah Valley in order to engage Early's portion of the 2nd Corps, ANV. Long speaks of a place called Cedar Creek, but Hummel indicates that the place has to be Cedarville. Long, 554; Hummel.

[725] Written on left margin, probably on or after 14 August 1864.

[726] The young speaker, born in 1844, had moved to St. George's Parish in Accomack by 1870; the census lists him as *Minister*, and does not give a first name. VA . Census, 1870. *VA Mag. of Hist. and Biog.*, vol 5 (1897): 207 gives name of Rev. E. Converse. Pitts notes that printing of Bibles and religious tracts was dominated by England and by northeastern cities; southern printers had to smuggle plates southward to begin printing Bibles and tracts, and even with those resources, relied heavily on English imports. Collections were necessary in order to pay for what was thus a more expensive proposition in the CSA than in the US. Pitts also notes a heightened interest in religion after the defeats at Gettysburg and Vicksburg, and this heightened interest manifested itself in greater demand for printed materials. He also notes that certain officers contributed sums of money to buy the printed tracts. Pitts, 31, 89, 110-13.

[727] Prof. Bean had written a study of Rev. Bevery T. Lacy, and describes the minister as a beneficiary of Jackson's and Lee's piety, for he was a favorite preacher for both men. Bean also

[CAMP WEST OF WOODSTOCK, SHENANDOAH CO.]

[MONDAY] AUG. 15 [1864]

At work on reports to-day.

— Rained at evening—no mail —

[John Henninger] Reagan the P.M. General [Postmaster General] and the Supt. [Henry Donald Whitcomb] of the VCRR [Virginia Central Railroad] are at loggerheads[728]

Wrote to Dr. Faris asking him to see the Hon. F[ayette]. McMullen[729] for me.

[CAMP WEST OF WOODSTOCK, SHENANDOAH CO.]

[TUESDAY] AUG 16– [1864]

Nothing. Dr. Hagy sent to Mt. Jackson [field hospitals, Shenandoah Co]. The body of Asst. Surg. Price, 38 Geo. was brought in—he was killed on the skirmish line near Strasburg [Shenandoah Co].[730]

No mail again to-day.

I wrote to MJC, Box 717 [Mary Camden in Richmond].

---

describes Lay as a gripping speaker with a real sense of humor, though the diarist does not note anything of that sort in this entry. Idem, "Stonewall Jackson's Jolly Chaplain, Beverly Tucker Lacy," *West Virginia History*, 29 (1968): 77-97.

[728] John Henninger Reagan (1818-1905) was a native Tennessean who moved to Texas, farmed, practiced law, and entered politics, becoming a judge. Lowell H. Harrison says, "He acquired samples of Federal postal materials and secured the services of a number of former Federal employees. The [CSA] Constitution required the department to be self-supporting after 1 March 1863, a goal he met by eliminating some routes and offices, increasing rates, and securing a sharp reduction in railroad costs." It is the latter reduction in rate charges that put the postmaster "at loggerheads" with H.D. Whitcomb, the superintendent of the main VA railroad. Idem, "Reagan," *Hist. Times.* Henry Donald Whitcomb was born in Eastport ME in 1826 and was married in VA in 1854 and subsequently became superintendent of Virginia Central Railroad during Civil War; of continuing importance to railroads in postbellum VA, he died in Richmond in 1910.

[729] Fayette McMullen (1805-1880), already identified, was a colorful but above all very influential politician in Smyth Co. before and after The War. Armstrong, *Hist.*, 61-67, and passim.

[730] In nearby Co. of Warren, Battle of Cedarville, 16 August 1864. "Also called Engagement at Front Royal, and Guard Hill." *A Register*, comp., Warriner.

[CAMP NEAR NEWTOWN, FREDERICKS CO.][731]

[WEDNESDAY] AUG 17– [1864]

Ordered to move—sent sick to Mt. Jackson [field hospitals]—Moved at 9 o'clock—The army falling back. [General Richard Heron] Anderson [732] has formed a junction by way of Front Royal [Warren Co]. Citizens estimate the enemy's force at 40,000. 6, 8, & 19 Corps are here—[Gen. Philip H.] Sheridan in command. The farmers have lost everything. The enemy has inaugurated a system of burning provisions. All the farms containing wheat are in ashes—hay and oats share the same fate. Cornfields are destroyed. [733]

We camped at Newtown—firing towards Winchester [Frederick Co].

[CAMP AT ANGUS MCDONALD FARM;
REV. WILLIAM MCELWEE, FOUR SPRING, FREDERICK CO.]

[THURSDAY] AUG 18– [1864]

Moved to Winchester. Raining rapidly. The enemy has returned towards Harper's Ferry [Jefferson Co., WVA] and Martinsburg [Berkeley Co., WVA].

In the engagement yester-day we lost, principally of [John Cabell] Breckinridge's command—about 150 killed and wounded.[734] At York House we found, much to our surprise that nothing had been disturbed.

We moved out to Four Spring [Frederick Co.] and began to pitch tents. I am in the hall of the [Angus] McDonald house. Mrs. Brady, the housekeeper, is an odd one.

I called on the Misses Miller this afternon and found them preparing for a party. I was invited—they having no escort I went. I found a very pleasant evening at Mr. Ichelberger's [sic][735]

---

[731] Newtown Stephensburg or Newtown Stevensburg, Frederick Co. Hummel, *A List.*

[732] Richard Heron "Fighting Dick" Anderson (1821-1879), already identified. These are the infantry reinforcements spoken of earlier; also reinforcing was Gen. Fitzhugh Lee (1835-1905, already identified), who brought major cavalry force. Gen. Philip H. Sheridan Middle Military Div. had moved eastward toward Berryville [Clarke Co.], down the Valley, and he left a force near Winchester. Gen. Jubal Anderson Early attacked the rear guard of Sheridan's Winchester forces, but these "held well," according to Long, 556 and *OR*, ser. 1, vol. 43, pt. 1, "Report of Sheridan," 16 August 1864.

[733] Maj. Gen. Philip H. Sheridan in his report to Lt. Gen. U.S. Grant on 17 August 1864, states: "I have burned all wheat and hay, and brought off all stock, sheep, cattle, horses & cetera , south of Winchester." *OR*, ser. 1, vol. 43, pt. 1, 822.

[734] Maj. Gen. Philip H. Sheridan in his report to Lt. Gen. U.S. Grant says, "after a very handsome cavalry fight the enemy were badly beaten, with a loss of 2 stand of colors, 24 officers, and 276 men prisoners, 17 August 1864, *OR*, ser. 1, vol. 43, pt. 1, 19.

Returned to camp about midnight.

[ON ROAD AT SCHULTZ'S HOME[736], WINCHESTER, FREDERICK CO.]

[FRIDAY] AUG. 19: [1864]

Dark and rainy to-day. Sent off train of wounded. At Mr. [John W.] Schultz's this evening. —

[ON THE ROAD NEAR SCHULTZ'S HOME, WINCHESTER, FREDERICK CO.]

[SATURDAY] AUG. 20 [1864]

Called on the Misses Wolf—had a very pleasant time.

[ON THE ROAD NEAR SCHULTZ'S HOME, WINCHESTER, FREDERICK CO.]

[SUNDAY] AUG. 21– [1864]

To-day is my birthday. 27 years have I lived, and I look back only to see them barren and fruitless. I went to church. The Lutheran minister, Mr. Dosh,[737] preached. Called at Mr. [John W.] Schultz's in the afternoon. Took tea and then at Misses Miller.

[ON THE ROAD NEAR SCHULTZ'S HOME, WINCHESTER, FREDERICK CO.]

[MONDAY] AUG. 22– [1864]

Nothing— 60 wounded of [Brig. Gen. George Pierce] Doles' Brigade were brought in[738] —our forces are at Charlestown [in eastern panhandle, not the 20th century capital city]. [Dr.] Ellsberg returned from Richmond.

---

735 Probably misspelled. Charles F. Eichelberger, born in 1836, owned a home and land in Winchester in Frederick Co. VA Census, 1870.

736 Probably John W. Schultz, born in 1826, who had a home and land in Stonewall Twp, Frederick Co. VA Census, 1870.

737 A civilian minister rather than a military chaplain, and thus not listed in Pitts. Probably the Rev. William Dosh, born in 1813, who had a home and land in Shenandoah Co. VA Census, 1870.

738 George Pierce Doles (1830-1864) was already identified. The Brig. Gen. was killed at Cold Harbor (2 June 1864). These are GA brigades attached to ANV. Long says: "Sheridan pulled out of Berryville [Clarke Co.], VA and headed toward Charles Town [Jefferson Co. in eastern panhandle], WV. Early, learning this, headed toward Bunker Hill, north of Winchester. Skirmishing was along Opequon Creek [18 August 1864]....Early and R.H. Anderson planned to hit Sheridan in a two-pronged attack. The drive failed for lack of coordination after fighting near Berryville, [Clarke Co.] VA, Charles Town [Jefferson Co., WV, Middleway [Smithfield, Jefferson Co., WV], and Summit Point [Jefferson Co., WV....Late at night Sheridan pulled back from

[ON THE ROAD NEAR SCHULTZ'S HOME, WINCHESTER, FREDERICK CO.]

[TUESDAY] AUG. 23—[1864]

Ladies in their goodness have been with us all day tenderly administering to the comforts of the wounded. Ambulances and wagon traings were sent off.

I wrote Mrs. Faris a long letter.

[There are no entries between 23 August 1864 and 19 September 1864. Long notes that Jubal Anderson Early continued to skirmish and to make demonstrations before Gen. Philip Sheridan. Prof. Bean says that Early became "over-confident, and in this fatuous frame of mind, he was later suprised by the aggressive type of warfare which Sheridan waged. And it was also unfortunate at that time that R.H. Anderson's and J.B. Kershaw's divisions were ordered back to the Richmond-Petersburg front by General Lee." Bean, notes. Long agrees with Bean's assessment, idem, op. cit., 571, as also borne out by *OR*, ser. 1, vol. 43, pt. 1, see esp. report, Sheridan, s.v.]

[TEMPORARY CAMP NEAR FISHER'S HILL, STRASBURG, SHENANDOAH CO.]

[MONDAY] SEPT. 19– [1864]

An awful day—Whipped and Driven away. Hosp't supplies were lost. Drs. Wilkerson and Duval left at Winchester[.] Marched all night. Camped at Fisher's Hill above Strasburg [Shenandoah Co., some 20 miles southwest of Town of Winchester]. Our army is totally disorganized.[739]

[EMERGENCY FIELD HOSPITAL, WOODSTOCK, SHENANDOAH CO.]

[TUESDAY] SEPT. 20 [1864]

Moved up to Woodstock. Every place is filled to overflowing with wounded. Worked all day. With Dr. Williams[740] at the jail and Court House.

Charles Town to Halltown [Jefferson Co., WV] near Harper's Ferry and the Potomac River, into a virtually impregnable position. Once more the Valley was largely free of Federals, but the area had been too much fought over to be of great value." Idem, 556-58.

[739] *OR* lists 697 Federal soldiers killed, 2,983 wounded, and 338 missing; 276 CSA troops killed, 1827 wounded, and 1818 missing or captured. "Report," *OR*, ser. 1, vol. 43, pt. 1, 19 September 1864. Long notes, "A mix-up in movement may have cost Sheridan an even more successful battle, but Early was badly beaten. Long, 571.

[740] I cannot locate a Dr. Williams in Cunningham, in VA regimental histories, or in *OR*.

[EMERGENCY FIELD HOSPITAL, WOODSTOCK, SHENANDOAH CO.]

[WEDNESDAY] SEPT 21 [1864]

Sent to Mt. Jackson [Shenandoah Co. field hospital] a large number of wounded. The probability is that the army will be quiet for a few days. Dr. Bosie, 3 Ala has been helping us—He is a good man. Capt. Lindock is with us.[741]

[ON THE ROAD NEAR EDINBURGH OR EDENBURG,[742] SHENANDOAH CO.]

[THURSDAY] SEPT. 22. [1864]

This evening worse than ever. Another stampede in the cavalry came first; then to wagons and ambulances. Reports say that the enemy turned our left, captured our artillery and many prisoners. Dr. B put Dr. Hagy in charge with a complement of attendants and ordered us to leave. We started on foot. Slept at Edinburgh in Dr. Blue's yard.[743]

I don't know what is to become of us. Can it be that we are to be driven about like so many sheep?

Our wagon train had left Woodstock before we started which necessitated our walking. We overtook it at Mt. Jackson [Shenandoah Co.], however.

[ON THE ROAD AT HARRISONBURG COURT HOUSE, ROCKINGHAM CO.]

[FRIDAY] SEPT. 23 - [1864]

We came on to Harrisonburg and began again. Took supper at Mrs. [Martha] Shands' with Mr. Russell.[744] Our office at the C.H.

[ON THE ROAD AT ELK RUN TOWNSHIP, ROCKINGHAM CO.]

[SATURDAY] SEPT. 24TH [1864]

The army is still falling back. Very few badly wounded were sent off to-day—no transportation.

---

[741] I cannot locate a Dr. Bosie of 3rd Alabama Regt. I cannot locate a Capt. Lindock in Cunningham, in VA regimental histories, or in *OR*

[742] According to Hummel, the prefered spelling was *Edenburg*. Idem, *A List*.

[743] No physician, and indeed no person, named *Blue* is listed as holding property in Shenandoah Co. in 1870 census. VA Census, 1870.

[744] Martha Shands, a widow born in 1822, had property in Rockingham Co. VA Census, 1870. I cannot identify a Mr. Russell, and do not know if he is a civilian in Harrisonburg or a fellow soldier.

Moved off at 8 o'clock P.M.—Wagon Train started before we did[.] Night dark and road rough—walked to near Port Republic, and slept in a barn of Mr. [William] Maiden's.[745]

[ON THE ROAD IN BROWN'S GAP ON BORDER BETWEEN ROCKINGHAM CO. AND AUGUSTA CO.]

[SUNDAY] SEPT. 25– [1864]

Came to Port Republic. Met the Wagon Train. I am much bothered about a valuable bundle I sent to Staunton [Augusta Co.]—No way to get it.

Crossed the ridge at Brown's Gap.[746] Stopped near Mr. Brown's Hotel at the foot of the ridge. Am tired[,] sleepy and distressed.

[ON THE ROAD IN NORTH CENTRAL AUGUSTA CO., NEAR BROWN'S GAP]

[MONDAY] SEPT. 26 ` [1864]

Firing began across the [Brown] Mountain. Orders to go to Mechum's Depot [Albemarle Co. to east and south of Brown's Gap]. [Thomas Lafayette] Rosser & [Joseph Brevard] Kershaw are said to have joined our army. Not much hope of doing anything with the small help.[747]

---

[745] William Maiden, born in 1786, owned land in Elk Run Township near Port Republic. His sons, James and John, also owned land there. VA Census, 1870.

[746] Brown's Mountain is in south central Rockingham Co., and the gap is an entryway into Augusta Co. N. Harvey Deal, "The Mountains of Virginia," Occasional Papers of Virginia Place-name Society, #1, 7 October 1964, 4.

[747] Actually, both men were more than a small help, for the nonce, in this early fall season. Thomas Lafayette Rosser (1836-1910) was known as "Savior of the Valley" because of his skilled generalship in these very campaigns in which he came to help Gen. Jubal Anderson Early's 2nd Corps. A native of Campbell City, VA., Rosser moved to Texas, attended West Point, and became friends there with George Armstrong Custer (already identified, 1839-1876). He left his studies to fight bravely at 1st Manassas. Assigned to 5th VA Cav., he distinguished himself, was promoted to Brig. Gen., reassigned to Laurel Brigade, and was sent to help Early in the Valley. Often he skirmished against his old friend Custer. Even after Custer soundly defeated Rosser in October, the gallant general was said by historian Phillip R. Rutherford to be "one of a small group of Southern cavalry commanders who made war seem glorious and noble." Idem, "Rosser," *Hist. Times.* Joseph Brevard Kershaw (1822-1894) was an attorney from the Camden, SC planter society. He served in Mexican War and later was elected to SC Gen. Assy. Distinguished in victories at Fredericksburg and Chancellorsville and in defeat at Gettysburg, he became Maj. Gen. and in 1864 was sent to help Gen. Early in last Valley campaign. Emory Thomas, "Kershaw," ibid.

[EMERGENCY FIELD HOSPITAL, MECHUM'S DEPOT [ALBEMARLE CO.]

[TUESDAY] SEPT. 27– [1864]

Got tents (5) from Maj. [Alex] Bell.[748] Some for Dr. Drane at Staunton [Augusta Co]. —No cooking utensils have been procured yet. All the Staunton [General Hospital] officers are here—Yankees took possession of Staunton yester-day.[749] Sending wounded and sick to Charlottesville as rapidly as possible. Drew a requisition for 2000$ [500 US greenback dollars; 100 gold dollars]. Did not get the hospital funds.

[NO ENTRY FOR SEPTEMBER 28, 1864]

[ON THE ROAD NEAR WAYNESBORO, AUGUSTA CO.]

[THURSDAY] SEPT. 29 [1864]

Broke camp at Mecham's Depot [Albemarle Co.] and started [toward] Waynesboro. Camped at the base of the mountain [Afton Mountain]. Much uneasiness has been felt in regards to a Yankee raid on the eastern side of the ridge. Gen. [Jubal Anderson] Early's order is to scatter.[750] We left with Dr. [Thomas Henry] Williams[751] some sick and several tents—the sick to be transferred and the tents to [be] brought us in W[aynesboro, Augusta Co].

---

[748] Apparently Maj. Alex T. Bell, a surgeon originally with 9th VA Inf. and then transfered to hospital staff of 2nd Corps ANV. No birth or death or other data. Benjamin H. Trask, *9th VA Inf.*, VA Regimental Histories Series, ed. H.E. Howard (Lynchburg, VA.: H.E. Howard, 1984) 54.

[749] CSA forces had abandoned Staunton in July, and Gen. Philip Sheridan actually took possession of Staunton, where there was an important general hospital and significant rail connections, on 25 September 1864. Long says, "in Richmond and elsewhere, news of Early's defeat gave rise to severe criticism." Idem, 574. Sheridan, "Report," 25 September 1864, *OR*, Ser. 1, vol. 43, Pt. 1.

[750] As Long notes, "this day saw action on all fronts," and Early did not "scatter" before Gen. Philip Sheridan attacked. On the same day, Lt. Gen. Grant sent a "two pronged" attack, one north of the James River and one west of Petersburg, while calling for pressure against Early. Long, 575-76.

[751] Thomas Henry Williams (1822-1904) was Medical Director of the CSA Army of Potomac, medical officer in the Office of Surgeon General, and sometime Medical Inspector and Medical Director for hospitals in the field. A native of MD, he studied medicine under Alexander Hamilton Bagby and attained the M.D. from the University of Maryland (1849) before joining US Army and serving in the medical corps in the western frontier. When War came, he joined the CSA medical corps, immediately becoming an important member of the staff of Surgeon General Samuel Preston Moore (1813-1889) and of the field directing staff of Medical Director Lafayette Guild. Williams dedicated himself to better communications between staff and line physicians, better communication between line officers in the field and medical staff so that medical

[TEMPORARY FIELD HOSPITAL, WAYNESBORO, AUGUSTA CO.]

SEPT. 30: [1864]

Arrived at Waynesboro in the afternoon. Pitched tents at the foot of the hill on the road east of town. The army is in camp near the village [Waynesboro] but under marching orders. Raining to-day.

This is a dreary, dismal looking place.

[No entries for 1 and 2 October 1864. During this time came news that Gen. William Tecumseh Sherman had conquered and burned Atlanta and was proceeding onward with a lengthy supply train that included many freed slaves. It is interesting that the diarist records this time as a time of defeat and even disarray for Jubal Anderson Early's wing of the 2nd Corps of ANV, but E.B. Long notes that northern public opinion was perplexed by the "continual threat of Early" to Philip Sheridan's forces—and possibly even the "continual threat of Early" to the US capital if the 2nd Corps again tried to march down the valley into D.C. See Long, 576-77.]

[ON THE ROAD IN FISHER'S DEPOT,[752] AUGUSTA CO.]

[MONDAY] OCT 3– [1864]

Unexpectedly sent to Staunton [Augusta Co.][753] with ten ambulances to bring away such sick as had been sent to Hospt there since the army moved to Mt. Sydney[754] [sic; Mt. Sidney in N.E. Augusta Co]. Started at 1/2 past 5- PM. Raining very rapidly. By the time I had travelled 5 miles the darkness became

---

personnel could be prepared for major casualties, and better coordination of medical services and medical transport. He is credited with some successes in all these efforts. After the War, he practiced medicine in Richmond and then in Cambridge, MD, where he organized Cambridge Hospital. Cunningham, 284-86 and passim; "Williams," *Biographical Dictionary of the Confederacy*, ed. Jon L. Wakelyn (Westport, CT: Greenwood Press, 1977).

[752] Prof. Bean contributes the information that today's Fishersville was then Fishers Depot. According to Humel, Fishersville was then called Fisherville. Bean, notes; Humel, ed., *A List.*

[753] There was a major General Hospital directed by Dr. A.M. Fauntleroy in Staunton. Cunningham, 284-86, and passim.

[754] Mt. Sidney is a town in N.E. quadrant of Augusta Co. on the main rail line later operated by Southern RR. Humel, ed., *A List.* It is not listed as a bona fide mountain in the mountain place-names compiled by VA Place Name Society, idem, "The Mountains of VA,"7 October 1964, Occasional Papers, No. 1.

almost impenetrable. I stopped in a wood above Fishers' Depot and spent the night. The roads are horrible.

[GENERAL HOSPITAL, STAUNTON, AUGUSTA CO.]

[TUESDAY] OCT 4– [1864]

Moved out at 5 [AM] and reached Staunton 7 1/2 [7:30 AM] Took breakfast at Mr. [Frank] Fuller's—got my bundles all right (sent to him July 24). Called at Mr. [Nathan E.] Lyman and got baggage for Drs. Black & Elsberg.[755]

The orders I had seemed not very agreeable to the Surgeon in Charge (Dr. [A.M.] Fauntleroy. The [general] hospitals are splendidly kept, but I am not sure but the number of attendants detained are very detrimental to the service. The Yankees took off about 1/2 the attendants and it seemed that there was a surplus now. And yet I had to wait nearly three hours to get 28 men in the ambulance.[756]

I called at Mr. B[aylor]—saw Miss L[Lizzie Baylor] and sister.[757] Took dinner. Miss L's sister packed my haversack with a good lunch.

Arrived at W[aynesboro] about dusk.

[TEMPORARY FIELD HOSPITAL, WAYNESBORO, AUGUSTA CO.]

[THURSDAY] OCT. 6– [1864]

borrowed [sic] 20$ [5 US greenback dollars; 1 gold dollar] from [William] Mohler. Took my clothes to Mr. Reed—had coat and pants cut. Paid 15$ [3.75

---

[755] Frank Fuller, born 1796, had land and slaves and received mail at Mt. Sidney P.O., Augusta Co. VA Census, 1870. Nathan E. Lyman, born in 1820, had a home and business in Staunton, Augusta Co. VA Census, 1870. This bundle had been sent to Dr. A.M. Fauntleroy as noted in diary, 24 July 1864.

[756] The sarcasm is a bit heavier than usual for the diarist; as Cunningham notes and Apperson demonstrates, the field-hospital stewards and physicians had considerable disdain for the putatively easy life of the general-hospital stewards and physicians in the towns and cities. Cunningham, 117.

[757] Three men old enough to have daughters the age of the diarist owned land in Augusta Co. and were registered in the Town of Staunton in 1870: David Baylor, born 1809; George Baylor, born 1803, and Jacob Baylor, born 1801. Elizabeth Baylor herself had either married or moved away from the county by 1870. VA Census, 1870.

US greenback dollars; .75 gold dollar] for same.[758] Made up Monthly Return of Med. Officers—sent off Semi-Annual Return of property.[759]

[ON THE ROAD NEAR HARRISONBURG, ROCKINGHAM CO.]

[FRIDAY] OCT. 7– [1864]

Started to move camp as soon as we were packed up[.] Rec'd orders to move to Harrisonburg. Reached "Willow Point" [apparently someone's farm] about 7 o'clock.

I had my coat & pants cut by Mr. Reed—let him have 3 yds cambric for 21$.[760]

[ON THE ROAD NEAR LACEY SPRING, ROCKINGHAM CO.]

[SATURDAY] OCT. 8– [1864]

Left camp early—The weather very cold for the season. Little snow fell. Camped above Lacey Spring 2 miles.

The enemy has burned everything edible in the Country. Many almost heartrending tales are told of their outrages—The[y] seem particularly fond of oppressing poor, helpless women.

[TEMPORARY FIELD HOSPITAL NEAR NEW MARKET, SHENANDOAH CO.]

[SUNDAY] OCT. 9– [1864]

Moved to New Market. The army in camp near the village.

Our cavalry had an engagement this evening [Tom's Brook, Shenandoah Co.] and was most shamefully stampeded. Lost 11 pieces of artillery and several wagons. Our loss in men very small. The Army came as far as Mt. Jackson

---

[758] I cannot locate a Reed soldier who was still living and serving in 4th or 7th VA. regiments, op. cit.; he seems to be a civilian, but I cannot locate anyone named Reed then living in Waynesboro. VA Census, 1870.

[759] Of this day, Long notes: "Confederate cavalry under Thomas L. Rosser [already identified] attacked two regiments of George A. Custer's cavalry at Brock's Gap, [Rockingham Co.]Va.,....Custer repulsed the attack, but it showed that the Southerners were still active in the Valley." Idem, 580.

[760] Twenty-one CSA dollars was Apperson's monthly pay, although he also received various allowances.

[Shenandoah Co.] and fell back. I think nearly our whole force of cavalry was engaged.[761]

Saw Ike St. John. He says, "I am a stampeded man" [sic][762]

The day looks gloomy enough for the Valley. The reins of discipline must be tightened.

[TEMPORARY FIELD HOSPITAL NEAR NEW MARKET, SHENANDOAH CO.]

[MONDAY] OCT. 10– [1864]

Was quiet to-day. Saw Pete Sanders.[763] Went to church. Heard Rev. Mr. [John] Landstreet preach to a crowded house.[764]

[No entry onf Monday, Oct. 12, but apparently still near New Market, Shenandoah Co.]

---

[761] Gen. Jubal Anderson Early's official report is vague on these points: He says "some" artillery pieces and wagons were lost, but that casualties were "slight." He also says that Gen. Thomas L. Rosser's men were retiring in "good order" and according to sound tactics; but that Gen. Lunsford L. Lomax's men "came back to this place in confusion." Early to Gen. R.E. Lee, 9 October 1864, *OR*, I, vol. 43, pt. 1, 561. The journal of Capt. Jed Hotchkiss, topographical engineer for ANV 2nd Corps is more precise, but different from Apperson: Hotchkiss says that Rosser's men lost five artillery pieces and Lomax's men lost three. Hotchkiss also lists the Rev. John Landstreet as the officiating minister. Hotchkiss, "The Shenandoah Valley Campaign," *OR*, I, vol. 43, pt. 1, 758.

[762] Possibly N.C. St. John of Smyth Co. who joined original Jankins Bde, which became 8th VA Cav. This unit was apparently dispersed into other units in 1864, not long after this engagement. Goodridge Wilson says that Gen. Fitzhugh Lee took N.C. St. John and others into his cavalry, but he does not say which unit. Wilson, 238.

[763] Apparently Augustus Owry Sanders, Sr. (1836-1909) of Smyth Co., prewar occupation unknown. An original member of Smyth Blues, which became Co. D of 4th, he was wounded in an "accident" at Malvern Hill (1 July 1862), recovered and became commissary sergeant. Robertson, *4th VA Inf.*, 71; Smyth, *Smyth Co.*, ed. Presgraves, 20; Wilson, 236-40. He remained in reorganized ANV 2nd Corps, and he was among the very few who lined up in the remains of the original 4th Inf. at Appomattox Courth House. He is buried in Elizabeth Cemetary of Marion, Smyth Co. with a CSA marker. Sturgill and Sturgill, 71.

[764] The Rev. John Landstreet, born in 1818, was by 1870 serving a church in Loudon Co. VA Census, 1870. He was apparently a civilian minister with no chaplaincy experience, since he is not listed in Pitts, and Hotchkiss also records him as a minister in a church in New Market and not as an officer. Hotchkiss.

[ON THE ROAD NEAR MT. JACKSON, SHENANDOAH CO.]

[TUESDAY] OCT. 12– [1864]

Moved to Mt. Jackson. Asst. Surgn. Glocker and Dickert are here.[765] Things are much confused.

[ON THE ROAD NEAR MT. JACKSON, SHENANDOAH CO.]

[NO ENTRIES FOR THURSDAY, OCTOBER 13; FRIDAY, OCTOBER14, 1864]

[ON THE ROAD IN WOODSTOCK, SHENANDOAH CO.]

[SATURDAY] OCT. 15– [1864]

Moved to Woodstock. The army is at Fisher's Hill [Shenandoah Co]. ~~Took the Hotel for our Hospital.~~[766]

[TEMPORARY FIELD HOSPITAL, WOODSTOCK HOTEL, SHENANDOAH CO.]

[SUNDAY] OCT. 16– 1 [SIC]

Took the [Woodstock] Hotel for our [field] Hospital.

[TEMPORARY FIELD HOSPITAL, WOODSTOCK HOTEL, SHENANDOAH CO.]

[NO ENTRIES FOR MONDAY, OCTOBER 17; TUESDAY, OCTOBER 18, 1864]

[ON THE ROAD AT NEW MARKET, SHENANDOAH CO.]

OCT. 19– [1864]

Gen. [Jubal Anderson] Early made an attack on the enemy in position at Cedar Creek at dawn this morning and routed the 8th and 19th Corps capturing the camps and all their equipage, 18 pieces of artillery and prisoners. All were in ecstacies of the victory up to dusk when news came of a shameful reverse to our

---

[765] I cannot locate doctors named Glocker or Dickert in 4th or 7th regiments, and neither is listed in Cunningham. As is often the case, physicians, especially assistant surgeons seem to be attached to entire corps and not a regiment. Neither is involved in any official reports from the Valley Campaign of 1864, *OR*, I, vol. 43, pt. 1, passim and index.

[766] Sic. Apparently the steward wrote this entry on 16 October or later, and corrected his chronology of establishing the field hospital in the Woodstock Hotel.

army. Our army broke down after pushing the enemy to beyond Middletown [Shenandoah Co.] and came back to Fisher's Hill, leaving a large number of wagons, ambulances, & c. to the mercy of the enemy[.] 32 pieces of artillery were left. This is the most shameful affair of the war. All for want of discipline. Men left the ranks to prowl about the Yankee camp.

We left Woodstock at 2 o'clock in the morning of the20– [sic][767] —

Drs. Hagy and [H.P.] Magruder [of Orange Co.] were left in charge.

Three most elaborately fitted out medical wagons were brought to Dr. [William H.] Taylor [field surgeon].[768] Dr. Black got one with its appurtenances. I paid Mr. White 5$ [25 cents in gold; 1.25 in US greenback dollars] —

---

[767] Apperson must be writing these entries on or after 20 October. Lt. Gen. Jubal Anderson Early's official report of 20 October 1864 says: "I attacked [Philip] Sheridan's camp on Cedar Creek before day yesterday morning, and surprised and routed the Eighth and Nineteenth Corps, and then drove the Sixth Corps beyond Middletown, capturing 18 pieces of artillery and 1,300 prisoners; but the enemy subsequently made a stand on the pike, and, in turn, attacked my line, and my left gave way, and the rest of the troops took a panic and could not be rallied, retreating in confusion. But for their bad conduct I should have defeated Sheridan's whole force. On the retreat back to Fisher's Hill the enemy captured about thirty pieces of artillery and some wagons and ambulances. The prisoners were brought off. My loss in men was not heavy. General [Stephen Dodson] Ramseur [1837-1864, already identified] was seriously wounded while acting with gallantry, and was captured by the enemy." Idem, "Report," *OR*, Ser. 1, vol. 43, pt. 1, 560. On 21 October Early officially reported: "My net loss in artillery on the 19th was twenty-three pieces. My loss in killed and wounded is less [than] 1,000. In the early part of the day it was not more than 100. I cannot say how many were captured, but I think very few. Many of the men scattered, and are still coming in. The enemy's infantry is very badly demoralized. My men ran without sufficient cause, and the capture of artillery, & c., was made by the enemy's cavalry. The enemy is not pursuing; his loss was very severe. I have sent off 1,300 prisoners." Idem, "Report," *OR*, Ser. 1, vol. 43, pt. 1, 560. Maj. Gen. George Armstorng Custer [already identified] for the victorious Federals filed a different version of the same day's events: "Seeing so large a force of cavalry bearing rapidly down upon an unprotected flank and their line of retreat in danger of being intercepted, the lines of the enemy, already broken, now gave way in the utmost confusion. Realizing the necessity of at once gaining the bridge, the disordered masses of the enemy, now completely panic-stricken, threw away their arms, and in a headlong and disgraceful manner sought safety in ignominious flight....Hastily forming the First Vermont and Fifth New York under cover of the high bluff on the south side of the [Cedar] creek, I ordered both regiments to advance upon the ridge....Hearing the charge sounded through our bugles the enemy only stood long enough to deliver one volley; then, casting away his arms, attempted to escape under cover of the darkness. This was the last attempt the enemy made to offer organized resistance. That which hitherto, on our part, had been a pursuit after a broken and routed army now resolved itself into an exciting chase after a panic-stricken, uncontrollable mob." Idem, "Report," *OR*, Ser. 1, vol. 43, pt. 1,524-26. Stephen Dodson Ramseur did not survive his wounds; Early was reassigned another of another command.

[768] Birth and death dates unknown. Identified by Cunningham, who notes further, "Taylor was known to exaggerate on occasion." Idem, 111, 148n.

We came to New Market and stopped.

[TEMPORARY FIELD HOSPITAL NEAR NEW MARKET, SHENANDOAH CO.]

[NO ENTRIES FOR THURSDAY, OCTOBER 20; FRIDAY, OCTOBER 21, 1864]

[TEMPORARY FIELD HOSPITAL IN LACEY SPRING, ROCKINGHAM CO.]

[SATURDAY] OCT. 22– [1864]

We left New Market and came to Lacey Spring [Rockingham Co.] with the purpose of establishing an Hospital.

I called at Mr. Z's [Samuel Zigler] [769]—

[TEMPORARY FIELD HOSPITAL IN LACEY SPRING, ROCKINGHAM CO.]

[NO ENTRIES BETWEEN SUNDAY, OCTOBER 23 AND THURSDAY, NOVEMBER 3, 1864]

[TEMPORARY FIELD HOSPITAL IN LACEY SPRING, ROCKINGHAM CO.]

[FRIDAY] NOV. 4– [1864]

Rec'd for [Dr.] Ellsberg supplies belong to Surgn. [Samuel Rush] Sayers

Coverlets 100[,] bedsacks 97[,] shirts 2

Rec'd for Carroll [770] from Capt. [John M.] Preston [already identified; 48th VA Inf.] $46 [2.3 gold dollars; 11.5 US greenback dollars] and paid [Samuel] Mohler $10 [1/2 gold dollar; 2.5 US greenback dollars] out of it —

---

[769] Samuel Zigler, born in 1814, had a home and farm in Plains Township, Rockingham Co. VA Census, 1870.

[770] I cannot identify Carroll, who may have been a field surgeon. He is not in Cunningham, nor VA regimental histories.

[TEMPORARY FIELD HOSPITAL, MT. JACKSON, SHENANDOAH CO.]

[THURSDAY] NOV: 10– [1864]

Moved to Mt. Jackson [Shenandoah Co]. All supposed we would go down [northward] the Valley but were ordered to stop an[d] establish a receiving hospital

[TEMPORARY FIELD HOSPITAL, MT. JACKSON, SHENANDOAH CO.]

[NO ENTRIES FOR FRIDAY, NOVEMBER 11; SATURDAY, NOVEMBER 12; SUNDAY, NOVEMBER 13, 1864]

[TEMPORARY FIELD HOSPITAL, LACEY SPRING, ROCKINGHAM CO.]

[MONDAY] NOV. 14 [1864]

Ordered to return to Lacey Spring [Rockingham Co.]—reached there just before night.

[TEMPORARY FIELD HOSPITAL, LACEY SPRING, ROCKINGHAM CO.]

[NO ENTRIES BETWEEN TUESDAY, NOVEMBER 15 AND THURSDAY, DECEMBER 15, 1864]

[TEMPORARY FIELD HOSPITAL, MT. SIDNEY, AUGUSTA CO.]

[FRIDAY] DECR. 16 - [18]64

Ordered from Lacey Spring [Rockingham Co.] Camped near Mt. Sydney [sic]. On account of a deficiency in transportation we had to leave 9 tents and 14 iron bunks at the [Lacey] Spring. Thomas [Spottswood] White[771] was left in charge of them. The whole army [2nd Corps ANV] is moving. [Brig. Gen. John Austin] Wharton's[772] Div. is all the Infantry in the Valley now.

---

[771] Thomas Spottswood White (born 1845) was a farmer from Charlottesville originally with 4th VA Inf. who in 1862 transfered to 1st VA Cav. Robertson, *4th VA Inf.*, 80.

[772] John Austin Wharton (1828-1865) was born near Nashville, grew up in Texas, and was educated at South Carolina College. Admitted to Texas bar, he was elected to Texas state secession convention and joined Texas Rangers. Promoted, he was moved to VA, rising to Maj. Gen., fought with distinction in VA, including Valley briefly, and then was transfered to trans-

Snow on the ground and we had a disagreeable night.

[ON THE ROAD NEAR FISHERSVILLE, AUGUSTA CO.]

[SATURDAY] DEC. 17– [1864]

Left camp before 6 o'clock. At Willow Point [Augusta Co.] Dr. B left me with the train with orders to bring [it] on through Staunton [Augusta Co.] to Fishersville [Augusta Co].

Got to camp [Fishersville] about 2 P.M.

The prospect here is anything but flattering. The artillery has preceded us and all the empty houses occupied. We are obliged to take it in the woods. Near our camp is a small house which has been appropriated as a sort of Storeroom. I shall occupy [it]. Rumors to-day are that the enemy have made a raid into S.W. Va. and succeeded in taking the S[alt] works [Saltville, on the border between Washington and Smyth Co].[773]

[TEMPORARY FIELD HOSPITAL, FISHERSVILLE, AUGUSTA CO.]

[NO ENTRIES BETWEEN SATURDAY, DECEMBER 18 AND WEDNESDAY, DECEMBER 21, 1864]

[TEMPORARY FIELD HOSPITAL, FISHERSVILLE, AUGUSTA CO.]

[THURSDAY] DEC. 22– [1864]

Let Stallings and [F.] Jeffries[774] have each a pair of shoes to be replaced—one of the medical lot and one of the small pox lot. Stallings a pair of stockings also.

Mississippi theatre for duration of War. He died in a shoot-out in a hotel room in Houston TX, in a fight with long-time rival Col. George W. Baylor . Patricia L. Faust, "Wharton," *Hist. Times.*

[773] The rumors are prophetic, portentous rather than inaccurate. Gen. George Stoneman (1822-1894; already identified from earlier encounters), on 10 Dec. 1864 began a long march through upper east TN and SW VA. He destroyed the saltworks on 20 December 1864. Stoneman also raided Marion and other parts of Smyth Co., capturing four cities, 900 prisoners, 19 cannon, 3,000 horses and mules, 25,000 rounds of artillery ammunition, and destroying businesses, including "four pestiferous secession printing presses." Edward G. Longacre, "Stoneman's Raid, SW VA," *Hist. Times.* See also Armstrong, 145, 150-55, 165.; and Wilson, 246-60.

[774] Prof. Bean identifies Stallings and Jeffries as orderlies, but could not supply first names or other data. David F. Riggs identifies F. Jeffries, no birth or death data, no occupation data, as a private who had enlisted at Stanardsville (Greene Co.) into Co. F, 7th VA Inf., and as one captured at Sayler's Creek (6 April 1865). If this is the orderly, "5'8", dark complexion, hazel eyes, brown

[TEMPORARY FIELD HOSPITAL, FISHERSVILLE, AUGUSTA CO.]

[NO ENTRIES BETWEEN FRIDAY, DECEMBER 23, 1864 AND THURSDAY, JANUARY 12, 1865]

[TEMPORARY FIELD HOSPITAL, PROBABLY GREENWOOD DEPOT, ALBEMARLE CO.]

[FRIDAY] JANY 13; '[18]65

Paid to Capt. John Preston [48th VA Inf.] AQM [Acting Quartermaster for 2d Corps] $780.00 CSA [15.6 gold dollars; 31.2 US greenbacks]—being the effects of deceased soldiers.[775]

[TEMPORARY FIELD HOSPITAL, PROBABLY GREENWOOD DEPOT, ALBEMARLE CO.]

[NO ENTRIES BETWEEN SATURDAY, JANUARY 14 AND SUNDAY, JANUARY 29, 1865]

[TEMPORARY FIELD HOSPITAL, PROBABLY GREENWOOD DEPOT, ALBEMARLE CO.]

[MONDAY] JAN'Y 30 [1865]

Sent to Med. Dir. [Lafayette] Guild one box of books by Dr. [Hunter Holmes] McGuire's Direction. Delivered it to G.T. Gibson, agent Southern Express[776] —Directed to Petersburg [Dinwiddie Co].[777]

Dr. Dunn's address Cole's Ferry, Charlotte Co., Va.[778]

---

hair." Imprisoned at Pt. Lookout, he took oath of allegiance to US and was freed on 28 June 1865. Idem, 81.

775 Capt. John M. Preston would then disburse the funds to heirs and assigns of the surviving soldiers. It is not much compensation to spread around. Richard Todd notes that CSA currency briefly stabilized in the early winter, and that US greenbacks briefly experienced slight loss of value. However, by March CSA currency would be almost incalculable in gold, and US greenbacks moved to solid respectability. Todd, 198.

776 I cannot locate a man named G.T. Gibson in Albemarle Co. in 1870 Census.

777 The railroad and shipping center 20 mi. south of Richmond was still under siege by Lt. Gen. Ulysses Grant and a huge force; it was the eighth month of the longest sustained operation of the entire War.

778 I cannot locate in Charlotte Co. in 1870 census rolls any man old enough to be this Dr. Dunn; there is a widow, Elizabeth Dunn, born in 1813, but it is not clear that her late husband was a physician.

[TEMPORARY FIELD HOSPITAL, PROBABLY GREENWOOD DEPOT, ALBEMARLE CO.]

[THERE ARE NO ENTRIES BETWEEN TUESDAY, JANUARY 31 AND THURSDAY, MARCH 2, 1865]

[ON THE ROAD BETWEEN GREENWOOD DEPOT, ALBEMARLE CO. AND LYNCHBURG, CAMPBELL CO.]

[FRIDAY] MCH 3– [18]65

Chased from Greenwood Depot. [779]

[ON THE ROAD BETWEEN GREENWOOD DEPOT, ALBEMARLE CO. AND LYNCHBURG, CAMPBELL CO.]

[NO ENTRY FOR SATURDAY, MARCH 4, 1865]

[ON THE ROAD IN LYNCHBURG, CAMPBELL CO.]

[SUNDAY] MCH 5– [1865]

arrived in Lynchburg.

---

[779] On March 2, 1865, the remains of Jubal Anderson Early's 2nd Corps ANV were soundly defeated by Gen. George Armstrong Custer in the Battle of Waynesboro; thousands of prisoners were taken, and the Corps depleted. The VA Bde, the remnants of the 4th Inf., now commanded by Col. William Terry (1824-1888) had already been shifted southwest of Petersburg to assist in the defense of that city. William Terry was a native of Amherst, and he had alredy been wounded three times. Robertson, *4th VA Inf.*, 34; 76. The Battle of Waynesboro in Albemarle Co. marks the end of the Valley Campaign. The diarist's temporary Field Hospital in Albemarle Co. had to be abandoned, and the ambulance wagon train then went on the run, toward CSA forces trying to defend Petersburg; but it is not a straight line of retreat.

[TEMPORARY HOSPITAL CAMP IN LYNCHBURG, CAMPBELL CO.]

*[NO ENTRIES BETWEEN MONDAY,
MARCH 6 AND SUNDAY, MARCH 12, 1865]*

[ON THE ROAD NEAR BIG LICK, ROANOKE CO.][780]

[MONDAY] MARCH 13– [1865]

left Lynchburg [Campbell Co.] for Big Lick —Roanoke Co.
Stopping at Mr. Thomas'.[781]

[FIELD HOSPITAL CAMP NEAR BIG LICK, ROANOKE CO.]

*[NO ENTRIES BETWEEN TUESDAY,
MARCH 14 AND WEDNESDAY, MARCH 22, 1865]*

[ON THE ROAD SOMEWHERE EAST OF BIG LICK, ROANOKE CO.]

[THURSDAY] MCH. 23 [1865]

Left Big Lick [Roanoke Co.] for Petersburg [Dinwiddie Co].

[AT DUNLOPS FARM, POSSIBLY IN DINWIDDIE CO.]

[FRIDAY] MCH 24– [1865]

arrive at Dunlops farm where Surgn [Samuel Rush] Sayers has charge of Hosp't 2d Corps.

---

[780] This railroad junction became the City of Roanoke after the war. Humel, *A List.*

[781] Probably a relative of one of the several Thomases who served in 4th VA Inf. but I cannot figure out which one. Also possibly Joseph M. Thomas, onetime Capt. of 4th Inf. who resigned in late 1862 because of "incipient pthisis" and later removed to St. Albin's, WVA, Robertson, *4th VA Inf.*, 76. The oddly spelled disease was likely *ptosis*, described by *Taber's* as "Gk., a dropping or drooping of an organ or a part, as the upper eyelid, from paralysis." Ibid. A final possibility is the surgeon William H. Thomas, or relatives of his.

[FIELD HOSPITAL NEAR DUNLOPS FARM, POSSIBLY IN DINWIDDIE CO.]

[THERE ARE NO ENTRIES BETWEEN SATURDAY, MARCH 25 AND FRIDAY, MARCH 31, 1865 [782]

[FIELD HOSPITAL NEAR DUNLOPS FARM, POSSIBLY IN DINWIDDIE CO.]

[SATURDAY] APL 1– [1865]

Surgn Black took charge of the Hospital. It is near Dunlop's Station at its junction [possibly the junction ten miles southwest of Petersburg].

[Another hand writes at top of diary page:]

Rec'd of J.S. Apperson Coat and Boots to be sold at $300 [less than 4 gold dollars; less than 5 US greenback dollars]

[illegible merchant signature]

[witnesses] W.H. Egerton[783]

W.H. Johnson[784]

[ON RETREAT FROM PETERSBURG, DINWIDDIE CO.]

[SUNDAY] APL 2: [1865]

Heavy engagement this morning. The enemy broke through our lines at [Cadmus Marcellus] Wilcox's Division [ANV 3rd Corps].[785] Ordered about 1

[782] On 25 March 1865 at Battle of Fort Steadman in Dinwiddie Co., William Terry of 4th VA Inf., now a Brig. Gen., was wounded a fourth time and was replaced by Capt. Hamilton David Wade, who was brevetted Col. for the remainder of fighting (1836-1908). William Terry after War made his home in Wytheville, and is buried there. Hamilton David Wade , who was from Groveton, moved to Christiansburg after War, and is buried there. Robertson, *4th VA Inf.*, 34-36; 76, 78. Note also two social facts in this March: The CSA congress authorized the use of African American troops; and CSA currency was inflated to more than 70:1 ratio to gold dollars, but actually could seldom be used, while the US greenback moved to 1.4:1.0 ratio to gold dollars. Long, 651; Todd, 198

[783] I cannot locate a soldier named W.H. Egerton, or Edgerton, in 4th Inf., 7th Inf., or in Scott's list of soldiers in other units, Scott, *Hist. of Orange Co.*, 264-77.

[784] Possibly William Johnson, no birth or death data, of Co. B, 4th VA Inf. Robertson, 58.

[785] Cadmus Marcellus Wilcox (1824-1890) was a native of Wayne City, NC, a West Point graduate, and one honored for bravery in Mexican War. He also instructed at West Point, and was author of a textbook on rifle practice. When War came, he joined Maj. Gen. James Longstreet's (already identified) division and quickly earned promotion, to Brig. Gen. in charge of Alabama troops. Unhappy with Longstreet's leadership, he appeared to be blocked from promotion despite bravery and wise leadership in battles from Seven Pines to Gettysburg. During

o'clock to move—Richmond & Petersburg have at last to be given up. The crisis is upon us and it remains to be seen how our people will bear it.

It is adversity that tries men's hearts—At 3 o'clock we moved off—some of our bedding and Hospital furniture could not be moved.

We took the "Woodpecker Road" and camped 3 1/2 miles from Chesterfield C.H. [Chersterfield Co].

The number of wounded reporting to us is not large—all sent to Surgn. [illegible; possibly J.S.D.Cullen.][786]

[TEMPORARY FIELD HOSPITAL, CHESTERFIELD COURT HOUSE, CHESTERFIELD CO.]

[MONDAY] APL 3– [1865]

Moved at day light to Chesterfield C.H. We took the road leading to Summit Station [Charles City Co.] on the Coal Road. Gen'l [R.E.] Lee & [James] Longstreet passed us several times with units.

At a Mrs. Baldwin's[787] Ge. Lee was stopped by the old lady to shake hands. She manifested very consdierable feeling. That good old man looked at her with a sort of benignant smile and spoke kindly to her. There were some pretty girls—there—daughters I suppose. She is a true Virginian.

We camped near "Goode's Bridge". News from the opposite side of the river at Appomattox.

[ON THE ROAD NEAR AMELIA COURT HOUSE [AMELIA CO.]

[TUESDAY] APL 4 [1865]

Started early this morning—Crossed the river [Appomattox] on an indifferent pontoon, and took the road to Amelia Court House and camped two or three miles below—some firing to our left. 2 Corps is up and in camp near

---

long siege of Petersburg, he took a division under Gen. Ambrose Powell Hill (already identified) in the 3rd Corps of ANV, and he fought stubbornly and well, holding his division together despite heavy losses in defeat at Fort Gregg. Broeck N. Oder, "Wilcox," *Hist. Times.*

786 Cunningham identifies J.S.D. Cullen as medical director in field for Longstreet's Corps, 1st Corps ANV. Idem, 284.

787 I cannot locate in Chesterfield Co. in 1870 census a woman named Baldwin old enough to be this person. There is a man, William Baldwin, born 1805, who may have had a wife who could be she; but I cannot find her name. Also William Baldwin is not listed as having daughters who would be in their twenties. VA Census, 1870.

the trains. I returned to write Dr. Faris but made a poor hand—H[enry]. Earhart [sic][788] starts to-morrow for S.W. Va.

[ON THE ROAD NEAR PAINEVILLE, AMELIA CO.]

[WEDNESDAY] APL 5 1865

Left camp at 8 o'clock and took a road to the right of one taken by the main train leading by a Mr. Barksdale. The main train was cut by the enemy and a number of wagons destroyed. A small party did the work. Our men, principally stragglers, ran in confusion over the Country. Our train seemed in imminent danger. A small guard was gotten up. We reached Paynesville [sic; Amelia Co.][789] in safety, crossing the line of the enemy.

Gen. [Thomas Lafayette] Rosser [already identified] is in pursuit of the party that attacked the train.

I am very tired to-night. Took supper at Daytonsville [Deatonsville, Amelia Co].[790] Saw Gen. [Bushrod] Johnston [sic][791] there. He gives a gloomy account of the rabble in Richmond on its evacuation.[792] In camp.

---

[788] Henry Earheart (1836-1892), occupation and birthplace unknown, joined Co. L Liberty Hall Volunteers [Rockbridge Co.] of 4th VA Inf. and was soon detailed as agent for hospital supplies. After War, he lived and worked in Blacksburg [Montgomery Co.] and is buried there. Robertson, *4th Va Inf.*, 49.

[789] Humel indicates that the town was always spelled *Paineville*. Idem, *A List.*

[790] Humel indicates that Deatonville was often spelled *Deatonsville* and pronounced *Daytonsville*. Ibid.

[791] Bushrod Rust Johnson (1817-1880) "was one of the many excellent but unsung commanders whose skill kept the Confederacy alive for 2 years after Vicksburg and Gettysburg," according to Robert D. Hofsommer. A native of Ohio, he attended West Point in company with Willliam Tecumseh Sherman (already identified) and George Henry Thomas (1816-1870). He served credibly in Mexican and Seminole fighting, and then taught in colleges in KY and TN. When War came, he joined corps of engineers, was captured (Fort Donelson), escaped, was wounded (Shiloh), and distinguished himself at Chicakamauga. Promoted to Maj. Gen., he left the TN theatre and joined Lee to defend Petersburg. After War, he was president of University of Nashville, but when it closed for financial reasons, he moved to IL, where he "became a semi-invalid...on his farm near Brighton." Idem, "Johnson," *Hist. Times*.

[792] President Abraham Lincoln came into Richmond on 4 April to tour the former CSA White House and there confered with John A. Campbell, onetime US Supreme Court judge and onetime CSA Assistant Secretary of War. The "rabble" may be the diarist's reference to the many freedmen who joyously gathered around Lincoln; but there also are reports of roustabouts in town who were looting and causing danger to all, including Lincoln. See Long, 666.

[ON THE ROAD NEAR PAINEVILLE, AMELIA CO]

THURSDAY, APL 6– [1865]

Roused about midnight to start but the order was countermanded and we rested till 3 o'clock [A.M.] Stopped for three hours after 6 miles travel. Soon after we started again, the enemy charged our train and captured the wagons and ambulance of our [Medical] Dept. and about 100 others. Nearly all the Hosp't boys were taken—myself included. I was taken back some two miles and escaped on a mule. All my clothing lost. My friend Drane was taken off which I regretted to see so much. I ran back to the captured wagons but they were then under fire, though the enemy had left. The Medical Wagon was taken out. Another large train on the left is burning.

Fighting is horrible—It seems doubtful about getting out.[793]

I followed with Surg'n [Samuel Rush] Sayers along with the wagon train and crossed the [Appomattox] river at High bridge. Surg'ns [Hunter Holmes] McGuire, Black, Stevens, Hinkel, and Wilkinson[794] came up and all of us stayed in a pine forest near Mr. Barksdale's.

[ON THE ROAD NEAR BUCKINGHAM COURTH HOUSE, BUCKINGHAM CO.]

[FRIDAY] APL 7 [1865]

Started about sunrise.

High Bridge [over Appomattox River] burning. Got a coloured woman to cook a snack—Ashbread and bacon were sweet enough for an epicure. Three miles from Farmville [Prince Edward Co.], with the wagons leaving that point, for what point no one knew, I determined to quit the path. All is confusion—chaos.

A dark day for the Confederacy. We [marginalia: Dr. Samuel Rush Sayers & myself] came on thinking we had left the train, but found it in the road again. Left it at New Store [Buckingham Co.] and took out for Buckingham C.H., hoping to get something for man and beast but failed after 15 miles riding except a little fodder. Slept in the wood five miles from C.H. [Buckingham Court House].

---

[793] Battle of Sailor's Creek or Saylor's Creek, Prince Edward and Amelia Cos. *OR* estimates that R.E. Lee lost 1/3 of his already decimated troops. 8000 CSA troops surrendered. It was the last engagement of the War in VA. *OR*, ser. 1, vol. 46, pt. 1, p. 1464.

[794] I cannot identify surgeons Stevens, Hinkel. They are not in Cunningham, nor in Scott's list of surgeons from Orange Co., nor in regimental histories. Wilkinson may be the former steward who earned a MD during the war.

[ON THE ROAD NEAR APPOMATTOX COURT HOUSE, APPOMATTOX CO.]

[SATURDAY] APL 8– [1865]

Started on the [Appomattox] C.H. road, turned to the left to Mr. Holderman's whom we found a hospitable man—breakfasted & took the Lynchburg road and fell in with wagon train below Appomattox C.H. I am very much dissatisfied in regard to not meeting Surgn Black—If he were to remain with any wounded I wish to be with him. We stopped at a Mr. Harris' above [Appomattox] C.H. for supper but failed to get it.

While there a heavy fire began in direction of Appomattox Depot.

Farther up the road at Mr. McKinney's we found an excellent man—got supper. The enemy attcked our artillery and captured a great many guns. The position he has must sadly embarrass Gen. Lee's Army. Men are running in all directions—Deciding that the point was unsafe we road [sic] a few miles above Ausville[795] and slept in a pine thicket—Surgn. Paxton and Mr. Cooke were with us.[796]

[ON THE ROAD NEAR LYNCHBURG, CAMPBELL CO.]

[SUNDAY] APL 9–[1865]

Firing began early; We took the "Ridgeroad" and met with Col. Haynes and Mr. Gibson,[797] who were going to the James River. We went—crossed on a ferry at Stonewall Ferry. Above at a mill procured corn for our horses. We then went on to Lynchburg through Amherst. Everything is worse than Confusion. A short time after our arrival news reached us that the Army had been surrendered[798]—our hopes are crushed. Order was soon issued for the evacuation of the place [Lynchburg]. Straglers [sic] & a small train of wagons were ordered to Liberty [Bedford Co]. We traveled 12 miles and slept in the woods.

---

[795] Prof. Bean indicates that it is a town in Appomattox Co. It is not listed in the *OR*, or in Humel's list of placenames.

[796] I cannot identify the surgeon or the civilian.

[797] I cannot identify the col. or the civilian, but I do not think they were with 7th or 4th, the remnants of which were in Appomattox Court House with R.E. Lee.

[798] Apperson's old unit the 4th Inf. formed itself one more time, minus the medical personnel, for surrender. Forty-six men were there under Capt. Hamilton David Wade, including five from Co. D. Robertson finds that 1,487 men had served with 4th over the course of War, and thus those surrendering were "a pitiful remnant." Even the fierce Grayson Daredevils were gone completely. Idem, 34-36. Note of course that Apperson as medical staff is detached from his old unit, and did not surrender on that occasion; note also this news is regarded as rumor.

[ON THE ROAD NEAR BUFORDVILLE, BEDFORD CO.]

[MONDAY] APL 10– [1865]

Turned from the main road to Mr. Bells and breakfasted. took a road by Kesler's Mill to Lisbon [Bedford Co]. Met Capt Degarnette & Mr. Lyles,[799] making our party five—Stopped at Mr. Davidson's near Bufords [sic; Bedford Co].[800]

[ON THE ROAD NEAR LAFAYETTE, MONTGOMERY CO.]

[TUESDAY] APL 11– [1865]

Traveled to Lafayette. Capt. D[egarnette] & Mr. L[yles] left us to-day. Stopped at Salem [Roanoke Co]. a few minutes—Saw Miss K[Keziah Shepherd, hostess of palmier times]. Met Gen. [John] Echols[801] . He is panic stricken. The condition of his army is deplorable in the extreme—perfectly demoralized. Stopped at Mr. Taylor's. Met Gen. [George Bibb] Crittendon [1812-1880; already identified] there.

[ON THE ROAD NEAR CHRISTIANSBURG, ROANOKE CO.]

[WEDNESDAY] APL 12– [1865]

Passed [Gen. John] Echols' army at Christiansburg. He is allowing his army to go where they please. Passively yielding to disbandment, which appears to me to be disgraceful beyond [illegible; context is *beyond acceptance*].

Any army of 6 or 8000 men to be turned loose upon the Country to ravage and spoil and not a Yankee in 50 miles. *O tempora O mores.* [the classic lament: O what times, O what habits, used by Edgar Allen Poe, ca. 1825].

At Christiansburg I met Capt. [James W.] Shields,[802] who furnished me a good horse.

---

[799] I cannot identify the officer or the civilian.

[800] Humel indicates that the town was sometimes called Bufordsville and sometimes Bufordville, but never Buford or Buford's. Humel, *A List.*

[801] Gen. John Echols (1823-1896), from Lynchburg and Washington College, already identified; was trying to leave engagements in southwestern VA in order to help R.E. Lee in Appomattox Court House. Learning of surrender, he turned toward NC to try to join up with Gen. Joseph Eggleston Johnston; but eventually joined the party of President Jefferson Davis and surrendered with him in Augusta, GA. Jeffrey D. Wert, "Echols," *Hist. Times.*

[802] Capt. James W. Shields was formerly on staff of 4th Inf. in charge of commissary, but was dropped from rolls in disgrace after investigation by Inspector General's office. See Robertson, 72.

The wagon trains of [Gen. John] Echols were turned aside to be burned—his artillery destroyed and the teams turned over to the scattered army.

On arriving at New River the ford could not be crossed. We turned left to Cecil's ferry—stopped at Mr. Miller's for the night.

Parts of the Command here profess to be going—some to Ky. Some to [Gen. Joseph Eggleston] Johnston in N.C. and others anywhere to disband and surrender.

[HOME OF MAJ. JOHN THOMPSON SAYERS, MAX MEADOWS, WYTHE CO.]

[THURSDAY] APL 13– [1865]

Crossed at Cecil's ford and came to Newbern [Pulaski Co]. The road is thronged with men stealing horses and anything else. A most deplorable state of affairs now exist in our Country.

We took dinner at Mr. John Drapers in Draper's Valley [Pulaski Co]. Met Gen. [William] Terry [invalided onetime commander of 4th Inf.] there—several Kentuckians were there.

Reached Maj. [John Thompson] Sayers at Max Meadows [Wythe Co.] just before dark. Found Lt. Jno [John Thompson]Sayers just from prison.[803] I found an excellent family.

[HOME OF MAJ. JOHN THOMPSON SAYERS, MAX MEADOWS, WYTHE CO.]

[FRIDAY] APL. 14 [1865]

Went to Wytheville this morning. We stopped at Dr. [Samuel] Crockett's.[804] He puts a gloomy face on affairs. Advises the men to prosecute the struggle no longer. He said a batch of officers started this morning to Tennessee to surrender themselves to the enemy. A most disgraceful affair[.] Confederate

---

[803] John Thompson Sayers [1831-death date unknown] was farmer from Wythe Co. who joined Wythe Greys, who became Co. A of 4th Inf. Promoted to 1st Sgt., he rose in rank to 1st Lt., but was captured at Gettysburg (3 July 1863) and imprisoned on Johnson's Island. He was exchanged in March, and would have been free barely three weeks at this writing. Robertson, 71. His father, Major John Thompson Sayers, born 1805, owned land in Max Meadows, Wythe Co., was a farmer with military experience. VA Census, 1870.

[804] Samuel Crockett, born 1810, had a practice and a farm in Wythe Co. near Ft. Chiswell Township. VA Census, 1870. This is not his onetime supervisor, who was killed in action.

officers who have been in position to act[,] in a fawning manner towards the Yankee.[805] I can scarcely believe it.

This morning we met Gen. [Gabriel Colvin] Wharton[806] & staff at Gen. [William] Terry's. The first decision was to start on the morrow. Now they decide to wait a few days. [Gen. Joseph Eggleston] Johnston's army in N.C. [near Durham] is one point of destination.

Returned to Maj. [John Thompson] Sayers. Surg'n [Samuel Rush] Sayers is very much affected by the remarks of Dr. [Samuel] Crockett.

[DR. WILLIAM FARIS'S HOME, SEVEN MILE FORD, SMYTH CO.]

[SATURDAY] APL 15– [1865]

Concluded to go home for a day or so. Stopped at Gen. [William] Terry's[.] Gen. [Gabriel Colvin] Wharton & he think they may try to organise the scattered army here.

At Marion I stopped with a message to Col. [William Elisha] Peters.[807]

Reached home about dusk.

[DR. WILLIAM FARIS'S HOME, SEVEN MILE FORD, SMYTH CO.]

[SUNDAY] APL 16– [1865]

At Church. R[ichard] Price preached.[808] Burial of Miss Martha Oury, one of my first friends in SW VA.[809]

---

[805] The diarist needed a comma, and perhaps even a dash, for the sense of his sentence is that the officers were in a position to act, viz., fight; but instead they behaved in a fawning manner toward the Federal troops.

[806] Gabriel Colvin Wharton (1824-1906) was born in Culpeper City, VA and graduated 2d in class from Viriginia Military Institute in 1847. He became a civil engineer, exploring and investing his own funds in mining in the far southwest, especially New Mexico Territory. When War came, he joined 45th VA Inf., then transfered to 51st VA Inf, which elected him its Col. He earned promotion to Brig. Gen., and he served with distinction throughout southwestern VA and upper east TN. He was part of the success at New Market (15 May 1864) and was very active in Valley campaign of Jubal Anderson Early, becoming a divisional commander. After War he moved to Radford (Montgomery Co.) and explored VA mines, developing a New South business in mining in the region. He was elected to VA gen. assy. John E. Stanchak, "Wharton," *Hist. Times.*

[807] William Elisha Peters, from Bedford (Bedford Co.) was a professor of languages and literature at Emory & Henry College who helped organize students and others into Gen. John Buchanan Floyd's Brigade (1806-1863, already identified) of mountaineers. He rose to high rank, though he shared the embarrassments of Gen. Floyd's losses in TN.; after Floyd's death, Col. Peters joined the 2nd Corps of ANV and served with Gen. Jubal Anderson Early in final Valley campaign. William Elisha Peters Papers, Archives of Emory & Henry College.

Some peple try to keep up—generally ladies

[DR. WILLIAM FARIS'S HOME, SEVEN MILE FORD, SMYTH CO.]

[MONDAY] APL 17– [1865]

At Mr. [Campbell B.] St. Johns, John L. Sanders & Col. [Robert] Beatie. [810]

[HOME OF MAJ. JOHN THOMPSON SAYERS, MAX MEADOWS, WYTHE CO.]

[TUESDAY] APL 18– [1865]

Went back to Wytheville[.] Found Gen. [William] Terry had gone Somewhere. Gen. [Gabriel Colvin] Wharton [had left Wytheville] to see his wife and the men in the Country where they please [Wharton's soldiers had largely dispersed in the general's absence]. At Maj. [John Thompson] Sayers

[HOME OF MAJ. JOHN THOMPSON SAYERS, MAX MEADOWS, WYTHE CO.]

[WEDNESDAY] APL 19: [1865]

At Maj [John Thompson] Sayers all day.

---

[808] Smyth Co. historians Armstrong, Smyth, and Wilson do not list any minister in Smyth Co. named *Price*, nor is any *Price* listed in the Co. in 1870. However, Richard Price, born 1815, maintained a home in Elk Garden, Russell Co., and seems to be the minister involved, since he was likely part of a Russell Co. family that produced a number of ministers. VA Census, 1870.

[809] The Oury family evidently moved from Smyth Co. late in 19th cent., as they are not recorded by local historians Armstrong, Smyth, and Wilson, and do not appear in the genealogical entries of *Heritage of Smyth Co.*; none are listed in the burial sites compiled by Sturgill and Sturgill, op. cit. Martha Oury is mentioned in diary and in "Reminiscences," and was likely the daughter of Robertson G. Oury, born 1815, who maintained a home in Marion Township at this time. VA Census, 1870.

[810] C[ampbell] B. St. John, born 1830, owned a business of some sort in St. Clair Township near Marion, and is listed as receiving compensation by the Co. for war expenses, Armstrong, 128; John L. Sanders had a farm with a spring house in the Marion area, and was of some prominence after War; he is listed as missing from a required slave patrol in 1859 and apparently did not serve in War, ibid., 84, 85; 173; Col. Robert Beatie, born 1795 was the first County Clerk of Smyth Co. [a stepping-stone political position in antebellum VA and early New South era] and active in Democratic politics before, during and after War, even as an octogenerian, Armstrong, op. cit., Wilson, op. cit.

[HOME OF JOHN CADDALL, DUBLIN TOWNSHIP, PULASKI CO.]

[THURSDAY] APL ~~19~~ 20 [1865]

Started to Blacksburg to see Dr. Harvey Black at his home]. Stopped at Caddells [sic; John Caddall's].[811]

[A note, possibly written 20 April 1865 "Portage Account" for transportation expenses owed "up to Mch. 13th" "the best of my knowledge, these were $830 and account lost at Waynesboro. I owe Dr. [Samuel Rush] Sayers $107 on portage account...[owe] Dr. [Harvey] Black 10 [CSA dollars] [also list 50 CSA dollars owed Dr. Black for subsequent portage] Apl 2 [list concludes, making a total of $940 CSA owed for portage account. A rough estimate of this debt in gold for late March would be 13.40 dollars, and in US greenbacks approximately $16.00]

*[AT HOME OF DR. HARVEY BLACK,
BLACKSBURG TOWNSHIP MONTGOMERY CO.]*

[FRIDAY] APL 21 [1865]

Reached Blacksburg. Found Dr. [Harvey] Black at home. He gave me good advice which I shall take I think.[812]

[SATURDAY] APL 22– [1865]

*[HOME OF MAJ. JOHN THOMPSON SAYERS,
MAX MEADOWS, WYTHE CO.]*

Returned to Maj. [John Thompson] Sayers. Dr. B gave me a good letter.

[SUNDAY] APL 23. [1865]

Returned home to Stay.

---

811 John Caddall, born 1800, owned a farm and home in Dublin Township, Pulaski Co. on the road between Marion and Blacksburg; his son John H. Caddall, born 1848, was then living with him there. VA Census, 1870. The son, a teacher and friend of the diarist, was discharged from 4th VA Inf. on 17 April 1862 according to Robertson, 43.

812 The "Reminiscences" and family oral history both indicate that Dr. Harvey Black advised Apperson to go home and begin a civilian career with plans to attend the University of Virginia medical college in Charlottesville whenever practicable. Dr. Black apparently wrote a general letter of introduction "to whom it may concern" and also promised to write on the diarist's behalf for admission to the medical lectures—the very thing that Dr. Black had denied the frustrated steward for three years. "Reminiscences." Interview: Mary Apperson Kent Elliott (28 April 2001), John Herbert Roper Papers, Southern Historical Collection of Library of University of North Carolina, Chapel Hill.

EPILOGUE

With the War at last done, John Samuel Apperson saluted a final time and seldom looked back at the Old South to whose martial misadventures he had repaired. He was instead almost the exact description of the New South business elite, newly risen from the antebellum middling class of farmers, as described by the late historian C. Vann Woodward.[1] With his characteristic firm resolution, he marched at the double quick into a postbellum region of business enterprise and industrial endeavors. Between 1868 and 1908, Apperson established himself as the country physician of choice, helped to build and run a professional institution for care of the insane, helped to start a railway line, helped to start a bank, raised funds for higher education, invested in mineral extraction and an ironworks manufactory, and generally "boosted" other business enterprises.

Immediately before starting this New South career, he completed his medical training. With help from his wartime supervisor, sometime nemesis, and fulltime benefactor Dr. Harvey Black, he attended medical lectures at the University of Virginia in Charlottesville in the years 1866 and 1867. He stood the examinations successfully and was duly licensed as a doctor of medicine in 1868, at which time he returned to Smyth County, settling in Chilhowie and taking as his wife Ellen Victoria Hull. She was a "fair one" whom he had admired before the War, but from a very proper distance. The Hulls, like their friends and associates the Copenhavers, Sheffeys, and Pendletons, owned the best lands in the county; their family living and working in "The Wheatlands" of Smyth. The young steward and apothecary running his errands around town in July of 1860 could read of Victoria Hull being crowned Maid of Honour by the Knights of Marion at a special gathering of the few families who lived most comfortably and who enjoyed the "fairest prospects." In 1860 and 1861, Apperson understood from his advisor the matronly Mary Tomlin that he must bide his time patiently until he had risen to the status of a Hull or a Copenhaver or a Sheffey and

---

[1] Comer Vann Woodward, *Origins of the New South, 1877-1913*, vol. 9, History of the South Series, ed., Ellis Merton Coulter and Wendell Holmes Stephenson (1951. Reprint ed. with rev. bibliography and essay by Charles B. Dew; Baton Rouge: Louisiana State University Press, 1987).

could properly "make his proclamation and declare his intentions" to the daughter of such a family.[2]

By 1868 he was a licensed physician and this was a new era. Now he was a fitting suitor for her, and the two made a good marriage in 1868 that lasted twenty years and produced eleven children. Victoria Hull Apperson too was literary minded and produced correspondence and recollections of a high and fine character; and like her husband, she had seen her own adventures during the War. In May of 1861, Victoria Hull had run to the town's railroad line to stop a trainload of Confederate troops from Mississippi before they crashed into a wrecked car around a blind bend of the tracks. To gain attention of the engineer, she ripped off her petticoat and waved it. In retelling the incident, she is said to stand on the rails, and the train stops only in the nick of time, and the petticoat is red. What is known for sure is that the officer in charge of the Mississippi regiment sent her an official letter of commendation and thanks. Later, in the fag end of the year 1864, Victoria Hull witnessed and survived Stoneman's Raid of 10-24 December when federal cavalry general George Stoneman—the same feared horseman seen in the diarist's accounts of piedmont and valley campaigns—swept through Smyth County, destroying the saltworks at Saltville and an ironworks and some private homes in his wake. Stoneman's campaign also featured the Battle of Saltville, at which a detachment of his black troops, cut off from the main body of federal forces, were savaged, many killed while attempting to surrender, in what African Americans have called ever after the Massacre at Saltville. Seeing all, and surviving, Victoria Hull recorded her dramatic observations in correspondence and in her own reminiscences.[3]

And so John Samuel and Victoria Hull Apperson made a new family and moved from the antebellum into the postbellum world of Virginia's highlands. Although much changed, the couple brought two things with them from one era to the next: Deep piety and a passion for education. Even these transcending values were not completely immutable, however, and both the

---

[2] Biographical data and the role of Mary Tomlin as matronly advisor are seen in "Reminiscences" and the Diary; also "Apperson," *Men of Mark in Virginia*, vol. 3 (1906), s.v. Information on Hull family and newspaper notice of Knights of Marion, Armstrong, *History of Smyth Co*., 77, 134 All data and anecdotes confirmed in correspondence and conversation with Mary Kent Apperson Elliott of Blacksburg.

[3] Armstrong, 133-34. Armstrong takes some pains to disentangle the melodramatic details of the railroad rescue from the plainer facts.

profession of religion and the concern for an education reflected changes wrought by the War and its million-footed casualties. There was now in the Apperson's piety a quiet intentionality characteristic of the region's Calvinists, a determination and drive whose irresistible force and power could scarcely be guessed by those who saw the exterior calm and heard the almost precious understatements and self-effacements. As for education, the New South wanted the practical, the knowledge and techniques needed in an industrial economy where capital and productivity and return on investment—*risk reward* and *quality quantity* and *innovation* were the new words for the new order—displaced land and slaves and tradition.

Socially there were two striking changes in Smyth County: The freeing of the approximately eight hundred slaves by the thirteenth constitutional amendment; and the enfranchisement by the fifteenth constitutional amendment of those newly freed men and the approximately seventy previously free "men of colour" such as his old Smyth Blue Confederate mates James Cooley and John Ross. In a county where the white men were almost evenly divided between Republican and Democrat, the voting bloc of African American men made a significant addition to a slight majority enjoyed by the Grand Old Party between 1868 and 1901. Indeed, Apperson's old regimental commander ex-Major Albert Galatin Pendleton very self-consciously sought these black voters for his Readjuster reformist party of Republicans and disaffected Democrats who held some power between 1879 and 1890. Pendleton ran for superintendent of schools, and promised James Cooley and other African Americans in the county that he would see that their public schools were funded by the county, albeit separately from the white public schools. Blacks voted overwhelmingly for Pendleton, he was elected, and the superintendent dutifully arranged for public support for the "free school" established on Needmore Street in the west end of Marion by James Cooley on land deeded them by the former Federal general Major George Smith. The Democratic Party had no truck with such biracial cooperation, and Dr. Apperson cast his lot with the professedly "conservative" and "white supremacist" Democratic Party of that day.[4]

---

[4] According to Wilson, approximately three hundred black men were voting in the county in the years 1868 to 1901; and in those same years the Republican Party prevailed by a majority of approximately three hundred votes. Major Alexander Galatin Pendleton is the only specific example cited by Wilson, but his case does seem starkly suggestive of biracial political cooperation for a season in the highlands. Wilson, 282; 261-65.

There are no recorded instances of negrophobic violence in Smyth County in this era, and it is hard to imagine Dr. Apperson—who as a diarist in 1864 objected to "making fun" of black people with the Jim Crow stunts in the auditorium in Orange Court House—participating in any such brutality. Yet in 1901, when Virginians rewrote the state constitution to produce Jim Crow laws that segregated public facilties and virtually disfranchised the black men, the Democrats were strongly in support of the revisions, and the physician was certainly a strong supporter of the Democrats throughout his postbellum political career. Whatever was intended, and whatever simply happened, by the end of Dr. Apperson's days, the black proportion of the county had steadily declined as African Americans left Marion and Chilhowie and the countryside in droves, and their percentage of the population fell to less than 5%, a remarkable drop in an otherwise stable population. Unlike other counties, Smyth did not lose its Republican Party as a result of black disfranchisement, and in fact Dr. Apperson and his fellow Democrats continued to find themselves approximately three hundred votes short of the Grand Old Party in local elections. Of course, in terms of state-level patronage, Dr. Apperson and his fellows enjoyed considerable support as Virginia's piedmont, southside, and tidewater counties became almost exclusively Democrat between 1902 and 1948.[5]

Apperson was pleased to see his old supervisor Dr. Harvey Black working with his people to develop a new state university in his old home village of Blacksburg. This university, proudly styled *polytechnic* in its curriculum, could train engineers and financial managers for the new factories and the new mining operations and the other new business enterprises of the new era. The farmers who still predominated in numbers if not in wealth in the mountain and valley regions were not ignored, but were served now in a new way, for the Virginia Polytechnic Institute in Blacksburg provided scientific training for farmers who must now *engineer* a farm and *manage* the land and *innovate* with their resources, all again new words for new people in a new order of things. Too, the new university looked proudly to the mountains and the valley and the people of the middling class of farmers and the new bourgeoisie of industrialists and entrepreneurs, and set its tone and its style by their lights and not by the faded aristocracy of the old regime

[5] Wilson, op. cit., 106-16; Valdimer Orlando Key, *Southern Politics in State and Nation* (1949. Rev. reprint ed; Knoxville, TN: University of Tennessee Press, 1990).

who still had their state universities in Charlottesville and Williamsburg and their private colleges "back east" or "down there," as it was also put in the highlands.

There remained the task of producing teachers and preachers, and that task was to be served in the region by Emory & Henry College, which too must change in the new era. Dr. Apperson joined the board of trustees supervising the former hilltop college that had produced his onetime correspondents. Since 1836, this place, always Methodist, had served a disproportionate percentage of sons of the planters, and while set among wheatlands and dairy country, had before the War featured a student body drawn from the planter class from the entire South, more so than any other antebellum college in Virginia. Classically trained ministers professed their Latin and Greek and Hebrew texts for boys who would return to run plantations—and secondarily they professed such texts for boys who would serve pulpits in congregations dominated by planters. Now, that tone and style and mission too must change, and the college bent to the task of training preachers from the highlands who would serve pulpits in the valley of the Holston River—and those congregations would be marked as middling farmers and the bourgeoisie of the new industries. The other task to do was to train teachers, a whole new class of schoolmasters who were to serve in public schools that were replacing the old field schools where Apperson himself had studied. The pietistic physician once of the middling class and now of the new bourgeois elite was delighted to raise money to help the college in these new tasks of training new preachers and teachers.[6]

In 1888 Dr. Apperson's personal and professional lives took turns that brought him yet more deeply into the new economy of the New South. Victoria Hull Apperson, his wife of twenty years, passed on, and he cast about to find his way in a new life without her. At the same time, one of Dr. Harvey Black's long-lived dreams became real: The Southwestern Asylum for the Insane was established, and it was one of the first such institutions in the

6 See George J. Stevenson, *Increase in Excellence: a History of Emory &Henry College* (New York: Macmillan, 1964); Board of Trustees minutes and correspondence, *Register* of Students, 1838-1861, Archives of Emory & Henry College; Stevenson talked with me about these things at some length, and I have filed my recollections of his insights in John Herbert Roper Papers, Southern Historical Collection of the Library of the University of North Carolina, Chapel Hill, hereinafter Roper Papers. Much of the interpretation comes from Woodward, op. cit., passim, but much also comes from his talking with me, interviews, Woodward (1978-1986), Roper Papers.

Commonwealth, or anywhere else, that actually sought to treat the insane as sick persons instead of chaining them up and virtually punishing them for "transgressions." Dr. Apperson had earnestly served on the building commitee that raised funds for his old mentor's project, and he had been pleased to see it actually set into place under the supervision of Dr. Black. To his surprise and pleasure, the widower was called on by the supervisor to serve the Southwestern Asylum as second assistant physician, effective the day of its opening. This new assignment took Dr. Apperson off the highlands country roads and gave him a professional status in a progressive institution. He moved to Marion with his ten surviving children and went at the new task with the same determination and high resolution that had defined his wartime stewardship and the first twenty years of his postbellum doctoring and business leadership in Chilhowie.

Suddenly in October of 1888, the patriarch Dr. Black passed on, and there was a new superintendent at the Southwestern Asylum, someone who presumably wanted his own "team" at the institution. There was also a void for the Black family with the sudden death of the dominant figure of male authority. No less abruptly, Dr. Apperson resigned from the asylum in November of 1888 and the following year he married Lizzie Black, the very eligible daughter of his old benefactor and boss. With his own large family now broadened to include his new wife's siblings, Dr. Apperson virtually left the service of Aesculapius while remaining very true to the broader sense of community mission preached and practiced by Dr. Black. The new patriarch helped to start the Bank of Marion, the county's first such institution, for which he served as major stockholder and officer for the remaining eighteen years of his life. With such resources, he put up much of the operating capital for the Staley Creek Manganese and Iron Works, one of the county's first ventures into heavy industry. Serving this firm as major stockholder and secretary treasurer, Dr. Apperson was generally regarded as one of the three entrepreneurs most responsible for building industry in the county. Although most attention in Virginia's postbellum industrialization focused properly on Richmond, he drew enough notice that in 1892 he was elected business executive commissioner to represent the Old Dominion at the World's Exposition in Chicago.

Still active in support of the new Virginia Polytechnic Institute and the revamped and reconfigured Emory & Henry College, Dr. Apperson further diversified his business enterprises in 1894 when he helped to found the Marion and Rye Valley Railroad, among other things a freight hauler for his own iron and manganese concerns. Chairman of the construction efforts, he put forward operating capital and persuaded Marion businessmen and some dairy farmers in the Smyth County countryside to invest in the new railroad. Once the engines actually rolled on the new rails, he became major stockholder and vice president and secretary of the treasury for the Marion and Rye Valley Railroad.

In 1908 Dr. Apperson passed on and thus lived out a little less than the time allotted in his Bible for a man—sixty eight years instead of seventy—but he had lived considerably longer than most people did in this time. When the quintessentially New South business publication, *Men of Mark*, issued its third volume, the editors proferred a biography of Dr. Apperson and noted him as one who had risen from modest antebellum circumstances into business and entrepreneurial leadership in a modern era. And, as Vann Woodward marked it of such New South leaders, the old Confederate in a new century had helped to bring changes in economics and society far more revolutionary than anything ever dreamed of by the old nemeses Abraham Lincoln, George Stoneman, or Ulysses Grant.

INDEX

"A," Mrs., *see* Mary Camden
abatis, 213; def., 213n
Abe, slave of Dr. Harvey Black, is sick and diarist treats, 240
Abingdon (city), 74, 107, 113
Abingdon Virginian, 74
Abolitionists, 6, 7, 8, 11, 13, 17, 35, 40, 49, 88, 248
abscesses, 55, 174
  operation, 186
acapnia, 110
acetate of copper, 71
acromion process, 264
Adams, S.W., operated on, 332
Aeolus, 157
aerophagia, 110
Aesculapius, 7, 16, 145
African American
  troops in CSA, 255, 608
  see also Racism, James Cooley,
  Henry Johnson, 339, 340
  John Ross
Afton Mountain, 227
Ahab, 181
Alabama, 4, 136,
Alburtis family, 101
alcohol, use and abuse, 21, 69, 84, 85, 108, 122, 133, 142, 149, 150, 156, 158, 162, 173, 181, 188, 269-70, 406; drunken soldier shoots at officer, 162; D. Trucks damaged by alcohol, 212; *see* also temperance pledge
Alexandria (city), 127, 129, 132, 133, 141
"Allegheny Ed"
  see Edward Johnson
"Allen, Mrs.," *see* Mary Camden
Allen, Nancy, hosts campsite, Clarke Co., 275-85
Allen, Sue, 74
Allen, Tinsley Lindsley, Lt., 352-3; 357-9; 413
Allison, William, 67
Almond, J.F., Orange Co. friends, 148
Almond, J.W. "Bud", 122, 124, 148
Alpine Depot, 180
Alsop, S., Orange Co. neighbor, 315
Alum Springs, field hospital, Feb 1862, 209
ambulances, 2, 19, 113, 118, 135, 144, 181
American Party, 26, 62n, 77n
American Philosophical Society, 59
Amos, Thomas, 58
amputation, 115; instruments, 304; diarist assists, 326
Anaconda (Lincoln's blockade policy and actions), 126, 137n, 337, 508
Anderson, Richard Heron (Fighting Dick), Gen., 590
Anderson, Robert, Maj., 78, 80
Anderson, Sherwood, 55
Andrews, James Osgood
anesthesia, 109, 130
angina, 54
angor animi, 293
anodyne, 130
Antietam, *see* Sharpsburg; *see* Emancipation Proclamation
antiphlogistic, def., 131n
Apocrypha, reading, 384
Appalachian mountains, 5, *see* highlands
Apperson, Alfred, 1, 2, 4, 155, 173, 261, 314, 315, 328
  attends church with diarist, 151-2
  hunting like Nimrod, 149
  tends diarist on sick furlough, 145
Apperson, Bettie (cousin), 39, 46, 68, 70, 76, 80, 111, 157, 161, 165, 176, 184, 187 188, 205, 220, 261, 265, 277, 285, 290, 314, 316, 328, 340
  342, 346; sends socks, 370; 390
  writes of father's misfortune, 164
Apperson, Charles (brother), soldier, 122, 124
Apperson, Cincinnatus (Nat), soldier, 113, 161, 166, 192, 200, 279, 365
  at Centreville campaign, 163, 183
  on sick furlough, 148

Pickett takes command of unit, 353
Petersburg, 394
Apperson, Eli (brother), suffers erysipelas, 314
Apperson family, sketch, 1-14, and passim
Apperson family, modern, ii, iii
Apperson, James (cousin), 54, 75, 126
Apperson, Jason, 54
Apperson, John Samuel, biographical sketch, 1-14; epilogue, i-xi
Apperson, Joseph (uncle), helps care for diarist, 145
Apperson, Livia (wife of Tom), 39
Apperson, Malinda Jones (mother), introd.
tends diarist on sick furlough, 145
Apperson, Malinda E. (sister), 45, 77
Apperson, Malinda (aunt), 40, 122, 142, 265
Apperson, Malvina (aunt), 73, 80
Apperson, Mary E. (sister), 34, 45, 78, 143, 165, 277, 348
Apperson, Matilda (aunt), 140
Apperson, Nathan (brother), at Williamsburg battle, 234
Apperson, Tom (uncle and benefactor), 39, 145, 146, 154, 163
takes care of diarist and provides sick furlough, 145-46, 152, 153
Apperson, William (uncle), introd., 3, 20, 28, 33, 38, 72, 75, 76
Apperson, William (cousin Bill), soldier, 122
Appomattox Court House (the city), introd., 21, 23
Appomattox Court House, battle, 12
April Fool's Day, 401
Argantes, 30, 31
Aristotle, on magnanimity, 258
Arkansas regt, 183
Arkansas (state), 179
Armada, Spanish (allegory), 126
Armida, 30
Armstrong, Joan Tracy, v and cited passim
Army of Northern Virginia, introd., 1, 15, and passim
Army of the Potomac, rumored moving toward Valley, 1862, 210
and passim
Arnold, Richard, Capt., 116n
aromatic spirits of ammonia, 68
aromatic sulfuric acid, 146 and 146n
Ashby, Turner, Gen., 179n; at Bunker Hill, 213, 215, 219; at Massanutton, 242n
Ashby's Gap, 284
Asheville Female Institute, 388
aspirin, 174n
Assyrians, Biblical analogy, 167
asthma, 128n
Auden, Wystan Hugh, quoted, 14
Augusta Co., 109n, 178n
Augusta, GA, 136n
Augusta Springs,
see Stribling Strings
Augustinian, introd.
Aury, Stuffle, 76, 77
auscultation, 278, 283

Ba'al, allusion, 127, 181n
Babel, allusion, 148n
Baber, David, iv, vii
Babylon, allusion, 154
bacterial pneumonia, misidentified, 131, 131n, 132
Bailey, patient, 98
Baker (civilian Dr.), 62
Baldwin, Robert Frederick, Dr. and surgeon, runs field hospital, Twin Springs, 1864, 582
Ballard, Maj., Commissary, 259
Baltimore American, newspaper"rampant" over McCausland's raid
Baltimore and Ohio R.R., 177n; rebuilding after CSA destruction, 209; indemnification by Federal government for war damages, 267
bandages, of era, 133
Bane, Eugene, ii
banjo,
as African American instrument, 156
Bank of Marion, 26n and epilogue

Banks, Nathaniel Prentiss, Gen., 179, 180n, 211n
Baptists, introd., 1, 5, 35, 56, 57n, 60, 64, 5, 84148, 375-7; 402, 425, 496, 529-31
  discussion of immersion, 151
Barbran (visiting French Dr.), 46, 47, 56, 57, 58, 59, 60, 66, 75, 84
Barger George Washington, 297
Barr, (minister and editor), 74
Barron, Samuel, CSA navy, 137n
Bartens, 79
Barton, hosts camp, Frederick Co., 1862, 217
Barton (anti-secession candidate), 36
Barton, Clara, introd., 13
Bates, patient, 96, 97
Bath campaign, 179n
Bath Co., 179
Bath (town), 177n, 178, 179, 180n, 181
  rumors of Federal reoccupation, 1862, 183
Bayley, John, 371
Baylor, Elizabeth (Lizzie), 585
Bean, George, Dr., 108; "flank" for dinner, 219
Bean, William Gleason, ii, iii
Bear, David W., officer and Dr., 123-4, 133, 138
  sick, 134
  introduces family, 141
Beattie family, Chilhowie, 135-6n
  and militia muster, 135
Beattie, C.B., Capt., 122
Beattie, Clairborne Watkins, officer and Dr., 122, 135, 160, 165; dies (?), 372n; books sold after death to Mrs. Faris, 412
Beattie, Dr. (Grayson Co.), 69, 70
Beattie, Robert, 135n
Beauregard, Pierre Gustave Toutant, Gen., 108, 112n, 113, 136n, 154n
Beck, Capt., GA, dates Mollie Graves, 352, 353, 354
Bedford Co., 154n
Beech Creek, battle
  see Somerset, battle
Bell, William Anderson, ambulance driver, 261
Benevolence and Education, reading, 370
Benjamin, Judah P., CSA Sec. of War;
  authorizes new arty. co. ,201
  petitioned by diarist, 210
Bennington, John, patient, 98
Benson, Francis, Master Sgt., 343; contracts variola, 345
benzene, 146
Berkeley Co., WV, 100 and 10ln
Berkeley Springs, WV, 179, 180
Berry's Ferry, WV, 112
Berry's Ford, engagement, 573
Berryville, 305-6
Beverly, WV, 132n
Bible, KJV, introd., 5, 6, 51n, 52, 56n, 62, 74n, 75, 76, 77n, 79, 82n, 119n, 122, 123n, 138n, 151n, 152, 180, 181n, 203, 259, 261, 273, 283-4
  resolution to read daily, 146
bichloride of mercury, 297
Big Spring (village)
Bishop, patient, 77, 97
Bishop, A.R., Sgt., loses election as Smyth Blues officer, 209
Bishop, John J., Lt., wounded at 2d Manassas and dies, 252; 253n; 259; late notice of death, 317
Black, Elizabeth (Lizzie), introd. and epilogue, 14
Black, Harvey, Dr., introd. and epilogue, 1, 10 -12, 14, 19-21, 89, 108, 110, 111, 112, 115, 117, 129, 132, 135, 139, 144, 162, 201-2, 204
  255, 263, 265, 266, 268, 279-80, 280, 283, 284, 286, 295, 297, 299
  302, 304, 310, 311, 313, 319, 328, 330, 333, 346, 355, 360, 364, 582
  diagnosing, 131, 132
  discusses infant baptism, 402
  dubious about CSA, 89
  duty, 249
  "Black Hospital," 144
  mentor and benefactor, 90; 210, 211; 218, 248, 268-9, 278, 342
  messes by himself, 270
  organizing efficiently, 200-06; restores order on return, 206
  performing surgery, 109, 139, 144;

amputation with diarist assisting, 232; becomes chief surgeon of Div., 252
returns from long leave, 382
scolds diarist for criticizing surgeon reports, 286
takes charge of general hospitals, Winchester
treats horse's hoof, 301
tries to discipline Mary Camden, 412
persuades diarist to surrender, 20 April 1865, Blacksburg, 617
and passim
Black Hospital, *see* Harvey Black
Blacksburg, introd. and epilogue, 89, 179n
black bean (unwelcome detail), 474
Black Flag, symbol for vicious fight, 253
bleeding, technique, *see* venesection
blister treatment, *see* vesication
blockade and blockade-resistance, *see* also Anaconda
bloodletting, treatment, *see* venesection
Bloomery Gap, WV, 183n
Bloomery, WV (town), 183-4
blue mass pill, *see* mercury
Blue, civilian, Hanging Rock Pass, WV; house burned by Federals, 189
Blue Ridge, introd., 16, 18, 89, 112, 113n, 155, 220, 225, 267, and passim
boils, 109
bonesetting, 21n
Bonaparte family,
Jerome (misidentified?), 125
Joseph Charles Paul (Plon-Plon), 125n
and visit to CSA camp, 125, 125-6n
Bonaparte, Louis (Emperor Napoleon III), 59, 125, 125n, 126, 132, 133, 172n; rumors of help after speech, 197-9; rumors of help, 253
Bonaparte, Napoleon, allusion, 108
Bonham, Milledge Luke, Gen., 136, 136-7n, 154
Bonham, Robert S., 82
Bordan, Charles M., 4th VA Inf., sick and dies, 399
Bordwine, Willie, iv
Boring, John (minister), 51, 79
Boteler, G.W., court martial, cleared, 362; visits, 401
Bowman, civilian, hosts in Edinburg, 219
Boyd, (elderly man, Smyth Co.), 78
Boyd, Belle, possibly in camp, 103
Bragg, Braxton, Gen., 251, 258, 266, 337, 341
Brahmin, allusion, 127
Brazil, 132n
Bridgewater (town), 238-39
Brock, Archibald and Sarah, Rockingham hosts, 239
bronchial diseases, 302, 303n
and passim
Brooks, William, patient, 109
dies, 111
Brown, Miss (civilian), Massanutton, 240
Brown, Bedford, Dr., character reference for Mary Camden, 380
Brown, Ellen Apperson, ii
Brown, Isaac, 289
Brown, John, 132n
Brown's Gap, 224-5
Brown's Mountain, 594
Brunot (visiting French Dr.), 35, 57, 65, 75
Brutus, 24, 49n
Buchanan, James, 170 and 171n
Buck, (civilian), 178
Buckles Town, WV, (Darkesville), 100
Buckner, Simon Bolivar, Gen., takes blame for Ft. Donelson, 206n
Buell, Don Carlos, Gen., 258, 259, 266, 270
Buffalo Gap, 228
Bull Pasture Mountain, *see* McDowell, Batle
Bull Run (battle), *see* First Manassas,
Bulwer, Edward, Baron Lytton, novelist, 396
Bunker Hill, WV, 249, 258n
camp, 259-65; camp, 268-77
skirmish, 213
battle, 1864, 577-8; casualties not accurately reported in OR, 578n
Burks, Jesse S., officer, 224

Burnside, Ambrose Everett, Gen., leads amphibious landing, Roanoke Island, NC, 198, 199n; 292, 301, 326, 327, 331, 332
Burton, Dr., 260
Butler, Benjamin Franklin, Gen., 137n; New Orleans "suffers," 250
Byron, George Gordon, Lord, *Don Juan*, 260 and 261n, 261-62

CC, Miss, 46
CSA (the government), introd., 9, 11, 12, 41n, 89, 100n, 113, 116, 117, 124, 125n, 131n, 135, 136n, 137, 142, 153, 167, 173n, 182
    bounty for reenlistment, 166
    Montgomery government, 41n, 43, 48, 82, 86
    treatment of soldiers, 137
Cabell, J.L., Dr., criticizes record reports, field hospitals, 410
Cablestown (village), 280
Caesar, Julius, 26, 157
    compared to Lincoln, 49
Caldwell, Jane, vii
Calhoun, John Caldwell,
calomel, 301
Calvinists, Calvinism, *see* Presbyterian
Camden, Mary , 340, 352, 353, 354, 355-9, 364-5, 368, 371, 373, 374 377, 378, 380; plans to *see* on his leave, March 1863, 382; 385, 388; leave denied, does not *see*, 390; 396; sends magnolia blossoms, 398; writes her short, cold note, 399; writes diarist and Bev Jones, 407; visits Caroline Co. field hospital again, April 1863, 412-15; writes letters to her, 571, 585, 589
    also called Mollie and Mrs. Allen and Mrs. A and MJC
Camp Carter, *see* Emily Carter
Camp Crenshaw, 307
Camp Harman, 137-42
Camp Maggot (First Manassas camp), 117
camp meetings, 16, 78
Camp Preston, 196-218
Camp Stephenson, 164-68, 173, 175, 333
    diptheria outbreak, 165
    parotitis outbreak, 165
Campbell, Gen., Cedar Creek Bridge, 243
Capon Depot Road, 183
Capon Mountain, 183n
Capon River, 183n
caput, 334n
Carlisle, John, unionist politician, Augusta Co., 178, 179n
castor oil, prescribed, 98
Caroline Co.,
    field hospital,
Carpenter, Joseph Hannah, officer, 263 and 264n
Carrington, William A., Dr., director of field hospitals, 321, 322n
Carter, Emily, hosts camp, Clarke Co., 296-305
castor oil, 23, 73, 74n, 110
catarrh, 53, 54, 128
cathartic, 73n, 110n, 113, 120, 136
    prescription, 115
Catherine, Princess of Wurtemberg, 125
Catlett family, Caroline Co., 365, 368, 372, 411, and passim
Catlett, Harriet, 365, 368, 372
Catlett, Sue, 411
Catlett, Thomas, the Rev., 368
caustic potash, 296
Cedar Creek Bridge, battle saves bridge, 243
Cedarville, battle, 589
Cemetary Hill, introd.
Cedar Mountain, 250
Cedar Run, battle, 258
Cemetary Ridge, introd., 171, 172n
Centreville, camp, 122-37; 137n, 163, 165, 173, 183
Chadduck, Catherine, hosts supper, Massanutton, 240; 241n
Chamberlain, Dr., ambulance duty, 323, 324, 329; passes course at Medical College of Virginia and returns to military duty, 381
    accepted as military surgeon, 403
Chancellorsville, battle, introd., 13

Chancelly, M., minister; visits Locust Grove, 148
  see Baptist
Chapel Road, 243
Chaplin Hill, KY, battle, 267
charity, churches, 535
Charleston, SC, 84
  rumors, 167
Charles Town, WV (panhandle), 112, 263
Charles Town, WV (capital)
Charlottesville, epilogue, 144
  general hospital
Chase, Salmon Portland, sec. of treasury, 332 and 333n
Chatham Hill, 160, 161n
Cheat Mountain, battle, 143
Chesapeake and Ohio Canal Co., 177
Chesterfield Co., 147
Chilhowie, introd. and epilogue, 4, 20, 22n, 25n, 18, 135n
Chilton, Robert Hall, inspector general, 279-80
chloroform, 109, 130n
  liniment, 130n
cholera, def., 134n
Chopart's amputation, 326
Christians, introd.,
  see also by Protestant sects and sermons
Christian Baptism, reading, 402
Christmas observations, 1862, 332-4
Civil War Day by Day; Almanac, vii and cited passim
Civil War Revival, 1864
  purchases of Bibles, 588-9
  see Beverly T. Lacy, John Johns, and Rev. E. Converse
Clarke Co., physical beauty noted, 275
Clayman, Jason, iv
Clemens, Sherrard, 41n,42, 45n, 58
Clyrie, the Rev., Lutheran minister, Woodstock, preaches 1864, 574
cocaine, as prescription, 115n
  and passim
Cole, Mrs., 29
Coleman, R.T., Dr., dreaded by diarist, 268; 287; 293, 294
  proffers theory about variola, 298; 353
colic, 40
  def., 131n
  cramp, 131, 133, 163; diarist treats soldier, 236
Collins, civilian, provides campsite, 177
Collins, Arthur E., army pharmacist, 343
Collins, C.E., hospital steward and clerk, 396
Collins, Van Buren, army pharmacist, 329, 365
Colston, R.T., Capt., 168-9
Columbus, KY
confinement, *see* pregnancy
Connecticut Peace Democrats,
Conner's Creek, 69
conscription, 166, 253469
  changes in law, 1862, 200; new law, May 1862, 222
  draft riots, 495
  exemptions and substitutes, 497
  inspection of draftees, 271-2
Constitution, US, 58n, 77
Continental Hotel, 16, 27, 139n
controlled experiments, (as diarist understood) 297
Converse, E., the Rev., sells Bibles, Civil War Revival, 588
convulsions, 110
Cooley, James, introd., 11, 255, 256n, 262, 269; returns to cook after discharge, 270; earns fees, 289; 290; 320, 330, 341, 344; is ill, and diarist expresses worry, 347; is well and borrows money, 365; becomes angry with, 367; returns, 368; 377; in trouble with Dr. Black, 379
Copenhaver, D. (customer/client), 55
Copenhaver, George, declines to host, Shenandoah Co., 308
Cornet, Troy C., officer, Dare Devils, wounded, 264; 265
corrosive sublimate, 301
coryza, 287
costal cartilege, 163n

court house events, 67
  court day, 84, 85
court martial (the place), 524
court martial (judgments), 256, 362
court martial (camp joke), 374
Courtz, civilian, hosts, Page Co., 312
Craige Co., 132
cramp colic, *see* colic
cramps, 110, 133n
Crayon, Porte
  see David Hunter Strother
Creek Native Americans, i
Creole, 112 and 112n
Crenshaw's Batt., 6th VA Cav., 31 and 32n
Crittenden Resolutions, 45n, 58
Crittenden, George Bibb, Gen., 191 and 192n
Crittenden, John J., Sen. and Gen., 57, 58, and 58n
Crockett, Joseph S., Dr., 91, 93, 94, 95, 97, 139, 204, 236, 241
  criticized for inefficiency and poor record-keeping, 158, 193, 200-06
  Crockett's Battalion X (the sick), 200-06; 226-7
  leaves sick and goes with diarist to front, Kernstown battle, 244-5
  supports diarist's prescriptions, 198
Crockett, Samuel, Dr., urges diarist to surrender, 614
Cross, William G., Methodist on baptism, 402
Crossman, Capt., 102
Crowell, D., patient, 94
Crump, Mrs., MS lady disfigured by variola, 392
Crusades, introd., allusions, 23n, 29, 30, 89
Crusoe, Robinson, allusion, 302
Culpeper Co., 39, 124, 153n
  field hospital, "Barracks Hospital," 144
  Lee's army hospital, 303
Cunningham, H.H., vi and cited passim
Cupid, allusion
"cupping," 109
Curtis, George J., 39n
Cush, allusion, 148n
Custer, George Armstrong, Gen., 594; defeats Early in Waynesboro, destroys Stonewall Bde., 606

D Company, *see* Smyth Blues, 1st VA Bde. 4th VA Inf.
Dabney, civilian visitor, identity unclear, 413
Dalton, Reese (Grayson Co. customer), 69
Daniel, Claudine, vii
Danville (city)
  seminary, 237n
Darden, GA soldier looks for relatives, 346
Darke, William, Gen., 100n
Darkesville, WV, 100, 101n,
Dave, Dr. F's slave, 63
Davis, J.W., Dr., runs field hospital, Mt. Jackson, 1864, 582
Davis, Jefferson Finis, 108, 113n, 125n, 126, 140n, 143, 395
  diarist guesses coastal defense strategy, 210
  enjoins penalties on liqour-makers, 212
  "harangued the people" after Bread Riot, 401
  inaugural, 22 Feb 1862, 207 and 208n
  tours "West" theatre and gives speech, January 1863, 344
Davis, John Bunnell, introd., 4, 42, 53n
  see also *Davis's*
Davis's, 4, 42, 53
Davis, Mrs., civilian,
Dawsey, James, vi
debate contests, camp, 1863, 349
Defoe, Daniel, 302
dehydration, 134n
Delaware Co., O., 132n
Democrats, introd. and epilogue; 26n, 132n, 179n, 266; northern gains, 1862, 267, 291
Department of WV, military, 178n
diarrhea, 123, 134n
Dick, Thomas, 370
Dickens, Charles, diarist reads and wants to buy complete works, 348

Dioscorides, *see Materia Medica*
Di Pietro, Bart, vii
diptheria, 21, 24, 36, 53n, 59, 65, 66, 68, 165
Diver, civilian, hosts, Page Co., 312
Dix, John Adams, US officer, 170
Dix, civilian, robbed by Frederal troops, 178
"Dixie," *see* popular songs
Doan's powders, 68
doctrine of restitution, 74, *see* sermons
Doles, George Pierce, Gen., 591
Doll, Margaret (Maggie), Hollingsworth Mills host, 580-81, 585
Dosh, William, the Rev., Lutheran minister preaches, 591
draft, *see* conscription
Drane, Dr., surgeon, 585
Dranesville, engagement, 172; 173n
dropsy, *see* edyma
Drummondtown, 132
dueling, introd.
Duff, F. (escort), 74
Dunbar, Joy, vii
Duncan, Blanton, officer, 103
Dungan, James V., 36, 55
Dungan, James W., 392
Dungan, John R., brother of Robert Henry visits, 388
Dungan, Robert Henry, student and officer, introd., 11, 25, 27, 36n, 55, 56, 57, 75, 137, 173, 177, 206, 230; wounded, 258, 261; 284, 338 382, 388
Dungan, Thomas, 79
Dungan, William, 81

Eads, James M., 307, 400
Earhart, Henry (Harry), Capt., paymaster, 287, 293, 338, 347, 379, 610
and passim
Early, Jubal Anderson, Gen., rumor of death, 234; identified, 235n; 306; 335, 352-3; 590; valley campaign, 554-604; loses battle of Waynesboro and loses Stonewall Bde, 606n
Easter, regional observances, 75
Echols, John, Gen., continues toward KY to fight after Lee's surrender, 613
Echol's Bde., 162n
economic downturn of 1857, 3
Edmondson, William, Capt., 162
edyma, 517
egg whites, prescribed, 71
Eichelerger, Charles F., hosts, Winchester, 591
Eleventh VA Inf., 335
Elijah, allusion, 52, 181n
Elliott, Greer, ii, iii
Elliott, Mary Kent Apperson, ii, iii
Ellsberg, Dr., army surgeon, 591 and passim
Elmwood farm, introd., 3
emetics, 131, def., 131n
Emancipation Proclamation, 248, 253
Emory & Henry College, introd. and epilogue, 5, 11, 17, 25, 27, 36n, 56, 57, 66, 89
as general hospital, 89
emphysema, 128n
England, *see* Great Britain
Enoch, and salvation, 52, *see* sermons
Enteric Fever, 128n
epigastriium, 32, 32n, 130n, 131, 133
epiplastic, def., 131-2n
Episcopalians, 118-9, 123, 127, 138, 140-41, 408, 496, 506, 508-9; 520-21, 528-30
pietists, 118-9, 123, 127, 138140-41, 533-34; 536-37; 587-8
see also John Johns, Gaines Miller, William Nelson Pendleton, St. Thomas', Orange, VA
Erichsen, John Eric, surgery textbook, 304 and 305n
Erminia, 30, 31n
Ernells, John, father of wounded soldier, 158
eruption, 109
erysipelas, 164, 174n, 314
erythemia (confounded with erythema), 405
ether, 131n
Euterpe, allusion to his lack of talent in music, 399

Evangelical Protestantism, introd. and epilogue; *see* pietism; *see* denominational sects
Evans, Randal, Winchester, hosts supper, 204
Evansport Batt., 164
Ewell, Richard Stoddert, Gen., joins Stonewall Bde on march, 238; identified, 239n; Cedar Creek Bridge, 243; Kernstown battle, 244-5; 271; 306, 307n
examining committee, diarist testifies, 322
excision, 264, 326
external ear, *see* helix

Fairfax Co., 122, 172n, 183
Fairfax Court House (town), 129, 133, 134, 136, 141, 144
Fairfax Station, 144
Faris, P., Mrs., Triford friend possibly related to Smyth Co. Farises, 142
Faris, William (antislavery Unionist), introd., 8, 36, 37, 38, 42, 47, 48, 50, 51, 57, 88
  Jonathan (son), 54
  Thomas (son), 54
  (unnamed son of antislavery Unionist), 36

Faris, William (Dr.), ii-xi, 4, 9, 16, 18, 19, 22, 23, 26, 27, 28, 30, 32, 33, 35, 42, 47, 49, 50, 51, 52, 53, 54, 55, 57, 63, 64, 65, 66, 69, 70, 71, 72, 73, 77, 78, 79, 81, 82, 84, 85, 120, 131, 134, 140, 146, 147, 156, 162, 164, 166, 170, 173, 182, 186, 191, 197, 205, 214, 217, 248, 261, 266, 328, 345, 368
  dubious about CSA, 88
  encourages diarist to remain in CSA army, 1862, 208
  informed by diarist of reenlistment, 209
  urges diarist to surrender, 18 April 1865, 616
  and passim
  Mrs. Faris, 35, 40, 68, 71, 77, 80, 84, 88, 111, 120, 129, 135, 141, 146, 157, 166, 167, 182, 183, 196; is very sick, 208; 256, 334 336, 337, 360
  Howard (son), 360
  Kate (daugher), 35
  Laura (daughter), 80, 81, 255, 256; starts attending Asheville Female Institute, 388; at school, 412
  Luther (son), 72
  William (son), 57
Farmville, 113n
Farrow, A.S., shows yard, Albemarle Co., 227
Faulkner, Charles James, Confederate sympathizer, Martinsburg, 266
Fauntleroy, A.M., Dr., director of general hospital, Staunton, 596
Fauquier Co., 112, 156, 179n
Faust, Patricia L., vii, and cited passim
Feldburg, civilian visitor, identity unclear, 414
"female diseases," 71
"female education," 161
femoral artery, 260, 263
fever, 129, 131n, 133, 143
field hospital, 1, 90
  contrasted with general hospital, 89, 306
field school, 2
Fifth VA Inf., at Newton Stephensburg, 243; at Kernstown, 244-5
Fifty-Eighth VA Inf., McDowell battle, 230; in Valley, 357
Fifty-Second VA Inf., McDowell battle, 230
Fillmore, Millard, 60n, 75n, *see* American Party
Findley, David, Smyth Blue wounded, McDowell, 232; Dr. Black performs amputation of thigh, 232
First Manassas, introd., 10, 15, 21, 88, 89, 90, 100n, 113, 114, 117, 134n, 152n, 250
  camp conditions, 117
First MD Inf., Federal and First MD Inf., CSA, fight, Page Co., 241

First Virginia Bde., 9, 10, 11, 88, 90
steal from civilian meat house in Valley, 182
Fishing Creek, battle, *see* Somerset, battle
fistula, 332
Fitzhugh, George, introd., 8
Fleming, Malcolm, Dr., surgeon, 272, 287
Fletcher, civilian, hosts camp, Monterey, 231
Floyd, John Buchanan, secessionist politician, 16, 26, 28, 84
as Gen., 162; severely wounded, 201; ineffective at Ft. Donelson, 206; diarist criticizes, 319
foot baths, *see* pediluvia
Foote, William Henry minister, Fairfax Co., preaches, 186
Ford, Sally Rochester, novel, 375
Foreman, William N., hospital orderly, 343; contracts variola, 345
Fort Alabama (Frederick Co.), 207; large guns, 214
Fort Clark, 137n
Fort Donelson, TN, lost, 197n, 198; diarist learns of disaster, 201; new rumors of victory, 204; finally learns true story of defeat, 205-7
Fort Hatteras, NC port lost, 137
Fort Henry, TN, lost, 197-8
Fort Macon, NC, lost, 198n
Fort Pickens, SC, 80
Fort Sumter, SC, introd., 9, 80, 83, 84, 88
Fort Steadman, battle, 608, 609
Foster, Gaines, vi
Forty-Fourth GA Inf., 352
Forty-Fourth VA Inf., McDowell battle, 230; Fredericksburg, 341
Forty-Eighth VA Inf., 33n, 133n, 179, 230
Forty-Seventh VA Inf., 409
Fourth Virginia Inf., (diarist's original unit) 10, 11, 102n, 112n, 113, 124n, 139n, 164n, 169, 178, 180, 181
surrender, Appomattox Court House, 612 (steward no longer
assigned there, continues in service and on run)
and passim
France, *see* Bonaparte family
Francisco, Robert Lafayette, QM, visits, 219; Stribling Springs visit, 237; 277, 286, 290, 392, 400; pays visit, 404, 411
Frayer's Farm, battle
see White Oak Swamp, battle
Frazer, Robert, Orange Co. friend, wounded, 325
Frederick Co., 156n, 165, 177
Fredericksburg, battle, introd., 13; shelled, 309
free agency, 385, 386
"freemen of color," introd., 10, 17
Fremont, John Charles, Gen., identified, 231n; reinforces Banks, 231-2
French, Samuel Gibbes, Gen., 169
Friend, the Rev., civilian minister, Caroline Co., preaches, 411-12
Front Royal, battlefield, 286
Fudge, Granville Henderson, visits camp, 164
Fugitive slave law, 58
Fulton, John Hall, officer, 321, 322n
Fulton, W.G., officer, 127-8, 321, 322n
Fulwider, Robert C., 289
Funsten, David, Col., 335
furlough denied diarist after Dr. Black enjoyed lengthy furlough, 380
furlough examination board, 263

Gaines Mill, battle, 91, 139n
Gallaher, Charles H., plays violin in parlor, 400
Gannaway, Robinson (Robertson), Lutheran minister, 78
Gardner, Robert Davidson, officer, 4th VA Inf., 321, 322n; wounded, 326
Garibaldi, Giusseppe, analogy to CSA,
Garland, Miss (school teacher), 78; prejudice against female education
Garnett, Richard Brooke, Gen., 192
comment on fighting without orders, 171
is sick on Valley Campaign, 1862, 188
Garnett, Robert Selden, Gen., 171n
general hospital
contrasted with field hospital, 306, 89
Genovese, Eugene Dominick, vi
Georgia (destination), introd., 3

German-American Federal troops, 101
Germans Bridge, 152
germs and disease, not understood, 89, 90
Gettysburg (battle), introd., 12, 13, 23, 135n, 136n, 171n; 482-87
retreat with ambulance train under siege, 486-7, *see*
Imboden
Gettysburg (town), 482
Gibbons, Col., killed at McDowell battle, 230
Gibson, Andrew E., officer, Smyth Co. Blues, granted furlough, 183; accompanies diarist to church, 202; unanimous election, Capt., 208 accompanies diarst for snack, 217; "flank" for dinner, 219; killed at 2d Manassas, 252; 259
Gibson, John Nelson, commissary, 6th VA Cav., 581
Gibson, J. St. P., Dr., commands ambulance train, 307
Gibson, Moses, clerk, 14th LA Inf., 287
Gibson, Moses, clerk, 4th VA Inf., 383
Giddings, E., medical purveyor, 338, 343
Gideon's Band, introd., 7
Gilkeson, J.B., Dr., 338
Gillespie, Dr., civilian, Page Co., 312
Glade Spring, introd., 4, 25, 26n, 27
Glaize, John, Capt., QM, valley campaign, 1863, 360, 372
glucose, admnistered, 109n
Goddess of Liberty, analogy, 122
Goins, William H., quarantined, 302
Goldsborough, Louis Malesherbes, USN officer, takes Roanoke Island, NC, New Bern, and Beaufort, 198, 199n
Gollohon, E. (Smyth Co. host and dry goods storeowner), 62, 67
Gollohon, James S., 75
Gollohon, John M., 75
Gollohon, Robert M., 75
gonorrhea, 64, 65, 72
Goode family, 152
Goodwin, Dr., 60
Goolsby, Robert, 30
Gordon, John B., Gen., 572
Gordonsville, 240; general hospital, 313
Gouchon, A.J., 48
gout, 128n
Grace Truman, reading religious novel
Graham, A.J., 38
Graham, Joseph Draper, Dr., 338, 340
Grandin, J. Marsdin, the Rev., chaplain preaches, July 1864, 572
Grant, US Ulyssess Simpson, introd., 20, 116n, 179n
Graves, Mollie, 341, 342, 351, 352, 354, 355, 372, 377
Graves' Road, 312
Grayson County country doctor, 69, 70, 71
Grayson County Daredevils, introd., 9, 10, 15, 16, 115n, 116, 132, 194; 301
feed diarist at McDowell battle, 233
See also First VA Bde.; Capt. Peyton N. Hale
suffer variola outbreak, 297
Great Britain, 126n, 132, 133n, 172, 176
policy on sea trade, 172n
rumors of helping CSA, 172, 199, 253
Great Cacapon Bridge, 180n
Greany, Patty, vii
Greeley, Horace, 37
Green, Charles Jones, Capt., 409
Green, James Williams, Maj. and commissary, drinking, 269
Greenhow, Dr. (textbook on diptheria), 65, 68
Greenwood Depot, 227
Gretz, Peter, iv
Griffin, J.H., inrod.; 6, 9, 10, 23, 23n
see also Torquato Tasso; *Jerusalem Delivered*
Griffith, William A., borrows money, 388
Grigsby, Andrew Jackson, Col., 243; *see* 27th VA Inf.; 256, 257n, 258n, 259, 265, 293; resigns commission, 296
Gross (author of surgery text), 163
Guild, LaFayette, Dr., surgeon general, 303; casualty report, Fredericksburg, 325-6n; orders move, 348; receives diarist's report,
381; scolds all for careless selection of patients for general
hospital, 419

Guinea's Depot (Guiney's), camp and field hospital, 315-24; receives wounded, Fredericksburg, 329
Gully Keeper, game, 2
Gweltillo, Joseph, Dr., 92

Hackler, Stephen, possibly stole horse, 239
Hagy, Dr., brings supplies, 323-4; messes with diarist, 330; 336; 342; unwell, 348; helps diarist study, 360-1, 366; passes surgeon's examination, February 1863, 365; 371; 407
Haiti, 318, 336
Hale, Gideon, wagonmaster, 227; 398
Hale, Peyton, Capt., Grayson Daredevils, 233n
Hall, H., Capt., 116
Hall, John N., 214, 215n; disciplined by Col. Ronald, 214
Hamburg, 240
Hamilton, Alexander M., Capt., accompanies diarist into McDowell battlefield, 230
Hamlet, allusion, 173
Hampshire Co., WV
Hams, Allen (Grayson Co. customer), 69
Hancock, MD, 180
Hanging Rock Pass, WV, 175; haven for CSA sympathizers and "malitia," 188
Hardy, Maj., QM for valley campaign, 581
Harman, John Alexander, Maj. and QM, 137n
Harper's Ferry, WV, 113n, 132, 166; surrender, 250
Harris, Isham, Gov., 208
Harris, James, examined by committee, 322
Harrison family, 101n
Harrisonburg, 236
Hart, Patrick S., 335
Hartford, CT, Peace Democrats,
Hatteras Island, NC, 137n, 141
Hawk's Bill, scenery, 312
Hawks, Wells Joseph, Maj., commissary, 342, 378
Hawkins, James D., 160, 167, 169, 176
Hawkins, Timothy, surgeon's assistant, 157
Haynesville, WV, 168
Hay, Dr., dinner, 219
Haynesville, skirmish, 1861, 168
Haynesville, MD, camp, 1864, 582
headaches, 123, 135, 139, 142, 143n, 150
Heankins, Pulaski Guards, 144
Heck, J.M., Col., 116n
helix, 73, 73n
Heim, W.H., Gen., 101
hemolysis, 109
Heniger, P.J., 82
Henrico Co.,
Henry, Patrick, introd., 8
hepatitis, misdiagnosed, 334
heroin, prescribed, 130, 130n
Hezekiah, Bible lesson, 203
Hicock, Samuel, possibly stole horse, 239n
Highland Co., 228
highlands, ii-xi, 14, 16, 55
  and wartime fervor, 89
  and pasim
Hill, A.P., Gen., 252, 275, 305-6, 315, 325-6; casualties, 335
Hill, Daniel Harvey, Gen., 271 and 272n, 273, 275, 280, 288; NC casualties, 335
Hinkle, C.C., Sgt., 271-2, 290
Hippocrates, introd., 5; 131n
Historical Times Illustrated, vii and cited passim
Hoffman's anodyne, def., 131-2n
Hogshead, George, hosts diarist and Dr. Crockett, 236
Holiday, civilian, hosts campsite, Caroline Co., 316
Holston River, 16
  Middle Fork, church, 56
  North Fork, 160n
  South Fork, 69, 79
Holt, John, 3
Holt, William A., Dr., briefly replaces Dr. Black, 1862, 316, 317n; 319, 321, 322n, 333
Home Circle, 76
Hood, John Bell, Gen., 387
  Hood's Texas Bde., 387n
Hoodville, introd., 3

Hooker, Joseph, Gen., 383
Hopkins, Abner Crump, chaplain, 2d VA Inf., 280
Horn, J.D., 29th VA Inf., messenger for Mary Camden, 412
horse, halter stolen, 275
horse hoof disease, 292, 298-302; 305-6; 313
Hotel Marion, *see* Continental Hotel
Houston, Dr., refuses diarist furlough, 144
Houston, Samuel, possibly stole horse, 239n
Howard, H.E., vi and cited passim
Howard, Norman DeV., Lt., 349, debates diarist, contest
Howard, Thomas R., Dr., surgeon, 369
Howe, Samuel, possibly stole horse, 239n
Howison, Robert Reid, historian of War, 364
Hull, John N., Smyth Blues, 294
Hummel, Ray O., Jr., vi and cited passim
Humphrey's Mill, Smyth Co., 55
Hunter, Edmund Pendleton, Confederate sympathizer, Martinsburg, 266
Hunter, John A., Dr., Medical Director, 256, 257n
hunting, 148
  rabbits, 148
  raccoons, 149
  see Nimrod
Hutchins, Thelma, ii-vii
Hutchinson, George H., sells horse, 262
Hymon, Samuel, possibly stole horse, 239n
hyperventilation, 110n
hysteria, *see* hyperventilation
Ichabod, allusion, introd., 10
identification of corpses, 410, 454
illiteracy, correllated with unionist support, 178
Illustrated News magazine, 360
Imboden, John Daniel, Gen., 184n; defends diairst and ambulance train on long retreat from Gettysburg, 485-7
inflammation of the brain, 59n, 65, 109
inflation, and money and supply
  317; 329, 492, 512n; 542 and ff.
  runaway for CSA, 512n; 606-08
  stabilized and moderated for US, 606-08, 617
International Red Cross, introd., 13, 20
intestinal colic, *see* colic
inventory of medicines, 120
Ireland, 141n
Irishmen in War, 169, 170
Israel, allusion, 181
Italy, analogy to independence struggle, 3352
Ithuriel, allusion, 300-01

Jackson, Andrew
Jacksonian Democrats, 170,
Jackson, Thomas Jonathan, introd., 9, 10, 11, 12, 88, 90, 91, 100n, 104
  137n, 143n, 162, 170, 171n, 177n, 179n, 180n, 181, 215; into MD, 251, 263, 264, 286, 287, 288, 325, 333
  "applauded most enthusiastically," 213
  at table in Winchester farmhouse, 190
  casualties at Fredericksburg, 335
  Cedar Creek Bridge, 243
  compared to Jehu, and criticized, 181
  criticized for 1862 Valley march, 183
  daring charge through defile, 231
  diarist learns of his death, 439
  honored with ceremonial sword, 162
  "hurry up, I am pressed," 229
  Kernstown campaign, 244-5
  marches to Fredericksburg, 323
  "mud march," 223-42
  rumors of resignation, 193-6
  strategy at Williamsport, MD, 170;
  strategy in Valley, 216-7; 224
  thought to be "partial" to 1st VA Bde and 4th VA Inf., 189
  takes over 2d Corps, 252
James, Ezekiel Martin, Dr., Smyth Blue, doctor and patient, 98, 320, 345
James Town, *see* Darkesville
Jameson, Harvey Allen, ambulance soldier, 323, 340; steward, 342, 343 369

Jehu, allusion, 181
Jenkins Bde., *see* Fourth VA Bde.
Jerusalem, introd., 9, 74
Jerusalem Delivered, introd., 6, 23, 28, 29, 30, 31n, 40, 66, 83, 89
Jesus Christ, introd., 8, 9, 11, 35, 40, 50n, 51, 74, 151,
Jewish peoples, analogy, introd., 9, 141, 154n
Johns, John, bishop, 140, 141n
Johns, John, Lt., commissary, 333
Johnson, patient, 97
Johnson, Andrew, wartime gov., TN, 250; postbellum pres., 41n
Johnson, Bradley Tyler, Gen., 586
Johnson, Bushrod Rust, Gen., 610
Johnson, Edward, Gen., "Allegheny Ed," wounded, 230; identified 231n
Johnson, F., tanner, 314
Johnson, Henry, African American works in camp, 341
Johnson, Thomas, tanner, 148
Johnston, author of *Chemistry of Human Life*, 215
Johnston, Albert Sydney, Gen., arrives with reinforcements, TN, 206
Johnston, Joseph Eggleston, Gen., 100, 101n, 104, 105, 106, 113n, 114, 143, 225
Jolley, Marc, i
Jones, patient, 98
Jones, Beverly Randolph, receives passionate letter from Mary Camden, 388; receives another letter, 407
Jones, Charles (uncle), introd., 3, 18, 28, 29, 72, 75, 76, 83, 135, 137, 147, 158, 170, 183; suffers from Federal invasion, 254; joins 1st MS Cav., 384; 386
Jones, Charles Lee, 258n
Jones, Jake (uncle), 75
Jones, John Robert, Gen., diarist is head nurse, 269; leads ambulance train, 270, 273, 274, 280, 291, 292, 309; sells books, 348
Jones, Richard M., 4th VA Inf., 413
Jones, Roger, Lt., Confederate sympathizer of Martinsburg, 266
Jones, William Edmundson "Grumble," Gen., 311
Jordan, Lafayette Hall, Dr., surgeon, 256, 257n; 304, 316, 321, 322, 345
Jordan, Richard A., soldier punished, 257
Jordan River, allusion and song, 149, 257
Jupiter, analogy, 57, 157n

Kanawha Valley campaign, 148
Kansas, 145
Kay, minister, Presbyterian, from England, 202
Kearneysville, WV, battle, 1862, 270-1
Kelley, Benjamin Franklin, 179n
Kelly's Ford, engagement, 1863, 387
Kemp, James H., hosts in Winchester, 1864, 581
Kennaman (?), Mrs., 80
Kennedy, James W., officer and editor, 39n, 102, 129, 140, 147, 153, 155, 156, 162, 164, 165
helps diarist draw up temperance pledge, 158
resigns comm., 212
sick and treated by diarist, 192
Kent, R.C., Maj., corr., 116, 171; promoted, 193; *see*ks election in Smyth
Blues, 194; refused commission and takes command of reserves,
Wythe and Carroll Cos., 194n;
returns home, 195
Kentucky, 58n, 102, 153; Kirby Smith and Braxton Bragg invade, 251
Kernstown, campaign, 90, 156, 244-45; "most exciting scene," 245
Kershaw, Joseph Brevard, Gen., 594
Kesner, Maggie, 55
Kimball, John A., 143n
Kite, Catherine, hosts, Columbia Bridge, 312
Know Nothing Party
see American Party
Knoxville, TN, 41n

Lacy, Beverly T., chaplain, ANV, 404-5; preaches in Early camp, 588
Civil War Revival, 588

LaFayette, Marquis de, 125n, 126
Landstreet, John, the Rev., preaches at New Market, 599
Language of Flowers, poetry reading, 349
Laprose, prisoner mistreated, 35, 171
laryngitis, 131; degrees and kinds, 294, 302
Laudanum, 29, 133
Laughlin, Capt., accompanies diarist into McDowell battlefield, 230
Laurel Hill, battle, 189n
Lawton, Alexander Robert, Gen., 314n
Lebby, B.M., Dr., general hospital, 313
Lee, Fitzhugh, 387
Lee, Robert Edward, introd., 11, 17, 20, 136n, 140n, 143n, 248, 264
criticized, called "Granny," 143-4, 144n; into MD, 251; 343; 351
Leesburg, 129
Leonard, Benjamin Franklin (Frank; Marion dry goods supplier), 130-1
as soldier, 175; is unwell, 363; suffers rheumatism, 384
Leonard, William, efforts to build school, 82
lesions, 131
Letcher, John, Gov., calls out "malitia," March 1862, 220; "harangued the people" after Bread Riot, 1863, 401
Levy family, 101n
Lewis, civilian, 71
Lewis, William (Baptist preacher), 35
Lewis, William Gaston, Gen., wound attended by diarist, 575
Leyburn, John, Dr., performing surgery, 139; 139n
Liberty Hall Guards, 109; *see* Smyth Blues, 4th VA Inf., 1st VA Bde.
ligature, 260
Light of the Harem, reading, 341
Lincoln, Abraham, introd., 11, 17, 39, 49n, 57, 61, 82, 84, 88,105, 125n 126, 141n, 166, 177n, 180n, 240, 246, 253, 318
called Despot, 125
compared to Julius Caesar, 49
compared to tyrant on VA flag, 105
personally occupies Richmond, 4 April 1865, 610
liniment, linimentum, 73, 109, 130n
linimentum saponis et chloroformis, 109
volar linimentum, 163n
lint, as particular bandage, 133n
Little, Harland, ii
Little, Nita Apperson, ii
Little Georgetown, MD, 168, 171
Livinard's (dry goods, Smyth Co.), 57
Locust Grove, introd., 2, 31
returns for sick furlough, 147-54
Logans Cross Roads, Battle, *see* Battle of Somerset
Long, Everette Beach, introd., vii; 177n, and cited passim
Longstreet, James (Pete), Gen., 136, 260, 285, 323, 370
Loring, William Wing, Gen., 143-5 and 144n, 179, 192; 196
Loring Command, 156, 165, 173, 174, 177, 178, 181, 186, 190; at Winchester, 195-6; leave for Manassas, 206
Loring-Jackson Dispute, 143-45; 192-3; 196
Loudon Co., 129
Louisa Co., 178
Louisiana, 112, 172n
Louisiana Tigers, 239, 242, 259-60; "depredations," 312-3
see also Wheat
Love, Robert V, Dr., 583
Lovelace, William (Grayson Co. customer)
69
Loving, Mrs., hosts in Clarke Co., 306 and 307n
"low dutch" troops, *see* Gen. W.H. Heim
Luker, Ralph, vi
Lutheran, 78, 576, 591
Luttrell, Marsha, vii
Lynan, William (Smyth Co. school), 68
Lynchburg, traveling, introd., 3; 60, 89
Lyon, patient, 97
Lyon's Gap, 37, 39, 67
Lyttle, Sherry, vii

McCall (Washington Co. civilian patient), 67
McCausland, John, Gen., wagon train, 572; loses battle, 586
McClellan, George Brinton, Gen., 100, 132n, 177n, 221; "easy," 252; 260, 272, 285, 292, 301
McCorkle, George Baxter, officer, 322
McCready, E.H., 115, 121
McDonald, Angus, 582
McDowell, battle, 1862, Dr. Black and diarist to front lines, 229; 250
McDowell, Iwin, Gen.,
McElwee, William D., the Rev., Associated Reform Presbyterian hosts Angus McDonald and 2d Corps field hospital, Four Springs
McGrew, Roderick, introd., vi, 21n, and cited passim
McGuire, Hunter Holmes, Dr., med. dir., ANV, 185; 186n; 195; 303, 324 328, 382
  criticizes steward, 267-8
  demands report, 341
  indifferent to diarist's petition, 211
  inspects and is pleased, 331
  orders hospital moved, 355
  orders reports, 254
McGuire, James, Dr., unidentified with regiment, 583
McLaughlin, Capt., 170
  see William Nelson Pendleton
McLemore, C.G., visits, 219
McMullen, Glenn, introd., iii; 103n
McMullen, LaFayette, 79, 589
Magruder, patient, 98
Magruder, H.P., Dr., assigned field hospital, Caroline Co., 406; 579-80
magnesium sulfate, 174n
Maiden, William, hosts, Port Republic, 594
Malvern Hill, battle, 221
Mammon, false gods, 127
Manassas Gap, 105, 112n, 113, 114, 115, 120, 121
Manassas Gap Railroad, 113n
Manassas junction, 117
Manassas Station, 146, 155
Manassas, town, 10, 122, 130, 144, 153, 154
Manassas, battle, *see* First and Second Manassas
Marion, introd., 4, 8, 15, 17, 18, 28, 32, 37, 39, 40, 47, 48, 50, 63, 67, 84, 108, 130, 139, 157, 164n, 165n, 174
  Co. secession debates, 27, 29
  Co. secession voting, 35, 36, 48
  Co. Home Guards, 130n
  and passim
Marion Visitor, introd., 39, 51, 129, 138, 140, 161
  diarist writes for, 140, 157, 165 and passim
  see also James W. Kennedy, Albert Gallatin Pendleton
Mark Anthony, 26
Marksdale (Marksville), scenery, 312
Marriage As It Is and As It Should Be, 371
Mars, allusion, 250; "sad blighting march," 269
Martinsburg, WV, 100-02, 103, 105, 106, 107, 171, 177
  camp, 168
  turnpike, 183
  "unsound and bitter enemies," 265
Maryland, 75, 169n, 170; Lee and Jackson invade, 251
Mason, A.P., 279-80
Mason, Don, ii
Mason, Fanny Apperson, ii
Mason, James Murray, ambassador, 172, 174
  see Mason-Slidell Case
Mason-Slidell Case, rumors, 172; discussed 172n; 176
Massachusetts, 151, 152n
Massanutton Mountain, 240n, 312
Massanutton (town), 240
Materia Medica, introd., 4, 43, 44, 47, 49, 53, 54, 57, 58, 59, 60, 61, 366
Mathews, Donald G., vi
Maury, Matthew Fontaine, CSA navy, 161
maxillary, 326
Meade, Francis B., civilian and rumors, 288

Meade, William, Bishop, 140n
Mechum's River Depot, 226 and 227n
Medical College of Virginia, introd., ii, 5, 10, 16, 17, 20, 28, 48, 76, 91, 198, 249
Medical College of Washington City (D.C.), 76, 83
medicine
  as career, 59, 69, 71-2, 81
  contrasted with law, 298-300
  country practice, 150
Meek, James, 207
Memphis, TN, surrender, 250
meningitis, 61
menstruation, case of early onset, 53
Mercer, Douglas, Maj., QM, 256, 257n, 262, 266; drinking, 269
Mercer, George W, possibly meets diarist, 219
Mercer, Hugh Weedon, identified, 220n
Mercer, Thomas H., possibly meets diarist, 219
Mercier, Edouard Henri, 391
mercurous chloride, 110n
mercury, prescribed as pill, 92-99, 143n
Meredith, Jaquelin Marshall, chaplain, 4th VA Inf., Episcopalian, 408
Mesopotamia, allusion, 148n
meteor, 1861 summer, 103
Methodists, introd., 1, 9, 13, 51, 52, 56, 74, 78n, 79, 346, 376, 402, 496, 513, 568
Mexican War, introd., 9, 15, 117n, 136n, 141n, 154n, 171n
Middlesex Co., 143n
Middletown, 156, 307, 308n; field hospital, 310
Midwest, 153n
midwifery, 62
Milam's Gap, 312
militia ("malitia"),
  as poor preparation for war, 82
  law and reenlistment, 1862, 200
  Orange Co., 124
  rumors of great success in Morgan Co., WV, 201
  TN activates "whole force of malitia," 1862, 206
  VA "malitia. . . trembling now," 1862,206
Miller, David, 156
Miller, David family, Opequon, July 1864, 574
Miller, Gaines (roving chaplain ANV), 118-19, 123, 127, 138, 141, 141n
  see also Episcopalians, pietism
Miller, James W., chaplain, 119
Mill Springs, battle, *see* Somerset, battle
Miller, David, hosts in Loudon Co., 310
Millwood, 112
Milton, John, reading, 290; 300 and 301n
Mississippi, destination, 1859, introd., 2; 28, 100, 113, 179n, 183
Missouri, 80
Mitchell's Station, 124
Mohler, Samuel, steward, 329-30, 383
Mohler, William, 571
Mollie, "Other Mollie," *see* Mary Camden
Moloch, false gods, 127
Monroe, Aron, Capt., 92
Montgomery, AL, 41n, 81, 167
Montgomery Co., 112n, 118, 119n, 179n
Montgomery, Capt., VA, QM, 577
Montgomery, Capt., LA, at Frances Thornton's party, 1863, 394
Moore, L.E., Lt. Col., 193
Moore, Samuel Preston, Dr., surgeon general, receives diarist's report, 381; 595
Moorefield, battle, 586
Morgan, Daniel, Gen., house, 289
Morgan Co., TN, skirmish, 201
Morgan Co., WV, skirmish, 201
morphine, 31
  prescribed, 97, 99, 109, 110, 115
  recognized as dangerous, 110
  sulphate m - , 23; prescription makes diarist ill, 142
Morphious, 31, 45
Morris, I.M., patient, 95
Mosby, John Singleton, Cav. officer, 405-6
Moses, allusion,
Motley, John L., hosts, Bowling Green Township, 407

Mott, David, Dr., civilian doctor paid by army for treatments, 572
Mount Airy (Rural Retreat), 4
Mt. Jackson, 173
Mt. Rogers, introd., 3, 10
Mt. Sidney, 596
Mt. Solon (village), 238
Mountain House, Highland Co., 229
Mouth of Wilson, 69
mucus, 131
Mulligan, James Adelbert, Col., wounded, Bunker Hill, 577-8
mumps, *see* parotitis
Muslims, introd., 6, 11, 12
mustard plaster, *see* sinapism

Napoleon, Jerome, 125
see Bonaparte family
narcotics, 109n
Nashville, TN, diarist learns of loss, 208
nativism, 77n, *see* American Party
nausea, 123
Neff, Samuel, Smyth Blue, patient, 98; dies, 295
"negro," *see* African American
Neill and Smith Compendium, surgery text, 254, 261, 360-1
Neligan, John Moore, on skin diseases, 407
Nelson County, crossing, 3; *see* White Oak Swamp, battle
Nelson, Horatio, biography, 347
Nelson, J.P., Sgt., 372
Nelson, Thomas A.R., 41, 43n
neuralgia, 31
New Bern, NC
New Castle, DE, 140n
New Hampshire, introd., 179n
New Hope (Orange Co.) church, 151-2
New Jersery, 170n
New Orleans, LA, surrendered and port reopened by Lincoln, 12 May 1862, 234, 250
New South, introd., 4, 15, 90
Newman, Conway, Lt., 289
Newtown, 165
New Year's observation, CSA, 336
New York City, 103n
New York State, 62, 115, 170n, 172, elections, 1862, 291
Nimrod, allusion, 148-9; identified, 148n
Ninth VA Inf., 343
Noah, 148n
Noland, James Henry, ambulance soldier, 323; "judge," 346, 368-9; borrows from diarist, 374; replaces diarist, 382; plays guitar, 400; "considerable flare-up," 418-9
Norfolk, surrendered, 12 May 1862, 234
North Carolina, 52, 136n, 141n
North Mountain, 267
Northern Methodist Church, Winchester; diarist attends, 1862, 203

Oakland, Louisa Co., unionists, 178
Odyssey, allusion, 157n
officers, election, 123-4
Official Records of the War of Rebellion, vii and cited passim
Ohio, 50, 141n
Old Dominion, *see* Virginia
Old Ringgold Cav.,
Old South, introd., 15,
oliguria, 134n
opium, prescribed, 29, 93, 98, 110, 115, 130n, 131, 134, 142
Orange Co., birthplace, introd., 1-14; 29n, 49n, 124, 147n, and passim
Orange Courthouse, 102n
Orange Rangers, *see* Sixth VA Cav.
osteopathy, 21n
Overby (Overbay?), patient, 97
Owry, R.G., officer, patient, 115
Owry, Thomas, dry goods supplier, 130
Ozenby, Spence, patient, 99

Pacific Northwest, 79n
Page Co., 312
Page, Mrs., civilian, host for campsite, Clarke Co., 286-92
Page Valley, 312
Pamlico Sound, NC
papule, 297
see variola

Parish, Smyth Co. Blue, granted furlough, 183
Paris (VA), 112, 113
Parkersburg, 143n
parlor games, 74
  "Sledge," 410
  "Tableau vivant," 417
  "Whist," 401
parotitis, 161, 162n, 163, 165
  diarist contracts, 166
paroxysms, 81, 131
Partisan Leader, 388-9
Patrick, Marsena Rudolph, Gen., 309 and 310n
patrols (required security), 57
Patterson, Elizabeth, 125n
Paxton, Elisha Franklin, Maj., reassignment, 293
Payne, Charles B., QM, 136, 193
Peace Conference, 49, 58
  see Crittenden Resolutions
Peake, C.W. (Smyth co. patient), 59
Peck, Col., 259
pediluvia, 62
Pegram, W.W., civilian, looks for soldier who died, 351
Pendleton, Albert Gallatin, editor and officer, introd., 10, 15, 78, 88, 102, 127-8, 131, 133, 138,161, 176, 193, 308
  assists diarist, 211
  hosts prayer meeting, 138
  in gen. hospital, 132-3
  tries to protect prisoner, 171
  wins controversial election in Smyth Blues, 194; promoted, 208
Pendleton, Alexander Swift ("Sandie"), ii, 382
Pendleton, Edward Starchan, Dr., surgeon, 585
Pendleton, William Nelson (priest and artillery commander), 133, 139, 170 324, 325n
penicillin, 174n
Pennsylvania state, 132n
  PA Volunteers, 101n
Pennsylvania University, 59n
percussion, 287 and 288n
peripneumonia, misdiagnosis of bacterial pneumonia, 131n 132
Perry, George H., in small pox ward, 392
Perryville, KY, battle, 267
personal liberty laws, 34
Peters, William Elisha, Col., former proffessor, Emory & Henry, 615
Petersburg, siege by Grant, 588, 595; eighth month of siege, 604
Phillip II, Holy Roman Empire, analogy, 125n
philopena (game), 417
Physician's Diary, book of era, 269
physic, *see* cathartic
Pickett, George, Gen., on move, 365
Pickett's Charge, 171
Piedmont Station, place, 112, 113, 155
pietism, 1, 5, 51, 52, 56, 74, 77, 78, 140-41, 168402, 496, 504, 508-9; 514; 516, 528-30; 534-5; 588-9
pill-making, duties of steward, 48, 63, 65, 78, 81, 101, 120
Pillow, Gideon Johnson, Gen., ineffective at Fort Donelson, 206n
Pirogoff's amputation, 326
Pitts, Charles F., vi and citted passim
plasma, 19th cent. med. def., 131-2n
Plato, quoted, 587
pneumonia, not distinguished, viral and bacterial, 55, 57, 68; post mortem, 334, 343
Poe, Edgar Allan, 161n; classical lament quoted as CSA collapses, 613
Point of Rocks, WV
poisoning, 71
Poland, analogy to CSA, 215
Poole, civilian, 144
Pope, Alexander, quoted, 70n
popular songs, 400, 409, 427
  "Dixie," 122
  "Fisher's Hornpipe," 393
  "Get Out of the Wilderness," 122
  "Good By," 400
  "Home, Sweet Home," 400
  "Jordan is a Hard Road to Travel," 257
  "Life is the Time to Serve the Lord,"

280
"Lone Starry Hour," 400
"Music in the Air," 400
"While it was Morning," 70
Port Republic, battle, 250
Port Royal, SC, assault, 154
Porter, John C., Capt.
Potomac Rier, 124, 127, 129, 167, 168, 170, 171
poultice, 73, 174, 177n; 296
Powers, Max, vii
"Prayer of Twenty Million," 37n, *see* Horace Greeley
pregnancy, 66
Presbyterians, introd., 7, 56, 109, 145, 280
New Light, 236-7; Stiles preaches New Light, 282-4
Old Light, 11, 90, 202, 248, 273, 274, 278, 280, 402, 496, 513, 516, 520, 528-30
predestination, 153
views on infant baptism, 145
Presgraves, James, v and cited passim
Preston, James Francis, officer, 112, 116; death, 190
Preston, John Montgomery, officer, 135, 574
distributes CSA funds to survivors of veterans, 605
sick, 141
Preston, Neuff (minister), 56
Preston, Robert T., officer, 102-03
Preston, Waller Redd, staff officer, 581
Price, Richard, the Rev., preaches at Seven Mile Ford, buries Martha Oury 615
Price, Sterling, Gen., 259n, 260
Prince Edward Co., 133n
Prince William City,
Princeton University, 140n
Progressive Era, 125n
Ptosis ("Pthisis"), incipient, 397
Pugh Town, 177
Pulaski Co., 118
Pulaski Guards, 144
purging, technique, 110n, 144
Purifoy, Dr., messmate, 330; 338, 345, 392
purulence, 131,
pus, 131n, 184n

quinine, as treatment, 145
Quisenberry, V. (Dr.), introd., 31, 49, 53, 110, 124-5, 133, 147, 149, 150, 156, 163, 166, 183, 186, 210, 220, 314, 406, 585
hosts on sick furlough, 147
Mrs. Quisenberry hosts, 149
quizing (courtship game), 46, 80

Raccoon Ford, 153
racism
in diarist, 156, 231, 318, 344, 379, 584
observed in others, 516, 531
railroads, 25, 106, 170n
see individual RR by name
Ralston, Samuel, Dr., theologian, 385
Ramseur, Stephen Dodson, Gen., 574
Rappahannock River, 152, 153n
Rarden, Joseph L., SC 7th officer, 154
Ray, patient, 97
Ready, David, 82
Reagan, John Henninger, CSA postmaster general, 589
Reamill, Dr., 108
record-keeping, field hospitals, criticized by LaFayette Guild, 410
Rector, James (neighbor of Dr. Faris), 36, 57, 73, 82
Mrs. James Rector, 63
sick child, 73
sons, 81
Rector, Jason, 57, 73, 82
reenlistment, inducements and furlough, 195
diarist reenlists, 5 March 1862, 212
religion and theology, 145-55; 384, 385, 386, 402, 496, 512-15, 528-30
Great Civil War Revival,
and passim
see sects by denomination
Religious Herald, introd., 5, 9
"Reminiscences," ii and passim
Revolutionary War, American, 125

Reynolds, Mrs., Orange Co. neighbor, 152
rheumatism (so-called), 128, 142, 143
Rhodes, artillery soldier and comrade, 133
Rhodes, Toulemiah, hosts campsite, Loudon Co., 571
Rich Mountain, battle, 189
Rich Valley, 37
Richards, Tazewell, 106
Richardson, George T., 585
Richmond, introd., 6, 12; 26n, 33, 35, 45, 48, 60n, 61
  bread riot, 401-02
  Lincoln's tour and "rabble," 610
  McClellan threatens, 1862, 221
  secession convention debates, 8, 48, 61, 64, 80
  studies, 5
Richmond Co., WV
Richmond Daily Dispatch, rumors of English recognition, 291
Richmond Examiner, sarcastic about Bread Riot, 404
Richmond Whig, rumors of English recognition, 291; exaggerates "shoeless soldiers," 307
Ripley, civilian, 283
ritualism, 402, 496, 534
Roach, H.D., Orange Co. neighbor, 152, 314
Roanoke Island, NC, falls to Federals
Roberts, John E., Capt., 322
Robertson, James I., vii and cited passim
Robinson, Joseph, civilian host, 134-5
Robinson, Mrs., Orange co. neighbor and hostess, 149, 152
Rockbridge Artillery, 324, 325
Rockbridge Rifles, 5th VA, 169
Rocky Mountains, introd., 11
Roman Catholic Church, introd., 9, 77n
Romney, WV, 167, 185, 196
  rumors of engagement, 174-5, 177
Ronald, Charles A., officer, 21, 238, 252, 263
  *see*ks election in Smyth Blues, 194
  assists diarist in petition, 211
  restores order in Winchester by disciplining Blues, 214
  scolds diarist and officers for flanking for dinner, 219
Rosecrans, William Starke, Gen., 132, 143-5, 144n, 258, 259n
Ross, John, introd., 6, 11
Rosser, Thomas Lafayette, Gen., 594; defends ambulance train, 610
Row, Dr., civilian doctor visited on sick furlough, 147
Rowan, Stephen Clegg, USN officer, 141n
rubifacient, passim; defined, 73n
Ruffin, Edmund, introd., 8
Ruffner, P.H., soldier, 122, 124
Russell, John, Sir
Russellville, KY
Rye Valley, 69

St. John, George W., 78, 79, 80
St. John, N.C.B., 35, 46, 75, 80, 83; "I am a stampeded man," 599
St. Louis, MO, 41n
salaries, adjusted, 124; deductions for clothing, 293, 405-6; 498; 500; 598
salt, cost inflated, 316
Saltville, destroyed by Stoneman, 604-5n
Sambo, *see* racism
Sanders (patient), 37
Sanders & Tate's (dry goods), 53
  see also L.N. Tate
Sanders, Alexander J., 36, 54, 56, 74, 118
Sanders, A.O., soldier, 155
Sanders, Andrew T.(Andy), 120, 144, 153, 284 and 285n; 340
  granted furlough, 183
  tells bad news of diarist's girlfriend (unidentified), 285
Sanders, Augustus Owry (Pete), 599
Sanders (dry goods), 53
  see Sanders & Tate's
Sanders, E.H., 124, 138
Sanders, E.W., 120, 121
Sanders, I.S., 53
Sanders, James P., 80
Sanders, John L., 28, 71, 72, 75n
  sick child, 71
Sanders, Mrs. (widow), 30, 49, 79
Sanders, Lauren, 80
Sanders, M.F. (escort), 56, 74, 80, 84

Sanders, Susan, 74, 348
Sanders, William A., 50
Sanders, William W., Smyth Blue, death, 190
Sanitary Commission, and variola, 307-8 and 308n
Sayers, John A., Lt., cruel treatment of prisoner, 171
see Laprose
Sayers, John Thompson, Maj. (ret.), hosts at Max Meadows, 614
Sayers, John Thompson, Lt., released from Federal prison, in
Max Meadows with father and diarist, April 1865, 614
Sayers, Samuel Rush, Dr., surgeon, 289, 316n; 322, 572, 581
Saylor's Creek (Sailor's Creek), battle, 611, Gen. Lee loses 1/3 of
remaining ANV troops, 611
scapulae, 264n
Scarborough, Dr., in charge of field hospital, Middletown, 308
"school for colored," introd., 10
school, Seven Mile Ford, 82, 83
chair of campaign, 82
Schultz, John W. hosts for dinner, Winchester, 578; hosts, 591
Schultz, Kate, 587
Schwartz, Thomas, sick soldier, unidentified unit, 197; diagnosed, pneumonia, 198-9; improves, 205
scientific method, (as diarist understood) 17, 299 and 300n
Scots Irish, 4, and passim
Scott, E.A., 25
Scott, Sir Walter, 6, 8, 363, 364, 366-7
Scott, Winfield, Gen., introd., 10, 13, 26
Scott, W.W., v and cited passim
Sealy, A.J., soldier visits, 196
Seates, Dr., 84
secession, introd, 7, 12, 17, 25, 26, 27, 29, 31, 34, 35, 36, 41, 42, 49n, 50, 61, 72
Second Manassas, 250
Second VA Inf., 243-5, Kernstown campaign; winter 1863, 350
seduction and revenge, debate, 350
Segus, L.W., patient, 142-43
Semmes, Raphael, "privateer," 335
sermons, 35, 51, 52, 56, 74, 79, 118-19, 120, 123, 127, 138, 140, 141, 147, 151-2; 167-8, 186-7, 202, 204; 236-7; 273, 274, 278, 280 386, 410-11, 423-4, 496, 503-4; 508-9,512-3; 514-5, 520; 521-2; 528-30; 534-35; 572, 576, 588-9, 591, 599; for funeral of Martha Oury, 616
Seven Days Campaign, 221
Seven Mile Ford, introd., 3, 4, 5, 8, 9, 16, 18, 19, 22n, 26n, 36n, 39, 54, 55n
and passim
Seven Pines, battle,
Seventh SC Vol. Corps,
Seventh VA Inf., 363-7
Severs, Thomas, hosts in Frederick Co., 1864, 579-80
Seward, William Henry, sec. of state, 332, 333n, "yawls" with Count Mercier, 391
Seymour, Horatio, Gov., 291
Sexton, Benjamin Franklin, "flanks" for a snack, 178; 205; visits, 206
Sexton, Charles McDonald, Smyth Blues, 294-5
Sexton, Joseph Carpenter, Smyth Blues commissary, 257, 258n, 259-60
Sexton, S.M., 258n; borrows money, 388
Sexton, T.L., Dr., Blues, 95, 116
Seymour, Thomas Hart, 391
Shakespeare, William, 26
Othello, diarist reading, "very affecting," 205
Rape of Lucerne, reading, 207
Shands, Martha, hosts, Rockingham Co., 593
Sharpsburg, battle, 248, 250; casualties from Smyth Co., 252 and 253n
Sheetz, George F., Capt., killed, Cedar Creek Bridge, 243; 245
Sheffey, James White, 16, 18, 25, 26n, 27, 33, 34, 36, 77n
Shelburn, minister preaches at Camp Stevenson, 167-8
Shelby, Dr., hosts in Rockingham Co., 222
Shenandoah River, 220

Shenandoah Valley, crossing, introd., 3
T.J. Jackson's Valley Campaign, 1862, 154-309
J.A. Early's Valley Campaign, 554-604
Shepherd, Keziah, (Aunt Kesey, Aunt K) 341, 349, 352, 353, 354, 357, 360, 369 370, 373, 374; buys religious books for her, 376; 398
Shepperdstown, WV, 252
Sheridan, Philip H., Gen., reports destroying crops and cattle in valley, 590; captures Staunton, 595; defeats Early, 596
Sherman, William Tecumseh, Gen., 116, 335; burns Atlanta, 596
Shields, James W., Gen., commissary, 277, 319; provides horse for escape from Federals, April 1865, 613
Shouttz, civilian, hosts company, Clarke Co., 292
Sigel, Franz, Gen., 276 and 277n
sillhouse, sillary, 269
Sims, Mr.; Orange Co. storekeeper, 148
sinapism, def., 131n; 62, 134, 176n
Sinclair's Bottom, 34
Sing, William, 63
Siry, William, 67
Sixth VA Cav., 311-12
Sixtieth GA Inf., casualties, Fredericksburg, 325
Sixty First GA Inf., casualties, Fredericksburg, 325
skin inflammation, *see* erysipelas
slavery, introd., 7, 10, 11, 12, 17, 18, 45n, 58n
extension of, 7
slaves, introd., 1, 4, 5, 11
captured at Kernstown trying to read Federal lines, 243-5
cooking in battle camp, 239
Archibald Brock's slvaes, 239
Dr. Faris's, 63
fugitive slave law, 58n
Slidell, John, ambassador, 172
see Mason-Slidell Case
small pox, *see* variola
Smith, A.C., Dr., general hospital, 303; 304-5; 319, 336, 345, 346
Smith, Edward Kirby, Gen., 251
Smith, Francis H., Gen. and Supt., V.M.I., 228n
Smithfield, 261
Smyth, Alexander, 17
Smyth Blues, introd., 9, 14, 15, 30,47, 78n, 88, 102, 115, 124n, 141, 142n, 154, 155, 170, 176n, 178, 186, 196, 216, 217n, 227, 234, 248n, 260n, 270n, 515n
conduct controversial election, 195n; 209
misbehave in Winchester, 1862, 214
take temperance pledge, 158
wounded and killed, Valley Campaign, 264
Smyth County, introd., ii-xi, 9, 14, 16, 18, 22n, 26, 37, 40, 47, 54, 55n 77n, 78n, 101, 102, 124n, 131n, 149, 162n, 167n, 176n, 203n, 206n, 209n, 222, 244n, 250, 253, 260, 263, 267, 270, 299n, 310n
and passim
Smyth County Heritage Book Commission, introd. and passim
v and cited passim
Smyth Greys, *see* First VA Bde; *see* Fourth VA Inf.
Smyth, Alexander, 17
Snapp, D.B., 120
see also Snapp & Graham store
Snapp & Graham store, 37
Snickersville, campsite, 573
Snidow, Dr., 129, 144, 223, 343
assisting at Centreville camp, 132, 133
sick, 142
Snodgrass, Henderson, soldier, Co. A, 4th VA Inf.
foot crushed, attended by diarist and not surgeon, 181; visited, 395 400
Somerset, battle, 191; 197n, 198
Sommerville, Dr., civilian Dr., Orange; 146
evaluated, 145
Presbyterian views, 145
South Carolina, 42, 154
Southern Literary Messenger, 363

South Mountain, introd., 12, 19
Southern Literary Messenger, 161
Southey, Robert, 347
southside, 8
speculators, blamed for inflation and shortages, 317
  see also inflation
Spenser, Edmund, 70n
splints, set, 21
Spotsylvania Co., introd., 2
squire's court, 16, 55, 56
Stainback, Robert H., 66
Stamper, Preston E., Lt., 4th VA Inf., killed, 264
State Rights, introd., 7, 11, 17
Staunton, 41n; falls to Philip H. Sheridan, 595
  General Hospital, 234, 236, 305-6, 315; abandoned, 596
Stephenson's Station Depot, skirmish, 1862, 215
Stevens, Dr., LA Bde, 274
Sterrit, James, testifies at preaching, 168
Stethoscope (Richmond), introd., 4, 60
Stewart, Jennifer, ix
Stiles, Joseph Clay, minister and roving chaplain, 273, 274, 277, 279
still-house, 20
Stirnberger Farm, on Shenandoah R., 221
Stoicism, classicism, 90
Stone, patient, 98
Stoneman, George, Gen., destroys saltworks and Saltville, 604, 605n
Stoneman's Raid, December 1864, through Smyth Co., 604, 605n
Stonewall (the man), *see* Jackson, Thomas Jonathan
Stonewall Bde., *see* First VA Bde
Story, David, merchant and host, Robertson Township, 313
Stowe, Steven, introd., vi, 17, 19n, 20, and cited passim
Straith, J.A., Dr., chief surgeon, 259, 262, 263, 272, 290, 571, 578
Strange Story, reading, 396
Strasburg, 165; field hospital, 308
Strasburg Pike, 295
streptococcus, Group A hemolytic, 128n
Stribling Springs, 237-8
Strickland, Mrs., looks for husband killed at Fredericksburg, 351
Stringfellow, Dr., civilian Dr.; evaluated, 145
Stringham, Silas, US navy, 137-8n
Strother, David Hunter, writer *Porte Crayon*, 179, 180n
  artwork destroyed by CSA troops, 179-80
Strother, James P., 16, 27
Strother, Wade S., 139-40, 141, visits camp, 140-42
Stuart, Alexander Hugh Holmes, 41, 45n, 58n
Stuart, J.E.B., Gen., 129, 141, 284, 311
  criticized, 136 and 136n
  rides around McClellan's army, 1862, 221; 260
  takes and deploys artillery to Fredericksburg, 1862-3, 323
Sturgill, Kenneth, v, and cited passim
Sturgill, Mack, iii, iv, v, and cited passim
Sulphur Springs, camp meetings, 78
Sulphur Springs church, 51, 79, 83
Summers, George William, 41, 45n, 58n
Summers, Lewis Preston, v and cited passim
Suphers, Dr., LA, 265
suppuration, 174, def. 174n
Swann, Dr. S.R., 310
"The Switch," (roadhouse), 54, 81, 84, 85
Sydnor, Dr., surgeon, ANV, 331, 341, 360; "El Cid," 362; 365; 367-8, 369, 371, 392, 404
Syme's operation, 326n
syphilis, confounded with variola, 298-302

Taber's Cyclopedic Medical Dictionary, vi
  and cited passim
tableau vivant, 415-6; 450
Taifer, Francis, gift of coat, 174
Talbot City, MD,
Taliafero's Bde.,

Taliafero, William Booth, Gen., 216, 216n, 224; Cedar Creek Bridge, 243
Talley, A.N., Dr., 366
Tammany Hall, 291
Tannan, patient, 98
tar and feathers, punishment by mob, introd., 9, 37
Tasso, Torquato, introd., 6, 8, 10, 12, 13, 23n, 28, 29, 30, 31, 35, 40, 43, 66, 75, 83, 88
Tate, L.N., 53, 65, 66
  sick child, 66
Tattaille, Mary, 377
taxes, 29, 34
Taylor (clerk, Lyon's Gap), 67
Taylor, Richard, Gen., Cedar Creek Bridge, 243; Patterson, LA fight, 405
Taylor, William, Dr., medical purveyor, 578-9, 585
telling needle, parlor game, 81
temperance pledge, among Smyth Blues, 158
Tennes*see* River, 41n
Tennes*see* state, 41n,
  Upper East, 16
Tennes*see* and Virginia R.R., 54, 162
Terry, William R., Capt., 92, 93, 271, 277, 321, 322n; becomes Gen., wounded fourth time and replaced, 608; recovers and attempts to reorganize ANV to join Joseph Eggleston Johnston in NC, 615
Thanksgiving Day observations
  CSA, 28 July 1861; 16 May 1862, 235n; 27 March 1863, 395-6
  US, 28 November 1861; 6 August 1863; current holiday set, 1864, 235n; 395-6
Thirteenth GA Inf., 346
Thirty-Seventh NC Inf., 334
Thirty-Seventh VA Inf., McDowell battle, 230; 295
Thirty-Third VA Inf., at Newton Stephensburg, 243; at Fredericksburg, 345
Thomas, GA soldier in incident, 335, 336
Thomas, Abijah, 54, 55, 121
Thomas & Summer's Factory
  see Abijah Thomas
Thomas, Columbia, sister of Joseph, 134
Thomas, James, soldier taking temperance pledge, 158
Thomas, Joseph M., officer, 123-4; 273, 289, 297, 342
  offers to pay for medical lectures, 198
  procures clothing for troops, 318, 322
  sickness, 126-28, 134, 137, 140
  recruits for artillery co., 176
  "treats" for election, 195-6
  elected 2d Lt., 208-9
  elected Capt., 252
  contracts "insipient Pthisis" and resigns commission, 397
Thomas, William H., Sgt., 404; visits Mollie Graves, 419
Thornton family, Caroline Co., 408
Thornton, Eve, 408, 414
Thornton, Frances (widow), hosts, Caroline Co., 385-6; hosts party, 393; 398
Thornton, Mollie, 311, 340, 411, 585
Thruston's Gap (Thurston's Gap), 309
Tibbs, Parson, 263, 3321, 322; to visit Quisenberry family, Orange Co., 406
Tomlin, Mary, 118-19, 127-8, 141, 153, 158, 163, 167, 175, 184, 195, 205, 207, 266, 273, 331, 332, 334, 351, 361, 372, 394, 585
  writes diarist about Mrs. Faris's illness, 206
tonsilitis, 73, 150
Treatise on Therapeutics, 59n
troop size estimates, overestimated, 179
Trucks, D., 4th VA Inf. soldier, damaged by alcohol, 212
Tucker, Nathaniel Beverly, 388-9
turacin cerate, 296-7
Turner (shoe-maker), 28, 29
Turner, B.T., GA soldier killed, 346
Tuscany, effort for independence, and CSA, 352
Twelfth GA Inf., McDowell battle, 230
Twenty-First VA Inf., McDowell battle, 230
Twenty-Ninth VA Inf., 412

Twenty-Second Fed. Cav.
Twenty-Seventh VA Inf., Newton
Stephensburg, 243; Kernstown, 244-5; 322
see also Andrew Jackson Grigsby
Twenty-Sixth AL Inf., 332
Twenty-Sixth GA Inf., 335
Twenty-Third VA Inf., 295
typhus, 277

Ulysses, allusion to high winds, 401 (possibly thinking of Agamemnon)
Umbarger, E.P., 62
Umbarger, Abram Newton, sick, 138; toe lacerated, 399
Underground Railroad, sarcasm about sneaking out whisky, 584
Unger's Store, Frederick Co., robbed by Federal troops, 178
campsite, 183
U.S. House of Representatives, 41n, 58n, 77n, 79
U.S. Military Academy, 9 and passim, notes
U.S.N. Diana, 405
U.S.N. Pawnee, rumors, 141
Unionists, introd., 8, 12, 13, 41, 42, 45n, 54n, 61178, 179n
see John Carlisle
Updyke, Capt., *see*ks and loses election in Smyth Blues, 194
Upshur, W.G., Dr., 310
uttering, 54

vaccination, 58, 66, 67, 271, 302, 304, 319, 345
see also variola
Valentine's Day, 43, 44
Valley Campaign, T.J. Jackson's, 1862, 154-309
J.A. Early's, 1863-4, 554-604
Van Buren, Martin,
Van Dorn, Earl, Gen., 258 and 259n, 260
variola, 60, 254; 297, 298-304; 307, 315-6; 319, 330, 331; 333-34, 335-6; 343; 345; 379, 394, 441, 447, 455, 501
outbreak in !st VA Bde, 271, 272n; 298
small pox ward, 307, 343, 345,392, 394, 441, 447, 455, 501
syphilis confounded with variola, 298-302
varioloid, *see* variola
Vass, Lachlan Cumming, Presbyterian chaplain, 27th VA Inf., preaches, 236; identified, 237n
Vaugh, Robert C., Lt., Smyth Co. Blue, granted furlough, 183; with fever, 397
Vejnar, Robert, vi, vii
Venable, Drury W. (possibly C.W. Venable), 133, 160, 175, 176, 192, 196-7, 262, 331, 351, 388, 411, 419
sends tobacco gift, 297
takes temperance pledge, 158
Venable, Marcellus, 175n, partner in *Marion Visitor*
Venable, R.J., 175n
venesection, 19, 21, 23, 31, 35, 66, 110
Vermillion, patient, 97
vesications, 9, 32
Vicksburg, MS, siege by Gen. Sherman and Grant, 335; falls to Federals,
Victoria, Queen, *see* Great Britain
Vilwig, John, cabinetmaker, Winchester, 308
Virginia and Monitor fight,
rumors, 217-8
facts, 218n
Virginia and Tennes*see* Railroad, 162
Virginia Central Railroad, 589, *see* Henry Donald Whitcomb
Virginia Military Institute, introd., 9, 15, 88, 89, 228
Virginia Place Name Society, vi and cited,
passim
Virginia Polytechnic Institute and State University, ii
Virginia Regimental Histories Series, vi and cited passim

Wainscott, Mrs., NC widow inquires about husband's death in battle, 378
"Walker, Miss," *see* Mollie Graves
Walker, R.L., Capt., 93

Walls, John Perry, Dr., surgeon, 264, 272, 364, 367, 369, 370, 376, 390
Ward, William, Dr., 288 and 289n
Washington County, introd., v, 7, 25, 67 and noted passim
Washington, D.C., 41n
Washington Peace Conference, Feb. 1861, 41n, 45, 49, 57
Washington Springs, 25
Washington Territory, and Gov. Fayette McMullen, 79
Watson textbook, unidentified, 59, 150
Watson, Edward S., Marion supplier, 130
Watson, Frank, 366
Watters, J.L., wounded, 139
Watts, Isaac, diarist reading, 173-4; 174n; quoted, 174
Improvement of the Mind, 173
Waverly novels, reading 362-4 366
Waynesboro, battle, March 1865, Stonewall Bde. destroyed, 606n
Webb, Eddy, soldier, 122, 148
Webb, Richard, Orange Co. neighbor, 151
Missionary Baptist, 151; *see* Baptists
Webster, Daniel, introd., 7, 10
Webster's Unabridged Dictionary, purchased, 348
Weems, Gen. 221
Weldon and NC Railroad, lost to Federals, 199
West Point, *see* U.S. Military Academy
West Virginia, 41; brought in as state, 336
Wharton, John Austin, Gen., remains in valley, 603; attempts to reorganize ANV army to meet Joseph Eggleston Johnston in NC, 615
Wheat, Chatham Roberdeau, 239; 242n
see also Louisiana Tigers
Wheeling, WV, 41n
Whig Interpretation of history, diarist, 49
Whig Party, 41n, 49n
whiskey, as painkiller, 585 and passim
Whitaker, 53
Whitcomb, Henry Donald, head of Virginia Central Railroad, 589
White, Hester, visits brother in hospital, 341; takes brother home, 342
White, Hugh R., Col., hosts diarist, 329
White, James J., Capt., 109
White, Julian Ivanhoe, soldier in hospital, 341; leaves for home, 342
White, Thomas Spottswood, in charge of hospital equipment, 603
White Hall, 226
White Oak Swamp, battle,
White Top, 3
Whitehead, Dr., 271
Whitescarver, Charles T., Capt., 179, 180n, 180-81, hosts diarist, 183; 191
Whiting, civilian hosts, Clarke Co., 1862, 275
Whittier, John Greenleaf, introd., 7, 10
Wilburn, James H., Smyth Blues, killed, 264
Wilderness, introd., 1, 4, 6, 7, 11, 20, 49n
Wilkerson, Dr., ambulance duty, 323; 331, 349, 374; goes to Richmond to "investigate" Mary Camden, 399-400; reveals Camden story to Mollie Thornton, 415
Wilkerson, Cadmus Marcellus, field officer, 608, 609
Williams, Maj., LA Tigers, 259
Williams, John M., officer 102
as patient, 97; permanently disabled, 252 and 253n
Williams, Mr., 31
Williams, Thomas Henry, medical director, Army of Potomac, CSA, 595
Williamsburg, battle, 1862, 234
Williamsport, MD, skirmish, 169, 179
Jackson attempts to destroy dam on Potomac, 169-70
Willmore, Bradley, soldier, 155
Wilson, Goodridge, introd., v, 10, and cited passim
Wilson, William James Erasmus, on skin diseases, 391
Wilson, William V., minister and chaplain, 206
Winchester, 104, 107, 175, 177, 191
battles (3), 110; Early loses "final" time, August 1864, 592
camp and field hospital, 109, 112, 156-62; 292-5

citizens criticized, 195
general hospital, 108, 182, 183; houses 3,200 wounded, 188; 265; 303; general hospitals in bad condition, 1864, 582
moving from general hospital, 306-7
outbreak of variola, 1862, 254
people much excited, 213
recaptured by T.J. Jackson, 25 May 1862, 245
skirmish, 308
Winder, Charles Sidney, Gen., 225, 229
Wise, Henry Alexander, Gen., 132, 148, 198
Wise, O. Jennings, officer, dies at Roanoke Island, 198n, 200
Wolf, Sampson, soldier and friend, death, 137
Wood, George (two textbooks), 59, 60, 62, 63 65, 68, 81, 83, 279, 287, 293, 302
Woodward, C[omer] Vann, introd. and epilogue; 10, 16, and passim
Wright, F.H., Dr., travels with diarist, 310
Wright, Grayson Co. Dare Devil, death, 132
Wyatt, Orange Co. neighbor, 315
Wythe Co. soldiers, *see* First VA Bde.

xiffoid cartilage, 32,

yellow fever, 83
Yerby, John P., hosts campsite, Cortland Township, 323

Zigler, Samuel, hosts, Plains Township, 602
Zoar Church, Chesterfield, visited on sick furlough, 147